T0229613

ASTHMA PREVENTION

LUNG BIOLOGY IN HEALTH AND DISEASE

Executive Editor

Claude Lenfant

Former Director, National Heart, Lung, and Blood Institute
National Institutes of Health
Bethesda, Maryland

*The opinions expressed in these volumes do not necessarily represent
the views of the National Institutes of Health.*

ASTHMA PREVENTION

Edited by

William W. Busse
University of Wisconsin
Madison, Wisconsin, U.S.A.

Robert F. Lemanske, Jr.
University of Wisconsin
Madison, Wisconsin, U.S.A.

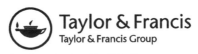

Taylor & Francis
Taylor & Francis Group

Boca Raton   London   New York   Singapore

Published in 2005 by
Taylor & Francis Group
270 Madison Avenue
New York, NY 10016

© 2005 by Taylor & Francis Group, LLC

No claim to original U.S. Government works
Printed in the United States of America on acid-free paper
10 9 8 7 6 5 4 3 2 1

International Standard Book Number-10: 0-8247-5409-3 (Hardcover)
International Standard Book Number-13: 978-0-8247-5409-9 (Hardcover)
Library of Congress Card Number 2005051484

This book contains information obtained from authentic and highly regarded sources. Reprinted material is quoted with permission, and sources are indicated. A wide variety of references are listed. Reasonable efforts have been made to publish reliable data and information, but the author and the publisher cannot assume responsibility for the validity of all materials or for the consequences of their use.

No part of this book may be reprinted, reproduced, transmitted, or utilized in any form by any electronic, mechanical, or other means, now known or hereafter invented, including photocopying, microfilming, and recording, or in any information storage or retrieval system, without written permission from the publishers.

For permission to photocopy or use material electronically from this work, please access www.copyright.com (http://www.copyright.com/) or contact the Copyright Clearance Center, Inc. (CCC) 222 Rosewood Drive, Danvers, MA 01923, 978-750-8400. CCC is a not-for-profit organization that provides licenses and registration for a variety of users. For organizations that have been granted a photocopy license by the CCC, a separate system of payment has been arranged.

Trademark Notice: Product or corporate names may be trademarks or registered trademarks, and are used only for identification and explanation without intent to infringe.

Library of Congress Cataloging-in-Publication Data

Asthma prevention / edited by William W. Busse, Robert F. Lemanske, Jr.
     p. cm. -- (Lung biology in health and disease ; v. 195)
  Includes bibliographical references and index.
  ISBN 0-8247-5409-3 (alk. paper)
    1. Asthma--Prevention. 2. Asthma in children--Prevention. I. Busse, W. W. (William W.) II. Lemanske, Robert F. III. Series.

RC591.A828 2005
616.2'3805--dc22   2005051484

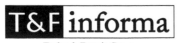

Taylor & Francis Group
is the Academic Division of T&F Informa plc.

**Visit the Taylor & Francis Web site at
http://www.taylorandfrancis.com**

PREFACE

For many asthmatic patients, the disease has its origins during infancy and early childhood. As such, much of the current research in asthma prevention has focused on events that occur early in life that contribute to asthma inception. The dramatic rise in prevalence of asthma throughout the world in the past few decades has underscored the importance of environmental factors interacting with a genetically susceptible host. Striking differences in prevalence rates in various parts of the world have drawn attention to characteristics of those macroenvironments that may modulate risk for disease expression. This is especially evident in so-called "Westernized" societies. Variations in these environments and their influence on asthma inception must be evaluated further in the context of genetic diversity in populations among various geographic and cultural boundaries that exist as well.

With these epidemiologic observations serving as an impetus for scientific inquiry, much new information has accumulated on the contribution of the environment, genetic background, gene–gene, and gene by environment interactions to the pathogenesis of asthma in the past decade. As a result, we have assembled a group of experts to review these advances in this evolving field of investigation. The first four chapters will review what is known regarding the natural history of asthma from birth to adulthood, with special emphasis on the characterization of various asthmatic phenotypes based on gender, age, ethnicity, and race within the context of various environmental exposures. The second set of chapters will review data on host immune responses and how they contribute to the immunoinflammatory events characteristic of allergic respiratory tract diseases. The third set of reviews will present an in-depth discussion of risk factors that have been determined to contribute to asthma pathogenesis. The final chapters will review treatment strategies, both currently available and under development, in the context of primary, secondary, and tertiary prevention of asthma and/or allergic diseases. Whenever possible, the authors have used translational approaches in reviewing basic science principles and relating them to asthma disease expression and its therapeutic modulation both short and long term.

This book should prove to be a valuable resource to those individuals desiring a comprehensive review of topics related to asthma prevention. Moreover, it is hoped that it will inspire novel research approaches and new directions for therapeutic interventions that will ultimately result in the primary prevention of this common respiratory tract disease.

Robert F. Lemanske, Jr., M.D.
William W. Busse, M.D.

EDITORS

William W. Busse, M.D., is chair of the Department of Medicine and a professor of medicine in the Section of Allergy, Pulmonary and Critical Care Medicine at the University of Wisconsin Medical School in Madison. He was named Charles E. Reed Professor of Medicine (WARF Professor) in 2001. He is board certified in internal medicine, allergy, and clinical immunology.

Dr. Busse has been funded by the National Institutes of Health (NIH) for research on the mechanisms of and the role of respiratory infections in asthma. His current research projects focus on mechanisms of virus-induced asthma, asthma from respiratory infections, cellular and molecular mechanisms of asthma, and mechanisms of severe asthma.

Dr. Busse is a past president and fellow of the American Academy of Allergy, Asthma and Immunology and holds memberships in several other professional societies, including the American College of Physicians, the American Thoracic Society, and the American Association of Physicians. He is an editor of *Allergy: Principles and Practice.* He is currently a deputy editor for the *Journal of Allergy and Clinical Immunology.*

Dr. Busse attended medical school at the University of Wisconsin at Madison. He completed his internship at Cincinnati General Hospital (University of Cincinnati) and residency in internal medicine at the University of Wisconsin, and was also a research fellow in allergy and clinical immunology at the University of Wisconsin.

Robert F. Lemanske, Jr., M.D. is a professor of pediatrics and medicine at the University of Wisconsin School of Medicine in Madison. He is also the head of the Division of Pediatric Allergy, Immunology, and Rheumatology and director of the Pediatric Asthma Center at the University of Wisconsin Hospitals. He earned his degree in medicine from the University of Wisconsin Medical School and completed his pediatric residency at the University of Wisconsin Hospitals.

He pursued allergy and immunology training at both the University of Wisconsin and the National Institute of Allergy and Infectious Diseases in Bethesda, Maryland.

Dr. Lemanske has written or co-written more than 130 articles published or accepted for publication in journals such as the *Journal of Immunology, Journal of Allergy and Clinical Immunology, New England Journal of Medicine, Journal of the American Medical Association, Pediatric Research, Journal of Pediatrics, American Review of Respiratory and Critical Care Medicine*, and *Immunology*. In addition, he has co-edited a text and contributed over 60 chapters to various textbooks.

Dr. Lemanske has served as an invited speaker on more than 300 occasions and is the recipient of the John M. Sheldon, M.D. (AAAAI) and Richard Talamo, M.D. (Johns Hopkins University) memorial lectureships, and the Sheldon Siegel, M.D. lectureship (AAAAI). He has served on the editorial boards of the *Journal of Allergy and Clinical Immunology* and *Pediatric Allergy and Immunology*, and was a director (1994–2000) and chairperson (2000) of the American Board of Allergy and Immunology. He also served on the expert panel for the development of guidelines for the treatment of childhood asthma in Canada and the United States (National Asthma Education Program). Dr. Lemanske is an appointed member to the Advisory Council of the National Heart, Lung and Blood Institute of the National Institutes of Health.

Dr. Lemanske is a fellow of both the American Academy of Allergy and Clinical Immunology and the American Academy of Pediatrics. He is also a member of the American Thoracic Society, the American Association of Immunologists, and the Society for Pediatric Research. Honors Dr. Lemanske has received include the NIAID Allergic Disease Academic Award and a membership in the Society for Pediatric Research. He is one of seven current principal investigators of the Asthma Clinical Research Network (ACRN) sponsored by the National Heart, Lung and Blood Institute, and one of six current principal investigators of the Childhood Asthma Research and Education (CARE) Network also sponsored by the institute. He is listed as one of the best 100 doctors in America by *American Health Magazine*. His research interests include the pathophysiology of late phase reactions, virus-induced airway dysfunction, and the origins and treatment of childhood asthma.

CONTRIBUTORS

Bengt Björkstén
Karolinska Institutet
Stockholm, Sweden

Larry Borish
Beirne Carter Center
  for Immunology Research
University of Virginia Health System
Charlottesville, Virginia, U.S.A.

John Britton
University of Nottingham
Nottingham, U.K.

David H. Broide
University of California San Diego
La Jolla, California, U.S.A.

G. Daniel Brooks
University of Wisconsin–Madison
Madison, Wisconsin, U.S.A.

Kristin M. Burkart
Boston University School of Medicine
Boston, Massachusetts, U.S.A.

Moisés A. Calderón-Zapata
National Heart and Lung Institute
Imperial College School of Medicine
London, U.K.

Lisa Cameron
University of Arizona
Tucson, Arizona, U.S.A.

Thomas B. Casale
Creighton University Medical Center
Omaha, Nebraska, U.S.A.

Christopher Clark
Creighton University Medical Center
Omaha, Nebraska, U.S.A.

Stephen R. Durham
National Heart and Lung Institute
Imperial College School of Medicine
London, U.K.

Elizabeth A. Erwin
University of Virginia
Charlottesville, Virginia, U.S.A.

C. Grüber
Charité-Humboldt University Berlin
Berlin, Germany

Theresa Guilbert
University of Arizona
Tucson, Arizona, U.S.A.

Peter W. Heymann
University of Virginia
Charlottesville, Virginia, U.S.A.

Sabine Hoffjan
University of Chicago
Chicago, Illinois, U.S.A.

S.T. Holgate
University of Southampton School
  of Medicine and Southampton
  General Hospital
Southampton, U.K.

P.G. Holt
Telethon Institute for Child
  Health Research and Centre
  for Child Health Research
University of Western Australia
Perth, Australia

P.H. Howarth
University of Southampton School
  of Medicine and Southampton
  General Hospital
Southampton, U.K.

Richard Hubbard
University of Nottingham
Nottingham, U.K.

S. Illi
Dr. v. Haunersches Kinderspital
Munich, Germany

Kunihiko Kitagaki
University of Iowa
Iowa City, Iowa, U.S.A.

Joel N. Kline
University of Iowa
Iowa City, Iowa, U.S.A.

Chakradhar Kotaru
University of Colorado Health
  Sciences Center
and National Jewish Medical and
  Research Center
Denver, Colorado, U.S.A.

Marzena Krawiec
University of Wisconsin–Madison
Madison, Wisconsin, U.S.A.

Peter N. Le Souëf
Princess Margaret Hospital
  for Children
Perth, Western Australia

S. Lau
Charité-Humboldt University Berlin
Berlin, Germany

Robert F. Lemanske, Jr.
University of Wisconsin–Madison
Madison, Wisconsin, U.S.A.

Sarah Lewis
University of Nottingham
Nottingham, U.K.

Richard J. Martin
University of Colorado Health
  Sciences Center
and National Jewish Medical and
  Research Center
Denver, Colorado, U.S.A.

Fernando D. Martinez
University of Arizona
Tucson, Arizona, U.S.A.

Paolo Maria Matricardi
Bambino Gesù Pediatric Hospital
  Research Institute
Rome, Italy

Tricia McKeever
University of Nottingham
Nottingham, U.K.

Alexander Möller
Princess Margaret Hospital
for Children
Perth, Western Australia

R. Nickel
Charité-Humboldt University Berlin
Berlin, Germany

Carole Ober
University of Chicago
Chicago, Illinois, U.S.A.

George T. O'Connor
Boston University School of Medicine
Boston, Massachusetts, U.S.A.

Thomas A.E. Platts-Mills
University of Virginia
Charlottesville, Virginia, U.S.A.

Jacqueline Pongracic
Northwestern University Feinberg
School of Medicine and
Children's Memorial Hospital
Chicago, Illinois, U.S.A.

J. Rowe
Telethon Institute for Child
Health Research and Centre
for Child Health Research
University of Western Australia
Perth, Australia

E.M. Salagean
University of Southampton School
of Medicine and Southampton
General Hospital
Southampton, U.K.

Megan T. Sandel
Boston University School
of Medicine
Boston, Massachusetts, U.S.A.

Malcolm R. Sears
St. Joseph's Healthcare and
McMaster University
Hamilton, Ontario, Canada

Jeffrey Stokes
Creighton University Medical
Center
Omaha, Nebraska, U.S.A.

Stanley J. Szefler
National Jewish Medical and
Research Center
and University of Colorado Health
Sciences Center
Denver, Colorado, U.S.A.

Donata Vercelli
University of Arizona
Tucson, Arizona, U.S.A.

Erika von Mutius
University Children's Hospital
Munich, Germany

U. Wahn
Charité-Humboldt University Berlin
Berlin, Germany

Judith A. Woodfolk
University of Virginia
Charlottesville, Virginia, U.S.A.

Anne L. Wright
Arizona Respiratory Center
University of Arizona
Tucson, Arizona, U.S.A.

Rosalind J. Wright
Brigham and Women's Hospital
and Harvard Medical School
Boston, Massachusetts, U.S.A.

CONTENTS

I

Epidemiology of Asthma

1

Epidemiology of Asthma

MALCOLM R. SEARS

St. Joseph's Healthcare and McMaster University
Hamilton, Ontario, Canada

I. Introduction

Of all respiratory diseases, asthma has one of the longest histories in recorded medicine, but it became increasingly problematic during the last century. The reported prevalence of asthma has increased substantially over recent decades among both children and adults.[1] Epidemics of mortality from asthma have occurred mainly among young people.[2] As the burden of disease has increased, so has the quest for understanding its genetic and environmental origins, pathogenesis, and immunology in the hope of ameliorating its severity and even preventing its occurrence. Reduction of the prevalence of the disease would relieve much anxiety and suffering, reduce direct and indirect health care costs, and decrease a not insignificant number of deaths.

II. Definition and Diagnosis of Asthma

In 1962, the American Thoracic Society proposed a definition of asthma that stated, "Asthma is a disease characterized by an increased responsiveness of the trachea and bronchi to various stimuli and manifested by a widespread narrowing of the airways that changes in severity either spontaneously or as a result of therapy."[3]

As the pathophysiology and immunology of asthma were further clarified, the definitions were modified to reflect these new understandings. The 1991 International Consensus Report on Diagnosis and Management of Asthma from the National Asthma Education Program Expert Panel provided a further description of common characteristics of the disease: "Asthma is a chronic inflammatory disorder of the airways in which many cells play a role, including mast cells and eosinophils. In susceptible individuals this inflammation causes symptoms which are usually associated with widespread but variable airflow obstruction that is often reversible either spontaneously or with treatment, and causes an associated increase in airway responsiveness to a variety of stimuli."[4]

The 1995 Global Initiative in Asthma (GINA) document defined asthma in similar terms with an expanded statement regarding symptoms: "Asthma is a chronic inflammatory disorder of the airways in which many cells play a role, in particular mast cells, eosinophils and T lymphocytes. In susceptible individuals this inflammation causes recurrent symptoms of wheezing, breathlessness, chest tightness, and cough, particularly at night and/or in the early morning. These symptoms are usually associated with widespread but variable airflow limitation that is at least partly reversible either spontaneously or with treatment. The inflammation also causes an associated increase in airway responsiveness to a variety of stimuli."[5]

One of the challenges in epidemiology is the need to translate mechanistic, cellular, physiological, and symptom-based descriptions of asthma such as those above into a working definition that can be used to establish the prevalence of the condition. This difficulty is compounded by the clear evidence for the heterogeneity of the disease, the lack of a single biological marker or clinical test for asthma, the variable expression of symptoms, multiple etiological factors, different responses to treatment, and variability in outcomes.

Prevalence studies have generally involved use of self-completed or administered questionnaires, and often include some form of objective assessment of airway function. Standardized validated questionnaires have been developed which record common symptoms of asthma, current or previously experienced. Accuracy of recall (recollecting events of years or decades ago), participation bias (those with disease may be more likely to be willing to respond to invitations to participate), and differing understandings of terminology (wheeze, chest tightness, and breathlessness) are issues that must be addressed in all questionnaire studies. Nevertheless the majority of reported prevalence rates for asthma are based on symptom reporting.

Requiring a diagnostic label of asthma provided by a physician rather than using the presence of symptoms suggesting asthma such as wheezing, dyspnea, or chest tightness results in lower prevalence rates.[6,7] The asthma label identifies those with more obvious disease, generally of sufficient severity to need repeated medical attention. In a recent monograph, Viegi et al. draw attention to the spectrum of terms used even in large epidemiological studies and the potential for noncomparability of results. For example, "asthma" questions include self-reported asthma, diagnosed asthma, current asthma, and ever-asthma. "Breathlessness" questions include breathlessness, wheeze and breathlessness, and breathlessness at night. "Wheeze" questions include wheeze, wheeze or whistling, wheeze without a cold, wheeze during exercise, wheeze and breathlessness, and others.[8]

III. Airway Hyperresponsiveness as an Epidemiological Tool

In many recent epidemiological studies of asthma, one or more objective tests to confirm that symptoms are indeed due to asthma or to validate a doctor's diagnosis of asthma have been included.[9,10] While spirometry with response to a bronchodilator (15 to 20% improvement in flow rate) is useful to establish the diagnosis in the setting of an acute episode of asthma, it is less useful in population studies because many individuals with asthma may be asymptomatic on the day of assessment and exhibit normal or near-normal function. Measurement of airway hyperresponsiveness (AHR) to a bronchoconstrictor such as methacholine or histamine has therefore been more widely used than the bronchodilator response. Bronchial challenge can be undertaken in population studies of adults and children over about 7 years old, both asymptomatic and symptomatic, with few exceptions (those who have recently used a bronchodilator or those with substantial degrees of bronchoconstriction at baseline such that challenge is not regarded as safe).

Population studies with AHR measurements have provided further insights into the nature of asthma. Some with AHR deny having had relevant symptoms suggesting asthma at any time; others have gone into remission but retain AHR; still others have symptoms suggesting asthma but without AHR on the day of assessment.[11] These latter individuals may have milder disease, may be using effective treatment to control AHR; their symptoms may have nonasthmatic causes; or they may have pre-asthmatic conditions. Measurement of AHR is useful in determining the range of severity of disease in a population. Generally, the more severe the disease (more frequent symptoms, greater variability in lung function, or greater need for medication to control symptoms), the greater is the degree of AHR (less bronchoconstrictor required to induce a predetermined degree of bronchoconstriction).

Toelle and colleagues first proposed using a combination of a recent history of symptoms consistent with asthma (within 12 months) and the presence of measurable AHR (provoking concentration of bronchoconstrictor agent below a defined cut point) as a useful definition of asthma for epidemiological purposes.[12]

While this has some advantages in defining a population with greater diagnostic certainty, a population with more obvious asthma, it has disadvantages similar to the use of a doctor's diagnosis of asthma. The definition of Toelle et al. excludes from the range of asthma in a population those with mild symptoms without sufficient AHR to reach the defined cut point and also those whose treatments may have made them asymptomatic or improved AHR beyond the defined limits. In their own study, those fulfilling their criteria for "current asthma" had more symptoms, greater variability in flow rates, and more atopy; they required more treatment than those with only symptoms without AHR or the few subjects who exhibited AHR without symptoms.[12]

While epidemiologists use AHR as a marker of asthma, it is not a "gold standard" for asthma without which the diagnosis is negated. Its measurement is more helpful for describing population characteristics and comparing populations than for adding great precision to a questionnaire survey of the prevalence of asthma. It may also be a predictor of increased risk of development of asthma.

In a birth cohort of 1037 New Zealand children followed to age 26, the clinical outcome of asymptomatic AHR to methacholine administration documented in study members at age 9 was determined.[13] Those with asymptomatic AHR at age 9 were more likely at follow-up to report asthma and wheeze, to have high IgE levels and eosinophils, and to demonstrate positive responses to skin allergen testing. Although AHR is a useful marker of current asthma, it may also represent a parallel pathological process that may lead to subsequent symptoms and clinical evidence of asthma.

IV. Atopy as an Epidemiological Tool

Measurements of atopy, whether via skin prick test or serum IgE, have also been included in many epidemiological studies. Clearly this is not a diagnostic tool — although the majority of children and many adults with asthma demonstrate positive skin tests, asthma does not depend on the presence of atopy. Similarly, subjects can demonstrate atopy on skin tests without having asthma or, indeed, any clinical manifestations of allergic disease. However, identifying the prevalence and spectrum of atopy is helpful in characterizing populations under study and may shed light on reasons for differences in prevalence rates among different communities, countries, and age groups.

V. Recent Trends in Asthma Epidemiology

A number of patterns are emerging from a multitude of epidemiological studies.[14] Surveys repeated over time in the same populations have shown that more individuals are presenting to their physicians with symptoms suggesting asthma. This pattern is evident worldwide; to date, no countries have reported decreases in the prevalence of asthma, although recent studies suggest the increase may have slowed or reached a plateau. Furthermore, substantially more asthma is evident in western countries compared with eastern countries, with a particular high prevalence in English-speaking countries.

"Westernization" in developing countries has been associated with increased prevalence of asthma within otherwise stable populations. The prevalences of other allergic disorders such as allergic rhinoconjunctivitis, eczema, and allergic dermatitis have also increased. Given the significant increases in incidence of all these allergic diseases, the increase in asthma is almost certainly a result of an increase in the prevalence of allergy.

In the United Kingdom, Morrison-Smith first reported a small increase in the prevalence of wheezing disorders in Birmingham from 1.8% in 1956 to 2.3% in 1968.[15] In New Zealand, Mitchell[16] repeated the study of Milne[17] in Lower Hutt schoolchildren after an interval of 13 years and found a substantial increase in prevalence from 7.1 to 13.5%. The prevalence of wheezing in 7-year-old children in Aberdeen doubled from 10 to 20%, and diagnosed asthma increased from 4 to 10% between 1964 and 1989.[18] The prevalence of hay fever and eczema also doubled, suggesting the increase in asthma and wheezing resulted from increased atopy.

Some 15 to 20 similar studies reported varying increases over various time periods. Some caveats apply to these studies; in some the impact of migration significantly changed the populations. Substantial evidence indicates that the rate of asthma is higher among immigrants than in the native population.[19] Additionally, a change in perception or understanding of asthma symptoms has occurred and diagnosis may be made more readily; wheezing symptoms are more commonly reported than ignored. Some studies involve methodological variations that may impact comparability of results; response rates may differ, leading to the possibility of participation by those with greater personal interests in the disease.

Other proxy measures for population prevalence of asthma include drug use.[20] However, drug use may increase with increased prevalence, increased treatment of the same number of subjects, or greater access to medical care with increasing prosperity, and is therefore not a reliable marker of change in prevalence. Hospital admission rates are also less reliable as admissions become more difficult and ambulatory treatments improve.[21,22] Most asthma admissions are of children under age 5. Changes in reported asthma admissions could also reflect greater acceptance of the label of asthma in young children than in the past.[23]

Increases in the prevalence of AHR may be more pertinent to understanding whether an increase in the prevalence of asthma is a reality. Such studies are more difficult to standardize than questionnaire studies[24] and fewer of this type have been performed to date. Increases in AHR have been demonstrated in several populations including residents of Australia[25] and Germany.[26]

Increases in the prevalence of atopy have also been documented, for example, in studies of hay fever in Scotland,[27] in an intergenerational study of parents and children over a 25-year interval. Increases in the prevalence of specific IgE by radioallergosorbent test (RAST) assays have been shown in many populations in disparate countries including Japan,[28] East and West Germany,[29] Denmark,[30] Finland,[31] and Greenland.[32]

VI. Epidemiological Trends in Asthma Mortality

Another striking feature of the epidemiology of asthma over the past 40 years has been the occurrence of two well-defined epidemics of asthma mortality among young people.[2] To a lesser extent, a gradual increase in asthma mortality was noted in many countries until very recently — a trend that is now apparently declining.[33–35] The first notable epidemic occurred in countries that marketed a high-strength formulation of isoprenaline (isoproterenol) that eventually was seen as the most likely cause of an epidemic in England, Wales, Australia, and New Zealand.[36] The cause of increased mortality was presumed to be cardiac arrhythmia,[37] although that was subsequently reconsidered.

A second more circumscribed epidemic of mortality from asthma occurred in New Zealand beginning in 1977, when high-strength fenoterol was introduced.[2,38] Following a series of three case-control studies, the link with fenoterol was established.[39–41] A concomitant clinical trial established that regular use of fenoterol increased airway responsiveness and decreased asthma control, making this a more likely mechanism explaining asthma deaths than cardiac arrhythmia.[42,43] The subsequent marked decrease in both mortality from asthma and hospital admissions for asthma when fenoterol was withdrawn in New Zealand[44] is striking testimony to the causal association with fenoterol and to the asthma severity mechanism that increased both admissions and mortality instead of cardiac arrhythmias which would have increased mortality only (Figure 1.1).

In the majority of countries, recent trends in asthma mortality have been downward, perhaps related to increased use of inhaled corticosteroids[45] and better overall management of chronic asthma and acute life-threatening episodes. Japan has had high mortality rates for decades, but the increase in sales of both inhaled corticosteroids and leukotriene receptor antagonists has been associated with a decrease in asthma death rates.[46]

VII. Incidence and Prevalence in Children

Studies of incidence are relatively few. Data documenting new cases prospectively in a cohort studied longitudinally have come from the Tucson Children's Study; the annual incidence rates were 11.3% before age 3 and 5% from ages 3 to

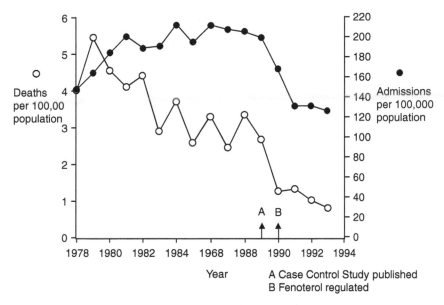

Figure 1.1 Admissions and deaths of 15- to 44-year olds in New Zealand, 1978 to 1993, showing an abrupt decline in both admissions and deaths following the marked restriction of sales of fenoterol. (From Sears, M.R., Epidemiological trends in asthma, *Can. Respir. J.*, 3, 261–268, 1996. With permission.)

6 years.[47] A national birth cohort in the United Kingdom estimated the annual incidence rates of asthma at ages 7, 11, and 16 years to be 2.6, 1.1, and 0.7%, respectively.[48]

Many local and regional cross-sectional studies of the prevalence of asthma in childhood have been conducted with differing methodologies of sampling frame, questionnaires, and interpretation, making valid comparisons of prevalence rates almost impossible. Further compounding this problem is a large proportion of undiagnosed frequent wheezing impacted by race and gender. Yeatts et al. found in a large adolescent survey in North Carolina that undiagnosed frequent wheezing was independently associated with female gender, current smoking, low socioeconomic status, and African-American ethnicity.[49] The gender differ-ence in asthma prevalence may have been influenced by such factors as how asthma was defined (diagnosed by a doctor, current wheeze in the past 12 months, or current wheeze with AHR).[50] Reliance on doctor-diagnosed asthma led to an underestimation of the prevalence of asthma, particularly among girls.

To determine more accurately the spectrum of asthma prevalence and the differences observed in prevalence rates within and between countries, the Interna-tional Study of Asthma and Allergies in Childhood (ISAAC) was developed jointly by investigators in New Zealand and Germany.[51] Phase I of the ISAAC study (questionnaires only) was undertaken in 155 centers in 56 countries around the world, the majority examining two childhood age groups (6- to 7-year olds and 13- to 14-year olds), with over 700,000 children participating. This study highlighted the marked geographic variability in prevalence rates of asthma and wheezing, and also of other allergic diseases such as hay fever, allergic rhinoconjunctivitis, and eczema (allergic dermatitis, urticaria).[52] In Hong Kong, the prevalence of wheezing among children aged 13 to 14 was 12.4%. In Australia, it was 29.4% with a range among four major urban centers of 24.7% (Sydney) to 33.5% (Adelaide). Differences within other countries were also noteworthy, for example, East and West Germany (17 versus 29%, respectively). In North America, wheezing among 13- to 14-year olds ranged from 19.8% in Chicago to 30.6% in Hamilton, Ontario.

Figure 1.2 illustrates variances in prevalence rates in different countries in 13- to 14-year olds.[52] The 12-month prevalence of self-reported asthma varied from 1.6% in Indonesia to over 30% in the United Kingdom, New Zealand, and Australia.[53] The reasons for the wide discrepancies in prevalence rates will be discussed elsewhere in this volume, in relation to known or suspected environmental risk factors for developing allergy and asthma.

Other factors may paradoxically provide protection against allergy and asthma, for example, living on a farm or exposure to childhood infections.[54,55] The major role played by environmental factors in determining prevalence rates is evident from the marked disparities between rates in populations of similar ethnic origins; for example, Chinese children in Hong Kong had a four-fold higher prevalence than their counterparts in Guangzhou, a mainland China city only 150 miles north of Hong Kong that uses the same language and has a similar climate.[53] The prevalence of asthma is related to affluence, but the mechanism remains to be elucidated. Other factors influencing prevalence rates in childhood include race; asthma in North America is more common among African-Americans.[56]

While the increasing prevalence of asthma may reflect increased incidence, the other possibility is increased persistence of asthma in childhood or from childhood to adulthood. Very few population-based studies focus on the persistence of childhood asthma. Most follow-up studies of asthma relating to children seen in specialty clinics for asthma introduce selection bias of more severe disease which by its nature is more likely to persist.[57,58]

Two Australian studies from Tasmania[59] and Melbourne[60] examined the natural history of asthma in population-based samples. Each study had limitations — the first because it included only a single follow-up some 20 years after the initial survey of 7-year olds, and the second because of the intermixing of an "enriched" cohort of subjects with severe asthma to provide sufficient data for determining outcomes in this end of the spectrum of asthma in the community.

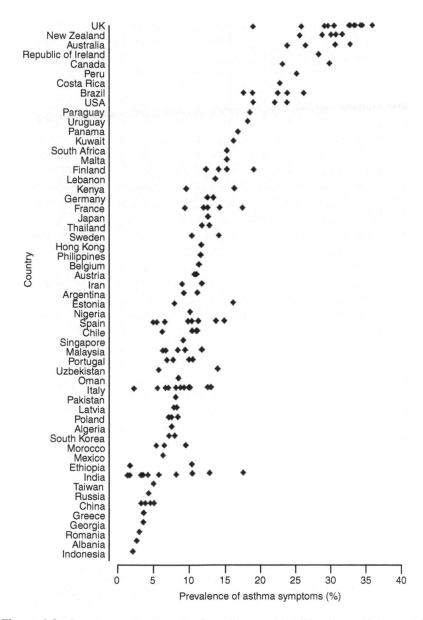

Figure 1.2 Prevalence of asthma in 13- to 14-year old children in multiple countries and centers within countries reported in the ISAAC Phase I study. (From International Study of Asthma and Allergies in Childhood [ISAAC] Steering Committee, Worldwide variation in prevalence of symptoms of asthma, allergic rhinoconjunctivitis, and atopic eczema, *Lancet*, 351, 1225–1332, 1998. With permission.)

The Tasmanian cohort reviewed after 20 years revealed that 25% of those with current asthma at 7 years of age had persistent asthma as adults, while 10% of those with no asthma at 7 had developed asthma by adulthood.[59] Risk factors for persistence to adulthood were female gender, childhood eczema, low lung function, and maternal and paternal asthma.

The Melbourne study was repeated at multiple ages (10, 14, 21, 28, 35, and 42 years), but with decreasing cohort retention and limited objective investigation. Nevertheless, the study yielded important information, reporting the outcome in mid-adult life of wheezing syndromes of childhood.[60–63] For instance, at age 35, 65% of those with mild wheezy bronchitis at age 7 were fully asymptomatic, compared with only 30% of those with diagnosed asthma at 7 years and only 10% of those with more severe asthma added to the cohort at age 10.[63]

The United Kingdom birth cohort study began in 1958 with a very large population sample exceeding 18,000 individuals seen at age 7; cohort retention decreased as subjects reached mid-adult life. Those who outgrew their childhood wheezing tended to return to normal pulmonary function, whereas those with persistent wheezing had reduced FEV1 (forced expiratory volume in 1 sec.) even after bronchodilator use.[64] Those with transient wheezing before age 7 continued to have abnormal lung function as adults, even if no symptoms were reported for the past year.[65] The lack of complete reversibility with bronchodilators suggests that early childhood illness may have set the scene for adult chronic airflow obstruction or possibly that those with transient childhood wheeze continue to wheeze because they have "permanently" smaller airways than average.

In Tucson, Arizona, a birth cohort commenced in 1980 and followed 1246 subjects from birth along with their families.[66] This study defined differing patterns of early childhood wheezing, including transient (wheeze in the first 3 years not persisting to age 6), late onset (no wheeze before age 3, then developing subsequently and persisting beyond age 6), and persistent (early onset before age 3 with persistence beyond age 6). Differing risk factors were associated with each form of asthma, or the same factors with differing strengths of association were considered. Transient wheeze was more often associated with smaller airways, while later onset or persistent wheeze was more commonly associated with a positive family history of asthma and allergies, higher IgE levels, and other allergic manifestations.

A New Zealand birth cohort has been followed to age 26 years, with frequent respiratory questionnaires, lung function tests, and measurements of airway responsiveness and atopy.[67] Wheezing commonly persisted from childhood to adulthood or relapsed after remission.[68] Factors predicting persistence or relapse after remission included house dust mite sensitization, AHR, female gender, smoking, and early age of onset. Lung function in those with persistent wheeze consistently tracked low from age 9 to age 26. These findings suggest that poor adult outcomes are primarily determined early in childhood. In this same cohort, a substantial fraction of this unselected population experienced hospitalizations for asthma.[69] Frequent respiratory symptoms, AHR, atopy, and low lung function were markers of severity that identified subjects at high risk for hospitalization for asthma.

VIII. Epidemiology of Adult Asthma

There are fewer studies of the prevalence and characteristics of asthma in adults than in children. Difficulties in obtaining a random sample in adults are greater than in childhood and asthma may be confused with other chronic lung diseases that cause airway obstruction. Studies using different population sampling frames and questionnaires have yielded widely differing prevalence rates for adult asthma.

The first National Health and Nutrition Examination Survey (NHANES-I) reported that 2.6% of American adults had asthma.[70] Repeated surveys found increasing prevalence rates; data from NHANES-III showed that 4.5% of U.S. adults had current asthma and 16.4% experienced wheezing within 12 months.[71] Perhaps some 10% of adult asthma is occupational in origin[72] and the distributions and types of industries within countries may impact adult asthma prevalence rates more than childhood rates. These issues are discussed in detail in a later chapter.

To overcome many of these methodological uncertainties in the study of adult asthma and to determine whether major differences in reported prevalence rates were real or represent artifacts of study design and differences in questions, the European Community Respiratory Health Survey (ECRHS) was developed as a standardized, multinational, multicenter survey of the prevalence, determinants, and management of asthma among adults aged 20 to 44.[73] Studies were initiated in Western Europe and subsequently undertaken in many countries. The prevalence rates of respiratory symptoms varied widely; they were generally lower in northern, central, and southern Europe and higher in the United Kingdom, New Zealand, Australia, and the U.S., but still showed significant within-country variations among centers. The lowest prevalence of wheeze in the previous 12 months was reported from Bombay, India (4.1%), and the highest rate was from Dublin, Ireland (32.0%).

Because the ISAAC and ECRHS studies were often conducted in the same countries, the opportunity arose to compare prevalence rates in adults and children.[74] A strong correlation was found between the ISAAC and ECRHS prevalence rates; 64% of the variation at the country level and 74% at the center level in the prevalence of wheeze in the previous 12 months in the ECRHS data was explained by variations in the ISAAC data. Similar correlations were seen for self-reported asthma, hay fever, and eczema. These findings support the validity of the two studies and also suggest a strong link between child and adult prevalence rates that has implications for understanding the persistence of childhood asthma into adulthood.

IX. Epidemiological Perspective on Prevention of Asthma

Few would debate the increase in the prevalence of atopy and therefore the prevalence of asthma over the past three decades. The causes are less clear than the evidence of the increase. Asthma is a classic example of a disease related to gene–environment interaction. What are the implications for prevention of asthma?

Can the genetics of the disease be altered? Not yet, and possibly not for a long time, if ever. What can be done in terms of environmental prevention? As discussed in the following chapters, many risk factors have been carefully studied. The contributions of exposure to environmental tobacco smoke in childhood and to occupational sensitizers in adulthood are well defined and represent potentially preventable risk factors for asthma.

Other issues such as the putative protective role of breast feeding are more controversial, but the weight of evidence now suggests that breast feeding is not protective against later development of atopy and asthma. The role of animal and farm exposures has proven to be counter-intuitive or paradoxical, with decreased risk of atopy and subsequent asthma among children raised on farms or exposed in early life to domestic animals. The effects of early childhood infections are also becoming clearer in that some infection along with the resulting Th1-type immune response appears protective against the dominant Th2-type allergic response characteristic of asthma.

Epidemiologically, the lowest risk for development of asthma should therefore be seen in communities with higher than average infection rates in early childhood, where exposure to farm or domestic animal is routine, where breast-feeding is not encouraged, and where smoking is uncommon. Such a community has yet to be identified. However the epidemiological data from the ISAAC and ECRHS international surveys provide some evidence that the geographic variability of the prevalence of asthma supports the importance of the first two scenarios.

The material presented in the remainder of this book explores in much more detail the evidence relating to these and many other risk factors for asthma. The challenge is to take the evidence as it unfolds and use it to devise and implement strategies that will prevent the development or reduce the burden of this increasingly troublesome disease.

References

1. Burney P. The changing prevalence of asthma. *Thorax* 2002; 57: ii36–ii39.
2. Sears MR and Taylor DR. The 2-agonist controversy: observations, explanations and relationship to asthma epidemiology. *Drug Safety* 1994; 11: 259–283.

3. Meneely GR, Renzetti AD, Steele JD, Wyatt JP, and Harris HW. Chronic bronchitis, asthma and pulmonary emphysema: a statement by the committee on diagnostic standards for nontuberculous respiratory disease. *Am Rev Respir Dis* 1962; 85: 762–768.
4. International Consensus Report on Diagnosis and Management of Asthma. *National Asthma Education Program Expert Panel Report*. U.S. Department of Health and Human Services, NIH publication 91-3042, Washington, D.C., 1991.
5. National Institutes of Health. *Global Initiative for Asthma*. National Heart Lung Blood Institute Publication 95-3659, Bethesda, MD, 1995, p. 6.
6. de Marco R, Cerveri I, Bugiani M, Ferrari M, and Verlato G. An undetected burden of asthma in Italy: the relationship between clinical and epidemiological diagnosis of asthma. *Eur Respir J* 1998; 11: 599–605.
7. Lundback B, Ronmark E, Jonsson E, Larsson K, and Sandstrom T. Incidence of physician-diagnosed asthma in adults: a real incidence or a result of increased awareness? Report from the Obstructive Lung Disease in Northern Sweden Studies. *Respir Med* 2001; 95: 685–692.
8. Viegi G, Annesi I, and Matteelli G. Epidemiology of asthma. *Eur Respir J.* 2003; 23: 1–25.
9. European Community Respiratory Health Survey II Steering Committee. The European Community Respiratory Health Survey II. *Eur Respir J* 2002; 20: 1071–1079.
10. Henriksen AH, Lingaas-Holmen T, Sue-Chu M, and Bjermer L. Combined use of exhaled nitric oxide and airway hyperresponsiveness in characterizing asthma in a large population survey. *Eur Respir J* 2000; 15: 849–855.
11. Sears MR, Jones DT, Holdaway MD, Hewitt CJ, Flannery EM, Herbison GP, and Silva PA. Prevalence of bronchial reactivity to inhaled methacholine in New Zealand children. *Thorax* 1986; 41: 283–289.
12. Toelle BG, Peat JK, Salome CM, Mellis CM, and Woolcock AJ. Toward a definition of asthma for epidemiology. *Am Rev Respir Dis* 1992; 146: 633–637.
13. Rasmussen F, Taylor DR, Flannery EM, Cowan JO, Greene JM, Herbison GP, and Sears MR. Outcome in adulthood of asymptomatic airway hyperresponsiveness in childhood: a longitudinal population study. *Ped Pulmonol* 2002; 34: 164–171.
14. Beasley R, Crane J, Lai CKW, and Pearce N. Prevalence and etiology of asthma. *J Allergy Clin Immunol* 2000; 105: 466–472.
15. Morrison-Smith J. The prevalence of asthma and wheezing in children. *Br J Dis Chest* 1976; 70: 73–77.
16. Mitchell EA. Increasing prevalence of asthma in children. *NZ Med J* 1983; 96: 463–464.
17. Milne GA. The incidence of asthma in Lower Hutt. *NZ Med J* 1969; 70: 27–29.
18. Ninan TK and Russell G. Respiratory symptoms and atopy in Aberdeen schoolchildren: evidence from two surveys 25 years apart. *Br Med J* 1992; 304: 873–875.
19. Ballin A, Somekh E, Geva D, and Meytes D. High rate of asthma among immigrants. *Med Hypothesis* 1998; 51:281-284.
20. Stafford RS, Ma J, Finkelstein SN, Haver K, and Cockburn I. National trends in asthma visits and asthma pharmacotherapy, 1978–2002. *J Allergy Clin Immunol* 2003; 111: 729–735.

21. Malmstrom K, Korhonen K, Kaila M, Dunder T, Nermes M, Klaukka T, Sarna S, and Juntunen-Backman K. Acute childhood asthma in Finland: a retrospective review of hospital admissions from 1976 to 1995. *Pediatr Allergy Immunol* 2000; 11: 236–240.

22. Korhonen K, Reijonen TM, Malmstrom K, Klaukka T, Remes K, and Korppi M. Hospitalization trends for paediatric asthma in eastern Finland: a 10-yr survey. *Eur Respir J* 2002; 19: 1035–1039.

23. Csonka P, Mertsola J, Kaila M, and Ashorn P. Regional variation in the diagnosis of asthma among preschool-age children. *Pediatr Allergy Immunol* 2000; 11: 189-192.

24. Peat JK, Toelle BG, Marks GB, and Mellis CM. Continuing the debate about measuring asthma in population studies. *Thorax* 2001; 56: 406–411.

25. Peat JK, van den Berg RH, Green WF, Mellis CM, Leeder SR, and Woolcock AJ. Changing prevalence of asthma in Australian children. *Br Med J* 1994; 308: 1591–1596.

26. Frye C, Heinrich J, Wjst M, and Wichmann H-E. Increasing prevalence of bronchial hyperresponsiveness in three selected areas in East Germany. *Eur Respir J* 2001; 18: 451–458.

27. Upton M, McConnachie A, McSharry C, Hart CL, Smith GD, Gillis CR, and Watt GC. Intergenerational 20-year trends in the prevalence of asthma and hay fever in adults: the Midspan Family Study surveys of parents and offspring. *Br Med J* 2000; 321: 88–92.

28. Nakagawa T, Nakagomi T, Hisamatsu S, Najagomi O, and Mizushima Y. Increased prevalence of elevated serum IgE and IgG_4 antibodies in students over a decade. *J Allergy Clin Immunol* 1996; 97: 1165–1166.

29. Weiland SK, von Mutius E, Hirsch T, Duhme H, Fritzsch C, Werner B, Husing A, Stender M, Renz H, Leupold W, and Keil U. Prevalence of respiratory and atopic disorders among children in the East and West of Germany five years after unification. *Eur Respir J* 1999; 14: 862–870.

30. Linneberg A, Nielsen NH, Madsen F, Frolund L, Dirksen A, and Jorgensen T. Increasing prevalence of specific IgE to aeroallergens in an adult population: two cross-sectional surveys 8 years apart. Copenhagen Allergy study. *J Allergy Clin Immunol* 2000; 106: 247–252.

31. Kosunen T, Hook-Nikanne J, Salomaa A, Sarna S, Aromaa A, and Haahtela T. Increase of allergen-specific immunoglobulin E antibodies from 1973 to 1994 in a Finnish population and a possible relationship to *Helicobacter pylori* infections. *Clin Exp Allergy* 2002; 32: 373–378.

32. Krause TG, Koch A, Friborg J, Poulsen LK, Kristensen B, and Melbye M. Frequency of atopy in the Arctic in 1987 and 1998. *Lancet* 2002; 360: 691–692.

33. Kumana CR, Kou M, Lauder IJ, Ip MSM, and Lam WK. Increasing use of inhaled steroids association with declining asthma mortality. *J Asthma* 2001; 38: 161–167.

34. Goldman M, Rachmiel M, Gendler L, and Katz Y. Decrease in asthma mortality rate in Israel from 1991–1995: is it related to increased use of inhaled corticosteroids? *J Allergy Clin Immunol* 2000; 105: 71–74.

35. Sly RM. Decreases in asthma mortality in the United States. *Ann Allergy Asthma Immunol* 2000; 85: 121–127.

36. Stolley PD and Schinnar R. Association between asthma mortality and isoproterenol aerosols: a review. *Prev Med* 1978; 7: 519–538.
37. Collins JM, McDevitt DG, Shanks RG, and Swanton JG. The cardio-toxicity of isoprenaline during hypoxia. *Br J Pharmac* 1969; 36: 35–45.
38. Wilson JD, Sutherland DC, and Thomas AC. Has the change to beta-agonists combined with oral theophylline increased cases of fatal asthma? *Lancet* 1981; 1: 1235–1237.
39. Crane J, Pearce N, Flatt A, Burgess C, Jackson R, Kwong T, Ball M, and Beasley R. Prescribed fenoterol and death from asthma in New Zealand, 1981–83: case-control study. *Lancet* 1989; 1: 918–922.
40. Pearce N, Grainger J, Atkinson M, Crane J, Burgess C, Culling C, Windom H, and Beasley R. Case-control study of prescribed fenoterol and death from asthma in New Zealand, 1977–81. *Thorax* 1990; 45: 170–175.
41. Grainger J, Woodman K, Pearce N, Crane J, Burgess C, Keane A, and Beasley R. Prescribed fenoterol and death from asthma in New Zealand, 1981–87: a further case-control study. *Thorax* 1991; 46: 105–111.
42. Sears MR, Taylor DR, Print CG, Lake DC, Li Q, Flannery EM, Yates DM, Lucas MK, and Herbison GP. Regular inhaled beta-agonist treatment in bronchial asthma. *Lancet* 1990; 336: 1391–1396.
43. Taylor DR, Sears MR, Herbison GP, Flannery EM, Print CG, Lake DC, Yates DM, Lucas MK, and Li Q. Regular inhaled β-agonist in asthma: effect on exacerbations and lung function. *Thorax* 1993; 48: 134–138.
44. Sears MR. Epidemiological trends in asthma. *Can Respir J* 1996; 3: 261–268.
45. Ernst P, Spitzer W, Suissa S, Cockcroft D, Habbick B, Horwitz R, Boivin J-F, McNutt M, and Buist AS. Risk of fatal or near fatal asthma in relation to inhaled corticosteroid use. *JAMA* 1992; 268: 3462–3464.
46. Suissa S and Ernst P. Use of anti-inflammatory therapy and asthma mortality in Japan. *Eur Respir J* 2003; 21: 101–104.
47. Martinez FD, Wright AL, Taussig LM, Holberg CJ, Halonen M, and Morgan WJ. Asthma and wheezing in the first six years of life. *New Engl J Med* 1995; 332: 133–138.
48. Anderson HR, Bland JM, and Peckham CS. Risk factors for asthma up to 16 years of age: evidence from a national cohort study. *Chest* 1987; 91: 127S–130S.
49. Yeatts K, Johnston Davis K, Sotir M, Herget C, and Shy C. Who gets diagnosed with asthma? Frequent wheeze among adolescents with and without a diagnosis of asthma. *Pediatrics* 2003; 111: 1046–1054.
50. Henriksen AH, Holmen TL, and Bjermer L. Gender differences in asthma prevalence may depend on how asthma is defined. *Respir Med* 2003; 97: 491–497.
51. Asher MI, Keil U, Anderson HR, Beasley R, Crane J, Martinez F, Mitchell EA, Pearce N, Sibbald B, Stewart AW, Strachan D, Weiland SK, and Williams HC. International study of asthma and allergies in childhood (ISAAC): rationale and methods. *Eur Respir J* 1995; 8: 483–491.
52. The International Study of Asthma and Allergies in Childhood (ISAAC) Steering Committee. Worldwide variation in prevalence of symptoms of asthma, allergic rhinoconjunctivitis, and atopic eczema. *Lancet* 1998; 351: 1225–1232.

53. The International Study of Asthma and Allergies in Childhood (ISAAC) Steering Committee. Worldwide variations in the prevalence of asthma symptoms. *Eur Respir J* 1998; 12: 315–335.

54. Leynaert B, Neukirch C, Jarvis D, Chinn S, Burney P, and Neukirch F, on behalf of European Community Respiratory Health Survey. Does living on a farm during childhood protect against asthma, allergic rhinitis, and atopy in adulthood? *Am J Respir Crit Care Med* 2001; 164: 1829–1834.

55. von Mutius E. Infection: friend or foe in the development of atopy and asthma? The epidemiological evidence. *Eur Respir J* 2001; 18: 872–881.

56. Fagan JK, Scheff PA, Hryhorczuk D, Ramakrishnan V, Ross M, and Persky V. Prevalence of asthma and other allergic diseases in an adolescent population: association with gender and race. *Ann Allergy Asthma Immunol* 2001; 86: 177–184.

57. Grol MH, Gerritsen J, Vonk JM, Schouten JP, Koeter GH, Rijcken B, and Postma DS. Risk factors for growth and decline of lung function in asthmatic individuals up to age 42 years: a 30-year follow-up study. *Am J Respir Crit Care Med* 1999; 160: 1830–1837.

58. Ulrik CS, Backer V, Dirksen A, Pedersen M, and Koch C. Extrinsic and intrinsic asthma from childhood to adult age: a 10 year follow-up. *Respir Med* 1995; 89: 547–554.

59. Jenkins MA, Hopper JL, Bowes G, Carlin JB, Flander LB, and Giles GG. Factors in childhood as predictors of asthma in adult life. *Br Med J* 1994; 309: 90–93.

60. McNicol KN, Williams HB, McNichol KN, Williams HE, McNichol KN, Williams HE, Allan J, and McAndrew I. Spectrum of asthma in children I: clinical and physiological components. *Br Med J* 1973; 4: 7–11.

61. Robertson CF. Long-term outcome of childhood asthma. *Med J Aust* 2002; 177: S42–S44.

62. Horak E, Lanigan A, Roberts M, Welsh L, Wilson J, Carlin JB, Olinsky A, and Robertson CF. Longitudinal study of childhood wheezy bronchitis and asthma: outcome at age 42. *Br Med J* 2003; 326: 422–423.

63. Oswald H, Phelan PD, Lanigan A, Hibbert M, Carlin JB, Bowes G, and Olinsky A. Childhood asthma and lung function in mid-adult life. *Pediatr Pulmonol* 1997; 23: 14–20.

64. Strachan DP, Butland BK, and Anderson HR. Incidence and prognosis of asthma and wheezing illness from early childhood to age 33 in a national British cohort. *Br Med J* 1996; 312: 1195–1199.

65. Strachan DP, Griffiths JM, Johnston IDA, and Anderson HR. Ventilatory function in British adults after asthma or wheezing illness at ages 0–35. *Am J Respir Crit Care Med* 1996; 154: 1629–1635.

66. Taussig LM, Wright AL, Holberg CJ, Halonen M, Morgan WJ, and Martinez FD. Tucson Children's Respiratory Study: 1980 to present. *J Allergy Clin Immunol* 2003; 111: 661–675.

67. Sears MR, Flannery EM, Herbison GP, and Holdaway MD. Asthma, in *From Child to Adult,* Silva PA and Stanton WR, Eds. Oxford: Oxford University Press, 1996, p 75.

68. Sears MR, Greene J, Willan AR, Wiecek EM, Taylor DR, Flannery EM, Cowan JO, Herbison GP, Silva PA, Poulton R. A longitudinal population-based cohort study of childhood asthma followed to adulthood. *N Engl J Med* 2003; 349: 1414–1422.

69. Rasmussen F, Taylor DR, Flannery EM, Cowan JO, Greene JM, Herbison GP, and Sears MR. Risk factors for hospital admission for asthma from childhood to young adulthood: a longitudinal population study. *J Allergy Clin Immunol* 2002; 110: 220–227.
70. McWhorter WP, Polis MA, and Kaslow RA. Occurrence, predictors, and consequences of adult asthma in NHANESI and follow-up survey. *Am Rev Respir Dis* 1989; 139: 721–724.
71. Arif AA, Delclos GL, Lee ES, Tortolero SR, and Whitehead LW. Prevalence and risk factors of asthma and wheezing among U.S. adults: an analysis of the NHANES III data. *Eur Respir J* 2003; 21: 827–833.
72. Blanc PD and Toren K. How much adult asthma can be attributed to occupational factors? *Am J Med* 1999; 107: 580–587.
73. European Community Respiratory Health Survey. Variations in the prevalence of respiratory symptoms, self-reported asthma attacks and use of asthma medication in the European Community Respiratory Health Survey (ECRHS). *Eur Respir J* 1996; 9: 687–695.
74. Pearce N, Sunyer J, Cheng S, Chinn S, Bjorksten B, Burr M, Keil U, Anderson HR, and Burney P. Comparison of asthma prevalence in the ISAAC and the ECRHS. *Eur Respir J* 2000; 16: 420–426.

2

The Natural History of Wheezing in Children

FERNANDO D. MARTINEZ

University of Arizona
Tucson, Arizona, U.S.A.

I. Introduction

Any potential strategy for the primary or secondary prevention of asthma has as a requirement a thorough knowledge of the natural history of the disease. Perhaps one of the most important obstacles affecting the development of such strategies has been, until recently, our limited knowledge of the most frequent ages of onset, its course, and the factors that determine remission and relapse. In addition, a lack of understanding of the heterogeneous nature of asthma made the factors associated with asthma initiation and progression more difficult to understand.

The publication during the last 10 years of the results of several longitudinal studies in which follow-up was initiated during the first years of life has considerably changed the way we understand the epidemiology of asthma. The results of these studies have been recently reviewed.[1] This chapter provides a summary of what we have learned from birth cohorts about the natural history of childhood wheezing and how this information may be relevant for the primary prevention of asthma.

II. Incidence

Several studies have shown that, at least in developed English-speaking countries, a very high proportion of subjects has at least one episode of wheezing during the first 20 to 30 years of life. Moreover, these high incidence rates seem to have markedly increased in the past 20 years. In the British National Child Development Study (1958 cohort), for example, 24% of all children developed wheezing illnesses by age 16 and 43% by age 33.[2] In the Dunedin Multidisciplinary Health and Development Study in New Zealand, researchers enrolled over 1000 children in 1972 and 1973 and followed them prospectively thereafter.[3] By age 26, 72.6% of study members (for whom data were available from longitudinal assessments started at age 9) had at least one episode of reported wheezing and 51.4% reported episodes of wheezing in more than one survey.

In both the British 1958 cohort and the Dunedin study, the majority of initial wheezing episodes occurred during the first 6 to 9 years of life. However, in both cohorts, information about the incidence of wheezing was obtained during the early school years and was based on parental recall.

A more accurate vision of the incidence of asthma in early life was revealed in a study by Yunginger et al.[4] These authors studied charts of patients seen at different ages for asthma-like episodes through late adult life in Rochester, Minnesota. They observed that the great majority of first episodes occurred during the first 6 years of life, and peak incidence occurred during the first 2 years of life. Similar results were reported for a birth cohort from Poole, England, in which detailed follow-up for a group of 100 children at high risk for asthma was started before they were born more than 25 years ago.[5]

III. Severity and Long-Term Prognosis of Early
Wheezing Episodes

The results discussed above clearly establish that first episodes of wheezing, when studied irrespective of prognosis, are more likely to occur in infancy and early childhood. Moreover, studies in which reliable information about wheezing episodes in early life was available for adult subjects with established asthma suggest that in this case also first episodes of asthma-like symptoms appeared early in life. These findings fail to clarify, however, the nature of the association between early life events and asthma. Studies were needed in which children with early episodes of wheezing were followed for many years to determine their outcomes. Results of such studies have only recently become available and what emerges from them is a remarkable pattern of heterogeneity of outcomes for infants and young children with very similar symptoms and clinical manifestations.

A first important observation was that a large proportion of children aged 3 or younger who wheeze have only one or two episodes (that can also be quite severe) and do not show any further manifestations of airway obstruction.[6] These episodes are usually associated with viral infections and the most common agent isolated is the respiratory syncytial virus (RSV),[7] although other agents such as rhinoviruses,[8] parainfluenza,[7] and the recently described metapneumovirus[9] can also trigger wheezing illnesses. No less than 60% of all children aged >3 years have this form of "transient early wheezing," and the proportion may be much higher for infants during the first year of life.[10]

One third of all children have at least one episode of wheeze before age 3. This means that approximately one fifth of all children will wheeze transiently in early life. An additional 10 to 12% will wheeze at an early age period and will continue to wheeze between the ages of 3 and 6 or 7 years. We propose these subjects be called "persistent wheezers."[6] Based on the observation noted earlier that a majority of older children and adults with chronic asthma symptoms had their first episodes during the first years of life,[4,5] it is plausible to conclude that many persistent wheezers will develop chronic asthma.

This conclusion is supported by our own continued follow-up of the children enrolled in the Tucson Children's Respiratory Study. When we studied transient early wheezers and persistent wheezers at age 11, we found that the latter were much more likely than transient early wheezers to have episodes of wheeze at both these ages.[11] Moreover, the former were not more likely to have episodes of wheeze or be diagnosed with asthma at age 11 than children who had never wheezed during the first 3 years of life. Therefore, it can be concluded based on these data that, at least through the adolescent years, transient early wheezers have very good prognoses.

Remarkably, parents seem to have arrived at the same conclusion. When asked in the year 11 questionnaires whether their children had "ever wheezed," many parents of transient wheezers had forgotten that their children had been taken to their pediatricians for lower respiratory illnessses (LRIs) in early life. The same thing was not true for parents of persistent wheezers, who usually did remember that their children had been wheezing since a very early age (unpublished results). This is an important observation from our view because it suggests that longitudinal studies based on retrospective questionnaires should be interpreted with great caution given the recall bias implicit in our findings.

Follow-up studies along with the benefit of hindsight have also allowed us to compare clinical symptoms during the first 3 years of life among transient early wheezers and persistent wheezers. In a study of over 1000 children followed from birth in the Isle of Wight in the United Kingdom, Kurukulaaratchy et al.[12] showed that future persistent wheezers, when compared with transient early wheezers, had significantly more physician-diagnosed asthma — a crude index of severity of symptoms — at ages 2 and 4 years.

Castro-Rodriguez et al.,[13] analyzing data from the Tucson Children's Respiratory Study, showed that children diagnosed with radiologically confirmed pneumonia in association with an LRI during the first 3 years of life were much more likely to continue wheezing at age 11 or 13 than those who had LRIs without pneumonia. The meaning of a diagnosis of pneumonia at this age is unclear because local atelectasis associated with severe bronchial obstruction may be radiologically undistinguishable from true inflammatory involvement of the lung parenchyma. Nevertheless, these studies suggest that despite considerable overlap between the two groups, the future persistent wheezers were much more likely to experience severe symptoms of airway obstruction in early life than transient early wheezers.

The fact that these two groups of children show different severities of acute episodes and very different prognoses in terms of future asthma-like symptoms begs the question as to the determinants of their wheezing episodes in early life and in what way these episodes are connected with their different prognoses. It is unlikely that these different prognoses are due to the types of viruses that triggered wheezing episodes in early life because no differences in the viral etiologies of the first episodes of LRI in these two groups were reported.[6] In fact, for both groups, RSV was the predominant virus isolated or cultured. Moreover, it is well known that all children are infected by RSV in early life, but only a small proportion develop any LRI symptoms. It is, thus, likely that more than the virus itself, the nature of the airway and immune response to the virus determines the development of an early LRI and possibly the subsequent development of persistent wheezing. This issue and its importance in asthma prevention will be discussed later in this chapter.

IV. Late Onset Wheezers

A third group of children also requires attention: those who do not have wheezing episodes in early life and experience their first episodes of wheeze after the first 3 years of life. It is a matter of great interest to determine whether these children have different outcomes than those who start wheezing during the first year of life. Recent data suggests that these "late onset wheezers" are as likely as persistent wheezers to continue wheezing in the preadolescent years.[12]

These data seem to suggest that at least in terms of the risk of having continued symptoms after the preschool years, persistent wheezers and late onset wheezers have similar long-term prognoses. A different picture emerges when indices of severity are also considered. The most detailed analysis was performed as part of the Isle of Wight study quoted earlier. When studied at age 10, persistent wheezers had significantly higher lifetime requirements for all levels of medical care with regard to their wheezing illnesses, as reported by their general practitioners, than late onset wheezers, and the latter did not differ from transient early wheezers. Moreover, persistent wheezers had the highest rates of asthma specialist referrals and hospital admissions. More than one fourth of all persistent wheezers had been admitted to hospitals at least once in their lifetimes for respiratory illnesses, compared with only 11% of late onset wheezers. When treatment received was assessed also at age 10, persistent wheezers showed significantly higher prevalence of inhaled corticosteroid use than late onset wheezers and over 61% of persistent wheezers required multiple courses of oral corticosteroids compared with 21% of late onset wheezers.[13]

These results clearly indicate that for children who will go on to develop asthma later in life, the timing of the initiation of symptoms is certainly not indifferent with respect to their outcomes. Persistent wheezers, whose first manifestations occur during the first 3 years of life, have more severe symptoms and require substantially more use of health care resources and prophylactic therapy than late onset wheezers. This is an important observation from the point of view of asthma prevention because everything seems to indicate that a successful intervention during the first 3 years of life could thwart the development of more severe cases of asthma.

V. Bronchial Hyperresponsiveness (BHR) and Lung Function in Early Wheezing Phenotypes

The results of the studies reported earlier suggest that, when studied in the preadolescent years, children with different wheezing phenotypes in early life show very different long-term clinical outcomes. It is thus of great interest to determine whether these different prognoses based on symptoms are corroborated by objective measures of lung function and bronchial responsiveness.

Our own studies in Tucson suggest that, by the age of 6 years, the patterns of lung function development for these different wheezing phenotypes are already clearly established.[14] We showed that, when maximal expiratory flows were measured shortly after birth with the chest compression technique and before any lower respiratory symptoms had developed, the future transient early wheezers had markedly lower levels of lung function when compared with children who never wheezed during the first 3 years of life. Conversely, persistent wheezers started life with levels of lung function that were slightly lower but not significantly different from those of "never wheezers." Even more interesting from the view of our discussion of differences in clinical outcomes of late onset and persistent wheezers, these two groups started life with almost identical levels of lung function.[6]

However, when we assessed maximal expiratory flows obtained with partial flow volume curves in the same groups at age 6, a different pattern was observed. Persistent wheezers had lower flows than all other groups, suggesting that this phenotype was associated with deficits in growth in airway function, whereas transient early wheezers showed catch-up growth relative to their peers, although their levels of lung function were still significantly lower at age 6 than those of children with no reports of wheezing during the first 6 years of life. Interestingly, late onset wheezers had maximal flows that had not changed their trajectories relative to those of children who never wheezed: they were still slightly but not significantly lower than those of the latter group. It is important to stress here that all children showed vast changes in absolute maximal flows and all comparisons were of the relative growth in airway functions of the different groups.

When we assessed lung function again at age 11 by use of maximal expiratory flow volume curves, we observed no changes in the relative positions of the different groups.[11] These striking results suggest no further deficits in growth of airway function among persistent wheezers between the ages of 6 and 11. Late onset wheezers also showed remarkable stability of airway function relative to their peers, whereas transient early wheezers showed maximal flows significantly lower than those of children who never wheezed, albeit still at the relative level that they had reached at age 6.

Very similar results from the Isle of Wight study quoted earlier were recently reported by Kurukulaaratchy et al.[12] In a similar manner to ours, these authors studied FEV1 (forced expiratory volume in one second), FVC (forced vital capacity), and peak flow at age 10 in children classified according to their early life symptoms. They showed that persistent wheezers had significantly reduced mean FEV1:FVC ratios when compared with children who never wheezed in early life and with transient early wheezers. The latter, on the other hand, had significantly reduced peak flows when compared with never wheezers, and late onset wheezers had levels of lung function that were slightly but not significantly different from those of children who never wheezed in early life.

Similar (albeit not identical) trends were reported by Lau et al. from another cohort study, the German Multicenter Allergy Study (MAS).[15] Contrary to the Tucson and Isle of Wight cohorts, the German MAS was enriched with newborns who had double-positive family histories of allergies or high cord serum IgE. By age 7, children in this cohort were also classified into the four wheezing phenotypes described earlier, and lung function and allergy status were assessed. Persistent wheezers had the lowest mean levels of FEV1:FVC ratios and maximal forced flows at mid and late expiration, and the levels were significantly lower than those of children who had never wheezed up to age 7.

Transient early wheezers showed levels of FEV1:FVC ratios that were slightly but not significantly diminished, whereas their maximal flows at mid expiration were significantly lower than those of never wheezers. Late onset wheezers, on the other hand, had levels of lung function that were between those of persistent wheezers and those of children who never wheezed. When they studied all children who were wheezing at age 7 as a group (that is, late and persistent wheezers combined), Lau et al. observed that time since the first wheezing episode was a significant determinant of lung function level.

This observation is very similar to that of Zeiger et al. from the Childhood Asthma Management Program (CAMP).[16] These authors found that baseline FEV1 levels among school age children with mild to moderate asthma were inversely related to time elapsed since asthma onset. Because data from the CAMP study were retrospective, it was not possible to determine whether the correlation observed was due to early onset or to duration of asthma. Our own observation that among late onset wheezers a remarkable stability of lung function was observed up to age 11 suggests that early age of onset rather than duration of asthma is an important determinant of the level of lung function attained during the school years.

The fact that late onset wheezers in this MAS study showed clearly diminished lung function levels — an observation that was not present in the other two cohorts — remains unexplained. It is tempting to speculate, however, that the enrichment of the MAS cohort with children at very high risk for the development of allergies early in life could account at least in part for these discrepant findings. (See below for further discussion of this issue.)

Of particular interest were the results of studies of methacholine BHR performed in the Isle of Wight study for the four early life wheezing groups.[12] When assessed at age 10, transient early wheezers had a prevalence of moderate or severe BHR that was very similar to that of children who never wheezed (15 and 10%, respectively), but approximately 50% of both late onset wheezers and persistent wheezers had moderate or severe BHR. Therefore, persistent wheezers and late onset wheezers had very similar prevalences of BHR and symptoms at age 10, but they had markedly different levels of lung function and more severe symptoms at that age.

As a whole, these results suggest that the patterns of development of lung function in the different wheezing phenotypes are already established by the early school years, and that these patterns are correlated with asthma severity even more strongly than with prevalence of BHR. The importance of this observation cannot be overstated, given the results of two longitudinal studies in which school-age children with asthma were followed up in mid-adulthood.[3,17] These studies showed that no further deterioration in FEV1:FVC ratio was observed after the ages of 7 to 9 years in children with asthma, even among those with severe disease and whose symptoms persisted into their fifth decade of life. These results thus suggest that intervention must occur very early in life if deterioration in lung function in asthma is to be prevented.

VI. Predicting Early Asthma

The conclusions proposed earlier suggest that an important task in the future development of any strategy for asthma prevention will be the capacity to identify during the first years of life those children who are having their first symptoms of airway obstruction and will go on to develop asthma later in life. In the data from the Tucson study, these children accounted for approximately 40% of all early life wheezers, a proportion that was very similar to that reported for the Isle of Wight study and more than twice as high as that of the MAS cohort (17%). The reasons for this discrepancy are not known. In any case, persistent wheezers constitute a minority of early life wheezers, and targeting prevention measures to all wheezers would not only be very expensive but would also subject many children and their families to unneeded therapies and unnecessary stress.

In order to determine whether predicting early asthma was possible, we searched for phenotypic markers in the Tucson study that could serve to identify among children who had developed recurrent symptoms of airway obstruction by age 3 those who would still have asthma during the school years.[18] We were particularly interested in markers that could be usable in any clinical setting. We devised an "asthma predictive index" (API) that had a positive predictive value of approximately 60 to 70% and a negative predictive value of approximately 90%. This meant that roughly two thirds of all children with positive APIs developed asthma later in life, whereas only 10% of those with negative APIs developed the disease.

To be included in the analysis, a child was required to have a wheezing frequency of at least 3 on a scale of 1 to 6. The index had two major criteria (eczema and parental history of asthma) and three minor criteria (eosinophilia >4% of circulating white blood cells, reports of wheezing without colds, and diagnosis of allergic rhinitis by a physician). Children with one major criterion or two minor criteria were considered positive. It is obvious from this description that most of these criteria point toward early development of allergic diatheses as important determinants of differential risk for asthma among children who wheeze during the first years of life. These findings have been corroborated by a study using the Isle of Wight cohort.[19]

VII. Early Development of T Helper-2 (Th2) Responses

The data thus confirmed and extended reports from the Poole birth cohort showing that early sensitization to aeroallergens is a strong risk factor for the development of persistent asthma in early adult life.[5] Data from the MAS study showed that early development of specific IgE against foods that is followed by sensitization against aeroallergens later in life is a very important risk factor for the development of asthma-like symptoms by the age of 7 years.[20] The finding that early sensitization to allergens is strongly associated with subsequent asthma may also explain the differences in the results observed between the MAS cohort and the other two birth cohorts (Tucson and Isle of Wight) in which enrollees were not selected for their asthma risks.

Having enriched their cohort with children who would have been classified as having positive APIs, the researchers on the MAS study may have identified a group of children with early life allergies at increased risk of developing lower levels of lung function during their first years of life regardless of the timing of initiation of their wheezing episodes. This was especially suggested by their finding that among current wheezers at age 7, those who had elevated cord blood IgE levels (a criterion for enrichment of the sample in this cohort) had markedly diminished FEV1:FVC ratios and maximal flows at mid expiration, and this was true for both persistent and late onset wheezers. For example, late onset wheezers with low cord serum had mean FEV1:FVC ratios of 91.3% at age 7, which is not greatly different from values of 92.9% observed among children who had never wheezed by age 7. Instead, late onset wheezers with high cord IgE had mean FEV1:FVC ratios of 84.7% — lower than those of persistent wheezers, regardless of cord IgE levels.

Because the prevalence of high cord IgE is low in the general population, it is likely that lung function results for late onset wheezers in the MAS cohort were influenced by the recruitment strategy chosen. Nevertheless, these results shed light on one aspect that could not be addressed in the other two cohorts: an important determinant of lung function during the school years may be early development of a T helper-2 phenotype. The MAS data suggest that this immune pattern may increase the risk of developing low levels of lung function regardless of the timing of initiation of asthma-like symptoms.

Strong support for this contention was provided by the results of a more recent birth cohort study, the Manchester Asthma and Allergy Study (MAAS).[21] Children were enrolled in this study at birth and classified into three groups according to their parents' allergy skin tests: high risk, if both parents were skin test-positive; medium risk if only one parent was positive; and low risk if neither parent was skin test-positive. Episodes of wheezing were assessed prospectively by questionnaires and allergy skin tests. Airway resistance using a whole body plethysmograph was measured at age 3.

The authors found that, even among children who had never wheezed, those who were skin-test positive to allergens or who had maternal histories of asthma had significantly higher specific airway resistance than those who had neither of these risk factors. It thus appears that either the early development of allergic sensitization or an inherited susceptibility to asthma may be associated with an alteration in airway function that is present even before any evidence of clinically overt airway obstruction. What determines this alteration is not presently known, but it is tempting to speculate that both these risk factors are associated with the early development of T helper-2-type responses in the airways that may interfere with normal airway growth. Cytokines associated with the T helper-2 phenotype are know to exert potent growth factor-like effects on fibroblasts and myofibroblasts.[22-24] These effects may be particularly influential between the ages of 1 and 6 years — a time in human life when lungs and airways grow at the fastest pace.

VIII. Conclusions

This paper reviews the findings of several asthma birth cohorts. These findings are changing our understanding of the natural history of asthma in a way that will certainly influence the development of strategies for asthma prevention. In summary, asthma is a disease that tends to start early in life, especially in the more severe and more persistent cases. Alterations in airway function in older children and adults with asthma are usually already established during the first 6 to 9 years of life; no further deteriorations are observed in these subjects as a group through the mid-adult years. Early development of T helper-2-type responses to aeroallergens appears to play a crucial role in the development of the chronic asthma phenotype.

References

1. Martinez FD and Godfrey S. *Wheezing Disorders in the Preschool Child.* New York: Taylor & Francis, 2003.
2. Strachan DP, Butland BK, and Anderson HR. Incidence and prognosis of asthma and wheezing illness from early childhood to age 33 in a national British cohort. *Br Med J* 1996; 312: 1195–1199.
3. Sears MR, Greene JM, Willan AR, Wiecek EM, Taylor DR, Flannery EM, Cowan JO, Herbison GP, Silva PA, and Poulton R. A longitudinal population-based cohort study: childhood asthma followed to adulthood. *New Engl J Med* 2003; 349(15): 1414–1422.
4. Yunginger J, Reed CE, O'Connell EJ, Melton LJ, O'Fallon WM, and Silverstein MD. A community-based study of the epidemiology of asthma: incidence rates, 1964–1983. *Am Rev Respir Dis* 1992; 146: 888–894.
5. Rhodes HL, Thomas P, Sporik R, Holgate ST, and Cogswell JJ. A birth cohort study of subjects at risk of atopy: twenty-two-year follow-up of wheeze and atopic status. *Am J Respir Crit Care Med* 2002; 165: 176–180.
6. Martinez FD, Wright AL, Taussig LM, Holberg CJ, Halonen M, and Morgan WJ. Asthma and wheezing in the first six years of life. *New Engl J Med* 1995; 332: 133–138.
7. Stein RT, Sherrill D, Morgan WJ, Holberg CJ, Halonen M, Taussig LM, Wright AL, and Martinez FD. Respiratory syncytial virus in early life and risk of wheeze and allergy by age 13 years. *Lancet* 1999; 354: 541–545.
8. Gern JE, Martin MS, Anklam KA, Shen K, Roberg KA, Carlson-Dakes KT, Adler K, Gilbertson-White S, Hamilton R, Shult PA, Kirk CJ, Da Silva DF, Sund SA, Kosorok MR, and Lemanske RF, Jr. Relationships among specific viral pathogens, virus-induced interleukin-8, and respiratory symptoms in infancy. *Pediatr Allergy Immunol* 2002; 13: 386–393.

9. Williams JV, Harris PA, Tollefson SJ, Halburnt-Rush LL, Pingsterhaus JM, Edwards KM, Wright PF, and Crowe JE, Jr. Human metapneumovirus and lower respiratory tract disease in otherwise healthy infants and children. *New Engl J Med* 2004; 350: 443–450.

10. Dodge R, Martinez FD, Cline MG, Lebowitz MD, and Burrows B. Early childhood respiratory symptoms and the subsequent diagnosis of asthma. *J Allergy Clin Immunol* 1996; 98: 48–54.

11. Stern DA, Morgan WJ, Taussig LM, Wright AL, Halonen M, and Martinez FD. Lung function at age 11 in relation to early wheezing. *Am J Resp Crit Care Med* 1999; 159: A148.

12. Kurukulaaratchy RJ, Fenn MH, Waterhouse LM, Matthews SM, Holgate ST, and Arshad SH. Characterization of wheezing phenotypes in the first 10 years of life. *Clin Exp Allergy* 2003; 33: 573–578.

13. Castro-Rodriguez JA, Holberg CJ, Wright AL, Halonen M, Taussig LM, Morgan WJ, and Martinez FD. Association of radiologically ascertained pneumonia before age 3 years with asthma-like symptoms and pulmonary function during childhood: a prospective study. *Am J Resp Crit Care Med* 1999; 159: 1891–1897.

14. Martinez FD. Development of wheezing disorders and asthma in preschool children. *Pediatrics* 2002; 109 (Suppl.): 362–367.

15. Lau S, Illi S, Sommerfeld C, Niggemann B, Volkel K, Madloch C, Gruber C, Nickel R, Forster J, and Wahn U. Transient early wheeze is not associated with impaired lung function in 7-yr-old children. *Eur Respir J* 2003; 21: 834–841.

16. Zeiger RS, Dawson C, and Weiss S. Relationships between duration of asthma and asthma severity among children in the Childhood Asthma Management Program (CAMP). *J Allergy Clin Immunol* 1999; 103 (Pt 1): 376–387.

17. Oswald H, Phelan PD, Lanigan A, Hibbert M, Carlin JB, Bowes G, and Olinsky A. Childhood asthma and lung function in mid-adult life. *Pediatr Pulmonol* 1997; 23: 14–20.

18. Castro-Rodriguez JA, Holberg CJ, Wright AL, and Martinez FD. A clinical index to define risk of asthma in young children with recurrent wheezing. *Am J Resp Crit Care Med* 2000; 162 (Pt 1): 1403–1406.

19. Kurukulaaratchy RJ, Matthews S, Holgate ST, and Arshad SH. Predicting persistent disease among children who wheeze during early life. *Eur Respir J* 2003; 22: 767–771.

20. Illi S, von Mutius E, Lau S, Nickel R, Niggemann B, Sommerfeld C, and Wahn U. The pattern of atopic sensitization is associated with the development of asthma in childhood. *J Allergy Clin Immunol* 2001; 108: 709–714.

21. Lowe L, Murray CS, Custovic A, Simpson BM, Kissen PM, and Woodcock A. Specific airway resistance in 3-year-old children: a prospective cohort study. *Lancet* 2002; 359: 1904–1908.

22. Doucet C, Brouty-Boye D, Pottin-Clemenceau C, Canonica GW, Jasmin C, and Azzarone B. Interleukin (IL) 4 and IL-13 act on human lung fibroblasts: implication in asthma. *J Clin Invest* 1998; 101: 2129–2139.

23. Doucet C, Brouty-Boye D, Pottin-Clemenceau C, Jasmin C, Canonica GW, and Azzarone B. IL-4 and IL-13 specifically increase adhesion molecule and inflammatory cytokine expression in human lung fibroblasts. *Int Immunol* 1998; 10: 1421–1433.

24. Zhu Z, Homer RJ, Wang Z, Chen Q, Geba GP, Wang J, Zhang Y, and Elias JA. Pulmonary expression of interleukin-13 causes inflammation, mucus hypersecretion, subepithelial fibrosis, physiologic abnormalities, and eotaxin production. *J Clin Invest* 1999; 103: 779–788.

3

Emerging Patterns of Asthma Worldwide

ERIKA VON MUTIUS

University Children's Hospital
Munich, Germany

I. Introduction

Not all languages include a word for "wheeze." Whether a missing term in certain languages indicates the lack of necessity to describe such a phenomenon remains a linguistic riddle. However, the spatial distribution of the prevalence of wheeze and asthma is extremely heterogeneous, ranging from almost nonexistent in some areas to an illness affecting almost half the population in other regions. The large variation in the occurrence of such symptoms and diagnoses is likely to be caused by a multitude of host and environmental factors and their specific interactions, most of which we do not understand or even recognize. Furthermore, wheezing syndromes do not represent a single entity, but most likely are the relatively uniform clinical manifestations of a wide array of various underlying pathological mechanisms affecting a multitude of systems such as the airways, immune responses, and neural systems, to name only a few.

Most studies to date have not been able to adequately take into account this large diversity of host and environmental factors. This criticism pertains to epidemiological studies in particular which must rely on solicited information and some measures of disease-associated traits due to the lack of a golden standard for asthma. Nevertheless, epidemiology has guided the thinking about the potential causes of asthma by initiating hypotheses and paradigms. In particular, descriptions of spatial and temporal variations in disease prevalence have greatly pressed the search for underlying determinants of this condition.

II. Worldwide Distribution of Wheeze and Asthma

The worldwide prevalence of allergic diseases was assessed in the 1990s by the large scale International Study of Asthma and Allergy in Childhood (ISAAC).[1] More than 700,000 children in 155 collaborating centers in 56 countries were studied. Children used one-page questionnaires to self-report symptoms of wheeze, allergic rhinoconjunctivitis, and atopic eczema. Between 20- and 60-fold differences were found among centers in the prevalence of symptoms of asthma, allergic rhinoconjunctivitis, and atopic eczema. The highest 12-month prevalences of asthma symptoms were reported from centers in the United Kingdom, Australia, New Zealand, and the Republic of Ireland. These were followed by most centers in North, Central, and South America. The lowest prevalences were reported by centers in several Eastern European countries, Indonesia, Greece, China, Taiwan, Uzbekistan, India, and Ethiopia. The self-reported 12-month prevalence of wheezing among 13- to 14-year olds among countries ranged from 2.1% in Indonesia to 32.2% in the United Kingdom.

The analysis showed consistently more variation among countries than within countries. However, the selected centers may not represent the prevalence of asthma symptoms throughout whole countries. No rural versus urban comparisons were made, nor were affluent areas contrasted with poor regions. The ISAAC collaboration agreed that the cardinal symptom of asthma would be the reflection of variable airway narrowing best described in English as "wheezing or whistling in the chest." More specific questions relating to the severity of asthma were also included. The proportion of wheezy children with severe asthma symptoms varied little with the increasing prevalence of wheezy children in a population, indicating that the high prevalences found in some centers were not explained by excessive inclusion of children with mild wheeze.

The validity of the ISAAC questionnaire is likely to have varied across cultures and languages. As mentioned earlier, certain languages have no equivalent of "wheezing" as understood by English speakers. However, spatial distribution using the video questionnaire was very comparable with the variations found with the written questionnaire. In general, centers with low asthma rates also showed low levels of other atopic diseases. However, countries with the highest prevalences of allergic rhinitis and atopic eczema were not the same countries that had the highest asthma rates (Figure 3.1).

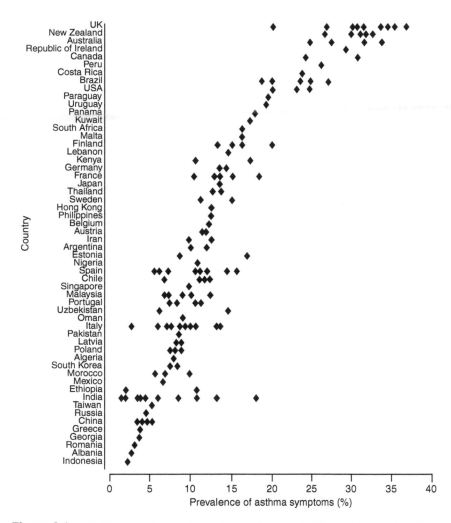

Figure 3.1 Worldwide variation of prevalence of wheeze in 13- and 14-year olds. (From International Study of Asthma and Allergies in Childhood (ISAAC) Steering Committee, Worldwide variation in prevalence of symptoms of asthma, allergic rhinoconjunctivitis, and atopic eczema, *Lancet*, 351, 1225–1332, 1998. With permission.)

The European Community Respiratory Health Survey (ECRHS) investigated young adults aged 20 to 44 years.[2] Data from over 13,000 men and women were obtained at the start of the study. A highly standardized and comprehensive study instrument including bronchial challenge using methacholine, and measurements of total and specific serum IgE antibodies was used by 48 centers in 22 countries predominantly in Western Europe, but also in Australia, New

Zealand, and the United States. Questionnaire findings documented a large variability of the prevalence of asthma across centers; the variability was supported by the results of the bronchial challenge test. High levels of responsiveness were seen in centers in New Zealand, Australia, the United States, and Britain. In turn, low levels of airway responsiveness were found in Iceland and Switzerland and in most centers in Sweden, Italy, and Spain.[3]

A strong correlation was found between the findings from children as assessed by ISAAC and the rates in adults as reported by the ECRHS.[4] Sixty-four percent of the variation at the country level and 74% of the variation at the center level in the prevalence of "wheeze in the last 12 months" in the ECRHS data was explained by the variation rates reported for children by the ISAAC. Thus, although differences in the absolute prevalences were observed in the two surveys, the good overall agreement added support to the validity of both studies (Figure 3.2).

III. Contrasting Results from Developing and Developed Countries

Some of the comparisons from the ISAAC are particularly informative. In China, the prevalence of asthma and other allergies among children living in Hong Kong was assessed and compared with prevalence among children living in mainland China, in Beijing and Urumqui.[5] Beijing children reported significantly more asthma symptoms than those living in Urumqui, and Hong Kong children had the highest prevalence of asthma and other allergic symptoms. Likewise, skin test reactivity as an objective assessment of atopy was also more prevalent in Hong Kong as compared with the other areas. Urumqui, Beijing, and Hong Kong represent communities at different stages of westernization and the results from these three cities reflect a worldwide trend of increasing prevalence of allergies as westernization intensifies.

Using another standardized methodology, the prevalence of symptoms and the rates of diagnosis and management of asthma in school-aged children in Australia were compared with those rates for Nigerian children.[6] Wheeze, asthma, and history of asthma medication use were less prevalent in Nigeria than in Australia. No significant differences were noted in the overall prevalence of atopy between the two countries, although atopy was a strong risk factor for asthma in both countries.

Dissociations between the prevalence of asthma and atopy have been found in other developing countries.[7] The dissociations suggest that asthma and atopy are only loosely linked phenotypes. Pearce and colleagues reviewed the available literature to assess the extent to which the development of asthma is attributable to atopy. The proportion of asthmatic and nonasthmatic subjects that were skin prick test-positive or showed elevated serum IgE antibodies to environmental allergens varied widely among study populations. The proportion of cases attributable to atopy

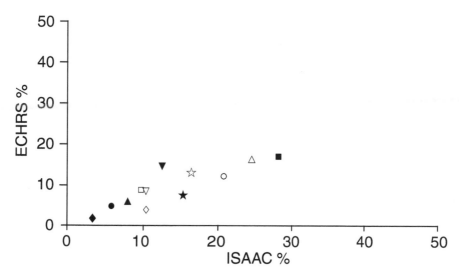

Figure 3.2 Relationship of asthma prevalence estimates of the International Study of Asthma and Allergies in Childhood (ISAAC) and European Community Respiratory Health Survey (ECRHS), Phase II by country. ■ = Australia. ▲ = Belgium. ◆ = Estonia. ▼ = France. ● = Germany. ★ = Ireland. □ = Italy. △ = New Zealand. ◇ = Spain. ▽ = Sweden. ○ = United Kingdom. ☆ = United States.

varied from 25 to 63% in cross-sectional studies investigating exclusively or mainly children. Similar numbers derived from studies of adults.

These findings suggest that the importance of atopy as a cause of asthma may have been overestimated because the high proportions found in high prevalence areas such as the United States or Britain were not seen in less affluent regions as in the developing world. Therefore, different phenotypes of wheeze and asthma may be encountered in different parts of the world. It seems likely that atopic asthma prevails among children in most westernized countries, whereas virus-associated wheeze is more likely to predominate in developing regions. For example, in the Fiji Islands, the prevalence of wheeze was identical for immigrant Indians and Fijians, but the prevalence of airway hyperresponsiveness in Indians was much higher than among Fijians who exhibited more prevalence of pneumonia and productive cough.[8,9]

The timing of exposures to certain environments may play a role in the development of asthma. Therefore, the relation between the prevalence of respiratory symptoms and time since arrival in Australia was studied in immigrant teenagers living in Melbourne. In subjects born outside Australia, residence for 5 to 9 years in Australia was associated with a two-fold increase in the odds of self-reported wheeze; after 10 to 14 years, this risk increased to three-fold. This time–dose effect on the prevalence of symptoms in subjects born outside Australia and living in Melbourne was independent of age and country of birth.[10]

IV. East–West Gradient across Europe

Another peculiarity of the variation in the prevalence of childhood asthma is the marked east–west gradient across Europe.[1] A number of reports have demonstrated large differences in the prevalence of bronchitis, asthma, airway hyperresponsiveness, hay fever, and atopy in children and adults between east and west European areas.[11-14] The prevalence of asthma was significantly lower in Eastern Europe as compared with Western Europe. Differences in the observed prevalence rates of physician-diagnosed asthma between West and East Germany may have reflected differences in medical practice and diagnostic labeling in the formerly separated states. However, when the relation of atopic sensitization, airway responsiveness, and respiratory illnesses was considered, wheezing illnesses other than those labeled as asthma were more strongly associated with atopy and airway responsiveness in West Germany than in the eastern part of the country. Likewise, the prevalence of bronchitis with atopy and airway hyperresponsiveness was higher in the western part of the country.

Children and adults living in West Germany showed significantly higher prevalences of airway hyperresponsiveness than those living in East Germany.[11,14] We acknowledge that the measurement of airway responsiveness by cold air hyperventilation is strongly dependent on the ventilation rate and thus on the compliance of the subject tested; however, similar results were obtained in adults using a methacholine challenge. Significantly lower prevalences of hay fever, nasal allergies, and atopy measured by skin prick tests or specific serum IgE antibodies toward environmental allergens were also found among children and adults living in Eastern European areas as compared with subjects living in Western Europe.[11,12,14]

When a cross-sectional survey of children was repeated in 1996 in East Germany, atopic sensitization measured by skin-prick tests had increased significantly although it did not attain the prevalence rates of atopy previously reported for Munich school children.[15] The children from East Germany who participated in this repeat survey were born 3 years before the downfall of communism and therefore were exposed to Western living conditions only after their third birthdays. This may indicate that factors present early in life are particularly important for the development of asthma and that environmental factors may influence the development of other allergic disorders after infancy. It remains to be seen whether the prevalence of asthma will increase in children who are born and raised according to a "western" lifestyle in formerly communist countries of Eastern Europe.

Recent data from the Eastern European ISAAC centers corroborated previous results and expanded findings to include such areas as Georgia and Uzbekistan.[16] Among the older age group of 13- to 14-year old children, the prevalence of wheezing was 11.2 to 19.7% in Finland and Sweden; 7.6 to 8.5% in Estonia, Latvia, and Poland; and 2.6 to 5.9% in Albania, Romania, Russia, Georgia, and Uzbekistan (except the city of Samarkand). The prevalence of itching eyes and flexural dermatitis varied in similar manners among the three regions. Among 6- to 7-year old children, the regional differences were less pronounced.

The reasons for these differences remain unknown. Wichmann and co-workers explored the potential role of allergen exposure by measuring concentrations in house dust samples of 405 homes in Hamburg, West Germany, and Erfurt, East Germany.[17] The homes were visited approximately 5 years after reunification. Three dust samples from the living room floor, bedroom floor, and mattress surface of each house were taken in a standardized manner. Higher levels of mite and cat allergens were found in Hamburg as compared with Erfurt, whereas cockroach allergens were only detected in 7.1% of all homes.[18] Differences in Der p 1 concentrations disappeared after adjusting for housing characteristics and indoor climate.

Two other studies from East Germany performed between 1992 and 1996 yielded similar concentrations of house dust mite allergen levels (Der p 1 and Der f 1) as studies from West Germany.[19] Interestingly, coal heating — the most common type of heating in former East Germany — was associated with higher house dust mite allergen concentrations. Because the allergen exposure studies were performed several years after German reunification and the ensuing rapid changes in indoor environments, exposure estimates for these years are more likely to reflect current rather than past exposures. According to questionnaire data collected in 1995 and 1996, almost a third of East Germany's coal heating furnaces had disappeared.[15] This suggests that exposure estimates from 1995 and 1996 are likely to significantly underestimate exposures in the former German Democratic Republic if the relation between coal heating and higher allergen levels holds true.

In the Estonian city of Tartu, 197 homes were visited in 1993 and 1994 for purposes of dust collection.[20] Three dust samples (bedroom floor, infant's mattress, and living room floor) were collected. The levels of house dust mite allergens in these homes were similar to those recorded in central Sweden and Norway in previous studies. Cat and dog allergens were also as commonly encountered in the Estonian as in Swedish homes, and the mean levels were similar.[20]

Dust samples from the 1995–1996 study in Hamburg and Erfurt were also assessed for viable molds.[21] No significant differences were shown for total and single genera (*Alternaria, Aspergillus, Cladosporium,* and *Penicillium*) in concentrations of spores of viable fungi in the settled dust samples. These findings suggest that neither allergen exposure nor mold exposure may explain the differences between Eastern and Western European exposures.

Nutritional intake has been incriminated as a potential cause of asthma and allergies. In a 1995–1996 survey in Leipzig, East Germany, changes in dietary habits since unification were explored.[15] In children whose parents reported increased consumption of margarine after the fall of the wall, the prevalence of hay fever was significantly higher (7.3%) than in children from households with equal (4.3%) or lower (1.6%) consumption (p <0.001). This relation remained significant after adjusting for potential confounding factors (odds ratio [OR] = 2.0; 95% confidence interval [CI], 1.1–3.5, p <0.05). No association was found, however, between changes in the intake of margarine and atopic sensitization, asthma, or bronchial hyperresponsiveness (BHR). Changes in the consumption of butter showed an inverse association with hay fever (higher intake, 4.3%; equal intake, 4.5%; lower intake, 6.5%) and atopic sensitization (higher intake, 16.7%; equal intake, 27.9%; lower intake, 28.8%). However, only the difference in atopic sensitization between those with higher and lower butter consumption levels reached statistical significance (p <0.05).

The mechanisms by which fatty acid consumption may influence the occurrence of atopic diseases are not clear. Linoleic acid is a precursor of arachidonic acid that can be converted into mediators such as prostaglandins and leukotrienes that play important roles in the pathophysiology of asthma and allergies.[22] It has been speculated that this process may be enhanced by higher intake of linoleic acid, while intake of omega-3 fatty acids such as linolenic or eicosapentanoic acid may inhibit this process.[23]

Margarine is, however, also a source of trans-fatty acids. Recent ecological analyses of the ISAAC data have shown a consistent association between intake of trans-fatty acids and the prevalence of atopic symptoms.[24] Interestingly, these associations were only seen for trans-fatty acids from predominantly industrial sources. The mechanisms by which such differences might be explained are not understood.

Strachan[25] showed a strong inverse association between the number of siblings and the prevalence of hay fever in British children and suggested that viral infections early in life may prevent the development of allergic sensitization. In the former German Democratic Republic, most women worked, thus exposing their children to day care settings and consequently to viral infections as early as at 12 months of age. In 1982 and 1983, day care settings were attended by 69 and 71%, respectively, of East German children aged 1 to 3 years, whereas in West Germany only 8.2 and 6.9% of all children in this age group had access to day care.[11] Moreover, children from East Germany had significantly (p <0.001) more siblings than those from West Germany.

In a large cross-sectional survey of East German children aged 5 to 14, Krämer and colleagues showed that children from small families, i.e., three family members at most, entering day nursery in the first year of life were at significantly lower risk to develop asthma, hay fever, and positive skin-prick tests than children beginning day care after their second birthdays.[26] A recent prospective study from the U.S. corroborated these findings.[27]

Attendance at day care in the first 6 months of life was associated with a significantly lower risk of asthma and atopy over the 13-year follow-up period. In fact, the risk of having asthma at school age and thereafter was decreased to one half to one third of previously expected dates. Likewise, a recent analysis of the German Multicenter Birth Cohort Study showed that repeated episodes of infectious rhinitis in the first year of life conferred protection from asthma at school age.[28] Interestingly, the magnitude of the effect was similar to the one demonstrated for the U.S. birth cohort study.

Immunization rates also differed between East and West Germany. BCG vaccination was routine in the eastern part of the country, whereas only a minority of children in Munich were immunized with BCG.

Shirakawa et al.[29] reported that among BCG-immunized Japanese school children aged 12 to 13, allergic and asthmatic symptoms were one half to one third as likely in positive tuberculin responders as in negative responders, and that remission of atopic symptoms between the ages of 7 and 12 years was six to nine times more likely in positive tuberculin responders. The interpretation of these findings has been debated intensively. The inverse association between allergic status and tuberculin reactivity may simply reflect the imbalance of Th1/Th2 responsiveness characteristic of atopic individuals who have been shown to express smaller delayed-type hypersensitivity skin reactions to recall antigens than nonatopic subjects.[30] All children in this study were vaccinated against BCG, suggesting that the vaccination per se did not account for the effects described in this paper. This notion is supported by findings from a Swedish study showing that a single application of BCG vaccination does not relate to the development of childhood asthma and allergies.[31]

V. Differences in Rural and Urban Populations

In some developing countries, lower prevalences of childhood asthma were reported from rural as compared to urban areas. Airway challenges performed in African urban and rural areas revealed that bronchial hyperresponsiveness (BHR) was almost nonexistent in some rural areas in the late 1980s and early 1990s.[32] Among the more affluent urban populations of South Africa and Zimbabwe, BHR reached prevalence rates of 3.2% and 5.9%, respectively. Similar results were reported by other African studies. However, over the last decade, BHR seems to have increased in rural Africa.[32] Similar findings were reported from urban and rural Saudi Arabia.[33] A significantly lower prevalence of allergic symptoms was found in rural as compared to urban children.

Differences in childhood asthma between rural and urban populations in Western countries were less pronounced. In a large British study, only marginal differences were observed in the prevalence of childhood asthma between rural and urban areas.[34] However, children from rural Scotland tended to show a lower prevalence of severe asthma symptoms.[35] Data from Sweden indicated a higher prevalence of atopic sensitization to aeroallergens in children from urban centers compared to those in rural areas, but no information was available for childhood asthma.[13] The increased risk for children to develop atopic diseases in an urban environment was attributed largely to increased levels of air pollution, particularly that related to heavy car traffic exposure. However, recent findings from Austria,[36] Finland,[37] Canada,[38] Southern Germany,[39] and Switzerland[40] suggest that the lower prevalences of atopic diseases in rural populations may be attributable to the presence of unspecified protective factors in a farm environment rather than to the absence of urban risk factors.

Several authors investigated rural populations and found that growing up on a farm confers significant protection against the development of asthma and atopy.[36,38–40] This protective effect was not detected in children raised in a rural environment by nonfarming parents. Several investigators observed that frequent contact with livestock conferred the protection associated with farm life. A dose–response relation between exposure to farm animals and the prevalence of atopic disease was reported among farmers' children in Southern Germany.[39]

The protective effect ascribed to exposure to livestock was not limited to children growing up on farms. Frequent contact with farm animals by children who did not live on farms and gained exposure through visits with peers living on farms likewise conferred significant protection.[36] The effects were pronounced when exposure to stables and raw milk from the farm occurred in the first year of life.[41] When maternal exposure to farm animals during pregnancy and lactation is considered and adjustments are made for potentially confounding factors, the odds of atopic sensitization were reduced to aOR = 0.18 (95% CI, 0.06–0.56), the odds of hay fever to aOR = 0.07 (95 % CI, 0.005–0.91), and the odds of asthma to null. This observation again supports the importance of timing with respect to the impact of environmental exposures on subsequent symptomatology.

Microbial exposures are manifold in these environments and microbial studies investigating stables reported a large variety of Gram-negative and Gram-positive germs as well as a diversity of molds and fungi. In addition, nonviable parts of microbes such as endotoxin from the outer walls of Gram-negative bacteria are found in abundance in stables and in elevated concentrations in indoor environments of farm houses.[42] Recent reports suggest that the environmental exposure to endotoxin as assessed in mattress dust levels significantly decreases the risks of hay fever, atopic sensitization, and atopic asthma in childhood.[43] This protective effect was observed among farm children and also among children from nonfarming rural families, indicating that the relatively low levels of exposure observed in nonfarm environments favorably influence the development of childhood atopic diseases.

Endotoxin exposure in house dust has been related to the development of atopic sensitization in infants enrolled in a cohort study in the U.S.[44] Among 61 children (9 to 24 months of age) of low socioeconomic status who suffered three physician-documented wheezing episodes, endotoxin levels in the house dust were inversely related to atopic sensitization. Interestingly, a strong relation between endotoxin exposure and interferon-gamma production by CD4- and CD8-positive cells was seen, suggesting a stimulation of the immune system toward Th1-like responses by environmental levels of indoor exposure to endotoxin.

Interestingly, endotoxin exposures were only inversely related to the atopic wheezing phenotypes, whereas for nonatopic wheezing, high levels of endotoxin exposure represented a risk factor. Because endotoxin levels are likely to be high in developing countries, the risk of nonatopic wheeze may be increased in such environments, whereas the development of atopy may be hampered.

High exposure levels to endotoxin may, however, be surrogates for other bacterial products such as nonmethylated cytidin–guanosin dinucleotides specific for prokaryotic DNA (CpG motifs) or cell wall components from atypical Mycobacteria or Gram-positive bacteria such as lipoteichoic acid that are known to affect immune responses in similar ways as endotoxin. The individual contribution of these different microbial or fungal exposures awaits further clarification.

Microbial stimulation, from both normal commensals and pathogens through the gut, may be another route of exposure that may have altered normal intestinal colonization patterns in infancy. As a consequence, the induction and maintenance of oral tolerance to innocuous antigens such as food proteins and inhaled allergens may be substantially hampered.[45,46] While they are intriguing, these hypotheses have not been supported to date by epidemiological evidence, mainly due to the significant methodological difficulties that arise in attempts to measure longitudinally the microbial patterns of intestinal flora in large numbers of children.

References

1. SAAC Steering Committee. Worldwide variations in the prevalence of atopic diseases: the International Study of Asthma and Allergies in Childhood (ISAAC). *Lancet* 1998; 351: 1225–1232.
2. Burney P, Luczynska C, Chinn S, and Jarvis D. European Community Respiratory Health Survey. *Eur Respir J* 1994; 7: 954–960.
3. Chinn S, Burney P, Jarvis D, and Luczynska C. Variation in bronchial responsiveness in the European Community Respiratory Health Survey (ECRHS). *Eur Respir J* 1997; 10: 2495–2501.

4. Pearce N, Sunyer J, Cheng S, Chinn S, Björkstén B, Burr M, Keil U, Anderson HR, Burney P, on behalf of the ISAAC Steering Committee and the European Community Respiratory Health Survey. Comparison of asthma prevalence in the ISAAC and the ECRHS. *Eur Respir J* 2000; 16: 420–426.
5. Zhao T, Wang A, Chen Y et al. Prevalence of childhood asthma, allergic rhinitis and eczema in Urumqui and Beijing. *J Paediatr Child Health* 2000; 36: 128–133.
6. Faniran A, Peat J, and Woolcock A. Prevalence of atopy, asthma symptoms and diagnosis, and the management of asthma: comparison of an affluent and a non-affluent country. *Thorax* 1999; 54: 606–610.
7. Pearce N, Pekkanen J, and Beasley R. How much asthma is really attributable to atopy? *Thorax* 1999; 54: 268–272.
8. Flynn MG. Respiratory symptoms, bronchial responsiveness, and atopy in Fijian and Indian children. *Am J Respir Crit Care Med* 1994; 150: 415–420.
9. Flynn MG. Respiratory symptoms of rural Fijian and Indian children in Fiji. *Thorax* 1994; 49: 1201–1204.
10. Powell C, Nolan T, Carlin J, Bennett C, and Johnson P. Respiratory symptoms and duration of residence in immigrant teenagers living in Melbourne, Australia. *Arch Dis Child* 1999; 81: 159–162.
11. von Mutius E, Martinez FD, Fritzsch C, Nicolai T, Roell G, and Thiemann HH. Prevalence of asthma and atopy in two areas of West and East Germany. *Am J Respir Crit Care Med* 1994; 149: 358–364.
12. Braback L, Breborowicz A, Julge K et al. Risk factors for respiratory symptoms and atopic sensitisation in the Baltic area. *Arch Dis Child* 1995; 72: 487–493.
13. Braback L, Breborowicz A, Dreborg S, Knutsson A, Pieklik H, and Bjorksten B. Atopic sensitization and respiratory symptoms among Polish and Swedish school children. *Clin Exp Allergy* 1994; 24: 826–835.
14. Nowak D, Heinrich J, Jorres R et al. Prevalence of respiratory symptoms, bronchial hyperresponsiveness and atopy among adults: West and East Germany. *Eur Respir J* 1996; 9: 2541–2452.
15. von Mutius E, Weiland SK, Fritzsch C, Duhme H, and Keil U. Increasing prevalence of hay fever and atopy among children in Leipzig, East Germany. *Lancet* 1998; 351: 862–866.
16. Björksten B, Dumitrascu D, Foucard T et al. Prevalence of childhood asthma, rhinitis and eczema in Scandinavia and Eastern Europe. *Eur Respir J* 1998; 12: 432–437.
17. Gross I, Heinrich J, Fahlbusch B, Jäger L, Bischof W, and Wichmann H. Indoor determinants of Der p 1 and Der f 1 concentrations in house dust are different. *Clin Exp Allergy* 2000; 30: 376–382.
18. Fahlbusch B, Heinrich J, Groß I, Jäger L, Richter K, and Wichmann H. Allergens in house dust samples in Germany: results of an East–West German comparison. *Allergy* 1999; 54: 1215–1222.
19. Hirsch T. Indoor allergen exposure in West and East Germany: a cause for different prevalences of asthma and atopy? *Rev Environ Health* 1999; 14: 159–168.
20. Julge K, Munir AK, Vasar M, and Bjorksten B. Indoor allergen levels and other environmental risk factors for sensitization in Estonian homes. *Allergy* 1998; 53: 388–393.

21. Koch A, Heilemann K-J, Bischof W, Heinrich J, and Wichmann H. Indoor viable mold spores: a comparison between two cities, Erfurt (eastern Germany) and Hamburg (western Germany). *Allergy* 2000; 55: 176–180.
22. Precht D and Molkentin J. Trans fatty acids: implications for health, analytical methods, incidence in edible fats and intake (a review). *Die Nahrung* 1995; 39: 343–374.
23. Black PN and Sharpe S. Dietary fat and asthma: is there a connection? *Eur Respir J* 1997; 10: 6–12.
24. Weiland SK, von Mutius E, Husing A, and Asher MI. Intake of trans fatty acids and prevalence of childhood asthma and allergies in Europe: ISAAC Steering Committee. *Lancet* 1999; 353: 2040–2041.
25. Strachan DP. Hay fever, hygiene, and household size. *Br Med J* 1989; 299: 1259–1260.
26. Krämer U, Heinrich J, Wjst M, and Wichmann H-E. Age of entry to day nursery and allergy in later childhood. *Lancet* 1998; 352: 450–454.
27. Ball T, Castro-Rodriguez J, Griffith K, Holberg C, Martinez F, and Wright A. Siblings, day-care attendance, and the risk of asthma and wheezing during childhood. *New Engl J Med* 2000; 343: 538–543.
28. Illi S, von Mutius E, Lau S et al. Early childhood infectious diseases and the development of asthma up to school age: a birth cohort study. *Br Med J* 2001; 322: 390–395.
29. Shirakawa T, Enomoto T, Shimazu S, and Hopkin JM. The inverse association between tuberculin responses and atopic disorder. *Science* 1997; 275: 77–79.
30. Hovmark A. An *in vivo* and *in vitro* study of cell-mediated immunity in atopic dermatitis. *Acta Dermatovenerol* 1975; 55: 181–186.
31. Alm J, Lilja G, Pershagen G, and Scheynius A. Early BCG vaccination and development of atopy. *Lancet* 1997; 350: 400–403.
32. Weinberg E. Urbanization and childhood asthma: An African perspective. *JACI* 2000; 105: 224–231.
33. Hijazi N, Abalkhail B, and Seaton A. Asthma and respiratory symptoms in urban and rural Saudi Arabia. *Eur Respir J* 1998; 12: 41–44.
34. Strachan DP, Anderson HR, Limb ES, O'Neill A, and Wells N. A national survey of asthma prevalence, severity, and treatment in Great Britain. *Arch Dis Child* 1994; 70: 174–178.
35. Strachan DP, Golding J, and Anderson HR. Regional variations in wheezing illness in British children: effect of migration during early childhood. *J Epidemiol Commun Health* 1990; 44: 231–236.
36. Riedler J, Eder W, Oberfeld G, and Schreuer M. Austrian children living on a farm have less hay fever, asthma and allergic sensitization. *Clin Exp Allergy* 2000; 30: 194–200.
37. Kilpelainen M, Terho E, Helenius H, and Koskenvuo M. Farm environment in childhood prevents the development of allergies. *Clin Exp Allergy* 2000; 30: 201–208.
38. Ernst P and Cormier Y. Relative scarcity of asthma and atopy among adolescents raised on a farm. *Am J Respir Crit Care Med* 2000; 161: 1563–1566.

39. von Ehrenstein O, von Mutius E, Illi S, Hachmeister A, and von Kries R. Reduced risk of hay fever and asthma among children of farmers. *Clin Exp Allergy* 2000; 30: 187–193.
40. Braun-Fahrländer C, Gassner M, Grize L et al. Prevalence of hay fever and allergic sensitization in farmers' children and their peers living in the same rural community: Swiss Study on Childhood Allergy and Respiratory Symptoms with Respect to Air Pollution. *Clin Exp Allergy* 1999; 29: 28–34.
41. Riedler JB-FC, Eder W, Schreuer M, Waser M, Maisch S, Carr D, Schierl R, Nowak D, von Mutius E, and ALEX Study Team. Early life exposure to farming provides protection against the development of asthma and allergy. *Lancet* 2001; 358: 1129–1133.
42. von Mutius E, Braun-Fahrländer C, Schierl R et al. Exposure to endotoxin or other bacterial components might protect against the development of atopy. *Clin Exp Allergy.* 2000; 30: 1230–1234.
43. Braun-Fahrländer C, Riedler J, Herz U et al. Environmental exposure to endotoxin, atopy and asthma in school-aged children. *New Engl J Med* 2002; 347: 869–877.
44. Gereda J, Leung D, Thatayatikom A et al. Relation between house-dust endotoxin exposure, type 1 T-cell development, and allergen sensitisation in infants at high risk of asthma. *Lancet* 2000; 355: 1680–1683.
45. Holt P. Mucosal immunity in relation to the development of oral tolerance/sensitization. *Allergy* 1998; 53: 16–19.
46. Wold A. The hygiene hypothesis revised: is the rising frequency of allergy due to changes in the intestinal flora? *Allergy* 1998; 53: 20–25.

4

Later Life Onset of Asthma

CHAKRADHAR KOTARU and RICHARD J. MARTIN

University of Colorado Health Sciences Center
and National Jewish Medical and Research Center
Denver, Colorado, U.S.A.

I. Introduction

Asthma is a syndrome rather than a specific disease entity. The presentations and courses of asthmatics differ in many aspects. Clinicians commonly encounter patients who present several varying features of the disease such as presence or absence of allergic disease, nocturnal symptoms, aspirin sensitivity, and response to anti-inflammatory therapy. Age of onset of symptoms is one such variation that is poorly understood. Whether the stage of life when disease manifests represents a fundamental difference in the pathogenesis is unknown.

Since asthma is a considered a complex genetic disease that requires interaction of inborn and environmental factors, one may presume that the age of onset simply represents the time at which a genetically predisposed individual is exposed to an external influence. However, available data suggest that such a view is probably simplistic. In this chapter, we review the available literature on adult onset asthma and attempt to distinguish the adult onset type from asthma that originates in early life.

II. Definition

In order to characterize a disease, it is important to first clearly define it. While the asthmatic symptom complex of episodic breathlessness, wheezing, and chest tightness is easy enough to recognize clinically, a standardized convenient definition to use in epidemiologic studies has been elusive. In 1995, the National Heart, Lung, and Blood Institute/World Health Organization (NHLBI/WHO) Global Initiative for Asthma Workshop[1] defined asthma as:

> A chronic inflammatory disease of the airways involving a variety of immune cells. This inflammation, in susceptible individuals, leads to airway hyperresponsiveness to a variety of stimuli and also leads to airflow limitation that causes the symptoms mentioned above, and is at least partially reversible either spontaneously or after treatment.

The complexity of this definition underscores the heterogeneity of asthma and the difficulty in estimating the prevalence of disease.

When it comes to distinguishing asthma based on age of onset, the issue becomes even more vague. No accepted age cutoff differentiates childhood asthma from asthma of later origin. Eighteen years is generally considered a point of transition from pediatric to adult medicine. However, such a cutoff is purely arbitrary. Perhaps it is more important to use age-related criteria that impact lung function. For example, hormonal changes associated with the onset of puberty likely influence airway physiology. Moreover, gender-specific differences in rates of lung growth and ages of peak maturity exist. Entering the workforce, usually after 18 years of age, for example, increases exposure to agents that can result in symptoms of asthma. Because of sparse data about the role that age of onset plays in the disease process and lack of a standardized definition for later onset asthma, we intentionally shy away from assigning a random numerical cutoff in this discussion. Instead, our focus is on analyzing the literature in an attempt to distinguish asthma originating in later life from childhood asthma.

III. Epidemiology

Most of what we know about the epidemiology of asthma comes from large population-based surveys. Whether such random questionnaires regarding the presence of symptoms of a disease accurately estimate its actual prevalence is debatable.[2,3] When such an approach is applied to a syndrome like asthma with its myriad manifestations, more caution is required in interpreting the results. Furthermore, retrospective questionnaires to assess self-reported age of onset of symptoms are subject to memory bias.

Three types of memory error are common in surveys: telescopic, false negative, and false positive.[4] Telescopic memory is reporting of the onset of the disease at an older age than the age at which it actually occurred; the reported age of onset increases as time passes. False negative memory or underestimation increases with time since the condition last occurred. Even though a false positive bias tends to compensate for a false negative, the net effect of reporting errors is difficult to predict.

Another factor that needs consideration during studies of the epidemiology of later onset asthma is that symptoms often go unrecognized.[5–7] Only three fourths of the adults who develop wheezing on lung auscultation in response to methacholine challenge perceive wheezing. Such under-perception increases with age; only 40% of adults above 65 years of age become aware of wheezing, and this can lead to significant underestimation of disease prevalence when symptom questionnaires are used.

Comparing survey instruments to the "gold standard" diagnostic test for a disease usually assesses their validity. However, in the case of asthma, a clearly standardized test is lacking. Toren and colleagues reported the test performance characteristics of asthma questionnaires in a review.[8] When self-reports of asthma symptoms were compared with physicians' clinical diagnoses, the overall sensitivity and specificity were 68 and 94%, respectively. This is not to suggest that a clinician's diagnosis of asthma is unassailable. In fact, clinicians tend to diagnose asthma more commonly in younger patients, nonsmokers, and women.[9,10] Older males and smokers who have the same symptoms as asthma patients are commonly labeled as having chronic obstructive pulmonary disease.

Objective measurements are occasionally used to improve diagnostic accuracy. Bronchial hyperresponsiveness,[11] a hallmark of asthma, is often used as a surrogate to identify asthma. When the responses about self-reported asthma were validated with bronchial challenge tests, mean sensitivity was only 36%.[8] Furthermore, measuring BHR is costly, subject to daily variability, and often impractical in large-scale epidemiological studies.[12] Nonetheless, objective airflow measures are useful adjuncts to questionnaires to enhance specificity and sensitivity.[12] Other complementary tools include assessment of atopy and serum immunoglobulin E and skin testing. However, such measurements likely estimate subgroups of asthma and their validity in studies aiming to define overall prevalence of asthma has been questioned.[13]

Despite the lack of a standard, convenient case definition, and potential problems with survey tools, a number of important advances in the epidemiological study of asthma have been made in the past several years. Studies such as the European Community Respiratory Health Survey (ECRHS) and those conducted by the National Center for Health Statistics (NCHS) of the Centers for Disease Control (CDC) in the United States have provided important information on variations in asthma prevalence rates and led to valuable insights regarding etiology and risk factors, [14] but data on the age of onset remain scarce. In the following sections, we report available data on the epidemiology of asthma in adults and attempt to shed some light on the magnitude of a subset of adult asthma: those whose symptoms appeared later in life.

A. Epidemiology: United States

The NCHS sector of the CDC conducted two large surveys that provide data on asthma prevalence: the National Health Interview Survey (NHIS) and the National Health and Nutrition Examination Survey (NHANES). The NHIS is an annual nationwide survey of the civilian population of the U.S. Information is obtained about health and other characteristics of each member of more than 100,000 households. A subset of these households is questioned about asthma.

From 1990 to 1992, the prevalence of asthma, based on the responses to "during the past 12 months, have you had asthma?" was 4.6%, affecting an estimated 11.5 million persons.[15] The age-adjusted prevalence of disease was higher for persons under 18 years of age (6.1%) than for older age groups (4.1% for adults 18 to 64 years of age). The prevalence rate in young males younger than 18 years old was particularly high (7.2%) compared with 4.4% for females of the same age group. However, a slight female predominance was noted when all age groups were included (4.8% in females versus 4.4% in males).

In 1997, NHIS questions were changed to measure the lifetime prevalence of a medical diagnosis of asthma.[16] An estimated 26.7 million people (96.6 people per thousand) reported physician diagnoses of asthma during their lifetimes. The estimated 12-month asthma attack prevalence was 11.1 million (40.7 people per thousand). Although data on age of onset of symptoms were not obtained, an estimated 7.9 million people 15 years or older reported asthma attacks in the preceding 12 months (36.2 per thousand).

Additional information has been obtained from another national survey using random-digit-dialed telephone surveys of noninstitutionalized adults (aged 18 years) and designated the Behavioral Risk Factor Surveillance System (BRFSS).[17] In 1999, two optional questions about asthma were added to the BRFSS; the lifetime prevalence of asthma was measured by asking respondents whether they had ever been told by their doctors that they had asthma. Current asthma was estimated by asking "do you still have asthma?" Based on more than 182,000 responses, the year 2000 lifetime prevalence of asthma was an estimated 10.5%; 7.2% of the sample or an estimated 14.6 million adults nationwide, reported "current asthma." Again, information regarding age of diagnosis or symptom onset is lacking.

The third NHANES is a cross-sectional multistage probability sample that is representative of the noninstitutionalized civilian population of the U.S. consisting of 20,050 adults aged 17 years or older. Along with questionnaires regarding physician diagnoses of asthma and respiratory symptoms, health and spirometry examinations were performed. The prevalence of doctor-diagnosed asthma among subjects 45 years of age or older was 2.7%.[18,19] Most striking was the large proportion of under-diagnosis of obstructive lung disease; about 12% of subjects with airflow limitations noted on spirometry did not carry diagnoses of asthma or chronic obstructive pulmonary disease (COPD).

An important survey that provides insight into age of onset was conducted in 59 primary care medical practices in Wisconsin.[20] A systematic sample (n = 14,127) of the practices' clinical populations was surveyed to obtain histories of physician-diagnosed asthma, presence of symptoms of wheezing and shortness and breath (undiagnosed asthma), age at diagnosis or at onset of symptoms, and current disease activity. Physician-diagnosed asthma that was active within the previous year was reported by 6.1% of patients (5.8% of patients younger than 20 years of age and 6.2% of adults). Undiagnosed asthma that was active within the previous year was reported by 3.3% (2.9% of patients younger than 20 years of age and 3.4% of adults). In about half the patients with physician-diagnosed asthma or patients with symptoms of asthma, onset of symptoms was later in life (20 years of age or later).

To provide information regarding the nature of asthma in the elderly, a subset of the general population in Tucson, Arizona enrolled in a longitudinal study were studied.[21] Of the 804 subjects who were 65 years of age or older, 46 admitted to current symptoms of asthma. Three fourths of asthmatics denied any respiratory problems prior to age 16 and about half reported their first attacks after age 40. In a similar report, annual incidence rates of asthma among the elderly were estimated from a general population-based cohort of 3,622 residents of Rochester, Minnesota.[22] The study reported 98 patients were identified diagnosed with asthma after age 65, resulting in an age-and-sex-adjusted incidence of 95 persons per population of 100,000 per year. Similar incidence rates (100 per 100,000 per year) were reported earlier from the same population sample when the onset of asthma from ages 15 through 30 was evaluated.[23]

In a follow-up survey to the first NHANES, the annual incidence of new onset adult (>25 years of age) asthma was estimated at 2.1 per thousand persons per year.[24] Broder et al. obtained a comparable rate of 2.0 per thousand persons per year when the epidemiology of asthma was studied on two separate occasions in about 6,500 adult residents of a community in Michigan.[25,26]

B. Worldwide Epidemiology

The European Community Respiratory Health Survey (ECRHS) investigation focused on asthma symptoms in adults aged 20 to 44 years in countries located primarily in Western Europe.[27] At each center, a representative sample of 3,000 adults in that age range completed Phase I screening questionnaires seeking information on asthma symptoms and medication use. Individuals who answered that they awoke with attacks of shortness of breath within the past 12 months,

Table 4.1 Epidemiology of Adult Onset Asthma

Data are scarce and subject to many limitations.

Asthma prevalence among adults in the U.S. ranged from 4 to 7%.

Large number of adults have undiagnosed obstructive lung disease.

At least half of adult asthmatics in the U.S. have onset of symptoms in adulthood (>18 years).

Annual incidence rates of asthma in adults range from 0.95 to 2.1 per thousand population in the U.S. and about 1.2 per thousand in other developed countries.

European Community Respiratory Health Survey suggests a progressive increase in incidence of asthma among adults in the western world.

experienced attacks of asthma within the past 12 months, or currently took asthma medications were defined as "asthmatic."

A random subsample of 600 subjects and an additional sample of up to 150 asthmatic individuals were then studied in more detail in Phase II. Measurements of skin prick reactions to common allergens, serum total and specific IgE, bronchial responsiveness to inhaled methacholine, and urine electrolytes were made. A more in-depth questionnaire on asthma symptoms and medical history, occupation and social status, smoking, home environment, and uses of medications and medical services was administered. Age of onset was established when subjects were asked, "How old were you when you had your first asthma attack?"[28] Although wide geographic variation exists, the overall yearly incidence rates were 3.3 per thousand for subjects aged 0 to 15 years and 1.2 per thousand for asthmatics older than 15 years. A progressive increase in the yearly incidence of childhood and later onset asthma by birth cohort was noted. When the cohort born in 1946 was used as baseline (relative risk = 1), the relative risks of developing asthma between ages 15 and 45 years were 1.22, 1.42, 2.53, and 3.51 for the cohorts born in the years 1951, 1956, 1961 and 1966, respectively.

Bodner et al. reported the prevalence of adult onset wheeze among individuals from a 1964 community survey of 2,511 children from Aberdeen in a subsequent investigation.[29] One hundred and seventy seven of 1,542 (11.5%) respondents reported onsets of wheeze after 15 years of age. Table 4.1 summarizes the conclusions that can be drawn regarding the epidemiology of adult onset asthma based on the above review.

IV. Genotypic Associations with Adult Onset Asthma

Observations that allergic diseases tend to cluster in families were first made almost a century ago.[30] Subsequent attempts at understanding the heritability of asthma using traditional methods like twin studies and segregation analyses hinted that simple Mendelian principles were not applicable.[31–33] With greater knowledge of the human genome, recent studies using linkage analysis identified specific genetic regions that potentially confer disease vulnerability.[34] As candidate genes within these loci and the potential roles of their gene products in the development of particular phenotypes of asthma are characterized,[35] the complex nature of the genetics of asthma becomes apparent.

It is increasingly clear that many genes confer susceptibility to disease and interaction with environmental factors determines disease expression. The interplay of genetic factors and external surroundings is particularly relevant when discussing the age of onset of asthma. If environmental factors are requisite for the inception of asthma, it follows that the onset of symptoms can only occur after interaction with that particular factor.

The role of such stimuli is suggested when the presence of disease is evaluated in family clusters of asthmatics. Holberg and colleagues reported greater concordance for asthma between siblings than between parents and off-spring in a familial aggregation and segregation analysis of physician-diagnosed asthma.[33] This implies a potentially greater role for environmental factors than for inherited factors. Examining the features of candidate genes identified for asthma to date also supports the necessity for external factors. A consistent aspect of these genes is their incomplete penetrance.[35] The mere presence of a predisposing polymorphism does not necessarily predict disease. It implies interaction with other appropriate factors, including those in the external milieu.

Some authors have suggested that the age of onset predicts the relative importance of genetic or external influences; the earlier the onset of asthma, the stronger the genetic predisposition and lesser need for outside influences. This hypothesis is in part based on findings that early onset asthma is more likely to be extrinsic[36] and a stronger correlation for a genetic basis for atopy.[35] In addition, the high phenocopy rate of asthma (environmental stimuli if strong enough can result in asthma even without predisposing genes) is typically described in adults with occupational asthma.

However, data to the contrary exist. First, while the association between atopy and asthma is greater in childhood onset asthma, a major proportion of adult onset asthmatics also have atopic features (*vide infra*). In addition, genetic variations have been associated with later age of onset. As a part of an epidemiological study of the Genetics and Environment of Asthma (EGEA) protocol, a sample of 107 French families with 2 siblings with asthma were analyzed for genetic influences on the age of onset of asthma.[37] A factor on chromosome 7q was identified and relative risks differed according to age at onset of disease.

In a study of 298 Japanese subjects, a functional polymorphism in the RANTES (regulated upon activation normal T-cell expressed) gene promoter (−28C/G allele) was significantly associated with the onset of asthma after 40 years of age [odds ratio = 2.033; 95% CI (confidence interval), 1.379–2.998; $p < 0.0025$].[38] The association was further supported by the release of higher levels of RANTES *in vitro* from monocytes of carriers of the −28 polymorphism. The same group also reported that a mutation (109T allele) in the promoter region of the high affinity immunoglobulin E receptor (FcRI) that mediates the IgE-dependent activation of mast cells and basophils was associated with increased total serum IgE levels among asthmatics.[39] The strongest evidence for such an association between total serum IgE levels and 109C/T polymorphism was obtained when age at onset of asthma was incorporated into the analysis.

Evidence for disease expression based on external influences on genetic backgrounds comes from a study by Barr et al. who explored the association of genetic polymorphism in the 2 adrenoreceptor in adult onset female asthmatics with body-mass indices and activity levels.[40] The presence of Gly16 allele is associated with adult onset asthma only in sedentary women, implying that the relationship between β2 adrenoreceptor polymorphisms in adult onset asthma is modifiable by environmental factors. A similar gene–environment interaction may exist between β2-adrenoreceptor polymorphisms and smoking.[41] The homozygous presence of arginine in codon 16 of the 2 adrenergic receptor gene markedly increased the risks of asthma in smokers compared with Gly-16 homozygotes who never smoked (odds ratio = 7.81; 95% CI, 2.07–29.5).

Such associations are also being identified in occupational asthma. Specific polymorphisms in serum proteins such as haptoglobin have been associated with a predisposition to development of asthma after exposure to industrial factors.[42] Similar associations between specific HLA genotypes and aspirin-induced asthma have been reported.[43]

As the complexities of genetics involved in asthma are slowly unraveled, valuable insights into the pathogenesis are being gained. It appears likely that all asthmatics have predisposing genetic variations. The culminating expression of a particular phenotype such as adult onset asthma probably requires a specific set of inheritable factors. However, these genetic factors are modifiable by the environment, including specific lifestyle choices (Table 4.2). This offers hope for potential interventions that may serve to quell the current epidemic of asthma.

V. Phenotypic Features of Later Onset Asthma

Asthma is generally considered a childhood illness that in some persons persists into adulthood. However, the magnitude of later onset asthma, its morbidity, and impact on health care resources are significant.[44] One fundamental question regarding asthma originating in adulthood is whether it is pathologically and clinically distinct from asthma of earlier onset. In other words, is adult onset asthma the same as childhood asthma and present in older people? Available data do not allow a clear distinction, but hint at the possibility of different pathobiologies.

Table 4.2 Predisposing Genetic Polymorphisms and Modulating Environmental Stimuli
Associated with Later Life Onset of Asthma

Genetic Polymorphism	Modulating Environmental Factor
-28C/G allele of the RANTES gene promoter	—
109C/T allele of high affinity IgE receptor promoter	—
Factor (markers D7S524, D7S527) on chromosome 7q	—
Gly16 allele of the β2 adrenoreceptor	Sedentary lifestyle
Arg16 allele of the β2 adrenoreceptor	Smoking
Several alleles of the HLA class II region	Diisocyanates, western red cedar, aspirin

A. Symptoms

The presentation of asthma is similar in both childhood and adult onset types,
although minor differences exist. Segala and colleagues reported the results of a
questionnaire survey of asthmatic adults who reported having (n = 84) or not
having (n = 235) asthma in childhood.[45] Childhood asthma that persists into
adulthood tended to present more often as an acute attack (60% of childhood
persistent asthma versus 42% of adult onset; p value not reported). In contrast,
38% of asthma originating in adults presented with wheeze as compared to only
29% of persistent childhood asthma (p = 0.03).

The circumstances of asthma onset and symptom exacerbations were significantly more likely to be allergy- and/or exercise-related in asthmatics who
developed asthma early in life. The presence of nocturnal symptoms was similar
in both groups. Asthmatics with childhood onset disease appeared to have a more
severe form of disease than those with adult onset asthma when the frequency
of acute attacks and lung function were considered. However, since this study
did not include childhood asthma that remitted before 18 years of age, the results
cannot be used to distinguish asthma based on age of onset.

B. Association with Atopy

Early onset asthma has been generally regarded to be extrinsic.[36] In contrast, the
association between atopy and later onset asthma is considered less rigorous.
However, such an association should not be underestimated. In a survey of 235
adult onset asthmatics in France, almost two thirds reported allergic symptoms
and had positive skin prick test reactions to common allergens.[45] Similar rates of
association between atopy and adult asthma were reported in studies conducted
in Finland and the United Kingdom.[46,47] About half the patients with adult onset
asthma had increased serum IgE levels >300 U/ml and positive radioallergosorbent test (RAST) results for house dust and mites compared to about 80%

positivity in childhood asthma.[48] In a nested case control study of a community cohort, risk factors for adult onset wheeze (onset after age 15) in 102 cases were compared with 217 controls.[49] The presence of atopy or a family history of atopic disease conferred significant risk of developing wheeze later in life.

C. Lung Function

Increasing data focus on the issue of whether age of onset predicts the severity and course of asthma. Several investigators have attempted to clarify the relationship of age of onset to severity of disease. Although the results are variable, most studies report no association between age of disease onset and severity of asthma.[6,21,50] Poor or incomplete reversibility of airway obstruction to bronchodilators has been suggested to be a feature of asthma in the elderly, but may be attributable to coexisting cardiopulmonary disease such as chronic bronchitis or congestive heart failure.[50]

As a part of the aging process, progressive decline in lung function occurs soon after peak lung growth is achieved. Several longitudinal studies report that a gradual decrease in 1-second forced expiratory volume (FEV_1) is more pronounced among asthmatics.[51,52] Since it has been proposed that adult onset asthma is most likely intrinsic, studying the association of decline in FEV_1 to atopic status may hint at the prognosis of lung function in later onset asthma. In a 10-year follow-up of 180 adult asthmatics, Ulrik and colleagues determined that decline in lung function is greater in intrinsic asthma (50 ml/yr) when compared to extrinsic (atopic) asthma (22.5 ml/yr).[53] However, some studies have failed to show such an association. In a 25-year follow-up of 181 subjects diagnosed with asthma based on symptoms and histamine challenges, a significant proportion outgrew their diseases.[11] While older asthmatics showed a small tendency to have persistent symptoms and BHR, it is interesting to observe that a shorter duration of untreated asthma, irrespective of age of onset, seemed to predict remission. Hence, early diagnosis and treatment may be critical in determining the course of asthma.

A recent investigation at our institution by Spahn and colleagues provided valuable insights into differences between severe childhood and adult onset asthmatics (Dr. Joseph Spahn, personal communication, 2003). One hundred twenty-five children with difficult-to-control asthma requiring large doses of inhaled or oral glucocorticoids for control of symptoms were compared to 150 adult asthmatics who had similar anti-inflammatory medication requirements. Of the adults, 42% (n = 63) had onset of symptoms after 18 years of age. Significant differences in lung function were identified between children and adults. Children were more likely than adults to have preserved airflows based on FEV_1 measurements, but were more prone to hyperinflation. It is intriguing to speculate that perhaps such disparities may represent differences in location of airflow limitation; children may have more distal or small airway obstruction, while adults may be limited

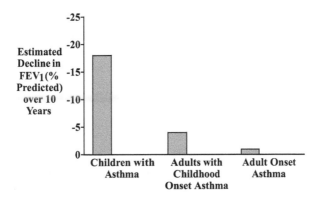

Figure 4.1 Relationship of decline in lung function to age of onset of severe asthma. (Dr. Joseph Spahn, personal communication.)

Table 4.3 Clinical and Physiologic Features of Early and Late Onset Asthma

	Symptoms				Lung Function			
	Initial Presentation	EIA	Nocturnal Symptoms	Atopy	FEV_1	TLC	BHR	Decline over Time
Early onset	Acute exacerbation	++	+	++	↓	? ↑↑	++	? ++
Late onset	Wheeze	+	+	+	↓	↑	+	+

EIA = exercise-induced asthma. Atopy based on symptoms, serum IgE levels, and skin test. FEV_1 = One-second forced expired volume. TLC = total lung capacity. BHR = bronchial hyperresponsiveness.

more proximally. No differences in lung function were noted between the childhood onset and adult onset asthmatics. However, when FEV_1 was related to duration of disease, large differences were noted (Figure 4.1). Children displayed the largest decrement, with a loss of 1.8% of predicted per year. Adults with asthma that originated in childhood had a 0.4% predicted decline per year. In contrast, lung function among adult onset asthmatics remained stable.

Oosaki reported the effect of age of onset of symptoms on response to histamine challenge.[48] Adults with asthma, whether new onset or childhood onset with adult relapse, required similar concentrations of histamine to decrease the FEV_1 by 20% (PC_{20}) and were significantly less responsive than childhood asthmatics. Similarly, Cuttitta and colleagues[6] reported no differences in BHR to methacholine among younger and older asthmatics when the severity and duration of disease were taken into consideration. Table 4.3 contrasts the clinical and physiologic characteristics of early and late onset asthma.

D. Pathology

While most data on the pathology of asthma are described in adults, the inflammatory responses have not been well characterized with respect to age of onset of disease. The scant information that exists reports similar patterns of persistent airway inflammation in childhood and adult onset disease.[54,55]

VI. Epidemiologic Associations

A. Infection

Increasing data suggest early life exposure to infectious agents may protect from inception of asthma. It appears that such a protective effect extends to adult onset asthma as well. Early exposure to measles has been associated with lower risk of adult onset asthma.[56] A similar prophylactic consequence was seen in subjects with two or more siblings, leading the authors to hypothesize that frequent exposures to infection as seen in large families may be important in defense against initiation of asthma.

Infection due to atypical bacterial like Chlamydia and Mycoplasma has been associated with chronic asthma. While the fact that such infections exacerbate asthma is well known, their role in inception of disease has been suggested only recently.[57,58] Hahn et al. reported that adult asthmatic patients had higher prevalences of elevated immunoglobulin titers against *Chlamydia pneumoniae* than did nonasthmatic control subjects.[57] Eighty percent of adults with asthma after respiratory tract infections and 100% of patients 40 years or older, with asthmatic bronchitis, had random titers of 1:64. Furthermore, a significant dose–response relationship between the antibody titer and the prevalence of wheezing was noted.

In a subsequent study, the same group reported a likelihood ratio of 3.7 (95% CI, 1.2–11.5) between specific IgA titers 10 against chlamydia and recent onset of asthma in adults.[59] Further corroboration of this association comes from trials of antichlamydial antibiotics in asthmatic patients with elevated antibody titers.[60] Nearly 50% of those treated showed improvement in asthma. However, data to the contrary have been reported as well. Routes and colleagues[61] measured specific IgG to chlamydia in 46 adult onset asthmatics and control subjects and did not find a correlation between seroreactivity and asthma.

Acute infection with *Mycoplasma pneumoniae* has been associated with onset of asthma as well.[62] Chronic infection with Mycoplasma has been implicated in stable asthma. Using polymerase chain reaction (PCR techniques), Mycoplasma was detected in bronchial biopsies of almost half of the chronic stable asthmatics studied compared to only 10% positivity in normal subjects.[63] Further evidence strengthening the hypothesized causal link between asthma and Mycoplasma infection comes from examining the nature of inflammation in both processes. The chronic inflammation of asthma involves TH-2 cytokines and immune cells.[64] The exact mechanisms of this TH-1/TH-2 imbalance are unclear, but similar changes in immune responses after Mycoplasma infection suggest a potential pathogenic role.

Koh et al. found significantly elevated interleukin-4 (IL-4) levels and IL-4/interferon (IFN)-γ in the broncho-alveolar lavage fluid of subjects with pneumonia from *M. pneumoniae* compared with normal controls or patients with pneumonia from *Streptococcus pneumoniae*.[65] The levels of IL-4 were even higher in a subgroup of children with family histories of atopy. IL-4 is known to stimulate IgE synthesis by B lymphocytes, and this may explain the increase in IgE noted in Mycoplasma infection. Martin et al. showed significantly greater numbers of mast cells in asthmatics who were PCR-positive than in PCR-negative patients.[63] Furthermore, treatment with macrolide antibiotics improved lung function in asthmatics with Mycoplasma in their airways.[66] Although data are lacking regarding age at initial infection and consequent onset of symptoms, this process can be conceivably initiated in adulthood.

Exposure to fungi has been linked with onset of asthma as well. In a survey of 521 adults with new onset asthma and 932 control subjects in Finland, the risk of disease was related to the presence of visible mold and/or mold odor in the workplace (odds ratio, 1.54; 95% CI, 1.01–2.32).[67] Furthermore, among the asthmatics, the presence of antibodies against specific fungi significantly correlated with risk of adult onset asthma.[68]

B. Diet

A change in western dietary habits is one of the reasons put forward to potentially explain the current epidemic of asthma in the developed world.[69] Lower consumption of antioxidants and mineral cofactors has been linked to increased risk of bronchial hyperreactivity.[45,70–72] Adult women with higher levels of vitamin E intake were modestly protected from developing asthma in a prospective study.[73] While several studies have evaluated the potential protective role of increased consumption of fish oils in the development of asthma, the results do not support a generalized recommendation that all asthmatics modify their dietary intakes.[74] Lower salt intake has been associated with better lung function[75,76] and decreased medication use.[77] Although firm data are lacking, it is certainly plausible based on available information that dietary habits influence manifestation of asthma in certain predisposed individuals.

C. Smoking Exposure

The ability of exposure to cigarette smoke to trigger symptoms in asthmatics is well known. Over the past few decades, increasing data link smoking to initiation of asthma. Significant correlation between passive smoke exposure from parental smoking and development of asthma in children has been reported by several investigators.[78–80] Similar association studies in adults are hampered by the so-called "healthy smoker effect."[81,82] Unlike exposures observed with children, smoking exposure in adults is more likely to be primary.

Adults who smoke and develop respiratory complaints are likely to quit. As a result, when surveys regarding symptoms of asthma are used to estimate the prevalence of asthma among current smokers, subjects who did not develop problems enrich the cohort somewhat. Consequently, a potential causal association between smoking and development of asthma will be underestimated. Reconstructing smoking history or studying the effects of environmental tobacco exposure can minimize such a bias.

Eisner examined the relationship of passive smoke exposure to lung function among adults.[83] Higher levels of serum cotinine, a biomarker of exposure to tobacco smoke, correlated with lower lung function in women, even among nonasthmatics. As a part of the ECRHS in Germany, passive smoke exposure in the workplace increased the relative risk of asthma (OR = 1.51; 95% CI, 0.99–2.32).[84]

Thorn and colleagues compared 174 adult onset physician-diagnosed asthmatics with 870 control subjects and reported an odd ratio for asthma of 2.4 (95% CI, 1.4–4.1) attributable to environmental smoke exposure.[85] The Swiss study on air pollution and lung diseases in adults known as SAPALDIA included more than 4,000 nonsmokers between the ages of 18 and 60 years and observed higher risks of asthma symptoms and physician diagnoses of asthma in those exposed to environmental tobacco smoke.[86] Similar correlations between smoke exposure among 7,882 nonsmoking adults and asthma symptoms and bronchial hyperresponsiveness were obtained from the analysis of surveys from 36 centers of the ECRHS from 16 countries.[87] Women may be more susceptible to the effects of smoking.[83,88]

D. Pregnancy and Menstrual-Related Conditions

Cyclic variation of asthma symptoms with menstruation is common. Symptoms, lung function, and bronchial hyperresponsiveness worsen in the late luteal phase of the menstrual cycle.[89] Concurrent variation in airway inflammation is suggested by changes in exhaled nitric oxide and sputum eosinophilia.[90] The exact pathogenesis of premenstrual asthma is not established, but hormonal fluctuations are believed to be important.[91,92] Association between exogenous hormones administered for hormone replacement therapy or for contraception and asthma symptoms further supports such endocrine influences on lung function.[93] However, the effects are mild and conflicting data exist.[94,95] It has been suggested that only severe asthmatics are susceptible to hormonal changes.[96] Such influences on only severe asthmatics hold true for asthma in pregnancy as well. The clinical courses of 20 to 40% of asthmatics worsen during pregnancy and women with poorly controlled asthma prior to pregnancy are more likely to deteriorate.[97,98]

It has been hypothesized that such hormonal factors bring on symptoms of asthma as well. The nurses' health study prospectively evaluated the risks of onset of asthma from hormone replacement therapy.[99] Having ever taken replacement therapy was associated with an increased incidence of asthma after controlling for age, body mass index, smoking, and previous use of oral contraceptive pills (incidence rate ratio = 1.49; 95% CI, 1.1–2.0). A dose–response relationship was noted between asthma incidence and current dose of estrogen and the duration of use. The association was present in women taking unopposed estrogens and those taking estrogens plus progesterone. However, a potential bias in this study may have been that women who take replacement therapy are more likely to seek medical attention, increasing the likelihood of diagnosis of other medical conditions, including asthma. At this time, unequivocal data linking female sex hormonal factors to onset of asthma do not exist.

E. Occupational Factors

An important consideration when dealing with new onset of symptoms in adults is potential workplace-related etiologies. The list of offending agents encountered in the workplace is long and both immunologic and nonimmunologic mechanisms have been implicated.[100] Work-related asthma is one of the most common occupational lung diseases worldwide.[101] Distinguishing occupational asthma (OA) from adult onset asthma without a workplace-related etiology is essential because of therapeutic, public health, and medicolegal considerations. However, clinical, functional and pathologic alterations in occupational asthma are indistinguishable from those of nonoccupational asthma.[102] Therefore maintaining a high degree of suspicion of OA in any adult with new onset symptoms is crucial.

How much of adult onset asthma can be attributed to workplace factors? Studies attempting to answer this question have yielded variable results, probably due to differences in methodology. Reijula and colleagues analyzed the national registry data in Finland on the incidence of new cases of asthma and compared it to new diagnoses of work-related asthma.[103] Occupational asthma was diagnosed by chest physicians or at the Finnish Institute of Occupational Health by careful clinical and immunologic examinations as well as by identification of a specific causative agent. The annual incidence rate of asthma among the 15- to 64-year old age group was 0.4%. Of that number, OA accounted for about 5% of the new cases.

As a part of the ECRHS, Kogevinas and colleagues estimated the incidence of OA among more then 15,000 subjects aged 20 to 44 from 12 industrialized countries[104] And 5 to 10% of the asthma found in this age group was attributable to occupation. Farmers, painters, plastic workers, cleaners, and spray painters had the highest risks. In a case control study of 321 adult onset asthmatics from Goteborg, Sweden, similar occupations were found to be at risk.[105] The occupation-attributable rate was 11%.

In a review of medical records of 79,204 health maintenance organization members between the ages of 15 and 55, the annual incidence of asthma was 1.3 per thousand.[106] Criteria for clinically significant asthma attributable to occupational exposure were met by 21% (95% CI, 12–32%) of cases, yielding an incidence of 71 per 100,000 (95% CI, 43–111). Using the ECRHS protocol, a survey of 383 asthmatics among 2,974 subjects in the 20- to 44-year old age group in Canada revealed a frequency of possible OA to be as high as 36%.[107] However, the presence of OA was not confirmed in this study. In a recent literature review of 43 reports on the incidence of occupational asthma, the median and mean attributable risk estimates were 9 and 13%, respectively.[108]

VII. Treatment and Prognosis

There are no data to suggest that the therapeutic options and responses to therapy in the late onset asthmatics are different from options and responses of patients with asthma that began in childhood. Clinical practice guidelines recommend the use of controller anti-inflammatory therapy for moderate and severe symptoms,[109] but under-treatment of asthma in the elderly is common. In a survey of asthmatics older than 65 years, less than a third were prescribed inhaled corticosteroids.[110] A higher degree of suspicion should be maintained for potential reversible causes in all new onset disease.

Work-related etiologies and medication-induced symptoms are of particular importance in adults. Unfortunately, cessation of exposure to an agent causing occupational asthma does not necessarily result in remission.[111] Atypical bacterial infection represents another potentially treatable cause of symptoms. However, diagnosis is not always straightforward. Present levels of evidence do not support empiric antibacterial therapy in all new onset or difficult-to-control cases of asthma.

While most asthma-related deaths occur in adulthood, no data link later onset of disease to increased mortality. Elderly patients with asthma have higher utilization of health services for asthma, but no differences in mortality attributable to disease diagnosed later in life have been noted.[22]

VIII. Conclusions

Asthma can originate at all stages of life, and a significant proportion of adult asthmatics do not report symptoms in childhood. The overall incidence of such a subset of patients appears to be increasing. As we begin to identify specific genetic factors that predispose to later onset disease, the pathophysiologic mechanisms are being unraveled. Further insights are made possible by resolving the roles of external stimuli in predisposed individuals. Behavioral and lifestyle modifications may actually be useful in prevention of asthma in such subjects.

Of particular importance is identification of potentially reversible conditions such as postinfectious or workplace-related asthma. Although strong data are lacking, available data suggest a milder course of asthma that began in adulthood. Treatment options and overall prognosis of adult onset asthma do not appear to be significantly different, but under-diagnosis and under-treatment are common. Lastly, more data are required to further characterize this poorly understood phenotype of asthma.

References

1. National Heart, Lung, and Blood Institute/World Health Organization. *Global Strategy for Asthma Management and Prevention*. National Institutes of Health 1995. Workshop Report: Publication 95-3659.
2. Burney P. Interpretation of epidemiological surveys of asthma, in Chadwick D and Cardew G, Eds. *Rising Trends in Asthma*. New York: Wiley. 1997; p. 111.
3. Peat JK, Toelle BG, Marks GB, and Mellis CM. Continuing the debate about measuring asthma in population studies (comment). *Thorax* 2001; 56: 406–411.
4. Stewart W, Brookmyer R, and Van Natta M. Estimating age incidence from survey data with adjustments for recall errors. *J Clin Epidemiol* 1989; 42: 869–875.
5. Connolly MJ, Crowley JJ, Charan NB, Nielson CP, and Vestal RE. Reduced subjective awareness of bronchoconstriction provoked by methacholine in elderly asthmatic and normal subjects as measured on a simple awareness scale. *Thorax* 1992; 47: 410–413.
6. Cuttitta G, Cibella F, Bellia V, Grassi V, Cossi S, Bucchieri S, and Bonsignore G. Changes in FVC during methacholine-induced bronchoconstriction in elderly patients with asthma: bronchial hyperresponsiveness and aging. *Chest* 2001; 119: 1685–1690.
7. Joo JH, Lim GI, Seo MJ et al. Perception of wheezing in the elderly asthmatics. *Korean J Int Med* 2001; 16: 260–264.
8. Toren K, Brisman J, and Jarvholm B. Asthma and asthma-like symptoms in adults assessed by questionnaires: a literature review (comment). *Chest* 1993; 104: 600–608.
9. Banerjee DK, Lee GS, Malik SK, and Daly S. Under-diagnosis of asthma in the elderly. *Br J Dis Chest* 1987; 81: 23–29.
10. Morris MJ. Difficulties with diagnosing asthma in the elderly (comment). *Chest* 1999; 116: 591–593.
11. Panhuysen CI, Vonk JM, Koeter GH, Schouten JP, van Altena R, Bleecker ER, and Postma DS. Adult patients may outgrow their asthma: a 25-year follow-up study. [Erratum appears in *Am J Respir Crit Care Med* 1997; 156: 674.] *Am J Respir Crit Care Med* 1997; 155: 1267–1272.
12. Toelle BG, Peat JK, Salome CM, Mellis CM, and Woolcock AJ. Toward a definition of asthma for epidemiology. *Am Rev Respir Dis* 1992; 146: 633–637.

13. Pekkanen J and Pearce N. Defining asthma in epidemiological studies. *Eur Respir J* 1999; 14: 951–957.

14. Beasley R, Crane J, Lai CK, and Pearce N. Prevalence and etiology of asthma. *J Allergy Clin Immunol* 2000; 105: 466–472.

15. Mannino DM, Homa DM, Pertowski CA et al. Surveillance for asthma: United States, 1960–1995. *MMWR* 1998; 47: 1–27.

16. Mannino DM, Homa DM, Akinbami LJ, Moorman JE, Gwynn C, and Redd SC. Surveillance for asthma: United States, 1980–1999. *MMWR* 2002; 51: 1–13.

17. Centers for Disease Control. *Behavioral Risk Factor Surveillance System User's Guide*. Atlanta, GA: U.S. Department of Health and Human Services, 1999.

18. Mannino DM, Gagnon RC, Petty TL, and Lydick E. Obstructive lung disease and low lung function in adults in the United States: data from the National Health and Nutrition Examination Survey, 1988–1994. *Arch Int Med* 2000; 160: 1683–1689.

19. Coultas DB, Mapel D, Gagnon R, and Lydick E. The health impact of undiagnosed airflow obstruction in a national sample of United States adults. *Am J Respir Crit Care Med* 2001; 164: 372–377.

20. Hahn DL and Beasley JW. Diagnosed and possible undiagnosed asthma: a Wisconsin Research Network (WReN) Study. *J Family Pract* 1994; 38: 373–379.

21. Burrows B, Barbee RA, Cline MG, Knudson RJ, and Lebowitz MD. Characteristics of asthma among elderly adults in a sample of the general population. *Chest* 1991; 100: 935–942.

22. Bauer BA, Reed CE, Yunginger JW, Wollan PC, and Silverstein MD. Incidence and outcomes of asthma in the elderly: a population-based study in Rochester, Minnesota (comment). *Chest* 1997; 111: 303–310.

23. Yunginger JW, Reed CE, O'Connell EJ, Melton LJ, 3rd, O'Fallon WM, and Silverstein MD. A community-based study of the epidemiology of asthma: incidence rates, 1964–1983 (comment). *Am Rev Respir Dis* 1992; 146: 888–894.

24. McWhorter WP, Polis MA, and Kaslow RA. Occurrence, predictors, and consequences of adult asthma in NHANES-1 and follow-up survey. *Am Rev Respir Dis* 1989; 139: 721–724.

25. Broder I, Higgins MW, Mathews KP, and Keller JB. Epidemiology of asthma and allergic rhinitis in a total community, Tecumseh, Michigan: IV. Natural history. *J Allergy Clin Immunol* 1974; 54: 100–110.

26. Broder I, Higgins MW, Mathews KP, and Keller JB. Epidemiology of asthma and allergic rhinitis in a total community, Tecumseh, Michigan: III. Second survey of the community. *J Allergy Clin Immunol* 1974; 53: 127–138.

27. Janson C, Anto J, Burney P et al. The European Community Respiratory Health Survey II: what are the main results so far? *Eur Respir J* 2001; 18: 598–611.

28. Sunyer J, Anto JM, Tobias A, and Burney P. Generational increase of self-reported first attack of asthma in fifteen industrialized countries: European Community Respiratory Health Study (ECRHS). *Eur Respir J* 1999; 14: 885–891.

29. Bodner C, Ross S, Douglas G et al. The prevalence of adult onset wheeze: longitudinal study. *Br Med J* 1997; 314: 792–793.

30. Cooke RA. Human sensitization. *J Immunol* 1916; 1: 201–205.

31. Edfors-Lubs ML. Allergy in 7000 twin pairs. *Acta Allergol* 1971; 26: 249–285.

32. Townley RG, Bewtra A, Wilson AF et al. Segregation analysis of bronchial response to methacholine inhalation challenge in families with and without asthma. *J Allergy Clin Immunol* 1986; 77: 101–107.

33. Holberg CJ, Elston RC, Halonen M et al. Segregation analysis of physician-diagnosed asthma in Hispanic and non-Hispanic white families. A recessive component? *Am J Respir Crit Care Med* 1996; 154: 144–150.

34. Wjst M and Immervoll T. An Internet linkage and mutation database for the complex phenotype asthma. *Bioinformatics* (Oxford) 1998; 14: 827–828.

35. Heinzmann A and Deichmann KA. Genes for atopy and asthma. *Curr Opin Allergy Clin Immunol* 2001; 1: 387–392.

36. Hendrick DJ, Davies RJ, D'Souza MF, and Pepys J. An analysis of skin prick test reactions in 656 asthmatic patients. *Thorax* 1975; 30: 2–8.

37. Dizier MH, Besse-Schmittler C, Guilloud-Bataille M et al. Indication of linkage and genetic heterogeneity of asthma according to age at onset on chromosome 7q in 107 French EGEA families. *Eur J Human Genet* 2001; 9: 867–872.

38. Hizawa N, Yamaguchi E, Konno S, Tanino Y, Jinushi E, and Nishimura M. A functional polymorphism in the RANTES gene promoter is associated with the development of late-onset asthma. *Am J Respir Crit Care Med* 2002; 166: 686–690.

39. Hizawa N, Yamaguchi E, Jinushi E, and Kawakami Y. A common FCER1B gene promoter polymorphism influences total serum IgE levels in a Japanese population. *Am J Respir Crit Care Med* 2000; 161: 906–909.

40. Barr RG, Cooper DM, Speizer FE, Drazen JM, and Camargo CA, Jr. Beta(2)-adrenoceptor polymorphism and body mass index are associated with adult-onset asthma in sedentary but not active women (comment). *Chest* 2001; 120: 1474–1479.

41. Wang Z, Chen C, Niu T et al. Association of asthma with beta(2)-adrenergic receptor gene polymorphism and cigarette smoking. [Erratum appears in *Am J Respir Crit Care Med* 2002; 166: 775.] *Am J Respir Crit Care Med* 2001; 163: 1401–1409.

42. Izmerov NF, Kuzmina LP, and Tarasova LA. Genetic-biochemical criteria for individual sensitivity in development of occupational bronchopulmonary diseases. *Central Eur J Public Health* 2002; 10: 35–41.

43. Dekker JW, Nizankowska E, Schmitz-Schumann M et al. Aspirin-induced asthma and HLA-DRB1 and HLA-DPB1 genotypes. *Clin Exp Allergy* 1997; 27: 574–577.

44. Kitch BT, Levy BD, and Fanta CH. Late onset asthma: epidemiology, diagnosis and treatment. *Drugs Aging* 2000; 17: 385–397.

45. Segala C, Priol G, Soussan D et al. Asthma in adults: comparison of adult-onset asthma with childhood-onset asthma relapsing in adulthood. *Allergy* 2000; 55: 634–640.

46. Huovinen E, Kaprio J, Laitinen LA, and Koskenvuo M. Incidence and prevalence of asthma among adult Finnish men and women of the Finnish Twin Cohort from 1975 to 1990, and their relation to hay fever and chronic bronchitis. *Chest* 1999; 115: 928–936.

47. Court CS, Cook DG, and Strachan DP. Comparative epidemiology of atopic and non-atopic wheeze and diagnosed asthma in a national sample of English adults. *Thorax* 2002; 57: 951–957.

48. Oosaki R, Mizushima Y, Kawasaki A, Hoshino K, and Kobayashi M. Clinical features of adult-relapse asthma in comparison with those of child-onset asthma and adult-onset asthma. *J Asthma* 1994; 31: 339–345.

49. Bodner CH, Ross S, Little J, et al. Risk factors for adult onset wheeze: a case control study. *Am J Respir Crit Care Med* 1998; 157:35-42.

50. Reed CE. Onset and outcome of asthma in older adults: a clinician's perspective. *Clin Rev Allergy Immunol* 2002; 22: 53–65.

51. Peat JK, Woolcock AJ, and Cullen K. Rate of decline of lung function in subjects with asthma. *Eur J Respir Dis* 1987; 70: 171–179.

52. Lange P, Parner J, Vestbo J, Schnohr P, and Jensen G. A 15-year follow-up study of ventilatory function in adults with asthma. *New Engl J Med* 1998; 339: 1194–1200.

53. Ulrik CS, Backer V, and Dirksen A. A 10-year follow-up of 180 adults with bronchial asthma: factors important for the decline in lung function (comment). *Thorax* 1992; 47: 14–18.

54. Molina C, Brun J, Coulet M, Betail G, and Delage J. Immunopathology of the bronchial mucosa in 'late onset' asthma. *Clin Allergy* 1977; 7: 137–145.

55. Aoki K, Ohtsubo K, Yoshimura K, Saiki S, Tai H, and Okano H. Histological evaluation of bronchial tissue from elderly individuals with bronchial asthma. *Jpn J Thoracic Dis* 1995; 33: 1421–1429.

56. Bodner C, Anderson WJ, Reid TS, and Godden DJ. Childhood exposure to infection and risk of adult onset wheeze and atopy. *Thorax* 2000; 55: 383–387.

57. Hahn DL, Dodge RW, and Golubjatnikov R. Association of *Chlamydia pneumoniae* (strain TWAR) infection with wheezing, asthmatic bronchitis, and adult-onset asthma (comment). *JAMA* 1991; 266: 225–230.

58. Allegra L, Blasi F, Centanni S et al. Acute exacerbations of asthma in adults: role of *Chlamydia pneumoniae* infection. *Eur Respir J* 1994; 7: 2165–2168.

59. Hahn DL, Anttila T, and Saikku P. Association of *Chlamydia pneumoniae* IgA antibodies with recently symptomatic asthma. *Epidemiol Infect* 1996; 117: 513–517.

60. Hahn DL. Treatment of *Chlamydia pneumoniae* infection in adult asthma: a before–after trial (comment*). J Family Pract* 1995; 41: 345–351.

61. Routes JM, Nelson HS, Noda JA, and Simon FT. Lack of correlation between *Chlamydia pneumoniae* antibody titers and adult-onset asthma (comment). *J Allergy Clin Immunol* 2000; 105: 391–392.

62. Yano T, Ichikawa Y, Komatu S, Arai S, and Oizumi K. Association of *Mycoplasma pneumoniae* antigen with initial onset of bronchial asthma (comment). *Am J Respir Crit Care Med* 1994; 149: 1348–1353.

63. Martin RJ, Kraft M, Chu HW, Berns EA, and Cassell GH. A link between chronic asthma and chronic infection. *J Allergy Clin Immunol* 2001; 107: 595–601.

64. Busse WW. Asthma: definition and pathogenesis, in *Asthma: Principles and Practice*. Middleton, E., Jr. and Ellis, E.F., Eds., St. Louis: Mosby-Year Book, 1998: 838–858.

65. Koh YY, Park Y, Lee HJ, and Kim CK. Levels of interleukin-2, interferon-gamma, and interleukin-4 in bronchoalveolar lavage fluid from patients with Mycoplasma pneumonia: implication of tendency toward increased immunoglobulin E production. *Pediatrics* 2001; 107: E39.

66. Kraft M, Cassell GH, and Pak J, Martin RJ. *Mycoplasma pneumoniae* and *Chlamydia pneumoniae* in asthma: effect of clarithromycin. *Chest* 2002; 121: 1782–1788.

67. Jaakkola MS, Nordman H, Piipari R et al. Indoor dampness and molds and development of adult-onset asthma: a population-based incident case-control study. *Environ Health Perspect* 2002; 110: 543–547.

68. Jaakkola MS, Laitinen S, Piipari R et al. Immunoglobulin G antibodies against indoor dampness-related microbes and adult-onset asthma: a population-based incident case-control study. *Clin Exp Immunol* 2002; 129: 107–112.

69. Hartert TV and Peebles RS. Dietary antioxidants and adult asthma. *Curr Opin Allergy Clin Immunol* 2001; 1: 421–429.

70. Schwartz J and Weiss ST. The relationship of dietary fish intake to level of pulmonary function in the first National Health and Nutrition Survey (NHANES-I) (comment). *Eur Respir J* 1994; 7:1821–1824.

71. Seaton A and Devereux G. Diet, infection and wheezy illness: lessons from adults. *Pediatr Allergy Immunol* 2000; 11: 37–40.

72. Soutar A, Seaton A, and Brown K. Bronchial reactivity and dietary antioxidants. *Thorax* 1997; 52: 166–170.

73. Troisi RJ, Willett WC, Weiss ST, Trichopoulos D, Rosner B, and Speizer FE. A prospective study of diet and adult-onset asthma (comment). *Am J Respir Crit Care Med* 1995; 151: 1401–1408.

74. Woods RK, Thien FC, and Abramson MJ. Dietary marine fatty acids (fish oil) for asthma in adults and children (update of *Cochrane Database Syst Rev.* 2000; CD001283; PMID 11034708). *Cochrane Database Syst Rev* 2002: CD001283.

75. Burney PG, Neild JE, Twort CH et al. Effect of changing dietary sodium on the airway response to histamine. *Thorax* 1989; 44: 36–441.

76. Carey OJ, Locke C, and Cookson JB. Effect of alterations of dietary sodium on the severity of asthma in men. *Thorax* 1993; 48: 714–718.

77. Medici TC, Schmid AZ, Hacki M, and Vetter W. Are asthmatics salt-sensitive? A preliminary controlled study. *Chest* 1993; 104: 1138–1143.

78. Harlap S and Davies AM. Infant admissions to hospital and maternal smoking. *Lancet* 1974; 1: 529–532.

79. Murray AB and Morrison BJ. The effect of cigarette smoke from the mother on bronchial responsiveness and severity of symptoms in children with asthma. *J Allergy Clin Immunol* 1986; 77: 575–581.

80. Martinez FD, Wright AL, Taussig LM, Holberg CJ, Halonen M, and Morgan WJ. Asthma and wheezing in the first six years of life (comment). *New Engl J Med* 1995; 332: 133–138.

81. Becklake MR and Lalloo U. The 'healthy smoker': a phenomenon of health selection? *Respiration* 1990; 57: 137–144.

82. Eisner MD. Smoking and adult asthma: a healthy smoker effect? (comment). *Am J Respir Crit Care Med* 2002; 165: 1566-1567.

83. Eisner MD. Environmental tobacco smoke exposure and pulmonary function among adults in NHANES III: impact on the general population and adults with current asthma. *Environ Health Perspect* 2002; 110: 765–770.

84. Radon K, Busching K, Heinrich J et al. Passive smoking exposure: a risk factor for chronic bronchitis and asthma in adults? *Chest* 2002; 122: 1086–1090.

85. Thorn J, Brisman J, and Toren K. Adult-onset asthma is associated with self-reported mold or environmental tobacco smoke exposures in the home (comment). *Allergy* 2001; 56: 287–292.

86. Leuenberger P, Schwartz J, and Ackermann-Liebrich U, et al. Passive smoking exposure in adults and chronic respiratory symptoms: Swiss Study on Air Pollution and Lung Diseases in Adults, SAPALDIA (comment*). Am J Respir Crit Care Med* 1994; 150: 1222–1228.

87. Janson C, Chinn S, Jarvis D et al. Effect of passive smoking on respiratory symptoms, bronchial responsiveness, lung function, and total serum IgE in the European Community Respiratory Health Survey: a cross-sectional study. [Erratum appears in *Lancet* 2002; 359: 360.] *Lancet* 2001; 358: 2103–2109.

88. Toren K and Hermansson BA. Incidence rate of adult-onset asthma in relation to age, sex, atopy and smoking: a Swedish population-based study of 15,813 adults. *Int J Tuberculosis Lung Dis* 1999; 3: 192–197.

89. Tan KS, McFarlane LC, Lipworth BJ. Loss of normal cyclical beta 2 adrenoceptor regulation and increased premenstrual responsiveness to adenosine monophosphate in stable female asthmatic patients (comment). *Thorax* 1997; 52: 608–611.

90. Oguzulgen IK, Turktas H, and Erbas D. Airway inflammation in premenstrual asthma. *J Asthma* 2002; 39: 517–522.

91. Pauli BD, Reid RL, Munt PW, Wigle RD, and Forkert L. Influence of the menstrual cycle on airway function in asthmatic and normal subjects. *Am Rev Respir Dis* 1989; 140: 358–362.

92. Eliasson O, Scherzer HH, and DeGraff AC, Jr. Morbidity in asthma in relation to the menstrual cycle. *J Allergy Clin Immunol* 1986; 77: 87–94.

93. Lange P, Parner J, Prescott E, Ulrik CS, and Vestbo J. Exogenous female sex steroid hormones and risk of asthma and asthma-like symptoms: a cross sectional study of the general population. *Thorax* 2001; 56: 613–616.

94. Hepburn MJ, Dooley DP, and Morris MJ. The effects of estrogen replacement therapy on airway function in postmenopausal, asthmatic women. *Arch Int Med* 2001; 161: 2717–2720.

95. Carlson CL, Cushman M, Enright PL, Cauley JA, and Newman AB. Hormone replacement therapy is associated with higher FEV1 in elderly women. *Am J Respir Crit Care Med Medicine* 2001; 163: 423–428.

96. O'Connor BJ. Premenstrual asthma: still poorly understood (comment). *Thorax* 1997; 52: 591–592.

97. Gluck JC and Gluck P. The effects of pregnancy on asthma: a prospective study. *Ann Allergy* 1976; 37: 164–168.

98. White RJ, Coutts, II, Gibbs CJ, and MacIntyre C. A prospective study of asthma during pregnancy and the puerperium. *Respir Med* 1989; 83: 103–106.

99. Troisi RJ, Speizer FE, Willett WC, Trichopoulos D, and Rosner B. Menopause, postmenopausal estrogen preparations, and the risk of adult-onset asthma: a prospective cohort study. *Am J Respir Crit Care Med* 1995; 152: 1183–1188.

100. Malo JL and Chan-Yeung M. Occupational asthma. *J Allergy Clin Immunol* 2001; 108: 317–328.

101. Beckett WS. The epidemiology of occupational asthma. *Eur Respir J* 1994; 7: 161–164.
102. Papi A, Corbetta L, and Fabbri LM. What can we learn from late-onset and occupational asthma? *Clin Exp Allergy* 1998; 28: 174–205.
103. Reijula K, Haahtela T, Klaukka T, and Rantanen J. Incidence of occupational asthma and persistent asthma in young adults has increased in Finland (comment). *Chest* 1996; 110: 58–61.
104. Kogevinas M, Anto JM, Sunyer J, Tobias A, Kromhout H, and Burney P. Occupational asthma in Europe and other industrialised areas: a population-based study. European Community Respiratory Health Survey Study Group. [Erratum appears in *Lancet* 1999;354: 166.] *Lancet* 1999; 353: 1750–1754.
105. Toren K, Balder B, Brisman J et al. The risk of asthma in relation to occupational exposures: a case-control study from a Swedish city. *Eur Respir J* 1999; 13: 496–501.
106. Milton DK, Solomon GM, Rosiello RA, and Herrick RF. Risk and incidence of asthma attributable to occupational exposure among HMO members (comment). *Am J Ind Med* 1998; 33: 1–10.
107. Johnson AR, Dimich-Ward HD, Manfreda J et al. Occupational asthma in adults in six Canadian communities. *Am J Respir Crit Care Med* 2000; 162: 2058–2062.
108. Blanc PD and Toren K. How much adult asthma can be attributed to occupational factors? *Am J Med* 1999; 107: 580–587.
109. Program NAEAP. Expert panel report 2: guidelines for the diagnosis and management of asthma. Bethesda, MD: National Institutes of Health, Publication 97-4051, 1997.
110. Enright PL, McClelland RL, Newman AB, Gottlieb DJ, and Lebowitz MD. Under-diagnosis and under-treatment of asthma in the elderly. Cardiovascular Health Study Research Group (comment). *Chest* 1999; 116: 603–613.
111. Paggiaro PL, Vagaggini B, Bacci E et al. Prognosis of occupational asthma. *Eur Respir J* 1994; 7: 761–767.

II

Immunology in the Early Development of Asthma

5

Ontogeny of the Immune Response

P.G. HOLT and J. ROWE

Telethon Institute for Child Health Research
and Centre for Child Health Research
University of Western Australia, Perth, Australia

I. Introduction

The human immune system is highly developed at birth relative to other mammalian species, and the majority of key effector mechanisms appear almost adult-equivalent in functional capacity. However, it is becoming increasingly clearer that subtle modification of a variety of cellular and molecular mechanisms is necessary to maintain immunological homeostasis in the intrauterine environment, and the persistence of these modifications into postnatal life has potential pathological implications in relation to a variety of diseases, including asthma and atopy. This review provides a broad summary of current understanding of immune ontogeny in humans, focusing in particular on issues of relevance to the etiology and pathogenesis of these latter two diseases.

II. Ontogeny of Fetal Immune System

In the human fetus, hemopoiesis initially occurs in the extraembryonic mesenchymal tissue and mesoderm of the yolk sac, with pluripotent and granulomacrophage progenitors detectable around 4 weeks' gestation. Between 6 and 8 weeks of gestation, CD7[+] T cell precursors and B cell precursors are detectable in the liver, followed by appearance in the thymus between 7 and 8 weeks' gestation.[1] After 15 to 20 weeks of gestation, T cells expressing alpha beta and gamma delta T cell receptors (TCRs) and mature B cells are present in the thymus.[2,3] Between 11 and 12 weeks of gestation, stem cells are detectable in the bone marrow; and by 13 to 15 weeks, T cells are found in the peripheral lymphoid organs.[4–6]

The gastrointestinal tract may be another site for extrathymic T cell differentiation in the fetus, as has been reported in mice.[7] The human fetal intestinal mucosa contains T cells from 12 to 14 weeks' gestation.[8] Many of these cells express the CD8αα phenotype, especially those located in the Peyer's Patches.[9] In mice, these cells appear to be thymus-independent and are believed to develop in the gut. While there is no direct evidence of this in humans, it has been demonstrated that many T cells in the intestinal mucosa of the human fetus proliferate in the absence of antigen, with an additional population of cells that are CD7[+] but CD3[-]. Furthermore, there is little overlap of gut- and blood-derived TCR-β transcripts.[10] For gamma delta T cells, rearrangement of TCR-δ genes is first detected between 6 and 9 weeks of gestation, in particular outside the thymus, in the liver and gut.[11,12]

It is well established that fetal cells have the capacity to respond to polyclonal stimuli as early as 15 to 16 weeks' gestation.[13] Furthermore, infection of a mother during pregnancy with a range of organisms including measles, helminths, malaria, and schistosomes results in transplacental priming of fetal responses; pathogen-specific responses are detectable at birth.[14–18] Conversely, maternal infection can also lead to the generation of tolerance in the fetus, as observed for toxoplasma infection.[19] It is noteworthy that maternal immunization with tetanus toxoid during pregnancy can lead to the development of active fetal immunity, with tetanus toxoid–specific IgM detected in cord blood samples, but no evidence of class switching to IgG.[20]

In addition to infectious agents, evidence suggests the possibility that environmental antigens to which a mother is exposed during pregnancy may prime fetal T cell responses transplacentally, and observations related to cord blood responses to seasonal allergens indicate that T cell priming may occur as early as 22 weeks' gestation.[21] Furthermore, cord blood proliferative responses to allergens are paralleled by a predominantly Th2-skewed cytokine response involving interleukin (IL)-4, IL-5, IL-6, IL-9, IL-10, and IL-13. The fetal origin of these apparently allergen-specific responder cells has been confirmed by genotyping of T cell clones derived from allergen-stimulated bulk cultures of cord blood cells.[22]

Recent studies from our group (Thornton, Holt et al., manuscript submitted) indicate that unlike the situation in allergen-stimulated adult peripheral blood mononuclear cell (PBMC) cultures, the fate of the majority of proliferating T cells in neonatal T cell cultures is rapid apoptosis. This argues against a conventional "memory" phenotype, and ongoing research in our lab focuses on the functional phenotype of these responding T cells in neonates.

During pregnancy, fetal cells have been detected in the maternal circulation as early as the ninth week of gestation,[23] and vice versa,[24] indicating bidirectional cell traffic between mother and fetus. This observation, along with the fact that the fetal immune system is at least partially competent, indicates that tight regulation must occur to protect the fetoplacental unit against the potentially toxic effects of T cell cytokines.[25]

The first line of defense that regulates the induction and expression of immune responses within the placenta appears to involve a series of overlapping nonspecific immunosuppressive mechanisms. The most potent of these involves generation of tryptophan metabolites that inhibit T cell activation and proliferation.[26] A second tier of immunosuppression is provided by trophoblast IL-10 production.[27]

Other mechanisms that act to down-regulate immune responses within the placenta include the high expression of FasL on trophoblasts that actively promotes apoptosis of locally activated T cells[28,29] and parallel mechanisms that selectively down-regulate the production of Th1 cytokines, particularly interferon (IFN)-γ. This cytokine plays a key role in implantation[30] and can also induce fetal resorption if produced in excess after implantation has occurred.[31] The production of progesterone during pregnancy directly inhibits IFN-γ gene transcription and stimulates progesterone-induced blocking factor that in turn stimulates the production of IL-10, IL-3, and IL-4.[32-34] Local production in the placenta by cells such as macrophages of PGE2 appears to play a similar role in damping Th1 responses[35] via promotion of Th2 cytokine secretion,[36,37] and this process may also be enhanced via the stimulatory effects of progesterone on fetal macrophage PGE2 secretion.[38]

III. Early Postnatal Development of Immune System

A. T Cell Function

Total lymphocyte numbers in peripheral blood are higher at birth than in adulthood, and a further doubling of lymphocyte counts occurs during the first 6 weeks of life.[39] During infancy, relatively high numbers of T cells express both CD4 and CD8; this is a hallmark of immaturity.[39-41] Infant T cells also express elevated levels of CD1,[42] CD38,[39,43,44] and peanut agglutinin receptor (PNA) antigen,[45] that are believed to mark mature thymocytes rather than mature naïve T cells. In contrast, the frequency of T cells that coexpress IL-2 and human lymphocyte antigen (HLA)-DR (indicative of recent activation), and CD57 (a marker of non-major histocompatibility complex (MHC)-restricted cytotoxic T cells) is low.[41] Paradoxically however, infant T cells also express low levels of several other activation markers including CD25, CD69, and CD154.[39]

Recent studies suggest that the majority of peripheral T cells at birth represent recent thymic emigrants (RTEs), as defined by the presence of T cell receptor excision circles (TRECs).[44] TRECs are extrachromosomal products generated during the process of V (D) J TcR gene rearrangement that are not replicated during mitosis and therefore become diluted with each round of cell division. These RTEs showed enhanced survival, entry into the cell cycle, and proliferation in the presence of IL-7, unlike mature long-lived naïve T cells obtained from adults, indicating that RTEs in early life represent an early stage in T cell ontogeny.[44,46]

The changing patterns of T cell CD45RA and CD45RO expression during postnatal life are particularly interesting in relation to the development of overall immune competence during this period. After leaving the thymus, T cells express the CD45RA isoform of the leukocyte common antigen CD45, which after activation, switches to CD45RO expression. Within the alpha beta and gamma delta T cell populations, the rate of postnatal increase of CD45RO expression is approximately equal and is slightly more rapid for CD4+ T cells as compared with CD8+ T cells. Within the CD4+ T cell compartment, the proportion of CD45RO+ cells increases from around 10% at birth to around 65% in adults, reflecting the age-dependent accumulation of antigenic experience.[39,41,47–52] The relative proportion of CD45RO+ memory T cells attains adult-equivalent levels within the teen years, although the rate at which this occurs is very heterogeneous within the population at large.[50]

The functional capacities of T cells during infancy differ both quantitatively and qualitatively from capacities in adults. Limiting dilution analysis has demonstrated that 90% of peripheral blood CD4+ T cells from adults can give rise to stable T cell clones as compared with less than 35% of CD4+ T cells in infants.[53]

It has also been observed that cloning frequencies are bimodally distributed within the infant population, with a significant proportion of apparently healthy individuals displaying cloning frequencies of 20%. In apparent contrast, cord blood T cells display higher proliferative rates shortly after stimulation with polyclonal mitogens when compared with adult T cells.[54] These initially high proliferative responses are not maintained, however, which may reflect the greater susceptibility of neonatal T cells to postactivation apoptosis (see Hassan and Reen[44] and discussion above) and/or their decreased production of IL-2.[55,56] In contrast, compared with adults, proliferative responses induced by TCR activation[57] and cross-linking CD2[56,58] or CD28[59] are reduced in infants.

Neonatal T cells have been demonstrated to be hyporesponsive to IL-12[60] and hyperresponsive to IL-4.[61] Furthermore, upon secondary stimulation with bacterial superantigen, cord blood T cells, unlike T cells isolated from adults, display hyporesponsiveness, even though vigorous primary responses are initially generated.[62] This anergy can be attributed in part to decreased responsiveness of cord blood T cells to IL-2,[63] although possible additional mechanisms may be involved including decreased activation of the Ras signaling pathway.[64] Other defects in intracellular signaling pathways identified in neonatal T cells include decreased activation of phospholipase C and expression of LcK,[65] decreased protein kinase C,[66] and reduced CD28-mediated signaling leading to dysfunctional FasL-mediated cytotoxicity[67] and reduced NFkB production.[59]

In addition, both cytotoxic effector functions[68,69] and ability to provide help for B cell immunoglobulin isotype switching[68–72] are low during infancy. These deficiencies may be attributed in part to attenuated expression of various cytokine receptors,[73] decreased expression of CD40L,[68,70,71] and reduced production of a variety of cytokines following stimulation including IL-10,[74] IL-15,[75] IFNγ,[76] IL-2, IL-4, and TNF-α.[77] The mechanisms underlying decreased cytokine production by cord blood T cells are unclear, although factors specific to both the T cells and accessory cells (discussed below) have been implicated.

Work from our laboratory has demonstrated that CpG methylation within the IFN-γ promoters of CD4+ CD45RO− T cells is higher than in their adult counterparts.[78] This hypermethylation correlates with the markedly decreased ability of these cells to produce IFN-γ. IFN-γ promoters in neonatal CD8+ CD45RO− T cells did not display comparable hypermethylation and produced levels of IFN-γ that were much closer to their adult counterparts. Furthermore, the differences in methylation patterns within the IFN-γ promoters of neonates and adults were not paralleled with respect to the IL-4 promoter, indicating that this methylation mechanism is not involved in developmental regulation of all cytokine genes.[78] In this context, it is also noteworthy that Mbawuike and colleagues recently demonstrated the capacity of infant CD8+ T cells to generate potent IFN-γ responses following respiratory syncytial virus (RSV) infection.[79]

B. B Cell Function

At birth, total B cell numbers in peripheral blood are high compared with numbers in adults, with further increases seen during the first year of life.[39] B cells expressing CD5 together with activational markers such as IL-2R and CD23[80] represent the major subset in cord blood. The subset decreases throughout childhood until adult levels equivalent to 25 to 35% of the overall B cell compartment are reached in late adolescence.[81] It has been hypothesised that CD5+ B cells act as a first line of innate defense in primary antibody responses in neonates, using a preimmune repertoire in contrast with CD5− B cells in which response patterns are acquired following antigen contact.

An additional B cell subset that is CD5 variable and expresses membrane IgM, IgD, CD23, and CD11b has been shown to secrete polyreactive IgM spontaneously against a range of autoantigens.[80] Neonatal B cells also express higher levels of CD1c and CD38 compared with adult cells[39] and have the capacity to proliferate in response to IL-4 and IL-2 in the absence of *in vitro* activation.[82]

As discussed above, neonates have reduced capacity for isotype switching that is believed to play a role in the inability of infants to mount sustained antibody responses following vaccination or infections, as compared with adults (see below). This defect in isotype switching may be explained in part by reduced cytokine production[55,74–77,83–85] and decreased expression of CD40L by neonatal T cells[68–72] because CD40L represents a critical signal for T helper cell–induced class switching.[86] With the addition of mature T helper cells or adequate soluble signals,[72,87,88] immunoglobulin production by neonatal B cells can be improved; however, production levels still fail to reach the adult range, suggesting that intrinsic B cell defects also exist in neonates.

C. Antigen-Presenting Cell (APC) Populations

In the context of this review, the major APC populations include dendritic cells (DCs), mononuclear phagocytes (MNPs), and B cells. The precise role of each of these cell types within individual immune responses is not completely understood, although it is clear from murine studies that DCs are the most potent APCs for priming of immunologically naïve T cells, in particular against environmental antigens that are typically encountered at very low concentrations.[89] Furthermore, the distributions and phenotypes of these cells appear comparable in both murine and human tissues, lending weight to the suggestion that DCs act as the primary links between innate and adaptive immunity in humans, as has been proposed in mice.[89–92]

DC seeding into peripheral tissues within a fetus is initiated relatively early during gestation.[93] DC networks are detectable at birth in a variety of tissues including the upper and lower respiratory tracts[94,95] intestinal mucosa,[96,97] and the epidermis.[93,98,99] DCs in these tissue networks are usually present at lower densities at birth than in adults, and express lower levels of MHC class II.[95,98,99] These differences suggest developmentally related variations in the functional phenotype of DC as demonstrated in recent studies. It has been shown in mice that the phenomenon of neonatal tolerance results primarily from the inability of neonatal DCs from central lymphoid organs to present efficient Th1-inducing signals to T cells, resulting in the preferential generation of Th2-biased immune responses.[100] Of relevance to the development of allergic disease in infancy, our group has demonstrated that the airway mucosal DC networks of neonatal rats develop surprisingly slowly after birth and do not reach adult equivalence in terms of density, MHC class II expression, and responsiveness to inhaled stimuli until after weaning.[95,101]

A paucity of data on the function of mucosal DCs in humans exists, but immunohistochemical studies of autopsied tissues suggest that the slow kinetics of postnatal maturation of respiratory tract DC networks may be comparable to the kinetics described in animal models.[102,103] The numbers of circulating

HLA-DR⁺ DCs are decreased at birth relative to adults and these cells display attenuated APC activity.[104] Furthermore, analysis of cord blood monocyte-derived DCs has demonstrated decreased expression of HLA-DR, CD40, and CD80, as well as decreased responsiveness to LPS and CD40 ligation as measured by production of IL-12p35.[105] The latter finding is consistent with recent reports of slow postnatal maturation of capacity of human peripheral blood DC to secrete bioactive IL-12p70 protein.[106]

As for DCs, ontogenic studies on human MNPs have been limited essentially to blood-borne populations. Neonatal monocytes have been shown to be approximately adult-equivalent in terms of numbers, phagocytic activity, and ability to present alloantigen.[107–109] However, monocytes isolated from cord blood expressed lower levels of a variety of surface markers, including MHC class II, CD11b, CD54, and CD14 when compared with monocytes isolated from adult peripheral blood.[110–112] Decreased CD14 expression has also been implicated in reduced production of TNF-α and IL-10 by cord blood monocytes after stimulation with LPS.[110] In this context, expression of Toll-like receptors 2 and 4 on monocytes are low at birth in mice and increase with age,[113] but systemic studies on the ontogeny of receptor expression in humans have yet to be reported.

Neonatal monocytes are also less responsive to IFN-γ due to decreased phosphorylation of STAT-1, an important component of the signalling pathway linked to the IFN-γ receptor.[114] Conversely, neonatal MNPs have been implicated as cofactors in the reduced IFN-γ responses of infant T cells to polyclonal mitogens such as phytohaemagglutinin (PHA),[115–117] possibly as a result of diminished elaboration of costimulator signals.[118]

Although no direct information is available on the APC functions of human neonatal B cells, studies in mice have demonstrated that neonatal B cells function poorly as APCs relative to their adult counterparts and maintain low levels of functional capacity until after the weaning period.[108,119]

D. Eosinophils and Mast Cells

Little information is available regarding the ontogeny of eosinophils. Low level eosinophilia is common in preterm infants, and inflammatory exudates in neonates commonly contain unusually high numbers of eosinophils.[120–122] This may reflect overall higher levels of constitutive IL-5 production within the "Th2-polarized" neonatal immune system. It has been suggested that the decreased expression of integrins such as Mac-1[123] and L-selectin[124] may contribute to developmentally related variations in eosinophil recirculation characteristics during early infancy. Additionally, the possibility that variations in eosinophil numbers in peripheral blood among infants may be predictive of susceptibility to subsequent inflammatory diseases is attracting growing interest. In particular, eosinophilia persisting to ≥3 months of age has been linked to subsequent diagnosis of atopy.[125]

In adults, two types of mast cells have been identified within mucosal tissues: mucosal mast cells (MMCs) that lie within the epithelia of the mucosae and connective tissue mast cells (CTMCs) located in the underlying laminar propria. It has been suggested that mast cells seed into human gut tissues during infancy in response to local stimuli,[126] although little direct information is available on the ontogeny of these cells. In rats, it has been shown that MMC and CTMC populations develop slowly in the respiratory tract between birth and weaning,[127] with increased levels of mast cell-derived proteases detected in the peripheral blood at weaning.[128] These increased levels of circulating mast cell-derived proteases suggest that the immature mast cell populations within tissues of rats undergo local stimulation during this period. Similar increases in levels of mast cell–derived tryptase have been detected in human serum during infancy.[129]

Direct information on the functional phenotype of human MMC populations during the neonatal period are lacking, but a recent study has demonstrated that cord blood–derived mast cells display marked decreases in the levels of FcεR1α transcripts compared with mast cells obtained from adult peripheral blood.[130] These decreases may serve to restrict IgE-mediated reactions during infancy,[130] but further studies are required to resolve this important question.

IV. Early-Life Immunity to Infectious Agents and Vaccines

As discussed above, there is a progressive maturation of the capacity to generate adult-like immune responses, both quantitatively and qualitatively, after birth. The development-related deficiencies in innate and adaptive immunological mechanisms described earlier appear to be collectively responsible for the transient high susceptibility to infection with a wide rage of pathogens[131-135] and accompanying high (relative) rates of mortality during infancy. Moreover, immune responses to microbial antigens encountered early in life when the immune system is immature can shape long-term immunological memory and thus influence the pathogenesis of infectious diseases in later life.

For example, Culley and colleagues demonstrated in mice that the age of primary infection with respiratory syncytial virus influences the cytokine phenotype of the host response to primary infection and also the type of memory response that develops upon reinfection. Thus, mice first infected as neonates in the early postnatal period, during which the adaptive immune system maintains expression of the Th2 bias characteristic of fetal life, generate Th2-biased antiviral responses compared with animals first infected at later ages that produce predominantly Th1-polarized responses.[136] Additionally, animals infected very early in infancy program Th2-biased memories that are recalled during postweaning reinfection,[136] a finding that has important theoretical implications for the pathogenesis of RSV disease in humans.[137]

For similar reasons, infancy also represents a period during which vaccine responses are attenuated, often requiring multiple boosters to achieve adequate levels of protection. In terms of the measles-mumps-rubella vaccine, it has been demonstrated that the age of vaccination in infancy affects the seroconversion rate, with infants vaccinated between 9 and 11 months having significantly lower antibody titers compared with those vaccinated between 15 and 17 months.[138] Similarly, Gans and colleagues demonstrated that while infants given the measles-mumps-rubella vaccine at 6 months had lower antibody responses compared with those vaccinated at 9 or 12 months, no differences were observed in IFNγ and IL-12 production after *in vitro* stimulation of PBMC with measles antigen. Compared with adults, however, these responses were significantly lower.[139] In mice, significant vaccine responses can be detected as early as the first week of life. However, these responses differed markedly from adults; neonates displayed decreased ratios of IgG2a:IgG1, increased vaccine-specific IL-5, and decreased IFN-γ responses after *in vitro* stimulation with the vaccine antigen.[140]

Our group recently examined the development of tetanus toxoid (TT)–specific responses after vaccination with the diphtheria-tetanus-acellular pertussis (DTaP) vaccine in a prospective cohort of 132 infants and compared the responses with age-related changes in systemic (polyclonal) Th1 and Th2 cytokine functions. We detected early Th1 and Th2 cytokine responses to the vaccine antigen. However, while the Th2 component of the vaccine response remained stable throughout the first 18 months of life, Th1 responses were transient and commonly declined after the final priming dose at 6 months.[141] Similar observations were reported in mice, with mixed Th1 and Th2 responses generated after vaccinations of neonatal animals. However, in animals first vaccinated as neonates, Th2-polarized secondary responses were seen after secondary vaccination, suggesting that Th1 memory may not be well maintained in early life.[142]

In our study on human infants, while vaccine-specific IFN-γ responses declined after the final priming dose at 6 months, we noted a marked resurgence of these IFN-γ responses between 12 and 18 months in the absence of further vaccination. This resurgent Th1 response coincided with a parallel increase in the overall capacity to produce IFN-γ as measured by polyclonal mitogen stimulation.[141]

With regard to the pertussis component of the vaccine, Ausiello and colleagues reported similar findings with age-associated spontaneous increases in pertussis-specific IFN-γ production detected in the absence of further vaccination. The authors attribute the increased pertussis-specific IFN-γ capacity to asymptomatic infection with *Bordetella pertussis*.[143] In light of our findings, it may be hypothesised that boosting by environmental antigens that cross-react with TT may account for the upswing of vaccine-specific IFN-γ production. However, given the parallel increased capacity to produce IFN-γ in response to polyclonal stimuli, a more likely explanation is that the maturation of accessory cell function may permit more efficient *in vitro* expression of IFN-γ memory responses by previously primed TT-specific Th1 cells.

In support of this hypothesis, it has been demonstrated that IFN-γ production in response to polyclonal mitogen stimulation of peripheral blood T cells can be boosted toward adult-equivalent levels if the cultures are supplemented with mature accessory cells.[116,117] Similarly, adult-like vaccine responses can be induced in early life with the use of powerful stimuli such as BCG[144,145] or CpG containing oligonucleotides[146] that exert potent effects on APC function; comparable boosting effects have been achieved employing plasmid DNA[147] and IL-12.[148] IL-12 may affect this process at a number of different levels, including promotion of overall Th1 differentiation[149] and stabilization of IFN-γ gene transcription in Th1-cells post-differentiation.[150]

V. Vaccination and Atopic Phenotype

As discussed in more detail below, high genetic risk for atopy is associated with delayed maturation of IFN-γ responses. Some evidence suggests that a further consequence of delayed maturation of Th1 function may be hyporesponsiveness to vaccination in infancy, notably Calmette–Guerin (BCG), DTaP, and pneumococcal vaccines. In terms of BCG, a Japanese study demonstrated that those who failed to develop long-lasting delayed-type hypersensitivity responses after vaccination in infancy were at increased risk for atopy at age 12.[151]

Our group has shown that TT-specific lymphoproliferative responses at 2 years of age were inversely related to the expression of the atopic phenotype.[22] More recently, children with atopic eczema had reduced capacities to respond to pneumococcal vaccination.[152] In our recent work, we observed that TT-specific responses remain constantly more skewed toward the Th2 phenotype in children up to 12 months of age. This is transient, however, and is no longer evident in these children at 18 months of age.[141] Similarly, no evidence of this was found in 6-year-old children who completed the standard priming and boosting schedules.[153] These studies suggest that infancy may be a period of high susceptibility to vaccine hyporesponsiveness, specifically in those at genetic risk of developing atopy. More studies are warranted to clarify this issue fully.

Conversely, vaccination has been hypothesized to be partially responsible for the increased incidence of allergy seen over the past few decades. As part of the hygiene hypothesis, exposure to potent Th1-stimulating infectious agents may help promote the maturation of the immune system away from the Th2-biased response seen at birth that is also associated with atopy. For example, measles infection has been associated with decreased risk for atopy,[154,155] prompting a suggestion that preventing measles infection with the use of vaccines may potentially increase the risk of atopy. However, Lewis and colleagues reported that both measles infection and vaccination were associated with decreased risk of subsequent development of hay fever.[156] A large retrospective study in Finland suggests that measles infections may be more frequent in atopics[157] (see further discussion below).

In addition to decreasing the levels of exposure of children to potent Th1-stimulating infectious agents, vaccines may also play roles in the development of atopy by stimulating vaccine-specific Th2 responses. This is the case for the DTaP vaccine which unlike natural infection or vaccination with whole-cell pertussis vaccine, stimulates a mixed Th1 and Th2 pertussis–specific response.[143] Furthermore, vaccine-specific IgE and IgG4 have been detected in humans[158–160] although no increases in allergen-specific IgE production or atopic disease were detected.[159,160]

VI. Postnatal Development of Immune Function and Susceptibility to Allergic Disease

Earlier studies from our laboratory[53] provided the initial evidence that genetic risk for allergic disease was associated with delayed postnatal maturation of Th1 function. This concept is now supported by a number of lines of independent investigation, but much remains to be elucidated in relation to the nature of the underlying mechanisms.

Our current working hypothesis to explain the operations of this process can be broadly summarized as follows:

1. The allergen-specific Th2-polarized memory that is the hallmark of atopy is in the majority of cases "programmed" by the end of the preschool years.[161,162] This occurs during the period when Th1 function is selectively up-regulated to redress the Th2-bias characteristic of the fetal immune system.

2. This process is driven by interactions among microbial pattern recognition receptors (notably CD14 and the TOLL family). The genes encoding these receptors are highly polymorphic and specific variants that modulate both Th1 function and risk for allergy in children are being identified.[163,164]

3. Children at genetic risk of atopy (and/or those who subsequently develop atopy) express lower levels of IFN-γ response capacity at birth and up-regulate this activity more slowly than the population at large.[53,162,165–169]

4. The relative paucity of Th1 feedback during the early phase of allergen-specific Th memory generation increases the likelihood that this process will default to the Th2 pathway.

A number of important issues underlying this hypothesis remain to be resolved. First, it is not clear precisely when allergen-specific T cell priming is initiated and which particular exposure routes are most important in this process. Earlier studies from a number of groups including ours identified putative allergen-responsive CD4+ T helper cells in cord blood.[170–173] T cell cloning and genotyping studies have established the fetal (as opposed to maternal) origin of these T-cells.[174] These findings suggest that transplacental priming against allergens may occur as a result of maternal exposure[174] consistent with precedents previously established in relation to maternal vaccination.[20]

This conclusion is challenged, however, by recent results from our laboratory indicating that unlike the situation in adults, the responses triggered by allergenic stimulation of cord blood CD4+ T-cells are rapidly terminated by large-scale apoptosis unless a complex mix of "rescue" cytokines is provided. Moreover, the responding cells express the naïve CD45RA+ phenotype (Thornton et al., manuscript submitted). Further research is clearly necessary to resolve the questions arising from these observations.

A second and perhaps more complex series of unanswered questions relates to the role and origin of the cytokines that control Th1 and Th2 switch regulation and Th memory development, during allergen-specific T-cell responses in infants. While it seems plausible that a transient developmental deficiency in IFN-γ production capacity may play a key role in the process, the molecular basis for the deficiency in at-risk children remains unclear. One possibility involves variations in IL-12 response maturation that display strong developmental regulation.[106] The principal sources of IL-12 are DCs. Human neonatal DCs display markedly diminished capacity to express the IL-12p35 gene.[105] The functions of other Th1-trophic cytokines such as IL-18 and IL-23 in this context also remain to be defined.

The contributions of different cell populations to Th1 and Th2 memory development are also unclear. Our recent studies indicate that unlike CD4+ T cells, neonatal CD8+ T cells express high IFN-γ response potential.[78] CD8+ T-cells are integral parts of allergen-specific Th memory responses in adult atopics,[175] but their roles in children are unknown.

An additional and possibly more important series of issues related specifically to disease *expression* also requires clarification via more intensive research. We know that development of persistent wheeze and/or airway hyperresponsiveness (AHR) among children sensitized to inhalant allergens is restricted to a relatively small subset (20 to 30% of the overall SPT+ population) and that >90% of sufferers are nevertheless sensitized.[176] This suggests that sensitization to inhalants may be necessary but not sufficient for the development of persistent airway disease.

What additional cofactors tip the balance toward symptom expression? Evidence from large scale epidemiological studies is continuing to shed light on this complex question. Notably, independent studies have reported that the risk of persistent wheeze among SPT⁺ children is inversely related to the age at which initial sensitization occurred.[177,178] This suggests that damage to an actively growing or remodeling airway may be central to long-term wheeze. Moreover, studies from our group on a birth cohort of ~2500 children established that maximal risk for persistent wheeze is present in those who suffer the combined effects of atopic sensitization and viral-induced wheezing illness during infancy.[179,180] We hypothesize that the synergistic effects of these two processes on the airways may in many cases be the end results of the operation of some family of genetic mechanisms responsible for the attenuated expression of Th1 function in early life, leading to concomitantly increased risk for development of atopy and severe viral infection.[137,179]

Another intriguing issue emerging from these studies is the potentially dualistic role of IFN-γ in diseases such as asthma. We and others have noted that the most common manifestation of CD4⁺ Th memory in atopic children is a mixed response comprising Th2 cytokines in combination with IFN-γ.[161] This implies that in relation to allergen-specific Th-memory responses, the Th2 inhibitory effect of IFN-γ may be restricted to a "gatekeeper" role during the early phase of memory development because T cells expressing Th1-polarized (IFN-γ-associated) and Th2-polarized (IL-4 and IL-5) immunity to inhalant allergens commonly coexist in the same individuals. Moreover, the magnitude of the Th1 component of allergen-specific[153,161,181] and vaccine-specific[141] responses in atopic children subsequent to infancy is typically higher than in their nonatopic counterparts. IFN-γ is highly toxic at high concentrations. Recent data from animal model studies suggest that hyperexpression of this cytokine during the host response to RSV may be an important component of viral-induced immunopathology.[182] Additionally, a series of studies in murine asthma models demonstrated the potential for Th1 cytokines expressed in the airways to induce AHR.[183,184] Hence, the apparent "rebound" in allergen-specific Th1 immunity in atopic children from hypoexpression to (in some cases) hyperexpression potentially has pathological consequences, and the maturation of these responses with age accordingly merits more detailed investigations in birth cohort studies.

References

1. Haynes BF, Martin ME, Kay HH, and Kurtzberg J. Early events in human T cell ontogeny: phenotypic characterization and immunohistologic localization of T cell precursors in early human fetal tissues. *J Exp Med* 1988; 168: 1061–1080.
2. Golby S, Hackett M, Boursier L, Dunn-Walters D, Thiagamoorthy S, and Spencer J. B cell development and proliferation of mature B cells in human fetal intestine. *J Leuk Biol* 2002; 72: 279–284.
3. Wilson CB, Penix L, Weaver WM, Melvin A, and Lewis DB. Ontogeny of T lymphocyte function in the neonate. *Am J Reprod Immunol* 1992; 28: 132–135.

4. Asma GEM, Van Den Bergh RL, and Vossen JM. Use of monoclonal antibodies in a study of the development of T lymphocytes in the human fetus. *Clin Exp Immunol* 1983; 53: 429–436.

5. Royo C, Touraine J-L, and De Bouteiller O. Ontogeny of T lymphocyte differentiation in the human fetus: acquisition of phenotype and functions. *Thymus* 1987; 10: 57–73.

6. Timens W, Rozeboom T, and Poppema S. Fetal and neonatal development of human spleen: an immunohistological study. *Immunology* 1987; 60: 603–609.

7. Fichtelius KE. The gut epithelium: a first level lymphoid organ? *Exp Cell Res* 1968; 49: 87–104.

8. Spencer J, MacDonald TT, Finn T, and Isaacson PG. The development of gut associated lymphoid tissue in the terminal ileum of fetal human intestine. *Clin Exp Immunol* 1986; 64: 536–543.

9. Latthe M and Terry L. High frequency of CD8 alpha alpha homodimer-bearing T cells in human fetal intestine. *Eur J Immunol* 1994; 24: 1703–1705.

10. Howie D, Spencer J, DeLord D, Pitzalis C, Wathen NC, Dogan A, Akbar A, and MacDonald TT. Extrathymic T cell differentiation in the human intestine early in life. *J Immunol* 1998; 161: 5862–5872.

11. McVay LD, Jaswal SS, Kennedy C, Hayday A, and Carding SR. The generation of human gamma delta T cell repertoires during fetal development. *J Immunol* 1998; 160: 5851–5860.

12. Wucherpfennig KW, Liao YJ, Prendergast M, Hafler DA, and Strominger JL. Human fetal liver g/d T cells predominantly use unusual rearrangements of the T cell receptor d and g loci expressed on both CD4+ CD8- and CD4- CD8- g/d T cells. *J Exp Med* 1993; 177: 425–432.

13. Stites DP, Carr MC, and Fudenberg HH. Ontogeny of cellular immunity in the human fetus: development of responses to phytohaemagglutinin and to allogeneic cells. *Cell Immunol* 1974; 11: 257–271.

14. Aase JM, Noren GR, Reddy DV, and St Geme JW. Mumps virus infection in pregnant women and the immunologic response of their offspring. *New Eng J Med* 1972; 286: 1379–1382.

15. Fievet N, Ringwald P, and Bickii J. Malaria cellular immune responses in neonates from Cameroon. *Parasite Immunol* 1996; 18: 483–490.

16. King CL, Malhotra I, Mungai P, Wamachi A, Kioko J, Ouma JH, and Kazura JW. B cell sensitization to helminthic infection develops *in utero* in humans. *J Immunol* 1998; 160: 3578–3584.

17. Novato-Silva E, Gazzinelli G, and Colley DG. Immune responses during human schistosomiasis mansoni: XVIII. Immunologic status of pregnant women and their neonates. *Scand J Immunol* 1992; 35: 429–437.

18. Sanjeevi CB, Vivekanandan S, and Narayanan PR. Fetal response to maternal ascariasis as evidenced by anti-*Ascaris lumbricoides* IgM antibodies in the cord blood. *Acta Pediatr Scand* 1991; 80: 1134–1138.

19. McLeod R, Mack DG, Boyer K, Mets M, Roizen N, Swisher C, Patel D, Beckmann E, Vitullo D, Johnson D, and Meier P. Phenotypes and functions of lymphocytes in congenital toxoplasmosis. *J Lab Clin Med* 1990; 116: 623–635.

20. Dastur FD, Shastry P, Iyer E, Awatramani V, Raut S, Mehta SD, and Irani SF. The foetal immune response to maternal tetanus toxoid immunization. *J Assn Phys India* 1993; 41: 94–96.

21. Jones AC, Miles EA, Warner JO, Colwell BM, Bryant TN, and Warner JA. Fetal peripheral blood mononuclear cell proliferative responses to mitogenic and allergenic stimuli during gestation. *Pediatr Allergy Immunol* 1996; 7: 109–116.

22. Prescott SL, Sly PD, and Holt PG. Raised serum IgE associated with reduced responsiveness to DPT vaccination during infancy. *Lancet* 1998; 351: 1489.

22a. Thornton, CA, Upham JW, Wikström ME, Holt BJ, White GP, Sharp MJ, Sly PD, and Holt PG. Functional maturation of CD4+CD25+CTLA4+CD45RA+ T regulatory cells in human neonatal T cell responses to environmental antigens/allergens. *J Immunol* 2004; 173: 3084–3092.

23. Lo Y-MD, Wainscoat JS, Gillmer MDG, Patel P, Sampietro M, and Fleming KA. Prenatal sex determination by DNA amplification from maternal peripheral blood. *Lancet* 1989; 9: 1363.

24. Ichinohe T, Maruya E, and Saji H. Long-term feto-maternal microchimerism: nature's hidden clue for alternative donor hematopoietic cell transplantation? *Int J Hematol* 2002; 76: 229–237.

25. Wegmann TG, Lin H, Guilbert L, and Mosmann TR. Bidirectional cytokine interactions in the maternal–fetal relationshiip: is successful pregnancy a Th2 phenomenon? *Immunol Today* 1993; 14: 353–356.

26. Munn DH, Zhou M, Attwood JT, Bondarev I, Conway SJ, Marshall B, Brown C, and Mellor AL. Prevention of allogeneic fetal rejection by tryptophan catabolism. *Science* 1998; 281: 1191–1193.

27. Roth I, Corry DB, Locksley RM, Abrams JS, Litton MJ, and Fisher SJ. Human placental cytotrophoblasts produce the immunosuppressive cytokine interleukin-10. *J Exp Med* 1996; 184: 539–548.

28. Guller S and LaChapelle L. The role of placental Fas ligand in maintaining immune privilege at maternal–fetal interface. *Sem Reprod Endocrinol* 1999; 17: 39–44.

29. Hammer A, Blaschitz A, Daxbock C, Walcher W, and Dohr G. Gas and Fas-ligand are expressed in the uteroplacental unit of first-trimester pregnancy. *Am J Reprod Immunol* 1999; 41: 41–51.

30. Ashkar AA, Di Santo JP, and Croy BA. Interferon gamma contributes to initiation of uterine vascular modification, decidual integrity, and uterine natural killer cell maturation during normal murine pregnancy. *J Exp Med* 2000; 192: 259–269.

31. Krishnan L, Guilbert LJ, Wegmann TG, Belosevic M, and Mosmann TR. T helper-1 response against *Leishmania major* in pregnant C57BL/6 mice increases implantation failure and fetal resorptions. *J Immunol* 1996; 156: 653–662.

32. Piccinni M-P, Giudizi M-G, Biagiotti R, Beloni L, Giannarini L, Sampognaro S, Parronchi P, Manetti R, Annunziato F, Livi C, Romagnani S, and Maggi E. Progesterone favours the development of human T helper cells producing Th2-type cytokines and promotes both IL-4 production and membrane CD30 expression in established Th1 cell clones. *J Immunol* 1995; 155: 128–133.

33. Szekeres-Bartho J, Faust Z, Varga P, Szereday L, and Kelemen K. The immunological pregnancy protective effect of progesterone is manifested via controlling cytokine production. *Am J Reprod Immunol* 1996; 35: 348–351.

34. Szekeres-Bartho J and Wegmann TG. A progesterone-dependent immunomodulatory protein alters the Th1/Th2 balance. *J Reprod Immunol* 1996; 31: 81–95.

35. Yagel S, Palti Z, and Gallily R. Prostaglandin E2-mediated suppression of human maternal lymphocyte alloreactivity for first-trimester fetal macrophages. *Obstet Gynecol* 1988; 72: 648–654.
36. Hilkens CM, Vermeulen H, Joost van Neerven RJ, Snijdewint FGM, Wierenga EA, and Kapsenberg ML. Differential modulation of T helper type 1 (Th1) and T helper type 2 (Th2) cytokine secretion by prostaglandin E_2 critically depends on interleukin-2. *Eur J Immunol* 1995; 25: 59–63.
37. Hilkens CM, Kalinski P, de Boer M, and Kapsenberg ML. Human dendritic cells require exogenous interleukin-12-inducing factors to direct the development of naïve T-helper cells toward the Th1 phenotype. *Blood* 1997; 90: 1920–1926.
38. Yagel S, Hurwitz A, Rosenn B, and Keizer N. Progesterone enhancement of prostaglandin E2 production by fetal placental macrophages. *Am J Reprod Immunol* 1987; 14: 45–48.
39. de Vries E, de Bruin-Versteeg S, Comans-Bitter WM, de Groot R, Hop WCJ, Boerma GJM, Lotgering FK, and van Dongen JJM. Longitudinal survey of lymphocyte subpopulations in the first year of life. *Pediatr Res* 2000; 47: 528–537.
40. Calado RT, Garcia AB, and Falcao RP. Age-related changes of immunophenotypically immature lymphocytes in normal human peripheral blood. *Cytometry* 1999; 38: 133–137.
41. Hannet I, Erkeller-Yuksel F, Lydyard P, Deneys V, and De Bruyere M. Developmental and maturational changes in human blood lymphocyte subpopulations. *Immunol Today* 1992; 13: 215–218.
42. Griffiths-Chu S, Patterson JAK, Berger CL, Edelson RL, and Chu AC. Characterization of immature T cell subpopulations in neonatal blood. *Blood* 1984; 64: 296–300.
43. Clement LT, Vink PE, and Bradley GE. Novel immunoregulatory functions of phenotypically distinct subpopulations of CD4+ cells in the human neonate. *J Immunol* 1990; 145: 102–108.
44. Hassan J and Reen DJ. Human recent thymic emigrants — identification, expansion and survival characteristics. *J Immunol* 2001; 167: 1970–1976.
45. Maccario R, Nespoli L, Mingrat G, Vitiello A, Ugazio AG, and Burgio GR. Lymphocyte subpopulations in the neonate: identification of an immature subset of OKT8-postive, OKT3-negative cells. *J Immunol* 1983; 130: 1129–1131.
46. Hassan J and Reen DJ. IL-7 promotes the survival and maturation but not differentiation of human post-thymic CD4+ T cells. *Eur J Immunol* 1998; 28: 3057–3065.
47. Bradley L, Bradley J, Ching D, and Shiigi SM. Predominance of T cells that express CD45R in the CD4+ helper/inducer lymphocyte subset of neonates. *Clin Immunol Immunopathol* 1989; 51: 426–435.
48. Gerli R, Bertotto A, Spinozzi F, Cernetti C, Grignani F, and Rambotti P. Phenotypic dissection of cord blood immunoregulatory T-cell subsets by using a two-color immunofluorescence study. *Clin Immunol Immunopathol* 1986; 40: 429–435.
49. Hassan J and Reen DJ. Neonatal CD4+ CD45RA+ T cells: precursors of adult CD4+ CD45RA+ T cells? *Res Immunol* 1993; 144: 87–92.
50. Hayward A, Lee J, and Beverley PCL. Ontogeny of expression of UCHL1 antigen on TcR-1+ (CD4/8) and TcR delta+ T cells. *Eur J Immunol* 1989; 19: 771–773.

51. Kingsley G, Pitzalis C, Waugh A, and Panayi G. Correlation of immunoregulatory function with cell phenotype in cord blood lymphocytes. *Clin Exp Immunol* 1988; 73: 40–45.

52. Sanders ME, Makgoba MW, and Shaw S. Human naïve and memory T cells; reinterpretation of helper–inducer and suppressor–inducer subsets. *Immunol Today* 1988; 9: 195–199.

53. Holt PG, Clough JB, Holt BJ, Baron-Hay MJ, Rose AH, Robinson BWS, and Thomas WR. Genetic risk for atopy is associated with delayed postnatal maturation of T-cell competence. *Clin Exp Allergy* 1992; 22: 1093–1099.

54. Pirenne H, Aujard Y, Eljaafari A, Bourillon A, Oury JF, Le GS, Blot P, and Sterkers G. Comparison of T cell functional changes during childhood with the ontogeny of CDw29 and CD45RA expression on CD4+ T cells. *Pediatr Res* 1992; 32: 81–86.

55. Hassan J and Reen DJ. Reduced primary antigen-specific T-cell precursor frequencies in neonates is associated with deficient interleukin-2 production. *Immunology* 1996; 87: 604–608.

56. Hassan J and Reen DJ. Cord blood CD4+ CD45RA+ T cells achieve a lower magnitude of activation when compared with their adult counterparts. *Immunology* 1997; 90: 397–401.

57. Bertotto A, Gerli R, Lanfrancone L, Crupi S, Arcangeli C, Cernetti C, Spinozzi F, and Rambotti P. Activation of cord T lymphocytes: II. Cellular and molecular analysis of the defective response induced by anti-CD3 monoclonal antibody. *Cell Immunol* 1990; 127: 247–259.

58. Gerli R, Agea E, Muscat C, Tognellini R, Fiorucci G, Spinozzi F, Cernetti C, and Bertotto A. Activation of cord T lymphocytes: III. Role of LFA-1/ICAM-1 and CD2/LFA-3 adhesion molecules in CD3-induced proliferative response. *Cell Immunol* 1993; 148: 32–47.

59. Hassan J, O'Neill S, O'Neill LAJ, Pattison U, and Reen DJ. Signalling via DC28 of human naïve neonatal T lymphocytes. *Clin Exp Immunol* 1995; 102: 192–198.

60. Shu U, Demeure CE, Byun D-G, Podlaski F, Stern AS, and Delespesse G. Interleukin 12 exerts a differential effect on the maturation of neonatal and adult human CD45RO⁻ CD4 T cells. *J Clin Invest* 1994; 94: 1352–1358.

61. Early EM and Reen DJ. Antigen-independent responsiveness to interleukin-4 demonstrates differential regulation of newborn human T cells. *Eur J Immunol* 1996; 26: 2885–2889.

62. Takahashi N, Imanishi K, Nishida H, and Uchiyama T. Evidence for immunologic immaturity of cord blood T cells. *J Immunol* 1995; 155: 5213–5219.

63. Macardle PJ, Wheatland L, and Zola H. Analysis of the cord blood T lymphocyte response to superantigen. *Human Immunol* 1999; 60: 127–139.

64. Porcu P, Gaddy J, and Broxmeyer HE. Alloantigen-induced unresponsiveness in cord blood T lymphocytes is associated with defective activation of Ras. *Proc Natl Acad Sci USA* 1998; 95: 4538-4543.

65. Miscia S, Du Baldassarre A, Sabatino G, Bonvini E, Rana RA, Vitale M, Di Valerio V, and Manzoli FA. Inefficient phospholipase C activation and reduced Lck expression characterize the signaling defect of umbilical cord T lymphocytes. *J Immunol* 1999; 163: 2416–2424.

66. Whisler RL, Newhouse YG, Grants IS, and Hackshaw KV. Differential expression of the α and β isoforms of protein kinase C in peripheral blood T and B cells from young and elderly adults. *Mech Ageing Dev* 1995; 77: 197–211.

67. Sato K, Nagayama H, and Takahasji TA. Aberrant CD3- and CD28-mediated signaling events in cord blood T cells are associated with dysfunctional regulation of Fas ligand-mediated cytotoxicity. *J Immunol* 1999; 162: 4464–4471.

68. Andersson U, Bird AG, Britten S, and Palacios R. Human and cellular immunity in humans studied at the cellular level from birth to two years. *Immunol Rev* 1981; 57: 5–19.

69. Hayward AR. Development of lymphocyte responses in humans, the fetus and newborn. *Immunol Rev* 1981; 57: 43–61.

70. Durandy A, De Saint Basile G, Lisowska-Grospierre B, Gauchat J-F, Forveille M, Kroczek RA, Bonnefoy J-Y, and Fischer A. Undetectable CD40 ligand expression on T cells and low B cell responses to CD40 binding antagonists in human newborns. *J Immunol* 1995; 154: 1560–1568.

71. Fuleihan R, Ahern D, and Geha RS. Decreased expression of the ligand for CD40 in newborn lymphocytes. *Eur J Immunol* 1994; 24: 1925–1928.

72. Splawski JB and Lipsky PE. Cytokine regulation of immunoglobulin secretion by neonatal lymphocytes. *J Clin Invest* 1991; 88: 967–977.

73. Zola H, Fusco M, MacArdle PJ, Flego L, and Roberton D. Expression of cytokine receptors by human cord blood lymphocytes: comparison with adult blood lymphocytes. *Pediatr Res* 1995; 38: 397–403.

74. Chheda S, Palkowetz KH, Garofalo R, Rassin DK, and Goldman AS. Decreased interleukin-10 production by neonatal monocytes and T cells: relationship to decreased production and expression of tumor necrosis factor-α and its receptors. *Pediatr Res* 1996; 40: 475–483.

75. Qian JX, Lee SM, Suen Y, Knoppel E, van de Ven C, and Cairo MS. Decreased interleukin-15 from activated cord versus adult peripheral blood mononuclear cells and the effect of interleukin-15 in upregulating antitumor immune activity and cytokine production in cord blood. *Blood* 1997; 90: 3106–3017.

76. Scott ME, Kubin M, and Kohl S. High level interleukin-12 production, but diminished interferon-γ production, by cord blood monoculear cells. *Pediatr Res* 1997; 41: 547–553.

77. Chalmers IMH, Janossy G, Contreras M, and Navarrete C. Intracellular cytokine profile of cord and adult blood lymphocytes. *Blood* 1998; 92: 11–18.

78. White GP, Watt PM, Holt BJ, and Holt PG. Differential patterns of methylation of the IFNg promoter at CpG and non-CpG sites underlie differences in IFNg gene expression between human neonatal and adult CD45RO⁻ T-cells. *J Immunol* 2002; 168: 2820–2827.

79. Mbawuike IN, Wells J, Byrd R, Cron SG, Glezen WP, and Piedra PA. HLA-restricted CD8⁺ cytotoxic T lymphocyte, interferon-γ, and interleukin-4 responses to respiratory syncytial virus infection in infants and children. *J Infect Dis* 2001; 183: 687–696.

80. Barbouche R, Forveille M, Fischer A, Avrameas S, and Durandy A. Spontaneous IgM autoantibody production in vitro by B lymphocytes of normal human neonates. *Scand J Immunol* 1992; 35: 659–667.

81. Bhat NM, Kantor AB, Bieber MM, Stall AM, Herzenberg LA, and Teng NN. The ontogeny and functional characteristics of human B-1 (CD5+ B) cells. *Int Immunol* 1992; 4: 243–252.
82. Punnonen J. The role of interleukin-2 in the regulation of proliferation and IgM synthesis of human newborn mononuclear cells. *Clin Exp Immunol* 1989; 75: 421–425.
83. Adkins B. T cell function in newborn mice and humans. *Immunol Today* 1999; 20: 330–335.
84. Kotiranta-Ainamo A, Rautonen J, and Rautonen N. Interleukin-10 production by cord blood mononuclear cells. *Pediatr Res* 1997; 41: 110–113.
85. Lee SM, Suen Y, Chang L, Bruner V, Qian J, Indes J, Knoppel E, van de Ven C, and Cairo MS. Decreased interleukin-12 (IL-12) from activated cord versus adult peripheral blood mononuclear cells and upregulation of interferon-γ, natural killer, and lymphokine-activated killer activity by IL-12 in cord blood mononuclear cells. *Blood* 1996; 88: 945–954.
86. Stavnezer J. Antibody class switching. *Adv Immunol* 1996; 61: 79–146.
87. Gauchat J-F, Gauchat D, De Weck AL, and Stadler BM. Cytokine mRNA levels in antigen-stimulated peripheral blood mononuclear cells. *Eur J Immunol* 1989; 7: 804–810.
88. Watson W, Oen K, Ramdahin R, and Harman C. Immunoglobulin and cytokine production by neonatal lymphocytes. *Clin Exp Immunol* 1991; 83: 169–174.
89. Steinman RM. The dendritic cell system and its role in immunogenicity. *Annu Rev Immunol* 1991; 9: 271–296.
90. Janeway CA. The immune response evolved to discriminate infectious self from noninfectious self. *Immunol Today* 1992; 13: 11–16.
91. Matzinger P. Tolerance, danger, and the extended family. *Annu Rev Immunol* 1994; 12: 991–1045.
92. McWilliam AS, Napoli S, Marsh AM, Pemper FL, Nelson DJ, Pimm CL, Stumbles PA, Wells TNC, and Holt PG. Dendritic cells are recruited into the airway epithelium during the inflammatory response to a broad spectrum of stimuli. *J Exp Med* 1996; 184: 2429–2432.
93. Foster CA and Holbrook KA. Ontogeny of Langerhans cells in human embryonic and fetal skin: cell densites and phenotypic expression relative to epidermal growth. *Am J Anat* 1989; 184: 157–164.
94. McCarthy KM, Gong JL, Telford JR, and Schneeberger EE. Ontogeny of Ia+ accessory cells in fetal and newborn rat lung. *Am J Respir Cell Mol Biol* 1992; 6: 349–356.
95. Nelson DJ, McMenamin C, McWilliam AS, Brenan M, and Holt PG. Development of the airway intraepithelial dendritic cell network in the rat from class II MHC (Ia) negative precursors: differential regulation of Ia expression at different levels of the respiratory tract. *J Exp Med* 1994; 179: 203–212.
96. Brandtzaeg P, Halstensen TS, Huitfeldt HS, Krajci P, Kvale D, Scott H, and Thrane PS. Epithelial expression of HLA, secretory component (poly-Ig receptor), and adhesion molecules in the human alimentary tract. *Ann NY Acad Sci* 1992; 664: 157–179.
97. Mayrhofer G, Pugh CW, and Barclay AN. The distribution, ontogeny and origin in the rat of Ia-positive cells with dendritic morphology and of Ia antigen in epithelia, with special reference to the intestine. *Eur J Immunol* 1983; 13: 112–122.

98. Mizoguchi S, Takahashi K, Takeya M, Naito M, and Morioka T. Development, differentation and proliferation of epidermal Langerhans cells in rat ontogeny studied by a novel monoclonal antibody against epidermal Langerhans cells, RED-1. *J Leuk Biol* 1992; 52: 52–61.

99. Romani N, Schuler G, and Fritsch P. Ontogeny of Ia-positive and Thy-1-positive leukocytes of murine epidermis. *J Invest Dermatol* 1986; 86: 129–133.

100. Ridge JP, Fuchs EJ, and Matzinger P. Neonatal tolerance revisited: turning on newborn T cells with dendritic cells. *Science* 1996; 271: 1723–1726.

101. Nelson DJ and Holt PG. Defective regional immunity in the respiratory tract of neonates is attributable to hyporesponsiveness of local dendritic cells to activation signals. *J Immunol* 1995; 155: 3517–3524.

102. Holt PG. Dendritic cell ontogeny as an aetiological factor in respiratory tract diseases in early life. *Thorax* 2001; 56: 419–420.

103. Stoltenberg L, Thrane PS, and Rognum TO. Development of immune response markers in the trachea in the fetal period and the first year of life. *Pediatr Allergy Immunol* 1993; 4: 13–19.

104. Hunt DW, Huppertz HI, Jiang HJ, and Petty RE. Studies of human cord blood dendritic cells: evidence for functional immaturity. *Blood* 1994; 84: 4333–4343.

105. Goriely S, Vincart B, Stordeur P, Vekemans J, Willems F, Goldman M, and De Wit D. Deficient IL-12(p35) gene expression by dendritic cells derived from neontal monocytes. *J Immunol* 2001; 166: 2141–2146.

106. Upham JW, Lee PT, Holt BJ, Heaton T, Prescott SL, Sharp MJ, Sly PD, and Holt PG. Development of interleukin-12-producing capacity throughout childhood. *Infect Immun* 2002; 70: 6583–6588.

107. Clerici M, DePalma L, Roilides E, Baker R, and Shearer GM. Analysis of T helper and antigen-presenting cell functions in cord blood and peripheral blood leukocytes from healthy children of different ages. *J Clin Invest* 1993; 91: 2829–2836.

108. Morris JF, Hoyer JT, and Pierce SK. Antigen presentation for T cell interleukin-2 secretion is a late acquistition of neonatal B cells. *Eur J Immunol* 1992; 22: 2923–2928.

109. Van Tol MJD, Ziljstra J, Thomas CMG, Zegers BJM, and Ballieux RE. Distinct role of neonatal and adult monocytes in the regulation of the *in vitro* antigen-induced plaque-forming cell response in man. *J Immunol* 1984; 134: 1902–1908.

110. Liu E, Tu W, Law HKW, and Lau Y-L. Changes of CD14 and CD1a expression in response to IL-4 and granulocyte–macrophage colony-stimulating factor are different in cord blood and adult blood monocytes. *Pediatr Res* 2001; 50: 184–189.

111. Stiehm ER, Sztein MB, and Oppenheim JJ. Deficient DR antigen expression on human cord blood monocytes: reversal with lymphokines. *Clin Immunol Immunopathol* 1984; 30: 430–436.

112. Varis I, Deneys V, Mazzon AM, De Bruyere M, Cornu G, and Brichard B. Expression of HLA-DR, CAM and co-stimulatory molecules on cord blood monocytes. *Eur J Haematol* 2001; 66: 107–114.

113. Harju K, Glumoff V, and Hallman M. Ontogeny of Toll-like receptors *Tlr2* and *Tlr4* in mice. *Pediatr Res* 2001; 49: 81–83.

114. Maródi L, Goda K, Palicz A, and Szabó G. Cytokine receptor signalling in neonatal macrophages: defective STAT-1 phosphorylation in response to stimulation with IFN-γ. *Clin Exp Immunol* 2001; 126: 456–460.

115. Lewis DB, Yu CC, Meyer J, English BK, Kahn SJ, and Wilson CB. Cellular and molecular mechanisms for reduced interleukin 4 and interferon-gamma production by neonatal T cells. *J Clin Invest* 1991; 87: 194–202.

116. Taylor S and Bryson YJ. Impaired production of γ-interferon by newborn cells *in vitro* is due to a functionally immature macrophage. *J Immunol* 1985; 134: 1493–1498.

117. Wilson CB, Westall J, Johnston L, Lewis DB, Dover SK, and Apert AR. Decreased production of interferon gamma by human neonatal cells: intrinsic and regulatory deficiencies. *J Clin Invest* 1986; 77: 860–867.

118. Holt PG. Regulation of antigen-presenting cell function(s) in lung and airway tissues. *Eur Respir J* 1993; 6: 120–129.

119. Muthukkumar S, Goldstein J, and Stein KE. The ability of B cells and dendritic cells to present antigen increases ontogeny. *J Immunol* 2000; 165: 4803–4813.

120. Bullock JD, Robertson AF, Bodenbender JG, Kontras SB, and Miller CE. Inflammatory response in the neonate re-examined. *Pediatrics* 1969; 44: 58–61.

121. Eitzman DV and Smith RT. The nonspecific inflammatory cycle in the neonatal infant. *Am J Dis Child* 1959; 97: 326–334.

122. Roberts RL, Ank BJ, Salusky IB, and Stiehm ER. Purification and properties of peritoneal eosinophils from pediatric dialysis patients. *J Immunol Methods* 1990; 126: 205–211.

123. Smith JB, Kunjummen RD, and Raghavender BH. Eosinophils and neutrophils of human neonates have similar impairments of quantitative up-regulation of Mac-1 (CD11b/CD18) expression *in vitro*. *Pediatr Res* 1991; 30: 355–361.

124. Smith JB, Kunjummen RD, Kishimoto TK, and Anderson DC. Expression and regulation of L-selectin on eosinophils from human adults and neonates. *Pediatr Res* 1992; 32: 465–471.

125. Borrese MP, Odelram H, Irander K, Kjellman NI, and Björkstén B. Peripheral blood eosinophilia in infants at three months of age is associated with subsequent development of atopic disease in early childhood. *J Allergy Clin Immunol* 1995; 95: 694–698.

126. Spencer J, Isaacson PG, Walker-Smith JA, and MacDonald TT. Heterogeneity in intraepithelial lymphocyte subpopulations in fetal and postnatal human small intestine. *J Pediatr Gastroenterol Nutr* 1989; 9: 173–177.

127. Wilkes LK, McMenamin C, and Holt PG. Postnatal maturation of mast cell subpopulations in the rat respiratory tract. *Immunology* 1992; 75: 535–541.

128. Cummins AG, Munro GH, Miller HRP, and Ferguson A. Association of maturation of the small intestine at weaning with mucosal mast cell activation in the rat. *J Cell Biol* 1988; 66: 417–423.

129. Cummins AG, Eglinton BA, Gonzalez A, and Roberton DM. Immune activation during infancy in healthy humans. *J Clin Immunol* 1994; 14: 107–115.

130. Iida M, Matsumoto K, Tomita H, Nakajima T, Akasawa A, Ohtani NY, Yoshida NL, Matsui K, Nakada A, Sugita Y, Shimizu Y, Wakahara S, Nakao T, Fujii Y, Ra C, and Saito H. Selective down-regulation of high-affinity IgE receptor (FceRI) a-chain messenger RNA among transcriptome in cord blood-derived versus adult peripheral blood-derived cultured human mast cells. *Blood* 2001; 97: 1016–1022.

131. Burchett SK, Corey L, Mohan KM, Westall J, Ashley R, and Wilson CB. Diminished interferon-γ and lymphocyte proliferation in neonatal and postpartum primary herpes simplex virus infection. *J Infect Dis* 1992; 165: 813–818.

132. Joyner JL, Augustine NH, Taylor KA, La Pine TR, and Hill HR. Effects of group B streptococci on cord and adult mononuclear cell interleukin-12 and interferon-gamma mRNA accumulation and protein secretion. *J Infect Dis* 2000; 182: 974–977.

133. Miller ME. Phagocyte function in the neonate: selected aspects. *Pediatrics* 1979; 64: 709–712.

134. Siegrist CA. Vaccination in the neonatal period and early infancy. *Int Rev Immunol* 2000; 19: 195–219.

135. Wilson CB. Immunologic basis for increased susceptibility of the neonate to infection. *J Pediatr* 1986; 108: 1–12.

136. Culley FJ, Pollott J, and Openshaw PJ. Age at first viral infection determines the pattern of T cell-mediated disease during reinfection in adulthood. *J Exp Med* 2002; 196: 1381–1386.

137. Holt PG and Sly PD. Interactions between RSV infection, asthma, and atopy: unraveling the complexities. *J Exp Med* 2002; 196: 1271–1275.

138. Klinge J, Lugauer S, Korn K, Heininger U, and Stehr K. Comparison of immunogenicity and reactogenicity of a measles, mumps and rubella (MMR) vaccine in German children vaccinated at 9–11, 12–14 or 15–17 months of age. *Vaccine* 2000; 18: 3134–3140.

139. Gans HA, Maldonado Y, Yasukawa LL, Bweeler J, Audet S, Rinki MM, DeHovitz R, and Arvin AM. IL-12, IFN-γ, and T cell proliferation to measles in immunized infants. *J Immunol* 1999; 162: 5569–5575.

140. Barrios C, Brawand P, Berney M, Brandt C, Lambert P-H, and Siegrist C-A. Neonatal and early life immune responses to various forms of vaccine antigens qualitatively differ from adult responses: predominance of a Th2-biased pattern which persists after adult boosting. *Eur J Immunol* 1996; 26: 1489–1496.

141. Rowe J, Macaubas C, Monger T, Holt BJ, Harvey J, Poolman JT, Loh R, Sly PD, and Holt PG. Heterogeneity in diphtheria-tetanus-acellular pertussis vaccine-specific cellular immunity during infancy: relationship to variations in the kinetics of postnatal maturation of systemic Th1 function. *J Infect Dis* 2001; 184: 80–88.

142. Adkins B and Du R-Q. Newborn mice develop balanced Th1/Th2 primary effector responses *in vivo* but are biased to Th2 secondary responses. *J Immunol* 1998; 160: 4217–4224.

143. Ausiello CM, Lande R, Urbani F, La Sala A, Stefanelli P, Salmaso S, Mastrantonio P, and Cassone A. Cell-mediated immune responses in four-year-old children after primary immunization with acellular pertussis vaccines. *Infect Immun* 1999; 67: 4064-4071.

144. Marchant A, Goetghebuer T, Ota M, Wolfe I, Ceesay SJ, De Groote D, Corrah T, Bennett S, Wheeler J, Huygen K, Aaby P, McAdam KP, and Newport MJ. Newborns develop a Th1-type immune response to *Mycobacterium bovis* bacillus Calmette–Guerin vaccination. *J Immunol* 1999; 163: 2249–2255.

145. Vekemans J, Amedei A, Ota MO, D'Elios MM, Goetghebuer T, Ismaili J, Newport MJ, Del Prete G, Goldman M, McAdam KPWJ, and Marchant A. Neonatal bacillus Calmete–Guérin vaccination induced adult-like IFN-g production by CD4⁺ T lymphocytes. *Eur J Immunol* 2001; 31: 1531–1535.

146. Kovarik J, Bozzotti P, Love-Homan L, Pihlgren M, Davis HL, Lambert PH, Krieg AM, and Siegrist CA. CpG oligodeoxynucleotides can circumvent the Th2 polar-

ization of neonatal responses to vaccines but may fail to fully direct Th2 responses established by neonatal priming. *J Immunol* 1999; 162: 1611–1617.

147. Martinez X, Brandt C, Saddallah F, Tougne C, Barrios C, Wild F, Dougan G, Lambert P-H, and Siegrist C-A. DNA immunization circumvents deficient induction of T helper type 1 and cytotoxic T lymphocyte responses in neonates and during early life. *Proc Natl Acad Sci USA* 1997; 94: 8726–8731.

148. Arulanandam BP, Van Cleave VH, and Metzger DW. IL-12 is a potent neonatal vaccine adjuvant. *Eur J Immunol* 1999; 29: 256–264.

149. Trinchieri G. IL-12 and its role in the generation of Th-1 cells. *Immunol Today* 1993; 14: 335–338.

150. Yap G, Pesin M, and Sher A. IL-12 is required for the maintenance of IFN-g production in T cells mediating chronic resistance to the intracellular pathogen, *Toxoplasma gondii*. *J Immunol* 2000; 165: 628–631.

151. Shirakawa T, Enomoto T, Shimazu S, and Hopkin JM. Inverse association between tuberculin responses and atopic disorder. *Science* 1997; 275: 77–79.

152. Arkwright PD, Patel L, Moran A, Haeney MR, Ewing CI, and David TJ. Atopic eczema is associated with delayed maturation of the antibody response to pneumococcal vaccine. *Clin Exp Immunol* 2000; 122: 16–19.

153. Holt PG, Rudin A, Macaubas C, Holt BJ, Rowe J, Loh R, and Sly PD. Development of immunologic memory against tetanus toxoid and pertactin antigens from the diphtheria-tetanus-pertussis vaccine in atopic versus nonatopic children. *J Allergy Clin Immunol* 2000; 105: 1117–1122.

154. Bodner C, Anderson WJ, Reid TS, Godden DJ, and Group WS. Childhood exposure to infection and risk of adult onset wheeze and atopy. *Thorax* 2000; 55: 383–387.

155. Shaheen SO, Aaby P, Hall AJ, Barker DJP, Heyes CB, Shiell AW, and Goudiaby A. Measles and atopy in Guinea-Bissau. *Lancet* 1996; 347: 1792–1796.

156. Lewis SA and Britton JR. Measles infection, measles vaccination and the effect of birth order in the aetiology of hay fever. *Clin Exp Allergy* 1998; 28: 1493–1500.

157. Paunio M, Heinonen O, Virtanen M, Leinikki P, Patja A, and Peltola H. Measles history and atopic diseases: a population-based cross-sectional study. *JAMA* 2000; 283: 343–346.

158. Dannemann A, van Ree R, Kulig M, Bergmann RL, Bauer P, Forster J, Guggenmoos-Holzmann I, Aalberse RC, and Wahn U. Specific IgE and IgG4 immune responses to tetanus and diphtheria toxoid in atopic and nonatopic children during the first two years of life. *Int Arch Allergy Immunol* 1996; 111: 262–267.

159. Grüber C, Lau S, Dannemann A, Sommerfeld C, Wahn U, and Aalberse RC. Downregulation of IgE and IgG4 antibodies to tetanus toxoid and diphtheria toxoid by covaccination with cellular *Bordetella pertussis* vaccine. *J Immunol* 2001; 167: 2411–2417.

160. Ryan EJ, Nilsson L, Kjellman N-IM, Gothefors L, and Mills KHG. Booster immunization of children with an acellular pertussis vaccine enhances Th2 cytokine production and serum IgE responses against pertussis toxin but not against common allergens. *Clin Exp Immunol* 2000; 121: 193–200.

161. Macaubas C, Sly PD, Burton P, Tiller K, Yabuhara A, Holt BJ, Smallacombe TB, Kendall G, Jenmalm MC, and Holt PG. Regulation of T-helper cell responses to inhalant allergen during early childhood. *Clin Exp Allergy* 1999; 29: 1223–1231.

162. Prescott SL, Macaubas C, Smallacombe T, Holt BJ, Sly PD, and Holt PG. Development of allergen-specific T-cell memory in atopic and normal children. *Lancet* 1999; 353: 196–200.

163. Baldini M, Lohman IC, Halonen M, Erickson RP, Holt PG, and Martinez FD. A polymorphism in the 5' flanking region of the CD14 gene is associated with circulating soluble CD14 levels with total serum IgE. *Am J Resp Cell Mol Biol* 1999; 20: 976–983.

164. Lauener RP, Birchler T, Adamski J, Braun-Fahrlander C, Bufe A, Herz U, von Mutius E, Nowak D, Riedler J, Waser M, and Sennhauser FH, Expression of CD14 and Toll-like receptor 2 in farmers' and non-farmers' children. *Lancet* 2002; 360: 465–466.

165. Liao SY, Liao TN, Chiang BL, Huang MS, Chen CC, Chou CC, and Hsieh KH. Decreased production of IFNγ and increased production of IL-6 by cord blood mononuclear cells of newborns with a high risk of allergy. *Clin Exp Allergy* 1996; 26: 397–405.

166. Martinez FD, Stern DA, Wright AL, Holberg CJ, Taussig LM, and Halonen M. Association of interleukin-2 and interferon-γ production by blood mononuclear cells in infancy with parental allergy skin tests and with subsequent development of atopy. *J Allergy Clin Immunol* 1995; 96: 652–660.

167. Rinas U, Horneff G, and Wahn V. Interferon-γ production by cord blood mononuclear cells is reduced in newborns with a family history of atopic disease and is independent from cord blood IgE-levels. *Pediatr Allergy Immunol* 1993; 4: 60–64.

168. Tang MLK, Kemp AS, Thorburn J, and Hill DJ. Reduced interferon-γ secretion in neonates and subsequent atopy. *Lancet* 1994; 344: 983–986.

169. Warner JO, Warner JA, Miles EA, Jones AC. Reduced interferon-gamma secretion in nenonates and subsequent atopy. *Lancet* 1994; 344:1516.

170. Holt PG, O'Keeffe PO, Holt BJ, Upham JW, Baron-Hay MJ, Suphioglu C, Knox B, Stewart GA, Thomas WR, and Sly PD. T-cell "priming" against environmental allergens in human neonates: sequential deletion of food antigen specificities during infancy with concomitant expansion of responses to ubiquitous inhalant allergens. *Ped Allergy Immunol* 1995; 6: 85–90.

171. Kondo N, Kobayashi Y, Shinoda S, Kasahara K, Kameyama T, Iwasa S, and Orii T. Cord blood lymphocyte responses to food antigens for the prediction of allergic disorders. *Arch Dis Child* 1992; 67: 1003–1007.

172. Piastra M, Stabile A, Fioravanti G, Castagnola M, Pani G, and Ria F. Cord blood mononuclear cell responsiveness to beta-lactoglobulin: T-cell activity in "atopy-prone" and "non-atopy-prone" newborns. *Int Arch Allergy Immunol* 1994; 104: 358–365.

173. Piccinni M-P, Mecacci F, Sampognaro S, Manetti R, Parronchi P, Maggi E, and Romagnani S. Aeroallergen sensitization can occur during fetal life. *Int Arch Allergy Immunol* 1993; 102: 301–303.

174. Prescott SL, Macaubas C, Holt BJ, Smallacombe T, Loh R, Sly PD, and Holt PG. Transplacental priming of the human immune system to environmental allergens: universal skewing of initial T-cell responses towards the Th-2 cytokine profile. *J Immunol* 1998; 160: 4730–4737.

175. Seneviratne SL, Jones L, King AS, Black A, Powell S, McMichael AJ, and Ogg GS. Allergen-specific CD8+ T cells and atopic disease. *J Clin Invest* 2002; 110: 1283–1291.
176. Woolcock AJ, Peat JK, and Trevillion LM. Is the increase in asthma prevalence linked to increase in allergen load? *Allergy* 1995; 50: 935–940.
177. Peat JK, Salome CM, and Woolcock AJ. Longitudinal changes in atopy during a 4-year period: relation to bronchial hyperresponsiveness and respiratory symptoms in a population sample of Australian schoolchildren. *J Allergy Clin Immunol* 1990; 85: 65–74.
178. Sherrill D, Stein R, Kurzius-Spencer M, and Martinez F. Early senstization to allergens and development of respiratory symptoms. *Clin Exp Allergy* 1999; 29: 905–911.
179. Holt PG and Sly PD. Interactions between respiratory tract infections and atopy in aetiology of asthma. *Eur Respir J* 2002; 19: 1–8.
180. Oddy WH, de Klerk NH, Sly PD, and Holt PG. The effects of respiratory infections, atopy, and breastfeeding on childhood asthma. *Eur Respir J* 2002; 19: 899–905.
181. Smart JM and Kemp AS. Increased Th1 and Th2 allergen-induced cytokine responses in children with atopic disease. *Clin Exp Allergy* 2002; 32: 796–802.
182. Ostler T, Davidson W, and Ehl S. Virus clearance and immunopathology by CD8+ T cells during infection with respiratory syncitial virus are mediated by IFN-gamma. *Eur J Immunol* 2002; 32: 2117–2123.
183. Hessel EM, Van Oosterhout AJM, Van Ark I, Van Esch B, Hofman G, Van Loveren H, Savelkoul HFJ, and Nijkamp FP. Development of airway hyperresonsiveness is dependent on interferon-γ and independent of eosinophil infiltration. *Am J Respir Cell Mol Biol* 1997; 16: 325–334.
184. Randolph DA, Stephens R, Carruthers CJL, and Chaplin DD. Cooperation between Th1 and Th2 cells in a murine model of eosinophilic airway inflammation. *J Clin Invest* 1999; 104: 1021–1029.

6

Inflammatory Features of Childhood Asthma

MARZENA KRAWIEC

University of Wisconsin–Madison
Madison, Wisconsin, U.S.A.

THERESA GUILBERT

University of Arizona
Tucson, Arizona, U.S.A.

I. Introduction

The definition of asthma has historically evolved over the past several decades. In 1958, asthma was defined as a primary disorder of airflow obstruction that reversed spontaneously or in response to therapy.[1] In the decade that followed, the American Thoracic Society used the adjective *episodic* rather than *chronic* to describe asthma, further emphasizing the role of acute bronchospasm at the core of asthma pathology.[2] Despite extensive histologic evidence of airway inflammation from autopsy specimens of fatal asthma dating back to 1922,[3] the definition of asthma did not include the concept of inflammation based on additional biopsy data until the 1970s.[4]

The importance of asthmatic inflammation was acknowledged in the 1980s and accepted as central to the disease in the 1990s.[5] During the past decade, more extensive investigation techniques have been employed to study the characteristics of this inflammatory process. They include bronchoscopy, bronchoalveolar lavage (BAL), and endobronchial biopsy (EBB). The results of these studies demonstrate ongoing evidence of airway inflammatory lesions with cellular infiltrates, submucosal wall edema, fibrosis, and epithelial cell (EPI) damage even in newly diagnosed, stable, and/or mild asthmatics.[6,7]

This historical progression led to our current appreciation of asthma as a chronic inflammatory disorder. As described by R.F. Lemanske, airway inflammation is the "underlying stimulus for the interaction of inflammatory cells with resident cells resulting in the activation of a cascade of pro-inflammatory events contributing to the maintenance of chronic inflammation."[8,11] Moreover, this inflammation can also worsen airway hyperresponsiveness (AHR) to various stimuli and activate various pathways leading to airway healing and repair. These mechanisms may lead to progressive, potentially irreversible airway damage and remodeling and subsequently to loss of lung function.[8,9]

Inflammation is now widely considered the cornerstone of asthma development, persistence, and progression,[10] and these processes may begin very early in life. Based on cohort studies of the natural history of the disease, most cases of persistent asthma have identifiable symptoms within the first several years of life.[11,12] Therefore, investigation of these processes early in life is critical because decline in lung function has been documented even in young children with persistent wheezing compared with normal controls in the Tucson Children's Respiratory Study.[11]

Initially, invasive techniques such as biopsy and BAL were used to characterize chronic airway inflammation in asthmatic adults. Studies demonstrating airway inflammation in children remain limited despite the focus on the onset of asthma in the first years of life. However, because asthma appears to be a complex disease involving several phenotypes in early life,[11,12] more research is needed to characterize the initiation of inflammation in the young asthmatic airway and its subsequent progression to persistent asthma. This chapter will briefly review the pathophysiology of airway inflammation in asthma, both allergic and nonallergic mechanisms, and mediators involved in these processes in adults and children. Data describing the early inflammatory features of asthma based on airway and systemic evaluations in children will ensue. Finally, future investigations for early identification of airway inflammation and their potential impact on prevention, treatment, and intervention of asthma will also be discussed.

II. Pathophysiology of Airway Inflammation in Children

Asthma is a heterogeneous disorder involving a wide spectrum of inflammatory cells and mediators. The interplay of activated infiltrating cells and mediators with resident airway cells and mediators is variable, leading to the complex phenotypic expression of this disease. The pathophysiology of asthma has been defined using broad categories based on various inflammatory mechanisms including antigen-specific versus nonspecific, pro- versus anti-inflammatory, and immunologic versus nonimmunologic.

In general, asthmatic inflammation progresses in the following manner: (1) an acute response resulting in airway edema, bronchospasm, and mucus hypersecretion; (2) a chronic response resulting from inflammatory cell and mediator influx and EPI activation and sloughing; and (3) chronic airway remodeling leading to potentially irreversible loss of lung function.[13] Consideration of airway inflammation based on these stages of progression provides a generalized and basic framework for the players, both cells and mediators, involved in the initiation and progression of asthmatic inflammation.

A. Allergic Sensitization

In a recent review, it was postulated that the development of childhood asthma was strongly dependent on allergic sensitization or atopy and characterized by elevated serum IgE levels or immediate skin hypersensitivity.[14] Atopy has been extensively linked to asthma, acute and chronic allergen-induced AHR to allergen- and IgE-dependent mechanisms.[15,16] The coexistence of elevated serum IgE levels and recurrent infantile wheeze results in a significantly heightened risk for the development of persistent asthma.[11,17]

It is unclear when the process of allergic sensitization begins. Initially it was thought that the immune system developed in response to environmental allergen exposures during the first several months of life. These early exposures would then result in allergic sensitization and the development of allergic disease in young children. However, allergen-specific IgE can be detected at birth,[18,19] thus suggesting that fetal exposure to allergens does occur and can affect the development of an infant's immune response prenatally.[20] In fact, fetuses of mothers exposed to various allergens including birch pollen, house dust mites, milk, and eggs demonstrated significant allergic proliferative cord blood mononuclear cell responses as early as 22 weeks' gestation.

This prenatal predisposition toward an atopic response is the basis for an imbalance in the TH_1 and TH_2 CD4+ lymphocytic responses at birth.[21,22] The naïve T cell becomes activated following allergen exposure and its cell surface receptor is then primed to recognize a complex of antigen and major histocompatibility complex (MHC). This activated T lymphocyte (LYM) can differentiate into one of two types of helper CD4+ cells, TH_1 or TH_2 based on specific cytokine influences during its priming.

Specifically, interferon gamma (IFN-γ) and interleukin (IL)-12 induce TH_1 LYM, while the presence of IL-4 results in TH_2 LYM cells (Figure 6.1).[23] TH_1 cells are involved primarily in cellular defense and preferentially secrete IL-2. Conversely, TH_2 cells are associated with the production of several pro-inflammatory cytokines including IL-4, IL-5, and IL-13. These three cytokines are central to the concept of allergic inflammation based on their interrelationships with IgE and eosinophils (EOS). More specifically, IL-4 and IL-13 are directly involved in IgE synthesis through B cell receptor binding, while IL-5 enhances EO survival. In addition to their individual roles, both cell classes participate in

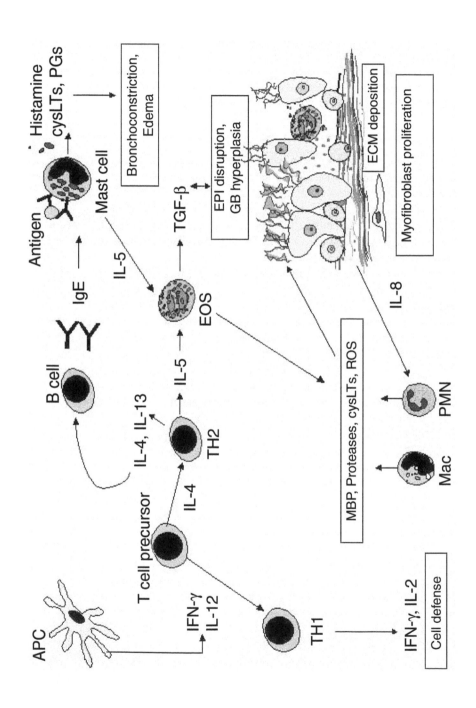

Figure 6.1 Asthma is a complex interplay of cells, cellular responses, and various inflammatory mediators. The resultant response is a progression from acute to chronic inflammation followed by irreversible airway remodeling. A naïve T cell recognizes a processed antigen presented by sensitized APCs. Based on the cytokine milieu, these precursor T cells are induced to elicit a TH2 response in the presence of IL-4 and a TH1 response in the presence of IL-12. TH1 cells produce IFN-γ, a critical cytokine in cell defense. Conversely TH2 cells are involved in both acute and chronic asthmatic response. An acute or early response is dependent on the interplay of IgE and mast cells to stimulate mediator release and onset of the acute features of asthma (smooth muscle bronchoconstriction and airway edema). A chronic or late response is multifactorial and heavily dependent on TH2 production and release of IL-5, a critical cytokine in EO recruitment and activation. EOs along with PMN cells and MACs produce significant amounts of pro-inflammatory mediators, resulting in significant airway obstruction, mucus hypersecretion, and disruption of the epithelium. EOs also produce significant amounts of TGF-β, a profibrotic cytokine critical in airway repair processes via fibroblast proliferation and ECM protein production. The interplay of such acute injury followed by chronic inflammation and profibrotic repair processes leads to the concept of airway remodeling and irreversible loss of lung function in asthmatic disease. (*Source:* Kiekhaefer, CA et al., Antigen-induced airway disease, in *Environmental Asthma*, Vol. 153, Bush, RK, Ed. New York: Marcel Dekker, 2001, p. 13. With permission.)

a reciprocal balance of the TH_1–TH_2 system that determines the numbers and types of cells and derived cytokines in the normal nonatopic host.

While a prenatal predisposition to a TH_2-predominant response is universal, nonatopic children rapidly suppress their TH_2 responses during the first year of life. Conversely, atopic children remain skewed toward a TH_2 pattern, potentially due to abnormalities in neonatal IFN-γ production.[24,25] Such innate abnormalities of IFN-γ production may be determined by a genetic predisposition to the development of asthma (refer to Chapter 8, this volume). In fact, genetic predisposition may play a critical role in the development of asthma; twin studies suggest genetic factors account for up to 75% of an individual's susceptibility to asthma.[26]

Although decreased production of IFN-γ has been associated with this prenatal atopic response, several *in vivo* studies in adult patients have demonstrated a correlation between increased IFN-γ with heightened EO activation and survival.[27] Therefore, the consistency of the TH_1–TH_2 hypothesis to explain both the inception and progression of asthmatic disease remains controversial. However, it appears to have predictive value in the development of allergic disease and/or asthma in early life.[28]

B. Inflammatory Cascade

1. Infiltrating Cells and Their Mediators

Classically, studies have documented the pivotal roles of mast cells, EOs, and LYM in adult and pediatric asthma.[29–31] Additional emphasis has been placed on the LYM influx as a principal feature of asthma especially in relation to a TH_2 phenotype as described above.[5] Finally, it has recently been postulated that other resident cells such as EPI may contribute to the chronic inflammatory changes of asthma leading to airway remodeling (Figure 6.1).[23]

Mast cells have been associated with both acute and chronic allergic inflammation and are resident cells of the airway mucosa.[32] They have been acknowledged as primary effector cells of allergic sensitization due to their high affinity surface receptors for IgE (FcεRI). Inhaled allergens are the primary triggers for mast cell activation through cross-linkage of membrane-bound IgE. This cross-linkage results in an explosive release of pro-inflammatory mediators including histamine, chymase, and tryptase. This activation also leads to up-regulation of arachidonic acid synthesis including the 5-lipoxygenase derived cysteinyl leukotrienes (cysLTs) and cyclo-oxygenase-derived prostaglandins (PGs), the most abundant being PGD_2.[33] The release of these mast cell products results in the pathologic features of acute asthma reflected by smooth muscle (SM) contraction, edema, and mucous hypersecretion by airway goblet (GB) cells. Various cytokines are also produced including IL-4, IL-5, IL-6, and tumor necrosis factor (TNF)-α; they are fundamental to chronic inflammation.[34]

Like mast cells, EOs are key participants in the development and maintenance of airway inflammation. Under the influence of several potent cytokines, especially IL-5, EOs originate and mature in the bone marrow and are then released, densely packed with inflammatory granules including major basic protein, into the circulation. These central effector cells and their array of mediators are prime markers of allergic asthmatic inflammation. Specifically, EO granule-associated protein, major basic protein (MBP), EO cationic protein (ECP), EO-derived neurotoxin, and EO peroxidase (EPX) have been directly linked to EO activation and airway EPI damage as seen in chronic airway inflammation.[35] In addition to pro-inflammatory proteins such as mast cells, EOs are rich sources for cysLTs (LTC_4, LTD_4, LTE_4).[36] These arachidonic acid-derived mediators were described by Kellaway[37] in the 1940s as "slow-reacting substance of anaphylaxis." They are 100- to 1,000-fold more potent bronchoconstrictors than histamine[38] and up to 10,000 times more potent than methacholine.[39] Additionally, they stimulate mucus hypersecretion more effectively than both PGs and/or histamine[40] and can induce significant increases in vascular permeability and inflammatory cell influx into asthmatic airways[41] and sputum.[42] EOs are therefore potent participants and likely central to the pathology of asthma.

Along with EOs, the infiltration of activated LYM into the airway is a critical feature of asthma.[5,43] As noted, LYM produce a vast array of cytokines involved in acute inflammation, specifically in relation to EO activation and survival, and also in the maintenance of chronic inflammation by inducing the expression of adhesion molecules, thereby further facilitating the movement of inflammatory cells from the circulation to the airway.[44]

While polymorphonuclear (PMN) cells are rich sources for proteases, lipid mediators, reactive oxygen species (ROS), and cytokines resulting in chronic airway inflammation and EPI injury,[45,46] their role in asthma remains controversial. Adult studies have suggested that they may play more critical roles in severe, steroid-resistant asthma[47] and status asthmaticus[48,49] than in allergic asthma. In a severe asthmatic patient, heightened airway PMN cells may reflect high-dose corticosteroid treatment, resulting in prolonged PMN survival by inhibition of apoptosis.[47]

In response to allergen challenge, an early PMN cell influx has been followed by more extensive and sustained EO infiltration.[50] However, while demonstrable recruitment of PMN cells occurred along with EOs in the BALs of both allergic and nonallergic asthmatic patients, airway PMN cell levels did not correlate with methacholine hyperresponsiveness or EPI injury.[52] Given the lack of association with airway PMN cells and AHR, the role of this cell in persistent asthma phenotypes remains unclear. As demonstrated in adult asthma literature, the role of the PMN cell in early pediatric airway inflammation is also unclear. Several studies have linked PMN cells to heightened symptom severity and inflammation in persistent childhood asthma,[53,54] infantile wheeze (IW),[55–58] and acute asthma exacerbation.[59–61]

2. *Resident Cells and Their Mediators*

The alveolar macrophage (MAC) derived from blood monocytes is the predominant resident cell of the lower airway. Following activation by allergen via low affinity IgE receptors,[62] the MAC plays several potential roles in airway inflammation:

1. An antigen presenting cell (APC) facilitating the activation of T LYM by engulfing foreign allergenic particles and presenting the processed fragments on its surface
2. An effector cell generating rich quantities of cysLTs, ROS, and various cytokines
3. An anti-inflammatory cell preventing allergic inflammation via reduction of LYM cytokine secretion, specifically IL-10[63] and IL-5[64]

Additionally, the MAC has also been linked to airway remodeling based on production of profibrotic factors such as transforming growth factor (TGF)-β and fibronectin.

In addition to serving as an important source for several pro-inflammatory mediators involved in the recruitment of inflammatory cells including EOS, LYM, and PMN cells,[65] the EPI also hosts several fibrogenic factors including TGF-β.[66] This profibrotic cytokine is a key player in the process of airway repair and remodeling. TGF-β is expressed in bronchial mucosa and controls the activities of various epidermal growth factor receptors (EGFRs).[67] These receptors are critical regulators of EPI function and repair in response to acute lung injury.[68,69] Holgate and colleagues demonstrated heightened EGFR apical expression in areas of EPI damage facilitating exposure to TGF-β and thereby enhancing repair. Remarkably, these same molecules involved in airway repair and remodeling are also involved in fetal lung development and airway branching. Therefore, a critical link may involve early life events, lung growth and maturation, acute injury, and the development of chronic asthma.[70]

C. Chronic Inflammation and Airway Repair

Individuals with asthma experience more aggressive declines in lung function compared with the gradual fundamental declines related to aging seen in nonasthmatics.[71] Therefore, it is possible that intrinsic abnormalities of the asthmatic airway may predispose it to chronic inflammation following acute injury despite early and aggressive intervention. In fact, one group reported increased subbasement membrane (SBM) collagen deposition and extracellular matrix (ECM) in children up to 3 years of age before they exhibited any clinical symptoms of asthma.[72] This progression is the basis for the concept of airway remodeling.

While acute inflammation results in the classic pathophysiologic triad of asthma, for the disease to develop and persist, chronic inflammation due to airway injury followed by repair must occur. Pathologically, airway remodeling is demonstrated by significant thickening of airway walls, increased SBM collagen density, and overall increases in SM.[73] The extent of this remodeling correlates with asthma severity and the degree of AHR[74] although histopathologic abnormalities are noted even in the face of mild disease.[7]

Recent focus has been placed on the role of EPI in airway remodeling. Airway EPI shedding is a characteristic feature of asthma and may contribute to the development of sustained AHR.[51] Such focus appears further warranted due to the impacts of viruses on recurrent wheeze and airflow obstruction during the first several years of life.[75] Overall, while the link between early viral infection and asthma development remains unclear, such an early viral insult in a genetically predisposed patient may pose a significant risk for the development of persistent wheezing and asthma.[76]

The epithelium forms the first barrier to external elements and thereby sustains the brunt of direct injury from allergens and viruses and indirectly from the influx and interplay of various cells and mediators in response to these stimuli. Following acute injury, EPI becomes activated and disordered.[66] Certain investigators have proposed that the bronchial EPI in asthma is intrinsically and structurally disordered and may exert an altered response to injury.[77,78] A fundamental defect may be present in EPI, resulting in an altered response to injury that is then further exaggerated by recurrent injury from allergen and virus, resulting in sustained and progressive damage. This results in a vicious cycle of acute injury and persistent inflammation followed by "profibrotic" repair. The end products of this cycle of inflammation are varying degrees of irreversible bronchial AHR, EPI permeability, and inflammatory cell influx, resulting in chronic inflammation and subsequent airway remodeling.[79–81]

III. Evaluation of Inflammation in Children

A. Airway Evaluation

1. Biopsy

Before the 1960s, biopsy data about asthma was limited to the pathologic examinations of postmortem adult airway specimens. Cutz and colleagues[30] were the first to present data on the histologic and ultrastructural pathology of the lungs in asthmatic children. They evaluated open-lung biopsy specimens from two children (age 12) with stable asthma compared with two age-matched children dying from status asthmatics. Light and electron microscopy demonstrated typical changes of bronchial asthma comparable in both groups including mucus plugging with dense material containing degenerate EPI, MAC and cellular fragments, GB hyperplasia, abnormal cilia, thickening of bronchial basement membranes (BMs), peribronchial SM hypertrophy, EO infiltration, and degranulated mast cells. These findings were critical because histopathologic abnormalities were evident even in the stable asthmatics, reinforcing the role of chronic inflammation in the pathophysiology of the disease.

Recently, Bai and colleagues provided clarity on the role and progression of chronic inflammation in their biopsy study comparing fatal young and older asthmatics with normal controls.[82] Biopsy data confirmed that SM area in both asthma groups was significantly greater, four-fold in the older subjects and two-fold in the younger group, compared with normal controls (p = 0.04 and 0.03, respectively). Furthermore, while histopathologic abnormalities were comparable in young (n = 14, 17 to 23 years) and older (n = 13, 40 to 49 years) asthma fatalities, the older group with a longer duration of asthma had increased airway wall areas and degrees of airway narrowing. In fact, a young child with fatal asthma did not have increased wall dimensions compared with age-matched normal controls. This suggests that while airway inflammation and histologic changes are present early, the age and severity of disease directly impact on the extent of airway remodeling.

Biopsy data do not exist from young children with mild persistent asthma; therefore, early inflammatory changes in airways have not been documented in this group. Laitinen and colleagues demonstrated that inflammation manifested by increased EO infiltration and a mild increase in subepithelial matrix proteins were present in adult asthmatic patients with only mild intermittent disease. Their findings suggest that inflammation and structural changes were initiated very early in the disease process.[79] Such early pathology based on adult data in mild disease could potentially be extrapolated to explain the loss of lung function documented in children with persistent wheezing by the age of 6.[11]

Finally, while the majority of both adult and pediatric biopsy data focuses on EO infiltration, a recent study reports LYM-dominated inflammation in 10 children with moderate atopic asthma (FEV_1 = 44 to 65% predicted and positive skin prick testing).[83] As noted in previous reports, thickening of the BM and degranulated mast cells were seen in most patients but EOs were seen in only one of the biopsies. Furthermore, this group did not report any correlation between the duration of asthma and the extent of BM thickening. They concluded that while the LYM was the predominant cell type, the inflammation might not be related to asthma severity compared with previous reports of EO inflammation.

Investigators also reported significant airway remodeling based on reticular BM thickening in 19 young children with difficult-to-treat asthma ($\geq$ 1600 µg/day of inhaled corticosteroids), comparable with that seen in adults with mild or life-threatening asthma and much greater remodeling than either adult or pediatric control subjects.[84] However, unlike the findings of Bai and colleagues, they found no association between the degree of airway remodeling and age, symptom duration, and/or severity based on lung function.

To summarize, while studies confirm the presence of significant airway remodeling very early even in mild disease, multiple factors may be involved in the progression of this process, leading to the heterogeneity of asthmatic disease, its duration and severity.

2. Bronchoscopy and BAL

Bronchial biopsy is the current "gold standard" for the evaluation of airway inflammation in asthma. Its role in the evaluation of children, however, is limited due to its invasive nature and ethical limitations of pediatric informed consent and minimum risk standards. Flexible fiberoptic bronchoscopy (FFB) and BAL have provided safe and useful alternatives for the evaluation of pediatric airway disease. Bronchoscopy was first introduced for adult use in 1915,[85] but pediatric use did not occur until 1979 with the availability of a pediatric FFB with a suction channel. The goal of BAL evaluations is to obtain aspirated fluid representing the EPI linings of the small airways and alveoli. The first reports of BAL data in children appeared in the late 1970s.[86] During the next decade, the use of BAL remained limited primarily to evaluation of respiratory symptoms in immuno-compromised patients.[87–89]

Multiple BAL evaluations have been performed to evaluate both pediatric asthma[29,53–55,59,90–98] (Table 6.1) and infantile wheeze (IW)[53,55–57,92–94,99,100] (Table 6.2). IW represents the earliest sign of obstructive disease and, potentially, airway inflammation. Most commonly, viral infection leading to inflammation of the medium and small bronchi is the stimulus for acute wheezing in the first several years of life. The difficulty in evaluating IW is the fact that 60% of children who wheeze in the first several years of life do so transiently and only about 40% develop persistent asthma.[11] Despite this limitation, BAL evaluations in young IW subjects have provided important insights into the earliest aspects of airway inflammation.

In vitro evaluations of BAL-acquired alveolar MACs from wheezing infants stimulated with A23187, a calcium ionophore, produced significant amounts of several arachidonic acid metabolites, specifically thromboxane (TXA_2) and LTB_4.[99] In a later study, alveolar MACs demonstrated significant spontaneous production of TNF-α, a pro-inflammatory cytokine, and TXB_2, another arachidonic acid metabolite, compared with normal controls.[100] This suggests that MACs are activated and contribute to the pathophysiology of airway inflammation in early wheezing disorders. Additionally, these BAL studies and several others confirm that arachidonic acid metabolites, the cysLTs, in particular, are characteristic of airway inflammation in recurrent IW.[56,99,100]

Interestingly, in previous studies of alveolar MACs from wheezing infants, *in vitro* dexamethasone challenge resulted in significant suppression of TXA_2,

Table 6.1 Summary of BAL findings in Children with Asthma

Ref. #	N	Description	BAL and Additional Evaluations	Conclusions
90	15	Biomarkers in 15 asthmatics compared with 24 NC	Adenosine deaminase, IL-1, IgA, lysozyme, α2-macroglobulin, α-1-antitrypsin	Primarily descriptive findings
91	22	BAL cellularity compared with PC20 histamine in stable AA	Cell differentials, PC20 histamine	1. PC20 histamine correlated with ↑EOS and MAC numbers and with EOS/MAC ratio 2. MACs may be important in the development of AHR directly and by EOS recruitment
29	17	EOS and mast cell markers compared with PC20 histamine in stable AA	Cell differentials, ECP, tryptase, PC20 histamine	1. EOS numbers and tryptase levels correlate with PC20 histamine 2. ECP levels had no correlation 3. Mast cells and EOS contribute to AHR
55	52	BAL cellularity using nonbronchoscopic lavage in 95 children (52 AA, 23 atopic, and 20 IW)	Cell differentials	EOS and mast cells were significantly ↑ and characteristic of AA compared with atopic children and IW
92	54	EOS, mast cells, and their mediators; nonbronchoscopic lavage in 161 children including 54 AA, 32 atopic, and 21 IW	ECP, histamine, tryptase	1. ECP levels were ↑ in stable AA suggesting ↑ airway EOS activation even at baseline 2. Histamine was ↑ in both AA and IW
53	14	BAL cellularity in 72 children including 14 AA, 26 IW, and 10 NC	Cell differentials, LYM subsets, cultures	1. ↑ EOS and EPI cells in AA 2. ↑ percent PMN cells associated with symptom severity 3. PMN cell-mediated inflammation contributed to AA

	N	Description	Measurements	Findings
93	77	Comparison of BAL cellularity using nonbronchoscopic lavage with serum EOS and mediators in 77 children (60 atopic AA and 17 IW)	Serum ECP and EOS, BAL cell differentials and ECP levels	1. Atopic AA had significantly ↑ percent BAL and serum EOS compared with IW 2. ↑ serum ECP levels in AA compared with IW ($p < 0.06$) 3. Serum ECP and percent EO are useful markers of EO airway inflammation
94	16	BAL cellularity and mediators in 68 children including 16 AA, 30 IW, and 10 NC	Cell differentials, sICAM-1,IFN-γ, LYM subsets, cultures	1. s-ICAM and IFN-γ levels in AA 2. ↑ s-ICAM correlated with LYM numbers and disease severity 3. s-ICAM and IFN-γ play a role in inflammation in AA
59	18	BAL cellularity in 18 acute AA compared with 20 infants with acute bronchiolitis and 14 NC	Cell differentials	Acute exacerbations in AA are characterized by ↑ EOS
95	19	Ig levels in 47 children with lung disease including 19 AA compared with 18 NC	Immunoprofiles, IgG subclasses	1. IgG was predominant in the lower respiratory tract and like IgM and IgA, were significantly ↑ in AA 2. IgG-1 and IgG-3 were significantly ↑ in AA
54	13	Retrospective study of BAL cellularity, ECP and MPO in 29 children (13 AA and 16 NC)	Cell differentials, ECP, MPO	1. AA had ↑ PMNs, ECP, and MPO levels 2. ↑ MPO and ECP levels and PMNs in mild-to-moderate persistent AA ≫ intermittent AA
96	16	BAL EOS and PMN cell mediators in 56 children (16 AA, 30 IW, and 10 NC)	Cell differentials, ECP, IL-8	1. No significant difference in ECP or IL-8 in AA vs. NC 2. EOS correlated with ECP and PMNs with IL-8 in AA 3. IL-8 levels correlated with symptom scores 4. PMN mediated inflammation reflects disease severity
97	79	BAL cellularity and cultures in 79 children including 41 atopic AA and 39 nonatopic AA	Cell differentials and cultures	1. Atopic AA is associated with ↑ EOS 2. ↑ alveolar PMNs correlate with persistent/chronic disease irrespective of bacterial infection
98	29	eNO and BAL cellularity using nonbronchoscopic lavage in 71 children (29 AA, 15 atopic, and 27 NC)	Cell differentials, ECP, histamine, eNO	eNO correlates with BAL percent EOS and ECP and is a useful noninvasive marker of airway inflammation

IW = infantile wheeze. AA = children with asthma. NC = normal controls. N = number of subjects.

Table 6.2 Summary of BAL findings in Children with Infantile Wheeze

Ref. #	N	Study Description	BAL and Additional Evaluations	Conclusions
99	13	*In vitro* evaluation of BAL acquired MACs from 13 IW compared with 6 NC	TxA2, LTB4; dexamethasone challenge	1. Arachidonic acid metabolites, TxB2 and LTB4, ↑ in IW compared with NC 2. Dexamethasone inhibited TxB2 but not LTB4 levels 3. Alveolar MACs are activated *in vivo* to release ↑ eicosanoids
55	14	BAL cellularity using nonbronchoscopic lavage in 95 children (20 IW, 52 AA, and 23 atopic)	Cell differentials	1. Total cells ↑ in IW group compared with AA 2. PMN cells ↑ in IW; EOS and mast cells did not
100	13	*In vitro* evaluation of BAL-acquired MACs from 13 IW compared with 7 NC	TNF-α, TxB2, PGE2; dexamethasone challenge	1. Alveolar MACs released significantly ↑ TNF-α and TxB2 2. Dexamethasone inhibited TNF-α, TxB2, and PGE2
92	21	Evaluation of EOS, mast cells, and their mediators with nonbronchoscopic lavage in 161 children including 21 IW, 54 AA, and 32 atopic	Cell differentials, ECP, histamine, tryptase	↑ histamine but not ECP in children with viral-induced IW
93	77	BAL cellularity using nonbronchoscopic lavage compared with serum EOS and mediators in 77 children (60 atopic AA and 17 IW)	Serum ECP and EOS, BAL cell differentials	Serum ECP and percent EOS weakly correlated with BAL percent EO in IW
53	26	BAL cellularity in 72 children including 26 IW, 14 AA, and 10 NC	LYM subsets, BAL cultures	PMN cell-mediated inflammation may be important in pathology of IW

	N			
94	30	BAL mediators in 68 children including 30 IW, 16 AA, and 10 NC	Soluble ICAM-1, IFN-γ, LYM subsets, BAL cultures	1. ↑ s-ICAM and IFN-γ correlated with LYM and disease severity 2. Significant linear correlation between sICAM-1 and IFN-γ in IW 3. s-ICAM and IFN-γ may play role in airway inflammation in IW
56	20	BAL cellularity, mast cell tryptase, and arachadonic acid metabolites in 20 severe, persistent IW compared with 6 NC	LTE4, LTB4, tryptase, PGD2, PGE2, 15-HETE; BAL cultures	1. EO, mast cell mediators, tryptase, and PGD2 were not ↑ in IW compared with NC 2. Leukotrienes (LTE4 and LTB4) were ↑ 3. ↑ EPI mediators — PGE2 and 15-HETE 4. Significant inflammation early in IW differs from patterns in adult asthmatics
57	36	BAL cellularity and ECP levels in 61 children (36 IW and 25 NC)	ECP	1. ↑ PMN cells but not EOS in IW 2. ↑ ECP correlated with PMN cells and not EOS in IW 3. Inflammation present in lower airways of IW and characterized by ↑ PMN cells and ECP
96	30	EOS and PMN cell mediators in 56 children (30 IW, 16 AA, and 10 NC)	ECP, IL-8, BAL cultures	1. IL-8 did not correlate with PMN cells or symptom scores; PMN-mediated inflammation did not reflect disease severity in IW 2. ECP correlated with percent PMN cells in IW and with percent EOS in AA 3. ECP >20 ng/ml may be indicator of persistent IW
58	83	Retrospective evaluation of BAL cellularity in 83 IW and 17 NC	BAL cultures	1. IW characterized by significantly ↑ total cell count and percent and total number of PMN cells 2. PMN cell-dominated inflammation better characterizes severe IW

IW = infantile wheeze. AA = children with asthma. NC = normal controls. N = number of subjects.

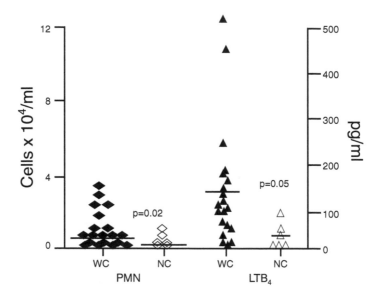

Figure 6.2 BAL PMN cells and LTB$_4$ in wheezing children compared with normal controls. Significant elevations in PMN cells ($\times$ 10^4/ml) and LTB$_4$, a potent chemoattractant, (pg/ml) were found in wheezing children. The median is shown as a single black line. Each diamond and triangle represents one individual. (*Source:* Krawiec, ME et al., *Am J Respir Crit Care Med* 2001; 163: 1338. With permission.)

TXB$_2$, and TNF-α, but not LTB$_4$.[99,100] Elevations in LTB$_4$, a potent PMN chemoattractant, and PMN cells were also reproduced in a recent study of 20 severe persistent wheezing children (WC; mean age, 14.9 mo; Figure 6.2).[56] Significant elevations in EPI (p = 0.03) and several EPI-derived mediators, PGE$_2$ and 15-hydroxyeicosatetraenoic acid (HETE), were also reported in WC compared with normal controls (p = 0.0005 and 0.002, respectively; Figure 6.3). Overall, investigations of airway inflammation in IW support the predominance of PMN cells, arachidonic acid metabolites, and potentially EPI-derived mediators, rather than EOs.

In 1997, Stevenson and colleagues investigated the spectrum of wheezing disorders in their nonbronchoscopic lavage study of 95 children including 52 with persistent asthma and 20 with IW.[55] They reported significant differences based on heightened levels of EOs (2.1 versus 0.2%, p <0.001) in children with persistent asthma compared with IW, suggesting distinct phenotypic differences in wheezing disorders.

Interestingly, however, a pilot study by Pohunek et al. reported that infants and young children with histories of recurrent lower respiratory illnesses, recurrent wheezing, and increased BAL EOs were more likely to develop persistent

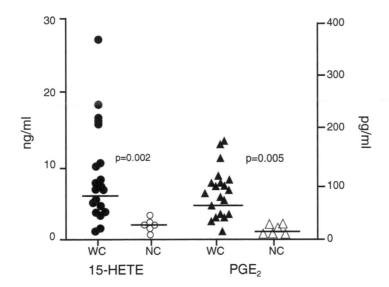

Figure 6.3 PGE$_2$ and 15-HETE levels in wheezing children compared with normal controls. PGE$_2$ (pg/ml) and 15-HETE (ng/ml) levels were significantly elevated in wheezing children. The median is shown as a single black line. Each circle and triangle represents one individual. (*Source:* Krawiec, ME et al., *Am J Respir Crit Care Med* 2001; 163: 1338. With permission.)

asthma.[101] Biopsy data from these children also demonstrated the presence of thickened BMs. Therefore, while the early pathophysiologic features of IW appear distinct from the features of persistent childhood asthma, evidence of early allergic airway inflammation may be a marker for progression to persistent obstructive disease.

Clearly, BAL evaluations of IW suggest that pediatric airway inflammation is present very early in life. In addition to multiple BAL studies consistently reporting elevated EOs, mast cells, and their mediators in atopic asthma,[29,55,92,97] several investigators suggested potential roles for additional cell types in the development of airway inflammation in persistent childhood asthma.[53,54,91] In a recent pediatric study that included 14 asthmatics and 26 IW subjects, one third of the asthmatic children and one half of the IW group had >10% BAL PMN cells that directly correlated to heightened symptom severity.[53] The investigators proposed that PMN cell–mediated inflammation may contribute to various wheezing disorders.

A more recent retrospective study of 29 children (13 asthmatics and 16 normal controls) reported significant elevations in BAL PMN cells and the PMN cell–derived mediator, myeloperoxidase (MPO), but not EOs.[54] Upon division of the asthmatic population into two groups based on disease severity (six children had mild-to-moderate persistent asthma and seven had intermittent asthma), PMN cell counts (p <0.06) and MPO levels (p <0.04) were higher in the mild-to-moderate persistent group compared with the intermittent group. This suggests a potential association between PMN cell-mediated inflammation and symptom severity.

In addition to PMN cells, both EPIs and MACs have been associated with the pathophysiology of persistent childhood asthma based on BAL studies. Marguet and colleagues reported significantly elevated EPI cell counts (13.5%) in their asthma group, supporting the association of EPI shedding with asthmatic inflammation.[53] Finally, evaluations of AHR based on histamine bronchial challenge in 22 chronic, stable asthmatic children correlated with elevated levels of both BAL EOs (r = –0.68; p <0.005) and MACs (r = –0.55; p = 0.006).[91] The investigators concluded that MACs were important in the development of AHR in asthma, both directly and indirectly via EO recruitment. In general, BAL studies in children broadened the understanding of the early presence of inflammation and the potential roles of various cell types and mediators in the spectrum of wheezing disorders from transient IW to persistent asthma.[102]

3. Sputum

Unlike biopsy and BAL, induced sputum provides a noninvasive means for evaluation of airway inflammation in children and can be performed successfully by children above the age of 6 years. The dominant cell in sputum from normal children is the MAC, with an upper limit of 2.5% sputum EOs.[102] Most sputum studies focused on cell differentials, with emphasis on EOs and EO mediators. In a study of 60 asthmatic children (aged 5 to 15 years) and 27 normal controls, sputum was induced using 4.5% hypertonic saline inhalation with a success rate of approximately 60% in both groups.[103] The investigators reported significantly higher sputum EO differential counts (p <0.004) and ECP levels (p <0.0001) in the asthmatic group compared with controls but found no correlation with asthma symptom severity and/or lung function. Conversely, Pin et al. reported reproducible elevations in sputum differential EO counts (mean of 18.5% versus 1.9%) that correlated directly with baseline FEV_1 in a study of 17 asthmatic patients (mean 30.3 years; range 11 to 69) compared with 17 normal controls.[104]

While sputum induction in young children presents limitations, the use of hypertonic saline challenge following pretreatment with a bronchodilator was well tolerated and achieved a high success rate (70%) in asthmatic children (aged 7 to 16 years with baseline FEV_1 levels >70%).[105] This combined procedure allowed simultaneous comparison of airway inflammation based on sputum cellularity and AHR. However, several limitations were uncovered:

1. Fewer children from the combined induction-and-hypertonic-saline group were able to provide adequate sputum samples compared with the sputum-induction-alone group (70% versus 92%; p = 0.03).
2. Sample contamination was more common (14 versus 6%; p = 0.02).
3. Significant differences in sputum cellularity were also noted (4% EOs in the induced sputum group versus 1.4% in the combined group; p <0.02).

In general, the inflammatory response in persistent childhood asthma is characterized by elevated numbers of sputum EOs and ECPs. Sputum EOs also appear to be quite specific for allergic asthma compared with potential variant asthma syndromes such as recurrent cough and bronchitis.[106] EO and ECP levels tend to be diminished in the presence of several asthma therapies including theophylline,[107] leukotriene modifiers,[108] and corticosteroid therapy[109,110] and correlate with disease severity, particularly in steroid-naïve children.[102]

However, one study in asthmatic children controlled on inhaled and/or oral corticosteroids demonstrated significant elevations in sputum EOs compared with normal controls, suggesting significant persistent airway inflammation at baseline in asthmatic children despite normal lung function and symptomatic control.[111] Furthermore, in a study evaluating sputum aspirates from young asthmatic children (≤ 4 years) obtained after coughing episodes, the investigators demonstrated that 33% of the children younger than 1 year, 55% at 1 year or age, and 80% at 2 to 3 years of age showed evidence of significant inflammation (>11 EOs per five microscopic fields).[112] These pediatric sputum studies reinforce the concepts of airway inflammation persisting even at asymptomatic baseline and occurring very early in the disease.

Sputum evaluation does appear to be reliable in the assessment of airway inflammation during acute asthma exacerbations. Two studies investigated sputum in children presenting with acute asthma in an urgent care setting. One examined 8 children (aged 8 to 15 years) and the other study described 38 children (aged 8 to 17 years). Children in both studies underwent sputum induction within 1 hr of presentation and again post-exacerbation. The smaller study revealed intense cellular infiltration comprised of EOs, PMN cells, and mast cells in the sputum during acute exacerbation, with significant resolution of the inflammation following recovery.[60,61]

In the second study, PMN elastase and EG_2-positive EOs were assessed along with ECP, MPO, IL-8, and IL-5.[60] Acutely, EG_2 positive cells correlated with the degree of acute airflow obstruction (r = –0.5; p = 0.02). ECP levels were also significantly elevated consistent with heightened EO activation during exacerbation. Similarly, MPO levels (220 to 1 ng/ml; p = 0.02) consistent with PMN cell activation and IL-8 (15.4 to 2.8 ng/ml; p = 0.004) were significantly acutely elevated with marked resolution at baseline. The investigators documented the intensity of airway inflammation in acute asthma, suggesting an exaggerated inflammatory process composed of both EO and PMN cell-mediated inflammation.

While EO-mediated airway inflammation may be demonstrated using sputum data, several additional limitations of detection particular to children remain. In a study involving three groups of children (15, first-time WC, 27 recurrent WC, and 56 with asthma), EOs were significantly elevated in the asthma group, but this elevation was not identified in the sputum of asthmatic children <1 year of age. In fact, accumulations of sputum EOs were not typical until children were >1 year of age, and rapid rises in sputum EOs were reported in asthmatic children as they aged to 5 years.[113] Because EOS are seen in BAL specimens in asthmatic children <1 year of age, these data suggest that sputum induction in these children may not accurately reflect lower airway inflammation.

Sputum evaluations may provide evidence of early airway inflammation, but techniques must be refined, particularly in young children, to overcome the difficulties surrounding sputum acquisition and the potential for sample contamination.

4. *Exhaled Measurements*

a. Exhaled Nitric Oxide (eNO)

eNO can be measured easily and noninvasively even in young children during flow-independent tidal volume breathing,[114] making it very attractive for the investigation of inflammation associated with asthma. NO is produced from the inducible form of NO synthase by a variety of cells including EPIs and MACs in the presence of acute inflammation. In general, this biomarker has been linked to heightened allergic sensitization[115] and is commonly elevated in pediatric asthmatic patients at baseline compared with normal controls.[116–118]

This marker may be significantly more useful in diagnosing asthma in corticosteroid-naïve patients compared with persistent asthma cases on inhaled corticosteroid (ICS) controller therapy. A recent study compared 36 children (aged 2 to 7 years) with mild intermittent asthma, 13 children (3 to 7 years) with moderate persistent asthma treated with ICS (200 to 800 µg budesonide), 20 nonasthmatic children (2 to 7 years) with chronic cough and recurrent pneumonia, and 15 normal controls. The corticosteroid-naïve intermittent asthmatics had significantly higher eNO levels (p <0.0001) compared with those with moderate persistent corticosteroid-treated asthma. Interestingly, no significant differences were noted in mean eNO in the treated moderate persistent asthmatics, the chronic cough group, or the controls. This suggests limited interpretative value of this marker in corticosteroid-treated asthma compared with other respiratory disorders and even normal controls.[119]

In a recent study, the effects of 4-week therapy with budesonide (100, 400, or 1600 µg/day) on sputum EOs, exhaled NO, and AHR to methacholine[120] were investigated. While eNO was exquisitely sensitive to ICS therapy and reached a plateau at a dose of ≥400 µg, sputum EOs and AHR demonstrated significant dose–response relationships with the varying doses. Therefore, this biomarker may be exquisitely sensitive to corticosteroid therapy that can decrease eNO even after a single dose.[121]

Similar findings of significantly higher eNO levels were reported in 12 subjects with intermittent asthma treated solely with β_2 agonists compared with 17 moderate persistent asthma subjects treated with 250 µg fluticasone priopri-onate/50 µg salmeterol twice daily for a minimum of 6 months prior to study inclusion and 6 normal controls.[122] However, unlike the previous study, a distinct subgroup of moderate asthma subjects was noted based on marked elevations in IL-8 and eNO levels. These "high-producers" experienced significantly more exacerbations compared with the "low producers" in the moderate persistent asthma group. This study emphasizes a redundant theme in that persistent inflammation may be present even in the face of appropriate controller therapy and that asthma is a very complex and heterogeneous disease with various phenotypes.

eNO measurements, while potentially useful markers, specifically of aller-gic inflammation in asthma, have several limitations. The first and most important factor limiting reliability and sampling in children is the actual eNO measurement (low flow versus high flow versus forced exhalation). In general, recommenda-tions concerning sampling techniques have markedly improved reliability but are still important considerations in the interpretation of eNO data.[123–125] Additionally, while significantly elevated in corticosteroid-naïve asthmatic patients, such increases may not be consistently disease-specific.[119,124] The applicability of eNO measurement to reflect airway inflammation has also been questioned because eNO has been found to correlate weakly with both biopsy[126] and sputum EOs.[120,127]

eNO levels appear to be most reflective of allergic inflammation based on significant elevations following acute allergen challenge,[128] but less consistently with nonallergen challenge.[129] Significant declines following exercise chal-lenge,[130] sputum induction,[131,] and airway methacholine challenge[132] were reported. Even β_2 agonist treatment and spirometry resulted in significant fluctu-ations in eNO levels, thereby limiting interpretation; specifically an 11 to 19% increase was reported post-bronchodilator and spirometry compared with pre-bronchodilator treatment levels in children with asthma.[133] As noted earlier, in addition to a significant eNO reduction in the face of ICS therapy, suppression has also been demonstrated in response to leukotriene antagonists.[134] Therefore, despite its ease of use and noninvasive nature, its overall applicability for the evaluation of inflammation in children remains controversial and requires ongoing study.

b. Exhaled Breath Condensates (EBCs)

Significant interest has arisen concerning the collection of EBCs for the mea-surement of various biomarkers in airways reflective of inflammation and/or oxidative stress. Barnes and Kharitonov hypothesized that "aerosolized nonvolatile particles exhaled in human breath reflect the composition of the bronchoalveolar extracellular lining fluid."[135] Based on this hypothesis, collection of EBCs may provide a direct and noninvasive approach to the evaluation of airway inflammation. This approach is potentially attractive for the evaluation of young children because it involves the passive collection of exhaled air during tidal volume breathing and does not affect airway caliber, thus allowing for repeated measurements. The exhaled air is cooled to $-20°C$ and collected as a condensate for approximately 15 minutes. The amount of condensate collected is dependent on the subject's minute volume ventilation, the exhaled air temperature, and the humidity.[136]

Typically, 1 to 3 ml of condensate are collected, then stored for analysis via chromatography and/or immunoassay. Although it is difficult to validate and reproduce the results, the methodology has been updated constantly to minimize saliva contamination and standardize analysis techniques such as pH monitoring. One limitation in children is that the procedure may require significantly more time to ensure adequate sample volume collection given their lower minute volume ventilation due to smaller tidal volumes.

EBCs have been used to study several biomarkers. EBC analyses in children have included nitrites,[137] leukotrienes,[138] and several cytokines, IL-4 and IFN-γ.[139] With results comparable with previous findings from airway and blood analyses,[28,140,141] Shahid and colleagues demonstrated the TH_1–TH_2 imbalance in their EBC study of 37 (11 normal controls, 12 corticosteroid-naïve children, and 14 corticosteroid-treated asthmatic) children.[139] EBC IFN-γ levels in both asthmatic groups were significantly lower compared with controls (3.7 ± 0.2 pg/ml; p <0.01 in the corticosteroid-naïve children and 4.1 pg/ml; p <0.05 in the corticosteroid-treated group compared with 5.1 ± 0.5 pg/ml).

Conversely, IL-4 levels were significantly elevated in the asthma groups compared with controls (p <0.05), but concentrations were lower in steroid-treated children (ICS dose >600 μg/day) compared with steroid-naïve participants (p <0.01) and did not reach statistical significance compared with controls. Furthermore, IL-4:IFN-γ ratios were most significant in the corticosteroid-naïve asthmatic population compared with both controls (p <0.05) and corticosteroid-treated asthma subjects (p <0.05). While these findings of cytokine dysregulation are not unique, the ability to replicate such findings using EBC is encouraging, valuable, and attractive because it has the potential to allow noninvasive and early assessment in young children.

In addition to baseline assessments, EBCs can be used effectively and safely in the evaluation of acute asthma. For example, Corradi et al. evaluated EBC in 12 children presenting with acute asthma exacerbations. They demonstrated significant elevations of aldehydes and reductions of glutathione, biomarkers of oxidant-induced damage and antioxidant status, respectively. Acutely, aldehyde levels were significantly higher in patients with asthma than in normal controls (p <0.002). Significant reductions were noted following corticosteroid therapy. Conversely, glutathione levels were significantly lower in the acutely exacerbating subjects compared with normal controls (p <0.0001) and significantly increased following therapy.[142]

Thus, the use of EBCs to evaluate asthma is a novel methodology to characterize airway inflammation in both acute and chronic diseases. Such non-invasive evaluation is particularly attractive for the evaluation of young pediatric patients, but requires more extensive assessment.

B. Systemic Evaluations

1. Serum

Serum markers to determine EOS counts and IgE and ECP levels have been consistently used in the evaluation of pediatric asthma, although evidence that suggests any correlation with airway inflammation is limited. Castro-Rodriguez and colleagues included ≥4% EOs as a minor risk factor in their asthma predictive clinical profile.[17] Similarly, heightened ECP levels at first IW episode[143] and during acute viral bronchiolitis[144] may be helpful in the identification of subjects with IW who are at risk for the development of persistent asthma phenotypes. In fact, in 48 infants (mean age 153.5 days) with acute bronchiolitis, the risk for developing persistent wheezing over the next 5 years was 9.73 times higher for infants with serum ECP levels ≥8 µg/L than for those who had levels <8 µg/L (p <0.0001).[144]

A similar predictive potential has been suggested for elevated IgE levels in recurrently wheezing infants and the development of persistent asthma at 6 years of age.[11] The most important role these biomarkers may play is providing a predictive index for asthma development in young children, but due to the multifactorial nature of asthma, these factors alone are neither sensitive nor specific enough to predict the risks of developing asthma.

2. Urine

Similar to serum markers, urinary biomarkers may be limited in their ability to reflect airway inflammation. Most urinary studies have focused on EPX (a marker of eosinophil activation) and more recently, cysLT evaluations.[145] Specifically, urinary LTE_4 levels have been used as markers of total cysLT production in adults and children. Elevations have been reported in both acute[146] and chronic asthma,[147] viral-induced wheeze,[148] and exercise-induced bronchospasm[149,150] and with allergen challenge.[146,149] However, both urinary LTE_4 and EPX levels, commonly reported as creatinine ratios, may not be reliable, particularly in children, due to the dilute natures of their urine and decreased creatinine levels.

In addition, serial measurements of urinary EPX over 6 months did not provide additional information for management in monitoring childhood asthma; no relationship existed between these biomarkers and the clinical severity of asthma in 14 children with mild persistent disease.[151] Thus, the sensitivity of this biomarker may be inadequate to support its routine use for clinical monitoring in asthmatic disease.[152]

IV. Conclusion

It is clear that inflammation is at the core of the pathogenesis of asthma and is determined both by environmental influences and genetic predispositions. Furthermore, inflammation in asthma may occur in early life and results in irreversible airway remodeling with subsequent loss of lung function. Wheezing may be the initial symptom of underlying airway inflammation associated with asthma. The airway inflammation associated with early IW is characterized predominantly by PMN cells and differs from findings in pediatric asthma characterized by increased EOs and LYMs.

The ability to identify a wheezing child at risk for the subsequent development of persistent asthma is both challenging and difficult because most early wheezing episodes are transient. Despite this challenge, it is critical to identify the approximately 40% of young children with recurrent wheezing and predispositions for persistent disease.[11] Various evaluations including invasive bronchoscopy, BAL, minimally invasive sputum induction, and noninvasive eNO and EBC measurements are able to assess airway inflammation. However, once airway inflammation is identified, it is unclear whether early anti-inflammatory intervention can alter the natural progression of the disease.[153] The benefits of such therapeutic interventions early in life remain questionable and are the foci of various multicenter trials.

References

1. Symposium C. Terminology, definitions, and classifications of chronic pulmonary emphysema and related conditions. *Thorax* 1959; 14: 286–299.
2. Society AT. Definitions and classifications of chronic bronchitis, asthma and pulmonary emphysema. 1962; 85: 762–768.
3. Unger L. The pathology of bronchial asthma. *Arch Int Med* 1922; 30:689–760.
4. Buranakul B, Washington J, Hilman B, Mancuso J, and Sly RM. Causes of death during acute asthma in children. *Am J Dis Child* 1974; 128: 343–350.
5. Barnes PJ. Frontiers in medicine: new aspects of asthma. *J Intern Med* 1992; 231: 453–461.
6. Wenzel SE. Abnormalities of cell and mediator levels in bronchoalveolar lavage fluid of patients with mild asthma. *J Allergy Clin Immunol* 1996; 98: S17–S40.

7. Chetta A, Foresi A, Del Donno M, Bertorelli G, Pesci A, and Olivieri D. Airway remodeling is a distinctive feature of asthma and is related to severity of disease. *Chest* 1997; 111: 8520–8527.

8. Lemanske RF, Jr. Inflammatory events in asthma: an expanding equation. *J Allergy Clin Immunol* 2000; 105: S633–S636.

9. Bousquet J, Chanez P, Lacoste JY, White R, Vic P, and Godard P. Asthma: a disease remodeling the airways. *Allergy* 1992; 47: 3–11.

10. Bousquet J, Jeffery PK, Busse WW, Johnson M, and Vignola AM. Asthma. From bronchoconstriction to airways inflammation and remodeling. *Am J Respir Crit Care Med* 2000; 161: 1720–1745.

11. Martinez FD, Wright AL, Taussig LM, Holberg CJ, Halonen M, and Morgan WJ. Asthma and wheezing in the first six years of life. *New Engl J Med* 1995; 332: 133–138.

12. Wolfe R, Carlin JB, Oswald H, Olinsky A, Phelan PD, and Robertson CI. Association between allergy and asthma from childhood to middle adulthood in an Australian cohort study. *Am J Respir Crit Care Med* 2000; 162: 2177–2181.

13. Lemanske RF, Jr. Inflammation in childhood asthma and other wheezing disorders. *Pediatrics* 2002; 109: 371–372.

14. Djukanovic R. Airway inflammation in asthma and its consequences: implications for treatment in children and adults. *J Allergy Clin Immunol* 2002; 109: S539–S548.

15. Varner AE and Lemanske RF, Jr. The early and late response to allergen, in *Asthma and Rhinitis*, Holgate ST, Ed. London: Blackwell Science, 2000, p. 1172.

16. Burrows B, Martinez FD, Halonen M, Barbee RA, and Cline MG. Association of asthma with serum IgE levels and skin-test reactivity to allergens. *New Engl J Med* 1989; 320: 271–277.

17. Castro-Rodriguez JA, Holberg CJ, Wright AL, and Martinez FD. A clinical index to define risk of asthma in young children with recurrent wheezing. *Am J Respir Crit Care Med* 2000; 162: 1403–1406.

18. Bergmann RL, Edenharter G, Bergmann KE, Guggenmoos-Holzmann I, Forster J, Bauer CP, Wahn V, Zepp F, and Wahn U. Predictability of early atopy by cord blood: IgE and parental history. *Clin Exp Allergy* 1997; 27: 752–760.

19. Croner S, Kjellman NJM, Eriksson B, and Roth A. IgE screening in 1701 newborn infants and the development of atopic disease during infancy. *Arch Dis Child* 1982; 57: 364–368.

20. Jones AC, Miles EA, and Warner JO. Fetal peripheral blood mononuclear cell proliferative responses to mitogenic and allergenic stimuli during gestation. *Pediatr Allergy Immunol* 1996; 7: 109–116.

21. Prescott SL, Macaubas C, Holt BJ, Smallacombe TB, Loh R, Sly PD, and Holt PG. Transplacental priming of the human immune system to environmental allergens: universal skewing of initial T cell responses toward the Th2 cytokine profile. *J Immunol* 1998; 160: 4730–4737.

22. Holt PG, Macaubas C, Stumbles PA, and Sly PD. The role of allergy in the development of asthma. *Nature* 2000; 402: 12–17.

23. Kiekhaefer CA, Kelly EA, and Jarjour NN. Antigen-induced airway disease, in *Environmental Asthma*, Vol. 153, Bush RK, Ed. New York: Marcel Dekker, Inc., 2001, p. 13.

24. Prescott SL, Macaubas C, Smallacombe TB, Holt BJ, Sly PD, and Holt PG. Development of allergen-specific T-cell memory in atopic and normal children. *Lancet* 1999; 353: 196–200.

25. Holt PG, Clough JB, Holt BJ, Baron-May MJ, Rose AH, Robinson BWS, and Thomas WR. Genetic risk for atopy is associated with delayed postnatal maturation of T-cell competence. *Clin Exp Allergy* 1992; 22: 1093–1099.

26. Harris JR, Magnus P, Samuelsen SO, and Tambs K. No evidence for effects of family environment on asthma: a retrospective study of Norwegian twins. *Am J Respir Crit Care Med* 1997; 156: 43–49.

27. Hartnell A, Robinson DS, Kay AB, and Wardlaw AJ. CD69 is expressed by human eosinophils activated *in vivo* in asthma and *in vitro* by cytokines. *Immunology* 1993; 80: 281–286.

28. Tang MLK, Kemp AS, Torburn J, and Hill DJ. Reduced interferon-γ secretion in neonates and subsequent atopy. *Lancet* 1994; 344: 983–985.

29. Ferguson AC, Whitelaw M, and Brown H. Correlation of bronchial eosinophil and mast cell activation with bronchial hyperresponsiveness in children with asthma. *J Allergy Clin Immunol* 1992; 90: 609–613.

30. Cutz E, Levison H, and Cooper DM. Ultrastructure of airways in children with asthma. *Histopathology* 1978; 1978: 407–421.

31. Hoekstra MO, Grol MH, Hovenga H, Bouman K, Stijnen T, Koeter GH, Gerritsen J, and Kauffman HF. Eosinophil and mast cell parameters in children with stable moderate asthma. *Pediatr Allergy Immunol* 1998; 9: 143–149.

32. Busse WW and Lemanske RF, Jr. Asthma. *New Engl J Med* 2001; 344: 350–362.

33. Lane SJ and Lee TH. Mast cell effector mechanisms. *J Allergy Clin Immunol* 1996; 98: S67–S72.

34. Bradding P, Roberts JA, Britten KM, Montefort S, Djukanovic R, Mueller R, Heusser CH, Howarth PH, and Holgate ST. Interleukin-4, -5, and -6 and tumor necrosis factor-α in normal and asthmatic airways: evidence for the human mast cell as a source of these cytokines. *Am J Respir Cell Mol Biol* 1994; 10: 471–480.

35. Richter A, Puddicombe SM, Lordan JL, Bucchieri F, Wilson SJ, Djukanovic R, Dent G, Holgate ST, and Davies DE. The contribution of interleukin (IL)-4 and IL-13 to the epithelial-mesenchymal trophic unit in asthma. *Am J Respir Cell Mol Biol* 2001; 25: 385–391.

36. Rothenberg ME. Eosinophilia. *New Engl J Med* 1998; 338: 1592–1600.

37. Kellaway CH and Trethewie ER. Liberation of slow-reacting smooth muscle stimulating substance of anaphylaxis. *J Exp Physiol* 1940; 30: 121–148.

38. Barnes NC, Piper PJ, and Costello JF. Comparative actions of inhaled leukotriene C4, leukotriene D4 and histamine in normal human subjects. *Thorax* 1984; 39: 500–504.

39. Adelroth E, Morris MM, and Hargreave FE. Airway responsiveness to leukotrienes C4 and D4 and to methacholine in patients with asthma and normal controls. *New Engl J Med* 1986; 315: 480–484.

40. Shimizu T, Hirano H, Majima Y, and Sakakura Y. A mechanism of antigen-induced mucus production in nasal epithelium of sensitized rats: a comparison with lipopolysaccharide-induced mucus production. *Am J Respir Crit Care Med* 2000; 161: 1648–1654.

41. Laitinen LA, Laitinen A, Haahtela T, Vikka V, Spur BW, and Lee TH. Leukotriene E(4) and granulocytic infiltration into asthmatic airways. *Lancet* 1993; 341: 989–990.
42. Diamant Z, Hiltermann JT, and van Rensen EL. Cell differentials in induced sputum after inhaled leukotriene D4 in subjects with mild asthma. *Am J Respir Crit Care Med* 1997; 155: 1247–1253.
43. Azzawi M, Bradley B, and Jeffery PK. Identification of activated T lymphocytes and eosinophils in bronchial biopsies in stable atopic asthma. *Am Rev Respir Dis* 1990; 142: 1407–1413.
44. Keramidaris E, Merson TD, Steeber DA, Tedder TF, and Tang ML. L-selectin and intercellular adhesion molecule 1 mediate lymphocyte migration to the inflamed airway/lung during an allergic inflammatory response in an animal model of asthma. *J Allergy Clin Immunol* 2001; 107: 734–738.
45. Fujisawa T, Kephart GM, Gray BH, and Gleich GJ. The neutrophil and chronic allergic inflammation. *Am Rev Respir Dis* 1990; 141: 689–697.
46. Hallahan AR, Artour CL, and Black JL. Products of neutrophils and eosinophils increase the responsiveness of human isolated bronchial tissue. *Eur Respir J* 1990; 3: 554–558.
47. Wenzel SE, Schwartz LB, Langmack EL, Halliday JL, Trudeau JB, Gibbs RL, and Chu HW. Evidence that severe asthma can be divided pathologically into two inflammatory subtypes with distinct physiologic and clinical characteristics. *Am J Respir Crit Care Med* 1999; 160: 1001–1008.
48. Lamblin C, Gosset P, Tillie-Leblond I, Saulnier F, Marquette CH, Wallaert B, and Tonnel AB. Bronchial neutrophilia in patients with noninfectious status asthmaticus. *Am J Respir Crit Care Med* 1998; 157: 394–402.
49. Tonnel AB, Gosset P, and Tillie-Leblond I. Characteristics of the inflammatory response in bronchial lavage fluids from patients with status asthmaticus. *Int Arch Allergy Immunol* 2001; 124: 267–271.
50. Metzger WJ, Zavala D, Richerson HB, Moseley P, Iwamota P, Monick M, Sjoerdsma K, and Hinninghake GW. Local allergen challenge and bronchoalveolar lavage of allergic asthmatic lungs. *Am Rev Respir Dis* 1987; 135(2): 433–440.
51. Barnes PJ. Pathophysiology of asthma, in *Asthma*, Vol. 8, European Respiratory Society Journals Ltd., 2003.
52. Frangova V, Sacco O, Silvestri M, Oddera S, Balbo A, Crimi E, and Rossi G. BAL neutrophilia in asthmatic patients: a by-product of eosinophil recruitment? *Chest* 1996; 110: 1236–1242.
53. Marguet C, Jouen-Boedes F, Dean TP, and Warner JO. Bronchoalveolar cell profiles in children with asthma, infantile wheeze, chronic cough, or cystic fibrosis. *Am J Respir Crit Care Med* 1999; 159: 1533–1540.
54. Barbato A, Panizzolo C, Gheno M, Sainati L, Favero E, Faggian D, Giusti F, Pesscolderungg L, and La Rosa M. Bronchoalveolar lavage in asthmatic children: evidence of neutrophil activation in mild-to-moderate persistent asthma. *Pediatr Allergy Immunol* 2001; 12: 73–77.
55. Stevenson EC, Turner G, Heaney LG, Schock BC, Taylor R, Gallagher T, Ennis M, and Shields MD. Bronchoalveolar lavage findings suggest two different forms of childhood asthma. *Clin Exp Allergy* 1997; 27: 1027–1035.

56. Krawiec ME, Westcott JY, Chu HW, Balzar S, Trudeau JB, Schwartz LB, and Wenzel SE. Persistent wheezing in very young children is associated with lower respiratory inflammation. *Am J Respir Crit Care Med* 2001; 163: 1338–1343.

57. Azevedo I, de Blic J, Vargaftig BB, Bachelet M, and Scheinmann P. Increased eosinophil cationic protein levels in bronchoalveolar lavage from wheezy infants. *Pediatr Allergy Immunol* 2001; 12: 65–72.

58. Le Bourgeois ML, Goncalves M, Le Clainche L, Benoist M, Fournet J, Scheinmann P, and de Blic J. Bronchoalveolar cells in children <3 years old with severe recurrent wheezing. *Chest* 2002; 122: 791–797.

59. Kim CK, Chung CY, Choi SJ, Kim DK, Park Y, and Koh YY. Bronchoalveolar lavage cellular composition in acute asthma and acute bronchiolitis. *J Pediatr* 2000; 137: 517–522.

60. Norzila MZ, Fakes K, Henry RL, Simpson J, and Gibson PG. Interleukin-8 secretion and neutrophil recruitment accompanies induced sputum eosinophil activaton in children with acute asthma. *Am J Respir Crit Care Med* 2000; 161: 769–774.

61. Twaddell SH, Gibson PG, Carty K, Woolley KL, and Henry RL. Assessment of airway inflammation in children with acute asthma using induced sputum. *Eur Respir J* 1996; 9: 2104–2106.

62. Lee TH and Lane SJ. The role of macrophages in the mechanisms of airway inflammation in asthma. *Am Rev Respir Dis* 1992; 145: S27–S30.

63. John M, Lim S, Seybold J, Jose P, Robichaud A, O'Connor B, Barnes PJ, and Chung KF. Inhaled corticosteroids increase interleukin-10 but reduce macrophage inflammatory protein-1, granulocyte–macrophage colony-stimulating factor, and interferon-γ release from alveolar macrophages in asthma. *Am J Respir Crit Care Med* 1998; 157: 256–262.

64. Tang C, Inman MD, van Rooijen N, Yang P, Shen H, Matsumoto K, and O'Byrne PM. Th type 1-stimulating activity of lung macrophages inhibits Th2-mediated allergic airway inflammation by an IFN-gamma-dependent mechanism. *J Immunol* 2001; 166: 1471–1481.

65. Polito AJ and Proud D. Epithelial cells as regulators of airway inflammation. *J Allergy Clin Immunol* 1998; 102: 714–718.

66. Holgate ST, Davies DE, Lackie PM, Wilson SJ, Puddicombe SM, and Lordan JL. Epithelial–mesenchymal interactions in the pathogenesis of asthma. *J Allergy Clin Immunol* 2000; 105: 193–204.

67. Polosa R, Prosperini G, Leir SH, Holgate ST, Lackie PM, and Davies DE. Expression of c-erbB receptors and ligands in human bronchial mucosa. *Am J Respir Cell Mol Biol* 1999; 20: 914–923.

68. Barrow RE, Wang CZ, Evans MJ, and Herndon DN. Growth factors accelerate epithelial repair in sheep trachea. *Lung* 1993; 171: 335–344.

69. Davies DE, Polosa R, Puddicombe SM, Richter A, and Holgate ST. The epidermal growth factor receptor and its ligand family: their potential role in repair and remodeling in asthma. *Allergy* 1999; 54: 771–783.

70. Holgate ST, Lackie PM, Davies DE, Roche WR, and Walls AF. The bronchial epithelium as a key regulator of airway inflammation and remodelling in asthma. *Clin Exp Allergy* 1999; 29 (Suppl. 2): 90–95.

71. Lange P, Parner J, Vestbo J, Schnohr P, and Jensen G. A 15-year follow-up study of ventilatory function in adults with asthma. *New Engl J Med* 1998; 339: 1194–1200.

72. Phunek P, Roche WR, Tarzikova J, Kurdmann J, and Warner JO. Eosinophilic inflammation in the bronchial mucosa of children with bronchial asthma (abstract). *Eur Respir J* 1997; 25: 160.

73. Ebina M, Takahashi T, Chiba T, and Motomiya M. Cellular hypertrophy and hyperplasia of airway smooth muscles underlying bronchial asthma: a 3-D morphometric study. *Am Rev Respir Dis* 1993; 148: 720–726.

74. Boulet LP, Laviolette M, Turiotte H, Cartier A, Dugas M, Maol JL, and Boutet M. Bronchial subepithelial fibrosis correlates with airway responsiveness to methacholine. *Chest* 1997; 112: 45–52.

75. Cypcar D, Stark J, and Lemanske RF, Jr. The impact of respiratory infections on asthma. *Pediatr Clin North Am* 1992; 39: 1259–1276.

76. Sears MR. Epidemiology of childhood asthma. *Lancet* 1997; 350: 1015–1020.

77. Laitinen LA, Heino M, Laitinen A, Kava T, and Haahtela T. Damage of the airway epithelium and bronchial reactivity in patients with asthma. *Am Rev Respir Dis* 1985; 131: 599–606.

78. Montefort S, Roberts JA, Beasley R, Holgate ST, and Roche WR. The site of disruption of the bronchial epithelium in asthmatic and non-asthmatic subjects. *Thorax* 1992; 47: 499–503.

79. Laitinen LA, Laitinen A, Altraja A, Virtanen I, Kampe M, Simonsson BG, Karlsson S, Hakansson L, Venge P, and Sillastu H. Bronchial biopsy findings in intermittent or "early asthma." *J Allergy Clin Immunol* 1996; 98: S3–S6.

80. Chetta A, Foresi A, Del Donno M, Consigli GF, Bertorelli G, Pesci A, Barbee RA, and Olivieri D. Bronchial responsiveness to distilled water and methacholine and its relationship to inflammation and remodeling of the airways in asthma. *Am J Respir Crit Care Med* 1996; 53: 910–917.

81. Jeffery PK, Wardlaw AJ, Nelson FC, Collins JV, and Kay AB. Bronchial biopsies in asthma: an ultrastructural, quantitative study and correlation with hyperreactivity. *Am Rev Respir Dis* 1989; 140: 1745–1753.

82. Bai TR, Cooper J, Koelmeyer T, Pare PD, and Weir TD. The effect of age and duration of disease on airway structure in fatal asthma. *Am J Respir Crit Care Med* 2000; 162: 663–669.

83. Cokugras H, Akcakaya N, Seckin I, Camcioglu Y, Sarimurat N, and Aksoy F. Ultrastructural examination of bronchial biopsy specimens from children with moderate asthma. *Thorax* 2001; 56: 25–29.

84. Payne DNR, Rogers AV, Adelroth E, Bandi V, Guntupalli KK, Bush A, and Jeffery PK. Early thickening of the reticular basement membrane in children with difficult asthma. *Am J Respir Crit Care Med* 2003; 167: 78–82.

85. Jackson C. *Perioral Endoscopy and Laryngeal Surgery.* St. Louis: Laryngoscope Co., 1915, p. 201.

86. Wood RE and Fink RJ. Applications of flexible fiberoptic bronchoscopes in infants and children. *Chest* 1978; 73: 737.

87. Pattishall EN. Use of bronchoalveolar lavage in immunocompromised children with pneumonia. *Pediatr Pulmonol* 1988; 5: 1–5.

88. Bye MR. Diagnostic bronchoalveolar lavage in children with AIDS. *Pediatr Pulmonol* 1987; 3: 425–428.

89. Frankel LR. Bronchoalveolar lavage for diagnosis of pneumonia in the immunocompromised child. *Pediatrics* 1988; 81: 785–788.

90. Hein J, Martens E, Bauer I, Dorfling P, Brock J, Gulzow HU, Breuel K, and Rudolph I. Bronchoalveolar lavage: a diagnostic method in chronic nonspecific bronchopulmonary diseases in childhood? Studies of cellular and humor parameters in BAL irrigation fluid. *Z Erkr Atmung* 1991; 176: 7–20.

91. Ferguson AC and Wong FWM. Bronchial hyperresponsiveness in asthmatic chldren; correlation with macrophages and eosinophils in broncholavage fluid. *Chest* 1989; 96: 988–991.

92. Ennis M, Turner G, Schock BC, Stevenson EC, Brown V, Fitch PS, Heaney LG, Taylor R, and Shields MD. Inflammatory mediators in bronchoalveolar lavage samples from children with and without asthma. *Clin Exp Allergy* 1999; 29: 362–366.

93. Shields MD, Brown V, Stevenson EC, Fitch PS, Schock BC, Turner G, Taylor R, and Ennis M. Serum eosinophilic cationic protein and blood eosinophil counts for the prediction of the presence of airways inflammation in children with wheezing. *Clin Exp Allergy* 1999; 29: 1382–1389.

94. Marguet C, Dean TP, and Warner JO. Soluble intercellular adhesion molecule-1 (sICAM-1) and interferon-γ in bronchoalveolar lavage fluid from children with airway diseases. *Am J Respir Crit Care Med* 2000; 162: 1016–1022.

95. Kitz R, Ahrens P, and Zielen S. Immunoglobulin levels in bronchoalveolar lavage fluid of children with chronic chest disease. *Pediatr Pulmonol* 2000; 29: 443–451.

96. Marguet C, Dean TP, Basuyau JP, and Warner JO. Eosinophil cationic protein and interleukin-8 levels in bronchial lavage fluid from children with asthma and infantile wheeze. *Pediatr Allergy Immunol* 2001; 12: 27–33.

97. Just J, Fournier L, Momas I, Zambetti C, Sahraoui F, and Grimfeld A. Clinical significance of bronchoalveolar eosinophils in childhood asthma. *J Allergy Clin Immunol* 2002; 110: 42–44.

98. Warke TJ, Fitch PS, Brown V, Taylor R, Lyons JD, Ennis M, and Shields MD. Exhaled nitric oxide correlates with airway eosinophils in childhood asthma. *Thorax* 2002; 57: 383–387.

99. Azevedo I, de Blic J, Scheinmann P, Vargaftig BB, and Bachelet M. Enhanced arachidonic acid metabolism in alveolar macrophages from wheezy infants: modulation by dexamethasone. *Am J Respir Crit Care Med* 1995; 152: 1208–1214.

100. Azevedo I, de Blic J, Dumarey CH, Scheinmann P, Vargaftig BB, and Bachelet M. Increased spontaneous release of tumour necrosis factor alpha by alveolar macrophages from wheezy infants. *Eur Respir J* 1997; 10: 1767–1773.

101. Pohunek P, Rocke WR, Turzikova J, Kudrmann J, and Warner JO. Eosinophilic inflammation in the bronchial mucosa of children with bronchial asthma. *Eur Respir J* 1997; 10: 160s.

102. Gibson PG, Henry RL, and Thomas P. Noninvasive assessment of airway inflammation in children: induced sputum, exhaled nitric oxide, and breath condensate. *Eur Respir J* 2000; 16: 1008–1015.

103. Wilson NM, Bridge P, Spanevello A, and Silverman M. Induced sputum in children: feasibility, repeatability, and relation of findings to asthma severity. *Thorax* 2000; 55: 768–774.

104. Pin I, Gibson PG, Kolendowicz R, Girgis-Gabardo A, Denburg JA, Hargreave FE, and Dolovich J. Use of induced sputum cell counts to investigate airway inflammation in asthma. *Thorax* 1992; 47: 25–29.

105. Jones PD, Hankin R, Simpson J, Gibson PG, and Henry RL. The tolerability, safety, and success of sputum induction and combined hypertonic saline challenge in children. *Am J Respir Crit Care Med* 2001; 164: 1146–1149.

106. Gibson PG, Simpson J, Chalmers AC, Toneguzzi RC, Wark PAB, Wilson AJ, and Hensley MJ. Airway eosinophiia is associated with wheeze but is uncommon in children with persistent cough and frequent chest colds. *Am J Respir Crit Care Med* 2001; 164: 977–981.

107. Tohda Y, Muraki M, Iwanaga T, Kubo H, Fukuoka M, and Nakajima S. The effect of theophylline on blood and sputum eosinophils and ECP in patients with bronchial asthma. *Int J Immunopharmacol* 1998; 20: 173–181.

108. Pizzichini E, Leff JA, Reiss TF, Hendeles L, Boulet LP, Wei LX, Efthimiadis AE, Zhang J, and Hargreave FE. Montelukast reduces airway eosinophilic inflammation in asthma: a randomized, controlled trial. *Eur Respir J* 1999; 14: 12–18.

109. Gershman NH, Wong HH, Liu JT, and Fahy JV. Low- and high-dose fluticasone propionate in asthma; effects during and after treatment. *Eur Respir J* 2000; 15: 11–18.

110. van Rensen EL, Straathof KC, Veselic-Charvat MA, Zwinderman AH, Bel EH, and Sterk PJ. Effect of inhaled steroids on airway hyperresponsiveness, sputum eosinophils, and exhaled nitric oxide levels in patients with asthma. *Thorax* 1999; 54: 403–408.

111. Cai Y, Carty K, Henry RL, and Gibson PG. Persistence of sputum eosinophilia in children with controlled asthma when compared with healthy children. *Eur Respir J* 1998; 11: 848–853.

112. Nagayama Y, Odazima Y, Nakayama S, Toba T, and Funabashi S. Eosinophils and basophilic cells in sputum and nasal smears taken from infants and young children during acute asthma. *Pediatr Allergy Immunol* 1995; 6: 204–208.

113. Nagayama Y, Tsubaki T, Toba T, Nakayama S, and Kiyofumi O. Analysis of sputum taken from wheezy and asthmatic infants and children with special reference to respiratory infections. *Pediatr Allergy Immunol* 2001; 12: 318–326.

114. Martinez T, Weist AD, Williams T, Clem C, Silkoff P, and Tepper RS. Assessment of exhaled nitric oxide kinetics in healthy infants. *J Appl Physiol* 2003; 94(6): 2348–2390.

115. Van Amsterdam JG, Janssen NA, De Meer G, Fischer PH, Nierkens S, Van Loveren H, Opperhuizen A, Steerenberg PA, and Brunekreef B. The relationship between exhaled nitric oxide and allergic sensitization in a random sample of school children. *Clin Exp Allergy* 2003; 33: 187–191.

116. Nelson BV, Sears S, Woods J, Ling CY, Hunt J, Clapper LM, and Gaston B. Expired nitric oxide as a marker for childhood asthma. *J Pediatr* 1997; 130: 423–427.

117. Byrnes CA, Dinarevic S, Shinebourne EA, Barnes PJ, and Bush A. Exhaled nitric oxide measurements in normal and asthmatic children. *Pediatr Pulmonol* 1997; 24: 312–318.

118. Baraldi E, Dario C, Ongaro R, Scollo M, Azzoli NM, Panza N, Paganini N, and Zacchello F. Exhaled nitric oxide concentrations during treatment of wheezing exacerbation in infants and young children. *Am J Respir Crit Care Med* 1999; 159: 1284–1288.

119. Avital A, Uwyyed K, Berkman N, Godfrey S, Bar-Yishay E, and Springer C. Exhaled nitric oxide and asthma in young children. *Pediatr Pulmonol* 2001; 32: 308–313.

120. Jatakanon A, Kharitonov S, Lim S, and Barnes PJ. Effect of differing doses of inhaled budesonide on markers of airway inflammation in patients with mild asthma. *Thorax* 1999; 54: 108–114.

121. Tsai YG, Lee MY, Yang KD, Chu DM, Yuh YS, and Hung CH. A single dose of nebulized budesonide decreases exhaled nitric oxide in children with acute asthma. *J Pediatr* 2001; 139: 433–437.

122. La Grutta S, Gagliardo R, Mirabella F, Pajno GB, Bonsignore G, Bousquet J, Bellia V, and Vignola AM. Clinical and biological heterogeneity in children with moderate asthma. *Am J Respir Crit Care Med* 2003; 167: 1490–1495.

123. Silkoff PE, McClean PA, Slutsky AS, Furlott HG, Hoffstein E, Wakita S, Chapman KR, Szalai JP, and Zamel N. Marked flow-dependence of exhaled nitric oxide using a new technique to exclude nasal nitric oxide. *Am J Respir Crit Care Med* 1997; 155: 260–267.

124. Kissoon N, Duckworth L, Blake K, Murphy S, and Silkoff PE. Exhaled nitric oxide measurements in childhood asthma: techniques and interpretation. *Pediatr Pulmonol* 1999; 28: 282–296.

125. Kharitonov S, Alving K, and Barnes PJ. Exhaled and nasal nitric oxide measurements: recommendations: European Respiratory Society Task Force. *Eur Respir J* 1997; 10: 1683–1693.

126. Lim S, Jatakanon A, Meah S, Oates T, Chung KF, and Barnes PJ. Relationship between exhaled nitric oxide and mucosal eosinophilic inflammation in mild to moderately severe asthma. *Thorax* 2000; 55: 184–188.

127. Berlyne GS, Parameswaran K, Kamada D, Efthimiadis A, and Hargreave FE. A comparison of exhaled nitric oxide and induced sputum as markers of airway inflammation. *J Allergy Clin Immunol* 2000; 106: 638–644.

128. Baraldi E, Carra S, Dario C, Azzolin N, Ongaro R, Marcer G, and Zacchello F. Effect of natural grass pollen exposure on exhaled nitric oxide in asthmatic children. *Am J Respir Crit Care Med* 1999; 159: 262–266.

129. Nightingale JA, Rogers DF, and Barnes PJ. Effect of inhaled ozone on exhaled nitric oxide, pulmonary function, and induced sputum in normal and asthmatic subjects. *Thorax* 1999; 54: 1061–1069.

130. Terada A, Fujisawa T, Togashi K, Miyazaki T, Katsumata H, Atsuta J, Iguchi K, Kamiya H, and Togari H. Exhaled nitric oxide decreases during exercise-induced bronchoconstriction in children with asthma. *Am J Respir Crit Care Med* 2001; 164: 1879–1884.

131. Piacentini GL, Bodini A, Costella S, Vicentini L, Suzuki Y, and Boner AL. Exhaled nitric oxide is reduced after sputum induction in asthmatic children. *Pediatr Pulmonol* 2000; 29: 430–433.

132. Piacentini GL, Bodini A, Peroni DG, Miraglia del Giudice M, Jr., Costella S, and Boner AL. Reduction in exhaled nitric oxide immediately after methacholine challenge in asthmatic children. *Thorax* 2002; 57: 771–773.

133. Kissoon N, Duckworth LJ, Blake KV, Murphy SP, and Lima JJ. Effect of 2-agonist treatment and spirometry on exhaled nitric oxide in healthy children and children with asthma. *Pediatr Pulmonol* 2002; 34: 203–208.

134. Bratton DL, Lanz MJ, Miyazawa N, White CW, and Silkoff PE. Exhaled nitric oxide before and after montelukast sodium therapy in school-age children with chronic asthma: a preliminary study. *Pediatr Pulmonol* 1999; 28: 402–407.

135. Barnes PJ and Kharitonov S. *Non-Invasive Monitoring of Airway Inflammation.* Hoechberg: Jaeger Information, 2001.

136. Kips JC, Kharitonov SA, and Barnes PJ. Noninvasive assessment of airway inflamamtion in asthma. *Asthma* 2003; 23: 164–179.

137. Formanek W, Inci D, Lauener RP, Wildhaber JH, Frey U, and Hall GL. Elevated nitrite in breath condensates of children with respiratory disease. *Eur Respir J* 2002; 19: 487–491.

138. Csoma Z, Kharitonov SA, Balint B, Bush A, Wilson NM, and Barnes PJ. Increased leukotrienes in exhaled breath condensate in childhood asthma. *Am J Respir Crit Care Med* 2002; 166: 1345–1349.

139. Shahid SK, Kharitonov SA, Wilson NM, Bush A, and Barnes PJ. Increased interleukin-4 and decreased interferon-gamma in exhaled breath condensate of children with asthma. *Am J Respir Crit Care Med* 2002; 165: 1290–1293.

140. Renzi PM, Turgeon JP, Marcotte JE, Drblik SP, Berube D, Gagnon MF, and Spier S. Reduced interferon-gamma production in infants with bronchiolitis and asthma. *Am J Respir Crit Care Med* 1999; 159: 1417–1422.

141. Hoekstra MO, Hoekstra Y, De Reus D, Rutgers B, Gerritsen J, and Kauffman HF. Interleukin-4, interferon-gamma and interleukin-5 in peripheral blood of children with moderate atopic asthma. *Clin Exp Allergy* 1997; 27: 1254–1260.

142. Corradi M, Folesani G, Andreoli R, Manini P, Bodini A, Piacentini G, Carraro S, Zanconato S, and Baraldi E. Aldehydes and glutathione in exhaled breath condensate of children with asthma exacerbation. *Am J Respir Crit Care Med* 2003; 167: 395–399.

143. Koller DY, Wojnarowski C, Herkner KR, Weinlander G, Raderer M, Eichler I, and Frischer T. High levels of eosinophil cationic protein in wheezing infants predict the development of asthma. *J Allergy Clin Immunol* 1997; 99: 752–756.

144. Pifferi M, Ragazzo V, Caramella D, and Baldini G. Eosinophil cationic protein in infants with respiratory syncytial virus bronchiolitis: predictive value for subsequent development of persistent wheezing. *Pediatr Pulmonol* 2001; 31: 419–424.

145. Severien C, Artlich A, Jonas S, and Becher G. Urinary excretion of leukotriene E4 and eosinophil protein X in children with atopic asthma. *Eur Respir J* 2000; 16: 588–592.

146. Taylor GW, Black P, and Turner N. Urinary leukotriene E4 after allergen challenge and in acute asthma and allergic rhinitis. *Lancet* 1989; 1: 584–588.

147. Westcott JY, Voelkel NF, Jones K, and Wenzel SE. Inactivation of leukotriene C4 in the airways and subsequent urinary leukotriene E4 excretion in normal and asthmatic subjects. *Am Rev Respir Dis* 1993; 148: 1244–1251.

148. Oommen A and Grigg J. Urinary leukotriene E4 in preschool children with acute clinical viral wheeze. *Eur J Pediatr* 2003; 21: 149–154.
149. Smith CM, Christie PE, Hawksworth RJ, Thien F, and Lee TH. Urinary leukotriene E4 levels after allergen and exercise challenge in bronchial asthma. *Am Rev Respir Dis* 1991; 144: 1411–1413.
150. Kikawa Y, Miyanomae T, Inoue Y, Saito M, Nakai A, Shigematsu Y, Hosoi S, and Sudo M. Urinary leukotriene E4 after exercise challenge in children with asthma. *J Allergy Clin Immunol* 1992; 89: 1111–1119.
151. Wojnarowski C, Roithner B, Koller DY, Halmerbauer G, Gartner C, Tauber E, and Frischer T. Lack of relationship between eosinophil cationic protein and eosinophil protein X in nasal lavage and urine and the severity of childhood asthma in a 6-month follow-up study. *Clin Exp Allergy* 1999; 29: 926–932.
152. Dahlen SE and Kumlin M. Can asthma be studied in the urine? *Clin Exp Allergy* 1998; 28: 129–133.
153. Childhood Asthma Management Program Research Group. Long-term effects of budesonide or nedocromil in children with asthma. *New Engl J Med* 2000; 343: 1054–1063.

III

Risk Factors in the Development of Asthma

7

Physiology

ALEXANDER MÖLLER and PETER N. LE SOUËF

Princess Margaret Hospital for Children
Perth, Australia

I. Introduction

The investigation of risk factors that impact the growing lung and hence the development of pulmonary function in newborns and infants requires accurate, objective measurements to be made early in life. Such measurements can also allow more meaningful comparisons with physiological outcome measurements used in epidemiological assessments later in life.

Most of these later outcome measures depend on active participation of the study subject, and therefore, a reasonable level of cooperation is needed for reproducible measurements. Infants and newborns cannot participate actively; their pulmonary function can only be assessed passively. Additionally, the several important physiological differences between adults and infants mean that existing techniques and equipment cannot be adapted easily for use with smaller lungs.

The first description of pulmonary function measurements in infants appeared at the end of the 19th century, but techniques originally used for adults were adapted and validated for use with newborns and infants only about 40 years ago.[1,2] During the 1970s, methods such as esophageal manometry and plethysmography were validated and used to investigate dynamic compliance, resistance, and lung volumes.[3,4] In the past 20 years, additional techniques for the assessment of respiratory mechanics have been specifically developed for use in infants.[5,6] The most important developments include techniques to induce forced expiration, and these produce outcomes similar to those provided by the well-established spirometry measures used in older children and adults.[7]

Further techniques such as oscillatory mechanics, gas dilution, and other methods have been devised to investigate tidal breathing parameters.[8,9] The most important problem related to all techniques used is the lack of standardized equipment — commercially available equipment as opposed to custom-made equipment used in some specialized centers. Results from different studies from different study centers are often difficult to compare, particularly when a need for a greater number of study subjects results in multicenter studies. Standardizing equipment remains a challenge for such studies.

Another important issue is the relatively large intersubject and intrasubject variation of infant lung function tests.[8] This has an impact on serial measurements throughout the whole development of a child from infancy through school age and on outcome measures including assessments of risk factors, early intervention studies, and clinical trials.

When measuring pulmonary function in infants and newborns, important issues of developmental physiology must be addressed. For example, a large proportion of total airway resistance (around 50%) is generated by the upper airways, mostly by the nose.[10] Because infants are preferential nose breathers, changes of minimal cross-sectional area in the nose exert important effects on most outcome measures of pulmonary function. Upper airway changes may mask lower airway changes due to risk factors or therapeutic intervention. Functional residual capacity (FRC) is unstable in infants and may change with different sleep stages, disease states, and dead space of the equipment used.[11,12] Another factor is the highly compliant chest wall that promotes a tendency to airway closure caused by too little outward recoil and hence less distention of the airways and lungs.[8]

An ideal technique for assessing lung functions in infants would be applicable to all age groups, operate independently of arousal state, and be reproducible and highly sensitive. Such a test would clearly distinguish between healthy and disease states and, therefore, reflect the clinical situation. Because no available test provides all the desirable information, combinations of different methods may be used, depending on information required.

II. Plethysmographic Measurements of Lung Volume and Airway Resistance

FRC is measured routinely in infants mostly using whole body plethysmography. The measurement of FRC is important both for estimating normal lung growth and for interpreting volume-dependent pulmonary mechanics (e.g., airway resistance, forced flows at standardized volumes [$V'_{max}FRC$]). The whole-body plethysmograph was adapted in the early 1960s for use with infants.[13] This technique is similar to the methods used in older children and adults. However, all maneuvers required to minimize changes in temperature and humidity of respired gas (e.g., panting) must be carried out without the infant's cooperation.

The child is placed in a supine position in a closed plethysmograph and breathes through a pneumotachograph via a face mask. Volumes are calculated by the integration of tidal flow. Temperature and humidity of the respired gas are maintained via rebreathing to a heated bag containing saturated gas at body temperature and pressure (BTPS). Airway resistance (R_{aw}) can be measured throughout the breathing cycle by occluding the airway opening for short periods using a remote-controlled shutter. During occlusion, the child attempts to exhale and this leads to compression of intrathoracic gas, whereas occlusion during inhalation leads to expansion of the thorax and hence decrease of alveolar pressure.

Volume can be calculated at the moment of occlusion, relating changes in alveolar pressure (measured as airway opening pressure during zero flow) to changes in alveolar volume (calculated by the plethysmographic signal). R_{aw} is calculated using the equation $R_{aw} = \Delta P/Flow$ when $\Delta P = P_a - P_{ao}$. In other words, a higher pressure is required to maintain the same flow when resistance rises. Hence, R_{aw} can be calculated to relate changes in alveolar pressure to changes in flow at the airway opening.

Using the Boyle–Mariott law that states that in a closed system under isothermic conditions the product of pressure (P) and volume (V) is constant (P * V = constant), the thoracic gas volume (TGV) can be calculated. In a volume-constant plethysmograph, the thorax expansion during attempted inhalation produces an increase in pressure measured at the box (P_{box}). The equation for the thoracic gas volume is TGV = f1 * $\Delta P_{box}/\Delta P_a$ * ($V_{box} - V_o$) where f1 is the water pressure of the breathed air and V_o is the volume of infant, pneumotachograph, and dead space. However, the only volume that can be determined reliably in infants is FRC when measured at the end of a tidal expiration (end expiratory resting volume). The outstanding problem of FRC measurement, and hence determination of lung function parameters in relation to lung volumes, is the substantial variation of end expiratory level over time.[6,14]

Intraindividual between-test variability also influences results of early intervention or longitudinal studies.[14–16] Despite certain limitations, whole-body plethysmography has an important place in the assessment of infant lung function and has been used to investigate developmental parameters and bronchopulmonary diseases.[17–20] However, its use is technically demanding and hence restricted to relatively few specialized laboratories.

III. Tidal Breath Analysis for Infant Pulmonary Function Testing

The assessment of tidal flow breathing movements provides the opportunity to study a range of physiological parameters related to respiratory control and pulmonary mechanical function, and has provided essential basic information regarding respiratory behavior in infants. A variety of parameters can be obtained from the flow signal, including tidal volume (V_t), respiratory frequency (f_R), inspiratory time (t_I), and expiratory time (t_E).

In 1981, Morris et al.[21] observed the distinct pattern of tidal flow versus time in patients with air flow obstruction compared with normal subjects who showed more sinusoidal appearances of flow–time curves. In order to quantify these differences, more complex timing indices have been devised from these basic parameters. Time to peak tidal expiratory flow (t_{PTEF}) can be related to time of expiration (t_E), time to peak expiratory flow divided by total expiratory time (t_{PTEF}/t_E), mean inspiratory flow (V_t/t_I), minute ventilation (V'_E), and duty cycle (t_I/t_{tot} [total breath time]).

Visual inspection of tidal breathing flow volume loops may provide information on airway obstruction. The technique is noninvasive and allows measurements in nonsedated newborns and infants. Most studies have been carried out using a pneumotachograph attached on a differential pressure transducer. Air flow is digitized and integrated to allow volume measurement. In healthy subjects, the parameters obtained via the breathing tidal curve and its shape reflect an integrated response of the entire respiratory system and show laryngeal, neural, and intrathoracic components, whereas the curve is mostly determined by intrathoracic airway mechanics during severe air flow limitation.

Tidal flow volume loops have been used in newborns and infants to assess developmental processes. T_{PTEF}/t_E and the corresponding volume to maximal forced expiration divided by total expiratory volume (V'_{PTEF}/V_E) are the most commonly used parameters to describe tidal flow breathing patterns. The t_{PTEF}/t_E ratio has been shown to decrease with age very early in life.[8,22,23] The lower ratios seen in newborn children may be explained by an increase in total expiratory time and decrease in respiratory rate.[24,25] The T_{PTEF}/t_E ratio calculated from tidal breathing flow curves predicts the development of recurrent wheezing over the subsequent 3 years of life.[26,27] Furthermore, the t_{PTEF}/t_E index has been demonstrated to distinguish between asthmatic and nonasthmatic children[28,29] and between children with cystic fibrosis and healthy children[29] and to show responses to methacholine, histamine,[25,30] and bronchodilators such as salbutamol[31] and adrenaline.[32]

IV. Tidal Forced Expirations

Infants and young children are unable to perform the forced expiratory maneuvers needed for assessment of maximum flow rates from maximal expiratory flow volume curves. In 1977, Taussig et al.[33] showed the feasibility of measurements of maximal expiratory flows at functional residual capacity ($V'_{max}FRC$) in 4- to 6-year-old children using partial forced expiratory flow volume (PEFV) curves.

This technique was adapted for use in infants. Pressure is applied around the body of an infant at end inspiration.[34] Another modification was placing an inflatable plastic bag around an infant's chest and abdomen.[35,36] This technique is usually referred to as the rapid thoraco-abdominal compression (RTC) or "squeeze" method. Tidal forced expirations are used widely to investigate lung growth and developmental changes, determine the effects of different diseases (e.g., asthma or cystic fibrosis) on lung functions in infants, and assess bronchial hyperreactivity via bronchial challenge tests or bronchodilator response.[9]

Infants are evaluated during spontaneous sleep or after sleep induced by chloral hydrate (70 to 80 mg/kg). Flow is measured with a heated pneumotachograph attached to an infant-sized face mask placed in a leak-free position over the child's nose and mouth. Volume is determined by digital integration of the flow signal. An inflatable jacket is wrapped around the infant's chest and abdomen. The jacket is connected via a tap to a reservoir containing air at pressures up to 10 kPa (100 cm H_2O). Forced expiration is achieved by rapid inflation of the jacket (70 to 100 msec to 95% peak pressure) at end inspiration by manual or computer-controlled opening of the tap of the reservoir that forces air from the infant's lungs.

The PEFV curve can be quantified by measuring the flow at FRC or end expiration. The forced expiratory maneuver is repeated with increasing reservoir pressures until $V'_{max}FRC$ is achieved, which means that flow limitation is achieved. The best $V'_{max}FRC$ obtained will be the highest value for that infant.

$V'_{max}FRC$ is thought to quantify peripheral airway function because it primarily reflects airway caliber upstream to the airway segment where flow limitation occurs.[8,37] A mean intrasubject coefficient of variation of 11% in the first year of life was reported for normal infants.[36] The shapes of PEFV curves in infants are important because they may reflect degrees of airway obstruction. Convex curves are associated with better respiratory function than concave curves.[11] The interpretation of PEFV curves and the derived parameters present certain limitations because FRC is actively controlled in infants. $V'_{max}FRC$ derives from partial forced expiratory flows curves only and is therefore strongly influenced by the lung volume at which it is measured.[38] This may lead to some increase of variability in the measurement of $V'_{max}FRC$ compared with measurements of forced expiratory flows in older children whose total lung capacity and residual volume are defined.[11,39]

V. Raised Volume Rapid Thoraco-Abdominal Compression (RVRTC)

In the further development of techniques using forced expiration, more reproducible and sensitive data were needed to allow better comparisons between infants and spirometric variables in older children. The most important change was passive inflation of an infant's lung toward total lung capacity (TLC) via a defined pressure before applying compression pressure.[7,40] This allows full forced expiratory maneuvers comparable with spirometric measurements such as forced vital capacity (FVC), forced expiratory volume in 1 second (FEV_t), and forced expiratory flow (FEF)% (e.g., maximal expiratory flow (MEF)50).[7,41] Flow at a given fraction of either absolute or forced lung volume can be measured.

In infants, forced expiration is usually completed in less than 1 sec. Therefore, measurements of $FEV_{0.5}$, $FEV_{0.75}$, and FEF25–75 may be more useful than measuring FEV_1 in this age group.

Recently, $FEV_{0.5}$ was noted to approach FVC in many infants less than 3 mo of age, hence the recommendation was made to report $FEV_{0.4}$ in newborns and small infants.[42] To determine TLC, the infant's lungs are inflated to a given airway pressure via a fan, diaphragm pump,[7] or an external gas source[43] before forced expiration begins. This has the advantage of allowing comparisons of raised volume breaths of different patients because lung volume can be standardized. Prior to forced expiration, the infant's lung volume is raised several times above tidal range.[43] This leads to a short apnea that may be induced by a minimal drop in PCO_2 due to augmented ventilation or induction of the Hering–Breuer inflation reflex (relaxation of respiratory muscles).

The Hering–Breuer inflation reflex is volume-dependent, and hence stronger and more consistently present at raised lung volumes. The apnea allows measurement of expiratory flows without interfering with respiratory muscle activity.[37] Preliminary clinical data show a good correlation with disease severity. However, this methodology is relatively recent and, therefore, the number of published studies is still small. However, evidence indicates that measurements using the RVRTC better distinguish healthy infants and those with recurrent wheeze or cystic fibrosis than the $V'_{max}FRC$.[37,41,44]

Flow limitation is more likely to be achieved in healthy infants with RVRTC than when using PEFV curves. The intraindividual variability of timed volumes from RVRTC measurement was found to be 5% and, thus, significantly lower than for $V'_{max}FRC$.[45] This may be mostly due to the fact that volume history and expiratory effort (compression pressure) are controlled. It has been shown that asymptomatic infants with recurrent wheeze have lower $FEV_{0.5}$ values than normal infants.[46]

The effects of bronchodilators have been investigated using the RVRTC technique, but the results are controversial.[45,47] Younger infants and those exposed to maternal tobacco smoking during pregnancy have been shown to have greater increases in forced expiratory flows after inhaling bronchodilators.[48] Two studies investigated responses to methacholine and showed decreases in forced expiratory flows.[49,50]

In a study of 155 healthy infants and toddlers 3 to 149 weeks of age, a high correlation of flow parameters (FEF_{50}, FEF_{75}, FEF_{85}, and FEF_{25-75}) and body lengths was reported, and maternal smoking during pregnancy was associated with significantly diminished flow parameters.[51] This study also provided reference values for measurements of full forced expiratory maneuvers in infants.[51]

VI. Measurement of Functional Residual Capacity by Gas Dilution

Gas dilution techniques used for adults have been modified for use in infants, mainly by adapting the size of equipment, reducing dead space, and increasing signal resolution.[52] Due to inherent technical difficulties, only functional residual capacity (FRC) has been routinely measured in infants. Different techniques are available to assess FRC apart from radiological estimation[53] and whole-body plethysmography. Gas dilution techniques include closed circuit helium dilution (FRC_{He}), open circuit nitrogen washout (FRC_{N2}), and the multiple breath inert gas washout using a gas mixture containing 4% sulfur hexafluoride (FRC_{SF6}).

Because gas dilution techniques measure only the volume of gas that communicates with the airway openings, gas trapped by obstructed airways or within cysts will not be measured, and hence FRC will be underestimated. Another reason for underestimation of FRC is very long time constants. Conversely, volumes measured by whole-body plethysmography may be overestimated because the technique assumes homogeneous pressures within all alveoli whether they communicate with airway openings or not. For this reason, trapped air is measured within both the thorax and the gastrointestinal tract. Time constants of lung areas can differ in infants because of structural instability or obstructions of distal airways, resulting in distal airway narrowing or collapses of terminal bronchioli. One consequence of these different time constants is uneven alveolar recruitment causing ventilation and perfusion mismatching.[54]

The volume of gas in the lungs at end tidal expiration can be measured by mass balance. The concentration of the gas is measured at the beginning and the end of the procedure. In the closed circuit helium dilution technique, the amount of the gas is initially known and the concentration is measured via the open circuit multiple breath nitrogen washout (MBNW). The initial fractional alveolar nitrogen (N_2) concentration is known when the infant breathes room air. When the infant breathes 100% O_2, all N_2 is washed from the lungs. After the amount of washed-out N_2 is measured, the lung volume at which the washout was initiated (FRC) can be calculated.[52,55]

With the closed circuit helium dilution method, the infant breathes from a known concentration and volume of helium. After equilibration between the spirometer and the lungs, the unknown lung volume can be calculated as the difference in helium concentration within the system.

Schibler et al.[56] developed a simple technique to measure FRC and ventilation inhomogeneities in spontaneously breathing infants using sulfur hexafluoride (FRC_{SF6}) multiple breath washin and washout. The technique uses an ultrasonic flow meter (Spiroson Scientific, ECO Medics AG, Dürnten, Switzerland) that allows measurement of the molar mass (MM) of the gas passing the flow meter; concentrations of different gases can be determined simultaneously. The measurement of FRC with this technique was highly accurate and reproducible in a tested lung model and also in healthy, unsedated infants, and indices of ventilation distribution such as alveolar-based mean dilution number (AMDN) and pulmonary clearance delay (PCD) could be calculated with this technique.[56]

Hjalmarson et al.[57] used the multiple breach nitrogen washout technique to show that preterm infants have moderately reduced FRC levels and more pronounced impairments of gas mixing efficiency when compared with infants born at term. This may be due to more efficient gas mixing efficiency in peripheral airways and by the volume and arrangement of terminal respiratory units, the development of which may be impaired in premature children.[57] The same group compared healthy, preterm infants and those with bronchial pulmonary dysplasia (BPD). The BPD group demonstrated reduced FRC and gas mixing efficiency.[58]

FRC measured by the MBNW method showed a linear correlation with body weight in healthy children from neonatal age up to 5 years.[59] Pulmonary inhomogeneity can also be assessed by measuring FRC using both the whole-body plethysmography (FRC_{pleth}) and multiple breath nitrogen washout (FRC_{N2}). The amount of air that is not communicating with airways (trapped air) can be measured by subtracting FRC_{N2} from FRC_{pleth}.[60,61]

VII. Measurement of Airway Mechanics Using Forced Oscillation

In 1956, DuBois et al.[62] introduced a minimally invasive forced oscillation technique to assess the mechanical impedance of the lungs or respiratory system. Mechanical impedance can be measured by forced oscillation; a sinusoidal pressure variation (P_{rs}) is applied to the respiratory system at the airway opening and the complex ratio of airway opening pressure (P_{ao}) to flow (V'_{ao}) is measured. The pressure–flow relationship is called impedance, Z ($Z = P_{ao}$ or P_{rs}/V'_{ao}).[63] The technique is noninvasive and does not require a patient's cooperation because oscillations are imposed on normal tidal breathing.

The respiratory system can be regarded as a group of airways and tissues separated by a volume of compressible alveolar gas. The mechanical structures of the airways and tissues are responsible for effective resistance, inertance, and compliance of the respiratory system and will influence the overall impedance spectrum.[63] For frequencies below approximately 2 Hz, the respiratory system can be considered mechanically as a series of resistance (R_{rs}) and compliance (C_{rs}) elements (e.g., a single balloon with a C_{rs} on a pipe with R_{rs}). For higher frequencies than that of spontaneous breathing, an additional term (inertance or I_{rs}) must be introduced into the model to account for pressure changes in phase with volume accelerations.[64]

The complex ratio P_{rs}/V'_{ao} is Z_{rs} defined by the amplitude ratio and phase angle between P_{rs} and V'_{ao}. Thus, R_{rs} is the "in phase" component of Z_{rs} and the respiratory system reactance ($-1/C_{rs} \cdot \omega = X_{rs}$) is the "out of phase" component. When the respiratory system is regarded as a linear model, the forced oscillation technique allows calculation of the same parameters as other techniques.[64] The limitation of this technique in spontaneously breathing infants is the inability to collect the low frequency data (below 2 Hz) that is necessary to adequately describe the mechanical properties of airways and tissues simultaneously. The superimposition of frequencies below 2 Hz (i.e., 0.5 Hz) requires the suspension of breathing via muscle paralysis or voluntary apnea.[65]

A modification of the RVRTC has been described. The technique is used to induce the Hering–Breuer reflex to produce a breathing pause. This allows an oscillatory signal to be superimposed with a lower frequency than the spontaneous breathing rate (0.5 to 21 Hz).[66] Both airway and tissue parameters have been shown to decrease in a quadratic relationship with increasing length in healthy infants from 7 weeks to 2 years.[67] In addition, a family history of asthma had a negative effect on airway resistance (R_{aw}) and elastance (H) measured with the low frequency forced oscillation technique.[67]

Another study from the same group revealed altered respiratory tissue mechanics in asymptomatic wheezy infants between 1 and 2 years of age. Z scores were significantly different for all assessed parameters: airway resistance (R_{aw}), tissue damping (G), and tissue elastance.[46] The low frequency oscillation technique is considered a suitable methodology to assess responsiveness of infants to bronchodilators.[68] In a group of 22 (9 healthy infants and 13 with recurrent wheeze), salbutamol decreased R_{aw} significantly although no statistical difference was observed between wheezy and healthy infants.[68] Although this technique is very promising in investigating developmental and risk factors in growing infants and children, the interpretation of results remains limited due to the wide range of values reported for healthy infants.

VIII. Assessment of Airway Responsiveness

A broad spectrum of different methods has been developed to investigate airway responsiveness. Both direct and indirect stimuli can lead to bronchoconstriction. Examples of direct stimuli are inhaled methacholine and histamine. Inhalation of adenosine monophosphate, hypertonic saline or mannitol, exercise, voluntary hyperventilation, and cold air are indirect stimuli. Most challenge tests require an outcome measure that reflects airway function, most importantly forced expiratory flow rate, although indirect outcome measures — transcutaneous oxygen levels and pulse oximetry — have been reported.

Positive responses to histamine were reported in 9 of 11 wheezy infants to doses smaller than 8g/l using partial forced expiratory flow volume curves.[69] However, in another study, histamine was shown to induce bronchoconstriction in all healthy infants studied; a decrease of more than 30% in $V'_{max}FRC$ was recorded.[70] The same result was shown after a cold dry air (CDA) challenge.[71] Lack of appreciation at that mass of the inhaled dose of histamine in infants (as opposed to the concentration of histamine in the nebulizer solution) led to the speculation that humans are born with "bronchial hyperresponsiveness" and that genetic or environmental factors determine which infants lose it thereafter.[70] This suggestion was withdrawn when a later publication by the same research group corrected the dose to make it appropriate to the size of the child.[72] This means, when a correction is made for dose, infants and older children appear to show similar responses to inhaled histamine.[72]

Young et al. used a decrease in $V'_{max}FRC$ greater than 40% to assess airway responsiveness. Increased airway responsiveness was demonstrated in healthy infants with positive family histories of asthma or parental smoking compared with infants with no family histories of asthma or smoking.[25] RVRTC has also been shown to be capable of assessing bronchial responsiveness to histamine or methacholine[50] and the forced expiratory volume–time parameters have been shown to detect histamine-induced bronchoconstriction.[73] The underlying physiological or structural factors responsible for producing the responses to histamine and methacholine in infants remain unclear.

IX. Factors Affecting Physiology in Infants and Children

A. *In Utero* Factors

1. *Maternal Smoking*

The influence of maternal smoking during pregnancy is the most important known environmental factor affecting the physiology of the developing lung and the likelihood of developing asthma in early life. The reasons for this are not clear. Tobacco smoke has so many toxic components that determining which ones

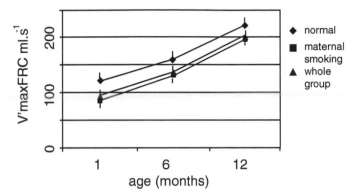

Figure 7.1 Maternal smoking and lung function in the first year of life in a cohort of unselected Australian infants recruited antenatally and followed longitudinally through the first year of life. $V'_{max}FRC$ represents maximal flow at functional residual capacity. (From Young, S. et al. *Eur Respir J* 2000; 15: 151–157. With permission.)

produce these adverse effects would be very difficult. The strength of the relationship of maternal smoking and outcome is likely to be driven to an extent by the high level of exposure that the fetus receives. Because tobacco smoke products including nicotine freely cross placental and tissue barriers, a fetus is exposed to the same levels as the mother. Cotinine is the principal break-down product of nicotine and has a long half-life. This makes it an ideal marker of tobacco smoke exposure.[74] Cotinine levels in mothers who smoke during pregancy were shown to reach the same levels as in nonpregnant smokers.[75] These data suggest that despite the knowledge of many pregant women that smoking will adversely affect their babies, the extent of the addiction means they do not cut down on smoking during pregnancy.

Many studies have shown that infants whose mothers smoked during pregancy are smaller at birth and their lung function is reduced compared with infants of nonsmoking mothers.[76–79] In a study of normal newborn infants from Norway, the level of reduction for the tPEF/tE ratio of offspring of smokers and nonsmokers was 0.023.[76] For compliance of the respiratory system, the reduction was 0.29 ml/cm H_2O.[76]

In another study of nonselected normal infants, $V'_{max}FRC$ levels at 1 month of age in infants whose mothers smoked during pregancy was a mean of 14.2 ml/sec (standard deviation [SD], 7.2) lower than in infants whose mothers did not smoke while pregnant (Figure 7.1).[79] In a U.S. study, $V'_{max}FRC$ levels in infants born to smoking mothers were lower than those found in infants whose mothers did not smoke during pregnancy (74.31 ml/sec [5.9 SD] versus 150.4 [8.9 SD]), respectively.[80] The differences remained significant when allowance was made for the size of each child.

In a more recent study from Manchester in which children determined to be at high risk of atopy were recruited at birth, maternal smoking during pregacny was associated with a mean V'_{max}FRC at 1 month of age of 99.0 ml.sec (53.2 SD) compared with 122.1 ml/sec (63.3 SD) in nonsmokers.[81] Although the difference between groups was not statistically significant, the direction was the same as in other studies. The timing of the effect of maternal smoking on developing lungs during pregnancy is not clear, but the effect is present in preterm infants.[82] At 1 year of age, several respiratory function parameters were adversely affected in infants of smoking versus nonsmoking mothers.[83] For example, mean airway resistance levels at end expiration were 3.03 (1.62 SD) and 2.10 kPa/L/sec (1.00 SD), respectively. Thus, many studies show reductions in respiratory function in infants of smoking mothers. Since many of these studies were performed soon after birth, the observed differences are unlikely to be due to passive inhalation of cigarette smoke after birth.

Maternal smoking is also an important risk factor for early wheeze and development of asthma in offspring. A large number of studies have shown that infants of smoking mothers are more likely to wheeze than infants of nonsmoking mothers.[77–79,81, 83–86] In the Manchester study, the odds ratio (OR) of developing wheezing for children of smoking versus nonsmoking mothers was 29.85 (95% confidence interval [CI], 2.46–36.2).[81] In another United Kingdom study, the odds ratio for wheezing in the first year of life was significantly increased in infants exposed to maternal smoking during pregnancy (4.9; 95% CI, 1.6–15.0; p = 0.005).[85] The impaired airway functions in infants of smoking mothers noted in some studies are likely to contribute to increased wheezing but unlikely to be the only contributing factor.

Maternal smoking is also associated with increased risk of diagnosis of asthma in early life[77,87] and in later childhood.[88] How much of the risk can be attributed to *in utero* exposure via the placenta compared with passive acquisition via inhalation of environmental tobacco smoke has always been difficult to estimate because most women who smoke during pregnancy continue to smoke after their children are born; very few mothers who did not smoke earlier take up smoking after their children are born. However, a recent analysis aimed at comparing risks of smoke exposure before and after birth concluded that *in utero* exposure accounted for most of the decrements in lung function seen in children of smoking mothers.[89]

a. Mechanisms by Which Maternal Smoking Causes Wheeze in Infants

Because airway function at or soon after birth is a strong predictor of wheeze and asthma in childhood[90] and a link between maternal smoking and low lung function in early life, a likely underlying link between smoke exposure and wheeze is that cigarette smoke impairs respiratory function during gestation.

Recent preliminary studies have suggested that maternal smoking triggers genetic factors that lead to asthma. These observations arose from genome screening studies in which large numbers of families were screened for asthma-related phenotypes. The single nucleotide polymorphisms that showed the greatest linkage scores were located in the cytokine cluster on chromosome 5,[91] but the linkage scores were much higher when children with nonsmoking mothers were excluded from the results. The important implication from these data is that maternal smoking acts strongly on genes in the region of the cytokine cluster to produce asthma in offspring. No other known environmental factor exerts such a strong influence on the genetics of asthma.

2. Preterm Delivery

Several factors are known to be associated with preterm delivery. However, preterm delivery is in itself a risk factor for wheeze in early life.[92,93] A large number of prospective studies have shown a long term reduction in respiratory function[94] that is proportional to the severity of respiratory problems experienced in the neonatal period[95] and inversely proportional to the time of gestation.[94] Whether it is also related to increased incidence of asthma is less clear.[94] A maternal history of asthma was also not associated with preterm delivery or chronic lung disease of prematurity,[96,97] but it was associated with increased duration of supplementary oxygen therapy.[97]

B. Genetic Associations

Few studies have shown genetic relationships with reduced respiratory function in childhood. There are likely to be several reasons for this. First, many genes have DNA variations that are related to asthma in various populations.[98] Indeed so many candidate genes have been identified that the effect of an individual genetic variation that exerts a small or moderate influence on respiratory function is unlikely to be seen unless a very large population is investigated. Even polymorphisms that exert large effects on pulmonary function may not be detected, particularly if the allele responsible is not common.

The β-2 adrenoreceptor gene has been studied more than any other gene in children, It is centrally involved in alteration of airway caliber and has several functional polymorphisms. The arg16gly polymorphism is not always related to respiratory function but is consistently associated with altered airway response to inhaled β-1 adrenergic treatment.[99,100] The arg16 allele is the more responsive variation to β-2 adrenergic therapy.[101] The same allele was also associated with a greater decline in respiratory function in adults after 16 weeks of treatment with adrenergic drugs compared with the gly16 allele.[102] The polymorphism at amino acid 27 is in linkage disequilibrium with arg16gly, but also appears to be independently associated with altered airway responsiveness. In a cohort of children, airway responsiveness was reduced in those with glu27 compared with gln27.[103]

Several other genes are associated with altered respiratory function in children. For example, for the CC16 A38G polymorphism, the 38A allele was associated with increased airway responsiveness in a cohort of German children.[104] For the leukotriene C4 synthase gene, asthmatic children with the –444C allele had lower FEV_1 values than those with the –444A allele (mean 97.4 versus 92.7% predicted, respectively).[105] Surfactant genes as causes of altered respiratory functions in infants have been noted.[106]

C. Gender

Several studies have shown that males have lower maximal expiratory flows than females during infancy.[107] In a study of unselected Australian infants, boys were found to have consistently lower $V'_{max}FRC$ values throughout the first year of life in comparison with girls. The boys' values demonstrated a mean of –21.05 mL/sec lower ($p < 0.05$).[107] Similar data were obtained in an English study in which $V'_{max}FRC$ was lower in boys than girls (mean 94 versus 115 ml/sec, respectively), although the difference in that study was not signficant.[108] In a U.S. study, forced expiratory flows at 75% of vital capacity were lower in males than in females.[51] The reason that males have lower expiratory flows is unclear. The difference between genders disappears by adolescence, due possibly to the greater general growth rates in males at that time.

The relatively reduced airway function in males in early life may be an important reason behind their increased respiratory morbidity. Boys are more commonly affected by most airway diseases than girls in the first few years of life. As no other predisposing risk factors unique to boys have been identified, this physiological disposition may be one of the more important factors responsible for the increased problems in males.

D. Race

Minor physiological differences in airway function have been demonstrated between infants of different races, but the differences appear to be of significance only in preterm infants. Respiratory resistance has been show to be lower in African than Caucasian boys in the United Kingdom.[109,110] These discrepancies are unlikely to contribute to the often major differences in respiratory moribidity seen among different races.

E. Bronchiolitis

Infants diagnosed with respiratory syncytial virus (RSV) bronchiolitis were formerly expected to develop impaired lung function, wheezing, and asthma due to damage of developing lungs caused by the virus.[111] Many studies confirmed this observation.[112,113] However, in a recent Australian study in a longitudinal cohort of unselected infants followed from birth to 11 years of age, lung function was measured at 1 month of age and again at 11 years. Participants who were diagnosed with bronchiolitis had impaired maximal expiratory flows both before they had bronchiolitis and at the 11-year follow-up (Figure 7.2a).[114] The degree of reduction of airway flow was similar at the two time points with respect to Z scores in those diagnosed with bronchiolitis (Figure 7.2b). The implication is that otherwise normal infants with airway function at the lower end of the spectrum develop similar degrees of reduced airway function in mid-childhood and that RSV does not, therefore, produce long-term damage to airways.

X. Early Physiological Factors as Predictors of Future Physiological Function and Asthma

The few longitudinal studies that assessed infant respiratory function soon after birth and then followed the infants into childhood produced results that have improved the general understanding of risk factors for asthma in children. In general, these studies show that initial levels of lung and airway function are associated with respiratory outcome through mid-childhood and establish an intrinsic level of airway function as an important risk factor for childhood respiratory problems and asthma.

A. Pulmonary Function Parameters

1. Forced Expiration Parameters

Studies of these parameters early in life have shown that the early level of function is associated with later respiratory outcome and airway symptoms. In a cohort of infants from Tucson, those destined to have recurrent viral-induced wheeze in the first 3 years of life demonstrated low $V'_{max}FRC$ levels in the first few months of life.[115] No other associations with reduced $V'_{max}FRC$ were demonstrated, as subjects who wheezed throughout the first 6 years of life and those who began wheezing in the latter half of this period did not demonstrate reductions in airway function. These results have been given broad applicability, although the early wheeze group contained a relatively small number of children, and as for any epidemiological study, the unique features of the environment where the study was performed must be considered.

Results from the Perth infant follow-up study differed from the Tucson data. In general, infant airway function assessed soon after birth in the Perth study was more predictive of long-term outcome than the Tucson cohort. In the Australian cohort consisting of 253 unselected infants recruited before birth, a

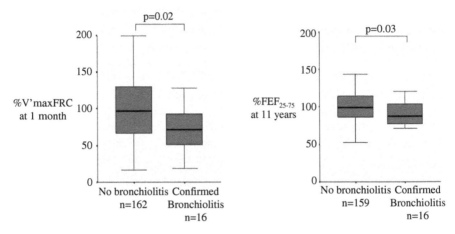

Figure 7.2a Box-and-whisker chart demonstrating reduced percent $V'_{max}FRC$ at 1 month and percent FEF_{25-75} at 11 years in cases with confirmed bronchiolotis. The smaller difference between groups at 11 years is a consequence of less variability in the measurement of FEF_{25-75}.

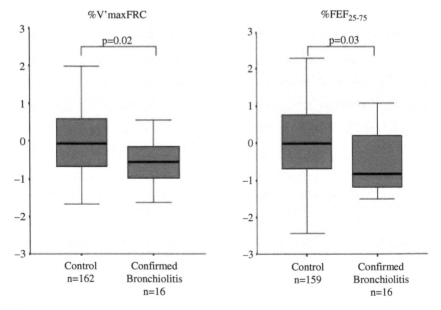

Figure 7.2b Box-and-whisker plot for z scores for $V'_{max}FRC$ at 1 month and FEF_{25-75} at 11 years. Note the absence of change in z score differences at 1 month and 11 years, indicating that the reduction in lung function is maintained over the years. (From Turner, S.W. et al. *Arch Dis Child* 2002; 87: 417–420. With permission.)

subgroup of 23 infants exhibited flow limitation on tidal expiration at their initial assessment at 1 month of age.[90,116] The majority of these infants were diagnosed by their local doctors as having asthma by the age of 2.[116] At 4 years of age, increased wheezing was noted in this subgroup compared with those who did not exhibit flow limitations.[90] At 6 years of age, they showed increased airway responsiveness to histamine and reduced FEV_1 and FEF_{25-75}. At age 11, the flow-limited group was still abnormal and exhibited increased airway responsiveness. Lung function was not statistically different compared with nonflow-limited children, although a trend to reduced FEF_{25-75} was observed.[90] The Perth data suggest that infants with the most impaired lung functions show increased symptoms and compromised respiratory functions that extend well beyond the first few years of life.

B.   Airway Responsiveness in Infancy

As noted earlier, factors that produce increased responsiveness to histamine or methacholine in infants remain unclear. However, the level of airway responsiveness in early life is highly predictive of respiratory outcome in the first 6 years of life. In the Perth study, infants with increased airway responsiveness at 1 month had highly significantly increased risk of diagnosis of asthma or wheezing before reaching 6 years of age or in the 12 months immediately preceding their 6-year assessments.[117] Airway responsiveness was observed to act independently of baseline respiratory function and atopy. Studies on the genetic variations associated with increased airway responsiveness in infancy are currently underway and may offer some clues as to the mechanisms involved in setting response level early in life.

C.   Predictive Values of Other Measurements of Infant Respiratory Function

The newer approaches to assessing airway and respiratory function in infants are likely to provide more accurate estimates of levels of physiological functions in early life and, therefore, may provide more accurate predictive data on outcomes in later life. Data to date are insufficient to indicate whether this is true. Studies assessing infant respiratory function are very labor-intensive and expensive, and many years must pass before data can be analyzed prospectively.

XI.   Summary

Over the past 20 years, improved methodologies for assessing respiratory function in infants have allowed more accurate measurements of function to be made in early life. The few studies that included these measurements and then followed subjects longitudinally have demonstrated that the level of respiratory function soon after birth is highly predictive of future physiological function and respiratory symptoms. The substantial differences in findings between studies may reflect the important impacts of environment on outcome.

References

1. Matthews LW and Doershuk CF. Measurement of pulmonary function in cystic fibrosis. *Bibl Paediatr* 1967; 86: 237–246.
2. Polgar G and Lacourt G. A method for measuring respiratory mechanics in small newborn (premature) infants. *J Appl Physiol* 1972; 32: 555–559.
3. Wohl ME, Stigol LC, and Mead J. Resistance of the total respiratory system in healthy infants and infants with bronchiolitis. *Pediatrics* 1969; 43: 495–509.
4. LeSouef PN, Lopes JM, England SJ, Bryan MH, and Bryan AC. Influence of chest wall distortion on esophageal pressure. *J Appl Physiol* 1983; 55: 353–358.
5. Beardsmore CS, Helms P, Stocks J, Hatch DJ, and Silverman M. Improved esophageal balloon technique for use in infants. *J Appl Physiol* 1980; 49: 735–742.
6. Lesouef PN, England SJ, and Bryan AC. Passive respiratory mechanics in newborns and children. *Am Rev Respir Dis* 1984; 129: 552–556.
7. Turner DJ, Stick SM, Lesouef KL, Sly PD, and Lesouef PN. A new technique to generate and assess forced expiration from raised lung volume in infants. *Am J Respir Crit Care Med* 1995; 151: 1441–1450.
8. Stocks J. Lung function testing in infants. *Pediatr Pulmonol Suppl* 1999; 18: 14–20.
9. Sly PD, Tepper R, Henschen M, Gappa M, and Stocks J. Tidal forced expirations: ERS/ATS Task Force on Standards for Infant Respiratory Function Testing. *Eur Respir J* 2000; 16: 741–748.
10. Stocks J and Godfrey S. Nasal resistance during infancy. *Respir Physiol* 1978; 34: 233–246.
11. Le Souef PN, Hughes DM, and Landau LI. Shape of forced expiratory flow-volume curves in infants. *Am Rev Respir Dis* 1988; 138: 590–597.
12. Stark AR, Cohlan BA, Waggener TB, Frantz ID, 3rd, and Kosch PC. Regulation of end-expiratory lung volume during sleep in premature infants. *J Appl Physiol* 1987; 62: 1117–1123.
13. Doershuk GF and Matthews LW. Airway resistance and lung volume in the newborn infant. *Pediatr Res* 1969; 3: 128–34.
14. Kosch PC and Stark AR. Dynamic maintenance of end-expiratory lung volume in full-term infants. *J Appl Physiol* 1984; 57: 1126–1133.
15. Malmberg LP, Pelkonen A, Hakulinen A, Hero M, Pohjavuori M, Skytta J, and Turpeinen M. Intraindividual variability of infant whole-body plethysmographic measurements: effects of age and disease. *Pediatr Pulmonol* 1999; 28: 356–362.
16. John J, Drefeldt B, Taskar V, Mansson C, and Jonson B. Dynamic properties of body plethysmographs and effects on physiological parameters. *J Appl Physiol* 1994; 77: 152–159.
17. Kraemer R. Whole-body plethysmography in the clinical assessment of infants with bronchopulmonary diseases. *Respiration* 1993; 60: 1–8.

18. Casaulta-Aebischer C and Kraemer R. Plethysmographic measurements in the clinical assessment of infants with bronchopulmonary disease. *Monaldi Arch Chest Dis* 1995; 50: 140–147.

19. Stocks J and Godfrey S. Specific airway conductance in relation to postconceptional age during infancy. *J Appl Physiol* 1977; 43: 144–154.

20. Beardsmore CS. Lung function from infancy to school age in cystic fibrosis. *Arch Dis Child* 1995; 73: 519–523.

21. Morris MJ and Lane DJ. Tidal expiratory flow patterns in air flow obstruction. *Thorax* 1981; 36: 135–142.

22. Lodrup-Carlsen KC and Carlsen KH. Lung function in awake healthy infants: the first five days of life. *Eur Respir J* 1993; 6: 1496–1500.

23. Lodrup Carlsen KC, Magnus P, and Carlsen KH. Lung function by tidal breathing in awake healthy newborn infants. *Eur Respir J* 1994; 7: 1660–1668.

24. Lodrup Carlsen KC, Stenzler A, and Carlsen KH. Determinants of tidal flow volume loop indices in neonates and children with and without asthma. *Pediatr Pulmonol* 1997; 24: 391–396.

25. Young S, Le Souef PN, Geelhoed GC, Stick SM, Turner KJ, and Landau LI. The influence of a family history of asthma and parental smoking on airway responsiveness in early infancy. [Erratum appears in *New Engl J Med* 1991; 325: 747.] *New Engl J Med* 1991; 324: 1168–1173.

26. Martinez FD, Morgan WJ, Wright AL, Holberg C, and Taussig LM. Initial airway function is a risk factor for recurrent wheezing respiratory illnesses during the first three years of life: Group Health Medical Associates. *Am Rev Respir Dis* 1991; 143: 312–316.

27. Martinez FD, Morgan WJ, Wright AL, Holberg CJ, and Taussig LM. Diminished lung function as a predisposing factor for wheezing respiratory illness in infants. *New Engl J Med* 1988; 319: 1112–1117.

28. Carlsen KH and Lodrup-Carlsen KC. Tidal breathing analysis and response to salbutamol in awake young children with and without asthma. *Eur Respir J* 1994; 7: 2154–2159.

29. van der Ent CK, Brackel HJ, van der Laag J, and Bogaard JM. Tidal breathing analysis as a measure of airway obstruction in children three years of age and older. *Am J Respir Crit Care Med* 1996; 153: 1253–1258.

30. Benoist MR, Brouard JJ, Rufin P, Delacourt C, Waernessyckle S, and Scheinmann P. Ability of new lung function tests to assess methacholine-induced airway obstruction in infants. *Pediatr Pulmonol* 1994; 18: 308–316.

31. Lodrup Carlsen KC, Halvorsen R, Ahlstedt S, and Carlsen KH. Eosinophil cationic protein and tidal flow volume loops in children 0–2 years of age. *Eur Respir J* 1995; 8: 1148–1154.

32. Lodrup Carlsen KC, and Carlsen KH. Inhaled nebulized adrenaline improves lung function in infants with acute bronchiolitis. *Respir Med* 2000; 94: 709–714.

33. Taussig LM. Maximal expiratory flows at functional residual capacity: a test of lung function for young children. *Am Rev Respir Dis* 1977; 116: 1031–1038.

34. Adler SM and Wohl ME. Flow-volume relationship at low lung volumes in healthy term newborn infants. *Pediatrics* 1978; 61: 636–640.

35. Taussig LM, Landau LI, Godfrey S, and Arad I. Determinants of forced expiratory flows in newborn infants. *J Appl Physiol Respir Env Exercise Physiol* 1982; 53: 1220–1227.

36. Tepper RS, Morgan WJ, Cota K, Wright A, and Taussig LM. Physiologic growth and development of the lung during the first year of life. [Erratum appears in *Am Rev Respir Dis* 1987; 136: 800]. *Am Rev Respir Dis* 1986; 134: 513–519.

37. Le Souef PN, Castile R, Turner DJ, Motoyama E, and Morgan WJ. *Forced Expiratory Maneuvers*. New York: Wiley–Liss, 1996.

38. Henschen M and Stocks J. Assessment of airway function using partial expiratory flow-volume curves: How reliable are measurements of maximal expiratory flow at frc during early infancy? *Am J Respir Crit Care Med* 1999; 159: 480–486.

39. Kosch PC, Davenport PW, Wozniak JA, and Stark AR. Reflex control of expiratory duration in newborn infants. *J Appl Physiol* 1985; 58: 575–581.

40. Stocks J, Sly PD, Tepper RS, and Morgan WJ. *Infant Respiratory Function Testing*. New York: John Wiley & Sons, 1996.

41. Turner DJ, Stick SM, Sly PD, and Le Souef PN. Respiratory function from raised lung volumes in normal and wheezy infants. *Am Rev Respir Dis* 1992; 145 (Abstr.): A248.

42. Ranganathan SC, Hoo AF, Lum SY, Goetz I, Castle RA, and Stocks J. Exploring the relationship between forced maximal flow at functional residual capacity and parameters of forced expiration from raised lung volume in healthy infants. *Pediatr Pulmonol* 2002; 33: 419–428.

43. Feher A, Castile R, Kisling J, Angelicchio C, Filbrun D, Flucke R et al. Flow limitation in normal infants: a new method for forced expiratory maneuvers from raised lung volumes. *J Appl Physiol* 1996; 80: 2019–2025.

44. Wildhaber JH, Dore ND, Devadason SG, Hall GL, Hamacher J, Arheden L et al. Comparison of subjective and objective measures in recurrently wheezy infants [comment]. *Respiration* 2002; 69: 397–405.

45. Modl M, Eber E, Weinhandl E, Gruber W, and Zach MS. Assessment of bronchodilator responsiveness in infants with bronchiolitis: a comparison of the tidal and raised volume rapid thoracoabdominal compression technique. *Am J Respir Crit Care Med* 2000; 161: 763–768.

46. Hall GL, Hantos Z, and Sly PD. Altered respiratory tissue mechanics in asymptomatic wheezy infants. *Am J Respir Crit Care Med* 2001; 164: 1387–1391.

47. Hayden MJ, Wildhaber JH, and LeSouef PN. Bronchodilator responsiveness testing using raised volume forced expiration in recurrently wheezing infants. *Pediatr Pulmonol* 1998; 26: 35–41.

48. Goldstein AB, Castile RG, Davis SD, Filbrun DA, Flucke RL, McCoy KS et al. Bronchodilator responsiveness in normal infants and young children. *Am J Respir Crit Care Med* 2001; 164: 447–454.

49. Hall GL, Hantos Z, Wildhaber JH, Petak F, and Sly PD. Methacholine responsiveness in infants assessed with low frequency forced oscillation and forced expiration techniques. *Thorax* 2001; 56: 42–47.

50. Hayden MJ, Devadason SG, Sly PD, Wildhaber JH, and LeSouef PN. Methacholine responsiveness using the raised volume forced expiration technique in infants. *Am J Respir Crit Care Med* 1997; 155: 1670–1675.

51. Jones M, Castile R, Davis S, Kisling J, Filbrun D, Flucke R et al. Forced expiratory flows and volumes in infants: normative data and lung growth. *Am J Respir Crit Care Med* 2000; 161: 353–359.
52. Tepper R, Merth IT, Newth CJL, and Gerhardt T. *Measurement of Functional Residual Capacity in Infants by Helium Dilution and Nitrogen Washout Techniques.* New York: Wiley–Liss; 1996.
53. Fumey MH, Nickerson BG, Birch M, McCrea R, and Kao LC. A radiographic method for estimating lung volumes in sick infants. *Pediatr Pulmonol* 1992; 13: 42–47.
54. Auld PAM. *Pulmonary Physiology of the Newborn Infant.* Philadelphia: Lea & Febiger; 1975.
55. Morris MG, Gustafsson P, Tepper R, Gappa M, and Stocks J. Testing EATFoSfIRF: the bias flow nitrogen washout technique for measuring the functional residual capacity in infants. *Eur Respir J* 2001; 17: 529–536.
56. Schibler A, Hall GL, Businger F, Reinmann B, Wildhaber JH, Cernelc M et al. Measurement of lung volume and ventilation distribution with an ultrasonic flow meter in healthy infants. *Eur Respir J* 2002; 20: 912–918.
57. Hjalmarson O and Sandberg K. Abnormal lung function in healthy preterm infants. *Am J Respir Crit Care Med* 2002; 165: 83–87.
58. Shao H, Sandberg K, and Hjalmarson O. Impaired gas mixing and low lung volume in preterm infants with mild chronic lung disease. *Pediatr Res* 1998; 43: 536–541.
59. Gerhardt T, Reifenberg L, Hehre D, Feller R, and Bancalari E. Functional residual capacity in normal neonates and children up to 5 years of age determined by N_2 washout method. *Pediatr Res* 1986; 20: 668–671.
60. Gappa M, Fletcher ME, Dezateux CA, and Stocks J. Comparison of nitrogen washout and plethysmographic measurements of lung volume in healthy infants. *Am Rev Respir Dis* 1993; 148: 1496–1501.
61. Wauer RR, Maurer T, Nowotny T, and Schmalisch G. Assessment of functional residual capacity using nitrogen washout and plethysmographic techniques in infants with and without bronchopulmonary dysplasia. *Intensive Care Med* 1998; 24: 469–475.
62. DuBois AB, Brody AW, Lewis DW, and Burgess BF. Oscillation mechanics of lungs and chest in man. *J Appl Physiol* 1956; 8: 587–594.
63. Lutchen KR. *Understanding Pulmonary Mechanics Using the Forced Oscillation Technique: Emphasis on Breathing Frequencies.* New York: Plenum Press, 1996.
64. Desager KN, Marchal F, and Van de Woestijne KP. *Forced Oscillation Technique.* New York: Wiley–Liss, 1996.
65. Hantos Z, Daroczy B, Suki B, Galgoczy G, and Csendes T. Forced oscillatory impedance of the respiratory system at low frequencies. *J Appl Physiol* 1986; 60: 123–132.
66. Sly PD, Hayden MJ, Petak F, and Hantos Z. Measurement of low-frequency respiratory impedance in infants. *Am J Respir Crit Care Med* 1996; 154: 161–166.
67. Hall GL, Hantos Z, Petak F, Wildhaber JH, Tiller K, Burton PR et al. Airway and respiratory tissue mechanics in normal infants. *Am J Respir Crit Care Med* 2000; 162: 1397–1402.

68. Hayden MJ, Petak F, Hantos Z, Hall G, and Sly PD. Using low-frequency oscillation to detect bronchodilator responsiveness in infants. *Am J Respir Crit Care Med* 1998; 157: 574–579.

69. Prendiville A, Green S, and Silverman M. Bronchial responsiveness to histamine in wheezy infants. *Thorax* 1987; 42: 92–99.

70. Le Souef PN, Geelhoed GC, Turner DJ, Morgan SE, and Landau LI. Response of normal infants to inhaled histamine. *Am Rev Respir Dis* 1989; 139: 62–66.

71. Geller DE, Morgan WJ, Cota KA, Wright AL, and Taussig LM. Airway responsiveness to cold, dry air in normal infants. *Pediatr Pulmonol* 1988; 4: 90–97.

72. Stick SM, Turnbull S, Chua HL, Landau LI, and Lesouef PN. Bronchial responsiveness to histamine in infants and older children [comment]. *Am Rev Respir Dis* 1990; 142: 1143–1146.

73. Turner DJ, Sly PD, and LeSouef PN. Assessment of forced expiratory volume-time parameters in detecting histamine-induced bronchoconstriction in wheezy infants. *Pediatr Pulmonol* 1993; 15: 220–224.

74. Bramer SL and Kallungal BA. Clinical considerations in study designs that use cotinine as a biomarker. *Biomarkers* 2003; 8: 187–203.

75. Foundas M, Hawkrigg NC, Smith SM, Devadason SG, and Le Souef PN. Urinary cotinine levels in early pregnancy. *Aust NZ J Obstetr Gynaecol* 1997; 37: 383–386.

76. Lodrup Carlsen KC, Jaakkola JJ, Nafstad P, and Carlsen KH. *In utero* exposure to cigarette smoking influences lung function at birth. *Eur Respir J* 1997; 10: 1774–1779.

77. Le Souef PN. Pediatric origins of adult lung diseases. 4. Tobacco-related lung diseases begin in childhood. *Thorax* 2000; 55: 1063–1067.

78. Lodrup Carlsen KC and Carlsen KH. Effects of maternal and early tobacco exposure on the development of asthma and airway hyperreactivity. *Curr Opin Allergy Clin Immunol* 2001; 1: 139–143.

79. Young S, Arnott J, O'Keeffe PT, Le Souef PN, and Landau LI. The association between early life lung function and wheezing during the first 2 yrs of life. *Eur Respir J* 2000; 15: 151–157.

80. Hanrahan JP, Tager IB, Segal MR, Tosteson TD, Castile RG, Van Vunakis H et al. The effect of maternal smoking during pregnancy on early infant lung function. *Am Rev Respir Dis* 1992; 145: 1129–1135.

81. Murray CS, Pipis SD, McArdle EC, Lowe LA, Custovic A, and Woodcock A. Lung function at one month of age as a risk factor for infant respiratory symptoms in a high risk population. *Thorax* 2002; 57: 388–392.

82. Hoo AF, Henschen M, Dezateux C, Costeloe K, and Stocks J. Respiratory function among preterm infants whose mothers smoked during pregnancy. *Am J Respir Crit Care Med* 1998; 158: 700–705.

83. Dezateux C, Stocks J, Wade AM, Dundas I, and Fletcher ME. Airway function at one year: association with premorbid airway function, wheezing, and maternal smoking. *Thorax* 2001; 56: 680–686.

84. Lux AL, Henderson AJ, and Pocock SJ. Wheeze associated with prenatal tobacco smoke exposure: a prospective, longitudinal study. *Arch Dis Child* 2000; 83: 307–312.

85. Dezateux C, Stocks J, Dundas I, and Fletcher ME. Impaired airway function and wheezing in infancy: the influence of maternal smoking and a genetic predisposition to asthma. *Am J Respir Crit Care Med* 1999; 159: 403–410.

86. Adler A, Ngo L, Tosta P, and Tager IB. Association of tobacco smoke exposure and respiratory syncytial virus infection with airways reactivity in early childhood. *Pediatr Pulmonol* 2001; 32: 418–427.

87. Yuan W, Fonager K, Olsen J, and Sorensen HT. Prenatal factors and use of anti-asthma medications in early childhood: a population-based Danish birth cohort study. *Eur J Epidemiol* 2003; 18: 763–768.

88. Martinez FD, Antognoni G, Macri F, Bonci E, Midulla F, De Castro G et al. Parental smoking enhances bronchial responsiveness in nine-year-old children. *Am Rev Respir Dis* 1988; 138: 518–523.

89. Gilliland FD, Li YF, and Peters JM. Effects of maternal smoking during pregnancy and environmental tobacco smoke on asthma and wheezing in children. *Am J Respir Crit Care Med* 2001; 163: 429–436.

90. Turner SW, Palmer LJ, Rye PJ, Gibson NA, Judge PK, Young S et al. Infants with flow limitation at 4 weeks: outcome at 6 and 11 years. *Am J Respir Crit Care Med* 2002; 165: 1294–1298.

91. Meyers DA, Bleecker ER, Jonepier H, Ampleford E, Koppelman GH, and Postma DS. Genetic susceptibility to asthma and exposure to passive smoking (abstract). *Eur Respir J* 2003; 22.

92. Greenough A, Maconochie I, and Yuksel B. Recurrent respiratory symptoms in the first year of life following preterm delivery. *J Perinat Med* 1990; 18: 489–494.

93. Thomas M, Greenough A, Johnson A, Limb E, Marlow N, Peacock JL et al. Frequent wheeze at follow-up of very preterm infants: which factors are predictive? *Arch Dis Child Fetal Neonatal Ed* 2003; 88: F329–F332.

94. Speer CP and Silverman M. Issues relating to children born prematurely. *Eur Respir J* (Suppl.) 1998; 27: 13s–16s.

95. Parat S, Moriette G, Delaperche MF, Escourrou P, Denjean A, and Gaultier C. Long-term pulmonary functional outcome of bronchopulmonary dysplasia and premature birth. *Pediatr Pulmonol* 1995; 20: 289–296.

96. Bracken MB, Triche EW, Belanger K, Saftlas A, Beckett WS, and Leaderer BP. Asthma symptoms, severity, and drug therapy: a prospective study of effects on 2205 pregnancies. *Obstetr Gynecol* 2003; 102: 739–752.

97. Hagan R, Minutillo C, French N, Reese A, Landau L, and LeSouef P. Neonatal chronic lung disease, oxygen dependency, and a family history of asthma. *Pediatr Pulmonol* 1995; 20: 277–283.

98. Hall IP. Genetics and pulmonary medicine 8: asthma. *Thorax* 1999; 54: 65–69.

99. Erickson RP and Graves PE. Genetic variation in beta-adrenergic receptors and their relationship to susceptibility for asthma and therapeutic response. *Drug Metab Dispos* 2001; 29: 557–561.

100. Taylor DR and Kennedy MA. Genetic variation of the beta-(2)-adrenoceptor: its functional and clinical importance in bronchial asthma. *Am J Pharmacogenomics* 2001; 1: 165–174.

101. Martinez FD, Graves PE, Baldini M, Solomon S, and Erickson R. Association between genetic polymorphisms of the beta-2-adrenoceptor and response to albuterol in children with and without a history of wheezing. *J Clin Invest* 1997; 100: 3184–3188.

102. Israel E, Drazen JM, Liggett SB, Boushey HA, Cherniack RM, Chinchilli VM et al. The effect of polymorphisms of the beta-(2)-adrenergic receptor on the response to regular use of albuterol in asthma. *Am J Respir Crit Care Med* 2000; 162: 75–80.

103. Ramsay CE, Hayden CM, Tiller KJ, Burton PR, Goldblatt J, and Lesouef PN. Polymorphisms in the beta-2-adrenoreceptor gene are associated with decreased airway responsiveness. *Clin Exp Allergy* 1999; 29: 1195–1203.

104. Sengler C, Heinzmann A, Jerkic SP, Haider A, Sommerfeld C, Niggemann B et al. Clara cell protein 16 (CC16) gene polymorphism influences the degree of airway responsiveness in asthmatic children. *J Allergy Clin Immunol* 2003; 111: 515–519.

105. Sayers I, Barton S, Rorke S, Beghe B, Hayward B, Van Eerdewegh P et al. Allelic association and functional studies of promoter polymorphism in the leukotriene C4 synthase gene (LTC4S) in asthma. *Thorax* 2003; 58: 417–424.

106. Cole FS, Hamvas A, and Nogee LM. Genetic disorders of neonatal respiratory function. *Pediatr Res* 2001; 50: 157–162.

107. Young S, Sherrill DL, Arnott J, Diepeveen D, LeSouef PN, and Landau LI. Parental factors affecting respiratory function during the first year of life. *Pediatr Pulmonol* 2000; 29: 331–340.

108. Dezateux C and Stocks J. Lung development and early origins of childhood respiratory illness. *Br Med Bull* 1997; 53: 40–57.

109. Stocks J, Henschen M, Hoo AF, Costeloe K, and Dezateux C. Influence of ethnicity and gender on airway function in preterm infants. *Am J Respir Crit Care Med* 1997; 156: 1855–1862.

110. Stocks J, Gappa M, Rabbette PS, Hoo AF, Mukhtar Z, Costeloe KL et al. A comparison of respiratory function in Afro-Caribbean and Caucasian infants: influence of ethnicity and gender on airway function in preterm infants. *Eur Respir J* 1994; 7: 11–16.

111. Pullan CR and Hey EN. Wheezing, asthma, and pulmonary dysfunction 10 years after infection with respiratory syncytial virus in infancy. *Br Med J* 1982; 284: 1665–1669.

112. Sly PD, Hibbert ME, Lin HC, Hwang KC, Yang YH, Lin YT et al. Childhood asthma following hospitalization with acute viral bronchiolitis in infancy: risk factors of wheeze and allergy after lower respiratory tract infections during early childhood. *Pediatr Pulmonol* 1989; 7: 153–158.

113. Hall CB, Hall WJ, Gala CL, MaGill FB, Leddy JP, Lin HC et al. Long-term prospective study in children after respiratory syncytial virus infection: risk factors of wheeze and allergy after lower respiratory tract infections during early childhood. *J Pediatr* 1984; 105: 358–364.

114. Turner SW, Young S, Landau LI, and Le Souef PN. Reduced lung function both before bronchiolitis and at 11 years. *Arch Dis Child* 2002; 87: 417–420.

115. Martinez FD, Wright AL, Taussig LM, Holberg CJ, Halonen M, and Morgan WJ. Asthma and wheezing in the first six years of life. *New Engl J Med* 1995; 332: 133–138.

116. Young S, Arnott J, Le Souef PN, and Landau LI. Flow limitation during tidal expiration in symptom-free infants and the subsequent development of asthma. *J Pediatr* 1994; 124: 681–688.
117. Palmer LJ, Rye PJ, Gibson NA, Burton PR, Landau LI, and Lesouef PN. Airway responsiveness in early infancy predicts asthma, lung function, and respiratory symptoms by school age. *Am J Respir Crit Care Med* 2001; 163: 37–42.

8

Genetic Factors

SABINE HOFFJAN and CAROLE OBER

University of Chicago
Chicago, Illinois, U.S.A.

I. Introduction

Asthma is a complex and multifactorial disease that affects nearly 155 million individuals worldwide.[1,2] A genetic component to asthma has long been suggested: the disease clusters in families and monozygotic twins show higher concordance rates compared with dizygotic twins,[3–7] but identifying asthma genes has been a daunting task. In contrast to monogenic disorders (e.g., cystic fibrosis) in which mutations in a single gene lead to the development of the disease in nearly all cases, the etiologies of common diseases such as asthma, coronary artery disease, and diabetes are complex (Figure 8.1), making genetic studies challenging.

First, the causes of these diseases are *multifactorial*, with environmental as well as genetic factors contributing to the expression of phenotypes. In fact, the rising incidence of asthma over the past decades underlines the importance of environmental and lifestyle factors.[8–11] Second, common diseases such as asthma are genetically *heterogeneous*, with variations in more than one gene influencing susceptibility. Furthermore, these susceptibility loci interact in complex (and often unknown) ways. The results of 12 genome-wide screens (see below) suggest that

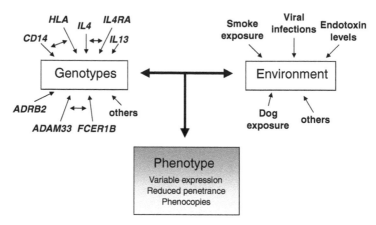

Figure 8.1 In complex genetic disorders such as asthma, the expression of the disease phenotype is influenced by variations in many genes and by many environmental factors. Unambiguously distinguishing affected and unaffected individuals is difficult because the expression of the phenotype is usually variable and phenocopies can exist (see text). Gene–gene and gene–environment interactions also play important roles in influencing disease expression. HLA-DRB1 = human leukocyte antigen DRB1. IL4 (13) = interleukin 4 (13). IL4RA = interleukin 4 receptor alpha chain. FCER1B = high affinity IgE receptor beta chain. ADRB2 = beta 2 adrenergic receptor.

at least 20 different asthma susceptibility loci exist and that each individually makes small contributions to overall asthma risk. As a result, susceptibility to asthma may be caused by different genes in different families, making traditional disease mapping approaches challenging.

It is often difficult to classify individuals unambiguously as "affected" and "unaffected" in family studies because the *expression of phenotypes can be variable.* The "asthma" phenotypes in individuals even with the same genetic susceptibilities may differ substantially with regard to age of onset, disease severity, and presence of associated phenotypes. For example, some family members may have severe asthma with onset in childhood, while others show only bronchial hyperresponsiveness (BHR) or atopy. Even ostensibly healthy individuals may carry the susceptibility gene because in complex diseases, mutations at susceptibility loci do not always lead to development of the disease (i.e., penetrance is always less than 100%).

To address this problem, many study designs use only clearly affected individuals in the analyses, ignoring apparently unaffected family members or sometimes even those with mild forms of the disease. Further, individuals in one family may even have the same phenotype (asthma) due to different underlying causes. Such individuals are called *phenocopies*. While one member of a family, for example, may exhibit asthma symptoms because he or she inherited a certain susceptibility allele (or alleles), another member may have aspirin-induced or another environmentally induced type of asthma. All these features of common diseases complicate gene mapping studies. While some can be taken into account in the analysis, all have the potential to reduce power and increase the error rate, often in unpredictable directions.

Gene–gene interactions likely play an important role in determining susceptibility, but such complex models have been considered in only a small number of genetic studies. For example, a variant in one gene may influence asthma susceptibility only if another variant in a different gene is also present. Thus, the effect of the first gene may be detected only if genotypes at both loci are considered simultaneously. In other cases, a susceptibility allele may cause asthma only in the presence of an environmental trigger (*gene–environment interaction*), such as viral infection, tobacco smoke exposure, or endotoxin exposure. Incorporating gene–gene and gene–environment interactions in genetic studies may lead to a better understanding of the complex factors underlying the development of asthma.[12–16]

Unraveling the genetics of complex disorders such as asthma has proven much more difficult than identifying genes for monogenic disorders. Despite the difficulties, steady progress has been made over the last decade, and some "asthma genes" have been identified. This chapter presents an overview of laboratory techniques, statistical methodologies, and the current status of asthma and atopy genome-wide screens, along with a review of candidate gene studies in biological pathways known to be important in asthma.

II. Laboratory Techniques and Study Designs

Although it has long been known that DNA provides an unlimited source of polymorphism,[17] recent advances in mapping and identifying asthma susceptibility loci can be attributed primarily to the development and automation of genotyping techniques and sophisticated analytical tools. Because only about 5 to 10% of the human genome contains functional genes, a large part of the genome can mutate (presumably) without functional consequences. A polymorphic locus is a site in the genome at which more than one allele is present in the population, with the frequency of the rarer (minor) allele at least 1%. Three types of polymorphic markers are primarily used for mapping studies (Figure 8.2).

Microsatellite markers (or short tandem repeat polymorphisms, STRPs) are composed of short DNA sequences that are repeated in different numbers from individual to individual. Insertion–deletion (In/Del) polymorphisms are fragments of one or more base pairs that are present (inserted) on some chromosomes and absent (deleted) on others. Single nucleotide polymorphisms

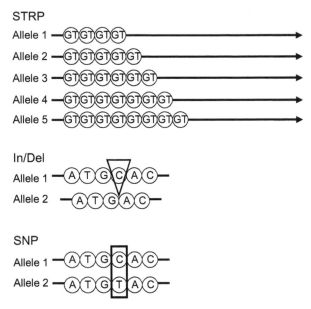

Figure 8.2 Genetic markers used in linkage and association studies. Short tandem repeat polymorphisms (STRPs) are composed of short DNA sequences (GT in this example) present in various copy numbers on different chromosomes in the population, representing the different alleles at this locus. In this example, alleles with four to eight repeats are shown. STRPs are generally found in noncoding regions of the genome. Insertion–deletion (In/Del) polymorphisms are short DNA fragments, in this example only a single base pair present (inserted) on some chromosomes and absent (deleted) on others. Single nucleotide polymorphisms (SNPs) are loci at which a single base pair differs between chromosomes in the population. A C/T SNP is shown in this example. While STRPs are usually multiallelic (more than two alleles present in the population), In/Dels and SNPs are biallelic (two alleles in the population).

(SNPs) are polymorphic loci at which one base pair at a certain position differs between chromosomes (e.g., adenosine [A] on some chromosomes and guanine [G] on others). In/Dels and SNPs are generally biallelic (two alleles present in the population). STRPs are usually multi-allelic, with as many as 10 or more alleles present at some loci. The work of many publicly funded consortia has made available in public databases a large — and rapidly increasing —number of known common polymorphisms such as dbSNP (http://www.ncbi.nlm.nih.gov/SNP) or SNPper (http://iipga:iipga@snpper.chip.org/bio/snpper-enter).

STRPs with multiple alleles are particularly useful for family-based linkage studies that examine whether alleles at certain marker loci are shared by affected individuals within families more often than expected by chance alone. Increased sharing of alleles among affected relatives indicates that a chromosomal region containing a marker locus also contains a gene that contributes to disease susceptibility. Placement of 400 or more STRP markers (or 10,000 SNPS) throughout the genome in a genome-wide screen makes it likely that "linkage" to a susceptibility locus anywhere in the genome can be detected.

The advantage of a genome-wide screen is that it can potentially identify all genes with detectable effects on asthma susceptibility regardless of any prior knowledge of the function of the susceptibility locus. Thus, novel genes may be identified as asthma susceptibility loci with this approach. Because genome-wide screens involve many hundreds of statistical tests, criteria for establishing a significant linkage have been debated.[18–20]

For example, Lander and Kruglyak proposed that suggestive evidence of linkage requires a p $\leq$0.002 (equivalent to LOD $\geq$1.9) and genome-wide significance requires a p $\leq$0.000049 (equivalent to LOD $\geq$3.3) in a linkage study of affected sibling pairs.[18] Once a candidate region is identified in a linkage analysis, positional cloning can be used to identify the disease-causing gene.[21] If candidate genes (see below) exist in the linked region, direct screening of these candidate genes is referred to as positional candidate cloning.

However, because complex diseases likely result from many genes with individually small effects, standard linkage analysis has limited power to detect all susceptibility loci.[22,23] *Association studies*, on the other hand, examine whether a certain allele is more common in affected individuals than in controls, and are most commonly used for *candidate gene studies*. In contrast to genome-wide linkage studies, the candidate gene approach focuses on known genes (candidates) chosen because their functions suggest that they may influence the disease phenotype (e.g., cytokines, cytokine receptors, and chemokines in asthma).

These studies are often conducted on samples of unrelated cases and unrelated controls. Significantly higher frequencies of alleles at candidate loci in cases compared with controls may indicate a causal relationship between a marker allele and a disease; for example, a variant may result in an amino acid exchange, modify exon–intron splicing, or affect transcription, and thereby directly affect function. Alternatively, the variant may be in linkage disequilibrium (LD) with the true susceptibility allele. LD, or allelic association, is the nonrandom association of alleles at linked loci in populations. As LD will be detected only over relatively small distances,[24–26] the disease-causing variant must therefore be close to the associated (marker) allele (usually less than approximately 60 kilobases).

Although association studies of candidate loci are simpler to perform than linkage studies, there are potential problems with with these studies. False positive results can occur due to population admixture. If, for example, one allele is more common in ethnic group A compared with ethnic group B, the allele frequency may be significantly higher in the cases than in the controls merely because the case group contains more people of ethnic group A than the control group.

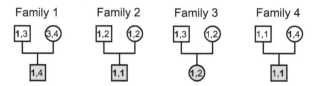

Figure 8.3 The transmission disequilibrium test (TDT) evaluates whether an allele at a marker locus is transmitted from heterozygous parents to an affected child more often than would be expected by chance alone. In this example, allele 1 is present in six heterozygous parents. We would expect this allele to be transmitted to three offspring and not transmitted to three, based on random segregation. However, in this example, it is transmitted to five children and not transmitted to only one child, consistent with evidence for an association with the 1 allele. In family 4, the homozygous father is not informative and not considered in the TDT.

This problem can be avoided by using *family-based association methods.* One example is the transmission disequilibrium test (TDT)[27] that evaluates whether a certain allele at a marker locus is transmitted significantly more often from heterozygous parents to an affected child than would be expected by chance alone (Figure 8.3). Because the nontransmitted allele serves as the control, these tests are robust to population admixture. However, although these studies only require genotyping trios (affected child and parents), they still require the collection of (small) families, making them more costly and time-consuming than sampling unrelated cases and controls. Further, only heterozygous parents are included in the analysis, so the TDT is less powerful than case-control studies of similar sample sizes. Finally, because many different markers, alleles, and haplotypes are often examined, spurious results may arise as a result of the large number of comparisons.

While thresholds of significance have been carefully considered for interpreting genome-wide linkage studies (see above), similar thresholds have not been determined for association studies. Using a standard Bonferroni correction for multiple comparisons is usually overly conservative because many tests are often correlated. Thus, many results of association studies are reported without correcting for multiple comparisons, and the significance of these studies is difficult to interpret. On the other hand, negative results may be due to a small sample size that reduces the power to detect an association. A complete survey of variations and the patterns of linkage disequilibrium must be examined before a negative study can truly exclude a gene. Because most association studies of asthma have been conducted in relatively small samples (<100 cases and controls) and have not surveyed all the variations in the genes, many negative studies may have prematurely dismissed a gene as contributing to susceptibility.

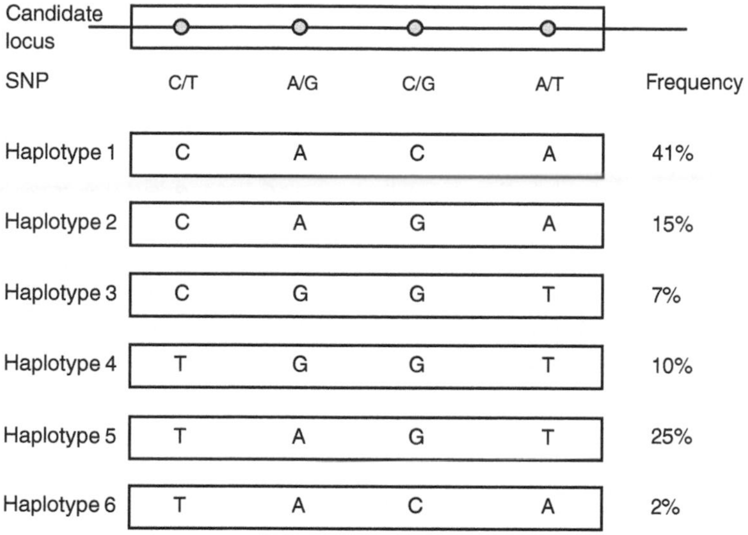

	Candidate locus				
SNP	C/T	A/G	C/G	A/T	Frequency
Haplotype 1	C	A	C	A	41%
Haplotype 2	C	A	G	A	15%
Haplotype 3	C	G	G	T	7%
Haplotype 4	T	G	G	T	10%
Haplotype 5	T	A	G	T	25%
Haplotype 6	T	A	C	A	2%

Figure 8.4 A haplotype is composed of alleles at different loci that are inherited together on the same chromosome. In this example, a candidate locus has four SNPs. Only 6 of 16 possible haplotype combinations are present in the population.

In fact, many recent studies indicate that considering multiple SNPs as *haplotypes* is preferable to single SNP analysis.[28–30] A haplotype is composed of alleles at different loci inherited together on the same chromosome (Figure 8.4). Thus, even if the disease-causing variant is not identified, a shared haplotype that contains the disease variant will be more common in cases than in controls. Overall, both linkage and association studies have proven useful for identifying asthma genes. The major results of these studies are presented below.

III. Genome-Wide Screens

Genome-wide screens for asthma and related phenotypes (including BHR, elevated total and specific IgE, eosinophil levels and positive skin prick tests [SPTs]) have been completed in 12 study populations to date (Table 8.1). Although many of the results vary among the studies, quite a bit of consensus was found overall. For example, 20 regions met the criteria for genome-wide significance in at least one study or suggestive evidence of linkage in at least two studies (Table 8.2). The five regions meeting genome-wide significance are on chromosomes 2p,[31] 2q,[32] 5q,[33] 7q,[34] and 11q.[35]

Table 8.1 Genome-Wide Searches for Susceptibility Loci for Asthma, Atopy, and Associated Phenotypes

Study	Sample	Ascertainment	Phenotypes
Daniels et al. [35]	172 sib pairs in 80 families from **Busselton**, Western Australia (primary sample); 268 sib pairs in 77 families from U.K. (replication sample)	Population-based	Slope BHR, atopy score, skin test index, total serum IgE, eosinophil count, asthma
CSGA [43, 181, 182]	266 families from three ethnic groups in the **U.S.**	Sib pairs with asthma	Asthma, total serum IgE
Ober et al. [32, 183, 184]	Inbred **Hutterite** pedigree; 693 individuals	Population-based	Asthma, BHR Symptoms, SPT to 14 allergens
Wjst et al. [185, 186]	156 affected sib pairs from 97 **German** families	Sib pairs with asthma	Asthma, BHR, slope BHR, peak flow, total serum IgE, RAST, eosinophil count
Dizier et al. [187]	297 affected sib pairs in 107 **French** families (46 families in primary sample; 61 in replication sample)	Sib pairs with asthma	Asthma, SPT, slope BHR, total serum IgE, eosinophil count
Xu et al. [34]; Koppelmann et al. [188]	1174 individuals in 200 **Dutch** families	Parent with asthma diagnosed between 1962 and 1975	Total serum IgE, specific IgE to aeroallergens and Der p 1, SPT to 16 allergens, eosinophil count
Yokouchi et al. [33]	65 affected sib pairs in 47 Japanese families (**Japanese 1**)	Sib pairs with mite-sensitive atopic asthma	Mite-sensitive atopic asthma

Reference	Sample	Ascertainment	Phenotype
Laitinen et al. [189]	220 affected individuals (asthma) in 86 **Finnish** pedigrees (primary sample); 80 affected individuals (asthma) in 22 French Canadian families (replication 1); 114 affected individuals (high IgE) in 29 families (replication 2)	Relative pairs with asthma (primary sample, replication 1) or high IgE (replication 2)	Asthma
Xu et al. [31]	2551 individuals in 533 **Chinese** families	Sib pairs with asthma	FEV_1, FVC, slope BHR, total serum IgE, eosinophil count, SPT to cockroach and house dust mite
Haagerup et al. [190]	33 affected sib pairs in 33 Danish families (**Danish 1**)	Sib pairs with allergic rhinitis	Allergic rhinitis
Haagerup et al. [191]	39 (asthma), 45 (total IgE) and 57 (specific IgE) affected sib pairs in 100 Danish families (**Danish 2**)	Sib pairs with asthma, increased total and specific IgE	Asthma, total serum IgE, RAST $\geq$ 1
Yokouchi et al. [192]	67 affected sib pairs in 48 Japanese families (**Japanese 2**)	Sib pairs with orchard grass–sensitive seasonal allergic rhinitis	Seasonal allergic rhinitis, orchard grass-specific RAST, total serum IgE
Hakonarson et al. [36]	596 affected individuals (asthma) in 175 **Icelandic** families	Proband with asthma, from a population registry	Asthma

Table 8.2 Regions with p Values ≤0.000049 or LOD Values ≥3.3 in at Least One Study or p ≤0.002 or LOD ≥1.9 in at Least Two Studies

Chromosome	Flanking Marker(s)	cM from pter^	Study Population+	Phenotypes	Linkage to Syntenic Regions in Mouse Models
1p	D1S468	4–20	Hutterites	Strict asthma (**p = 0.0002**)	
	D1S2667		Japanese 2	SAR, total IgE (**p <0.002**)	
			Danish 2	Asthma (**LOD = 2.02**)	
2p*	D2S1780	~10	Chinese	Slope BHR (**p = 0.00002**)	
2q*	D2S2944	173–210	Hutterites	SPT cockroach (**p = 0.00004**)	
	D2S116		German	Total IgE (**p = 0.0016**)	
	D2S1776–D2S1391		Dutch	Total IgE (**LOD = 1.96**), eosinophils (LOD = 1.49)	
3p	D3S3564	52–68	Hutterites	Loose asthma (**p = 0.0004**)	
			Japanese 2	Total IgE (**p <0.001**)	
4q	D4S1647	104–117	Chinese	SPT (**p = 0.0003**)	
			Danish 1	Allergic rhinitis (**LOD = 2.83**)	
4q	D4S2417–D4S408	181–207	Japanese 1	Mite-sensitive asthma (**p = 0.0002**)	
	D4S426		Busselton	Slope BHR (**p <0.0005**)	
5p	D5S268	33–45	French	Slope BHR (**p = 0.001**)	
	D5S1470		Hutterites	BHR (**p = 0.001**)	
5q*	D5S820–D5S1471	105–172	Japanese 1	Mite-sensitive asthma (**p = 0.0000013**)	BALBc×BP$_2$ F$_2$: eosinophil infiltration in brochial epithelium (**LOD = 2.5**) [40]
	D5S2014		Hutterites	Asthma symptoms (**p = 0.0009**), asthma (**p = 0.0007**)	
	D5S666–D5S402		Dutch	Total IgE (**LOD = 2.73**)	
	D5S410		Japanese 2	Total IgE (**p <0.001**)	
			Danish 2	Asthma (**LOD = 2.20**), total IgE (**LOD = 2.12**)	
6p	D6S276, D6S291	34–60	Busselton	Eosinophils (**p <0.0001**), atopy (p <0.005), total IgE (p <0.05)	BALBc×BP$_2$ F$_2$: BHR (**LOD = 2.1**) [40]
	D6S1281		CSGA (Caucasians)	Asthma (**p = 0.003, LOD = 1.91**)	(A)×C3H/HeJ)F$_1$×C3H/HeJ: BHR (**LOD = 1.7**) [38]
	D6S276–D6S291		German	Total IgE (**p = 0.0012**), RAST (**p = 0.0011**), eosinophils (**p = 0.0005**), asthma (p = 0.0081)	C57BL/6J×A/J) F$_1$× C57BL/6J: BHR (**LOD = 2.83**) [37]
	D6S1959–D6S2439		Japanese 1	Mite-sensitive asthma (**p = 0.0009**)	
			Danish 2	Asthma (**LOD = 2.41**)	

Chromosome	Marker	Distance (cM)	Population	Finding	Animal model
7p	D7S484–D7S2250	50–67	Busselton	BHR (p <0.0005), total IgE (p <0.005), eosinophils (p <0.05)	
	D7S817–D7S2436		Finnish	IgE, asthma (p = 0.02[a])	
	D7S484		French	Eosinophils (p = 0.002)	
7q*	D7S820–D7S821	98–09	Dutch	Total IgE (LOD = 3.36, SPT aeroallergens (LOD = 1.04)	
10q	D10S581	75–82	German	PEFR (p = 0.0017)	
			Icelandic	Asthma (LOD ≅ 2.0)	
11q*	FCERB	58–60	Busselton	Skin test index (p <0.00005), total IgE (p <0.005)	
	D11S1985		U.S. (African American)	Asthma (LOD = 2.00)	
12q	D12S366	111–134	French	Eosinophils (p = 0.0003)	
	D12S78–D12S79, D12S86		Japanese 1	Mite-sensitive asthma (p = 0.001)	
	PAH–D12S2070		Dutch	Total IgE (LOD = 2.46, p = 0.0004)	
	D12S86		Japanese 2	Total IgE (p <0.001)	
13q	D13S787	6–45	Hutterites	Asthma symptoms (p = 0.0006)	
	D13S175–D13S217, D13S153		Japanese 1	Mite-sensitive asthma (p = 0.0004, p = 0.001)	
	D13S1493–D13S218, D13S788		Dutch	Total IgE (LOD = 2.28), SPT (LOD = 1.27)	
	D13S270–D13S153		Busselton	Atopy (p <0.001)	
	D13S153		French	Eosinophils (p = 0.002)	
14q*b	GATA193A07	75–108	Hutterites	Asthma (p = 0.0001 TDT)	
	D14S588–D14S603		Icelandic	Asthma (LOD = 2.66[b])	
16p	D16S412	40–42	Chinese	FVC (p = 0.0006)	
	D16S3046		Japanese 2	RAST orchard grass (p <0.001)	
16q	D16S289	105–125	Busselton	Total IgE (p <0.0005), slope BHR (p <0.05)	
	D16S539		Hutterites	SPT molds (p = 0.0008)	
17q	D17S250	62–100	French	SPT (p = 0.001), asthma (p = 0.003)	
			Dutch	Eosinophils (LOD = 1.97), SPT mite (LOD = 1.21)	BALBc×BP$_2$ F$_2$: BHR (LOD = 3.8) [40]

Table 8.2 (continued) Regions with p Values ≤0.000049 or LOD Values ≥3.3 in at Least One Study or p ≤0.002 or LOD ≥1.9 in at Least Two Studies

Chromosome	Flanking Marker(s)	cM from pter^	Study Population+	Phenotypes	Linkage to Syntenic Regions in Mouse Models
19q	D19S900–D19S540	52–70	Hutterites	BHR (**p <0.001**)	(AJ×C3H/HeJ)F₁×A/J: allergen-induced AHR (**LOD = 1.9**) [39]
	D19S433		Chinese	BHR (**p = 0.002**)	(AJ×C3H/HeJ)F₁× C3H/HeJ: BHR (**LOD = 3.8**) [38]

Note: Regions identified by markers showing evidence for linkage that were ≤20 cM apart.

^ Genetic (cM) distance based on Marshfield map: http://research.marshfieldclinic.org/genetics/

+ See table 1 for references.

* Regions showing genome-wide significant evidence for linkage. Modified from Hoffjan S and Ober C. *Curr Opin Immunol* 2002; 14: 709–717. With permission.

a After adding additional marker, p = 0.0001.

b After adding additional markers, LOD = 4.00.

In one additional study, genome-wide significance was achieved on chromosome 14q after additional markers were added in the linked region with the highest LOD score.[36] The most consistently identified were regions on 5q (five studies), 6p (five studies), 13q (five studies), and 12q (four studies). The syntenic regions to 6p and 12q were additionally linked to BHR and the 5q region to eosinophilic infiltration in bronchial epithelium in mouse models.[37–40] However, the fact that at least 20 regions that likely house asthma susceptibility genes were identified emphasizes the great amount of heterogeneity that underlies this disease. Further, some of the linked regions are very broad and likely contain more than one susceptibility locus.

Despite the challenges of identifying asthma susceptibility loci, the first positional cloning success in asthma was recently reported by Van Eerdewegh et al.[41] Following a genome-wide screen and fine mapping on chromosome 20, they identified *ADAM33* as the asthma susceptibility gene in this region. ADAM (a disintegrin and metalloproteinase domain) proteins are membrane-bound enzymes that mediate cleavage of proteins as well as cell–cell adhesion. *ADAM33* is expressed in bronchus tissue, bronchial smooth muscle cells, and MRC-5 fibroblasts,[42] and could potentially play a role in small airway remodeling in asthmatic patients.[41] However, these functional implications have yet to be proven.

Interestingly, the region on 20p where *ADAM33* is located showed only modest evidence of linkage in the published genome-wide screens[32,43] and is not among the 20 linked regions cited in Table 8.2. The results of the Van Eerdewegh study are difficult to interpret because haplotypes rather than single SNPs within *ADAM33* were associated with asthma, different haplotypes were associated in different populations, and the haplotypes were defined by SNPs in the noncoding regions.

The identification of *ADAM33* clearly demonstrates the importance of the positional candidate cloning approach: *ADAM33,* a gene barely noticed earlier, would probably not have been examined as a candidate gene. It is likely that *ADAM33* is only a minor susceptibility locus for asthma in the general population, similar to other common disease genes identified through positional cloning, for example the calpain-10 gene for type 2 diabetes.[44] Positional cloning studies in many other regions linked to asthma are currently ongoing in laboratories worldwide, and it is likely that many more asthma susceptibility loci will be discovered.

IV. Candidate Gene Studies

Numerous association studies of asthma or atopy susceptibility loci have been performed since the early studies of HLA and specific IgE responses. It is noteworthy that variants in 52 genes have been associated with asthma-related phenotypes in at least one study (Table 8.3). These studies differ considerably

Table 8.3 Genes Associated with Asthma- or Atopy-Related Traits in at Least One Study

Gene	Chromosomal Location	Locus	Phenotype	Association?	Population	Influence on Function?§	Ref.
HNMT	1p32	Thr105Ile	Asthma	Yes	Caucasian	Yes	193
			Atopic asthma	No	Japanese		194
IL10	1q31	−571C/A	Elevated total IgE	Yes	American	Yes 195	196
			Asthma	No	Japanese		197
			Eosinophil count	Yes	German		198
			Atopic asthma	No	Icelandic		103
			Eosinophil, total IgE	Yes	Finnish		199
CHRM3	1q41–44	Haplotypes	SPT cockroach	Yes	Hutterite	Unknown	200
CTLA4	2q33	Haplotypes	Asthma/atopy	No	German	Yes 201	202
		−318C/T	Atopic asthma	No	Japanese		203
			Elevated IgE in asthmatics	Yes	Japanese		204
			Asthma severity	Yes	Korean		205
		49A/G	Asthma/atopy	No	German	Yes 201, 206	202
			Atopic asthma	No	Japanese		203
			IgE, asthma	No	Japanese		204
			Total IgE	Yes	American		207
			BHR	Yes	Korean		205
		−1147C/T	BHR, asthma	Yes	American	Yes	207
		(AT)$_n$ 3'UTR	Total IgE	Yes	American		207
CCR3	3p21	51T/C	Asthma	Yes	British	Unknown	208
			Asthma	No	Japanese		208
CCR5	3p21	32	Reduced asthma risk	Yes	British	Yes 209	210
			Asthma/atopy	No	Australian, British		211
			Atopy	No	Hungarian		212
			Asthma	No	Canadian		213

Gene	Location	Polymorphism	Phenotype	Replicated	Population	Functional	Reference
			Asthma/atopy	No	Hungarian		214
			Reduced asthma risk	Yes	English		215
			Reduced childhood asthma	Yes	British		216
TLR9	3p21.3	−1237C/T	Asthma	Yes	European American		217
				No	African American		217
EDNRA	4q31	His323His	Atopic asthma	Yes	British		218
IRF2	4q35.1	Haplotypes	AD	Yes	Japanese	Unknown	219
CSF2	5q31	Ile117Thr	Atopic asthma	Yes	Swiss	Unknown	220
			Atopic asthma	No	Icelandic		103
			AD	Yes	Canadian		221
		545G/A	Childhood asthma	Yes	Canadian	Unknown	221
		3606T/C	AD, atopy	Yes	Canadian	Unknown	221
IRF1	5q31	(GT)$_n$ intron 7	Atopic asthma	Yes	Japanese	Unknown	222
IL4	5q31	−590C/T	Total IgE	Yes	American	Yes	105
			Specific IgE HDM	Yes	Australian		106
			AD	Yes	Japanese		109
			Asthma	Yes	Japanese		107
			FEV$_1$	Yes	Caucasian		111
			Asthma/atopy	No	Hutterite		32
			Childhood asthma, rhinitis	Yes	Canadian		79
			Childhood asthma	No	Japanese		112
			Asthma severity	Yes	Canadian		108
			Atopic asthma	No	Icelandic		103
			AD	No	Australian		113
			AD	No	Japanese		114
			Extrinsic AD	Yes	German		110
		+33C/T	Total IgE	Yes	Japanese	Unknown	116
			AD	No	Australian		113

Table 8.3 (continued) Genes Associated with Asthma- or Atopy-Related Traits in at Least One Study

Gene	Chromosomal Location	Locus	Phenotype	Association?	Population	Influence on Function?§	Ref.
IL13	5q31	Haplotypes	Asthma	Yes	Japanese		223
		-1112C/T	Allergic asthma	Yes	Dutch	Yes	94
			Atopic asthma	No	Icelandic		103
			Asthma, BHR, SPT	Yes	Dutch		95
			AD	No	Japanese		99
		Arg110Gln	IgE, AD	Yes	German	Yes 102	96
			Total IgE	Yes	American, German		97
			Asthma	Yes	British, Japanese		100
			Asthma, atopy	No	Hutterite		32
			Total and specific IgE	Yes	Chinese		98
			Atopic asthma	No	Icelandic		103
			Asthma, total IgE	No	Costa Rican		104
			AD	Yes	Japanese		99
			Atopy	Yes	American		101
			Total IgE	Yes	Hutterite		16
CD14	5q31	-159C/T	Total IgE, sCD14 level	Yes	American	Yes 158	157
			Asthma, atopy	No	British, Japanese		224
			SPT	Yes	Hutterite		32
			Total IgE, SPT	Yes	Dutch		159
			Atopic asthma	No	Icelandic		103
			Asthma, AD, IgE	No	German		160
UGRP1	5q31-34	-112G/A	Asthma	Yes	Japanese	Yes	225
IL12B	5q31-33	-4475 4insG	Asthma severity	Yes	Australian	Yes	226

Gene	Location	Polymorphism	Phenotype		Population		
ADRB2	5q32-34	1188A/C	AD	Yes	Japanese	Yes 227	228
			Asthma, allergic rhinitis, IgE	No	Japanese		229
		Arg16Gly	Steroid-dependent asthma	Yes	American	Yes 166	168
			Nocturnal asthma	Yes	American		169
			Total IgE	No	British		172
			Response to formoterol	Yes	British		177
			Response to albuterol	Yes	American		175
			Childhood asthma	No	British		174
			Total and specific IgE	No	German		230
			Response to salbutamol	Yes	Japanese		176
			Response to formoterol	No	British		180
			Response to salmeterol	No	New Zealand		179
			FEV1, FVC	Yes	Hutterite		171
			Response to albuterol	Yes	American		178
			Nocturnal cough	Yes	Korean		231
			Asthma severity	Yes	New Zealand		170
			Asthma, atopy	No	Hutterite		32
			Atopic asthma	No	Icelandic		103
			Status asthmaticus	Yes	American		232
		Gln27Glu	BHR	Yes	British	Yes 166	173
			Nocturnal asthma	No	American		169
			Total IgE	Yes	British		172
			Response to formoterol	Yes	British		177
			Response to albuterol	No	American		175
			Childhood asthma	Yes	British		174
			Total and specific IgE	No	German		230
			Asthma onset	Yes	Japanese		176
			Response to formoterol	No	British		180
			Asthma, atopy	No	Hutterite		32
			Asthma severity	No	New Zealand		170

Table 8.3 (continued) Genes Associated with Asthma- or Atopy-Related Traits in at Least One Study

Gene	Chromosomal Location	Locus	Phenotype	Association?	Population	Influence on Function?§	Ref.
			Response to albuterol	No	American		178
			Atopic asthma	No	Icelandic		103
			Status asthmaticus	No	American		232
		Haplotypes	BHR	Yes	Italian		233
			BHR	Yes	German		234
			Response to albuterol	Yes	Caucasian	Yes	30
			Asthma, atopy	No	Hutterite		32
SPINK5	5q32	Glu420Lys	Atopy, AD	Yes	British	Unknown	235
LTC4S	5q35	−444A/C	Aspirin-intolerant asthma	Yes	Polish	Yes	236
			Aspirin-intolerant asthma	No	American	No	237
			Aspirin-intolerant asthma	Yes	Japanese		238
			Asthma	No	Japanese		197
			Atopic asthma	No	Icelandic		103
			FEV$_1$	Yes	Caucasian		239
HLA	6p21	DRB1	Specific IgE to Amb a 5	Yes	Caucasian	Yes 240	48
			Specific IgE to Amb a 6	Yes	Caucasian		49
			Specific IgE to Lol p 1 and 2	Yes	Caucasian		50
			Specific IgE to Lol p 3	Yes	Caucasian		241
			Specific IgE to Bet v 1	Yes	Austrian		51
			Specific IgE to Ole e 1	Yes	Spanish		54
			Specific IgE to Fel d 1, Alt a 1	Yes	British		52
			Atopy	No	British		66
			Specific IgE or IgG to Par o 1	Yes	Italian, Spanish, Bulgarian		55

Phenotype		Ethnicity	Ref.
Atopy	No	Israelian	55
Soybean epidemic asthma	Yes	French	62
Isocyanate-induced asthma	Yes	Spanish	63
Aspirin-induced asthma	No	German	67
Asthma, atopy	No	British	68
Specific IgE to Der p	Yes	British	64
Cockroach sensitization	Yes	German	242
	Yes	Hutterite, African American	56
Citrus red mite-sensitive asthma	Yes	Korean	65
Specific IgE to Der p 5	Yes	Taiwanese	58
Total IgE	Yes	Spanish Gypsy	243
Total IgE, asthma	Yes	Polish	60
Total IgE, specific IgE to Der p 1, 2, and Fel d 1	Yes	Australian	53
Atopy	Yes	Turkish	57
Specific IgE to Der p 1 and 2	Yes	Korean	59
Total IgE, specific IgE to HDM	Yes	Aboriginal Australian	61
Atopic athma	Yes	Italian	244
Occupational sensitization to rat allergens	Yes	British	245
Haplotypes			
Asthma, BHR	Yes	Australian	85
Atopic asthma	Yes	Venezuelan	246
Specific IgE to Der p 1	Yes	Spanish Gypsy	243
Atopic asthma	Yes	Polish	60

Table 8.3 (continued)   Genes Associated with Asthma- or Atopy-Related Traits in at Least One Study

Gene	Chromosomal Location	Locus	Phenotype	Association?	Population	Influence on Function?§	Ref.
		DPB1	Specific IgE to Der p	Yes	German		242
			Specific IgE to Der p 5	Yes	Taiwanese		58
			Atopy	No	French		62
			Atopy	No	British		66
			Aspirin-induced asthma	Yes	British		68
TNF	6p21	−308G/A	Asthma	Yes	Australian	Yes 70	71
			Childhood asthma	Yes	Australian		72
			Asthma, atopy	No	Italian		78
			Asthma	Yes	Canadian		73
			BHR	Yes	British		76
			Asthma	No	Singapore		247
			Atopic asthma	No	Italian		81
			Childhood asthma	No	Canadian		79
			Atopy	Yes	Spanish		77
			Asthma	No	Caucasian		80
			Childhood asthma	Yes	British		74
				No	South Asian		74
			Asthma	Yes	American		75
			Asthma	No	Taiwanese		82
			Atopic asthma	No	Czech		83
			Childhood asthma	No	American		248
		−857C/T	Atopic asthma	Yes	Japanese	Unknown	249
		Haplotypes	Asthma, BHR	Yes	Australian		71, 85
			Asthma, SPT	Yes	Italian		244
LTA	6p21	NcoI (intron1)	Asthma	Yes	Australian	Unknown	71
			Childhood asthma	Yes	Australian		72

Gene	Location	Polymorphism	Phenotype		Population		Ref.
			BHR	No	British		76
			Total IgE	Yes	Italian		81
			Asthma	No	Singapore		247
			Total IgE	Yes	Italian		78
			Atopy	No	Spanish		77
			Atopy	No	Czech		84
			Asthma, atopy	No	German		198
			Asthma	Yes	American		75
			Atopic asthma	No	Czech		83
			Childhood asthma	No	American		248
		Haplotypes	Asthma, BHR	Yes	Australian		71, 85
			Asthma	Yes	Taiwanese		82
TAP1	6p21	Gly637Asp	Atopy	Yes	Tunisian	Unknown	250
		AccI	Asthma/atopy	No	Czech		84
PAFAH	6p21	Val279Phe	Atopic asthma	Yes	Taiwanese	Unknown	251
			Asthma, asthma severity	Yes	Japanese	Yes	252
			Asthma	No	Japanese		253
			Atopic asthma	Yes	Japanese		254
		Ile198Thr	Total IgE, atopic asthma	Yes	German, British	Yes	255
		Ala379Val	Specific IgE, asthma	Yes	German, British	Yes	255
EDN1	6p24	4124C/T	Asthma	Yes	Caucasian	Unknown	198
			Atopic asthma	No	British, Japanese		218
IFNGR1	6q23	Intron 2	Total IgE	Yes	British	Unknown	256
		Val14Met	Atopy	No	Japanese	Unknown	256
			Atopic asthma	No	Japanese		222
EOTAXIN2	7q11.23	1265 A/G	Asthma	Yes	Korean	Unknown	257
CFTR	7q31.2	F508	Reduced asthma risk	Yes	American	Yes	258

Table 8.3 (continued) Genes Associated with Asthma- or Atopy-Related Traits in at Least One Study

Gene	Chromosomal Location	Locus	Phenotype	Association?	Population	Influence on Function?§	Ref.
			Reduced asthma risk	No	British		259
			Asthma	Yes	Danish		260
			Asthma	No	Italian		261
			Asthma	No	French		262
			Atopic asthma	No	Icelandic		103
		Combination of missense mutations	Asthma	Yes	Spanish		263
NOS3	7q36	Haplotypes	Asthma	Yes	Greek		264
		STRP intron 4	Asthma	Yes	Korean	Unknown	265
			Total and specific IgE, SPT	Yes	Czech		266
		Glu298Asp	Asthma, total IgE	No	British	Unknown	267
			Asthma, atopy	No	Czech		266
NAT2	8p22	Slow acetylation genotype	Atopy	Yes	Polish	Yes	268
			Atopy	Yes	Polish		269
			Extrinsic asthma	Yes	Turkish		270
			Reduced asthma risk	Yes	Russian		271
ALOX5	10q11.2	(GGGCGG)$_n$ promoter	Drug response	Yes	American	Yes 272	273
			Drug response	No	British		274
CCI6/CCI0	11q12–13	38A/G	Asthma	Yes	Australian	Unknown	147, 275
			Asthma	No	Britrish, Japanese		276
			Asthma	Yes	Dutch		277
			Atopic asthma	No	Icelandic		103

Gene	Locus	Variant	Phenotype	Association	Population	Linkage	Ref.
FCER1B	11q13		Asthma	No	Caucasian		278
			BHR	Yes	German		148
		STRP intron 1	Asthma	No	Japanese	Unknown	279
		Ile181Leu	Atopy	Yes	British	No 280, 281	133
			Total and specific IgE, asthma	Yes	British		134
			Asthma	Yes	White South African		135
			Atopy	No	French Canadian	No	142
		Leu181/Leu183	Atopic asthma	No	Icelandic		103
			Atopy, BHR	Yes	Australian		282
			Asthma	Yes	Kuwaiti Arab		283
			Atopy	Yes	Italian		128
		Gly237Glu	SPT, specific IgE, BHR	Yes	Australian	No 280, 281	139
			Atopic asthma, total IgE	Yes	Japanese		140
			Asthma	No	Swiss		284
			Atopic asthma	No	Japanese		285
			Nasal allergy, total IgE	Yes	Japanese		141
			Atopy	Yes	French Canadian		142
			Asthma severity	No	Canadian		108
			Atopic asthma	No	Japanese		112
			Childhood asthma	No	Canadian		79
			Atopic asthma	No	Icelandic		103
		Rsalin2	Asthma, total IgE	Yes	Australian	Unknown	143
			AD, asthma	Yes	British		144
			Atopy	No	Spanish		286
			Atopy, asthma	Yes	Swedish		145
		Rsalex7	Total IgE, eosinophil	Yes	Australian	Unknown	143
			Atopy, specific IgE	Yes	Swedish		145

Table 8.3 (continued)   Genes Associated with Asthma- or Atopy-Related Traits in at Least One Study

Gene	Chromosomal Location	Locus	Phenotype	Association?	Population	Influence on Function?§	Ref.
GSTP1	11q13	−109C/T	AD, asthma	Yes	British		144
		Ile105Val	Total IgE	Yes	Japanese	Unknown	146
			Asthma, IgE, SPT	Yes	British	Yes 287	149
			Atopic asthma	No	Icelandic		103
			Isocyanate-induced asthma	Yes	Italian		151
			Lung function growth, FVC, FEV$_1$	Yes	American		150
IL18	11q22	−656T/G	Total and specific IgE	Yes	German	Unknown	288
		−137G/C	Total and specific IgE, rhinitis	Yes	German	Unknown	288
		113T/G	Total and specific IgE, rhinitis	Yes	German	Unknown	288
		127C/T	Total and specific IgE, rhinitis	Yes	German	Unknown	288
		−133C/G	Total and specific IgE	Yes	German	Unknown	288
AICDA	12p13	7888C/T	Asthma, total IgE	Yes	Japanese	Unknown	289
STAT6	12q13	2964C/A	Mild atopic asthma	Yes	Japanese	Unknown	290
			Asthma, atopy	No	British		290
			Nut allergy	Yes	British		291
		(GT)$_n$ intron 1	Allergic diseases	Yes	Japanese	Unknown	292
			Eosinophil count	Yes	German		293
		1570C/T	Total IgE	Yes	German		293
IFNG	12q21	(CA)$_n$ intron 1	SPT	Yes	Hutterite	Unknown	32
			Atopic asthma	Yes	Japanese		222
			Total IgE	Yes	Indian		294
NOS1	12q24	(CA)$_n$ exon 29	Asthma	Yes	Caucasian	Unknown	295
		STRP intron 2	Asthma	Yes	British	Unknown	267
		(AAT)$_n$	Asthma, atopy	No	Hutterite		32
		3391C/T	Eosinophil count	Yes	Caucasian	Unknown	198
		5266C/T	Total IgE	Yes	Caucasian	Unknown	198

Gene	Location	Polymorphism	Phenotype	Association	Population	Replication	Ref
TCRA/D	14q11	VA8.1	Specicfi IgE to Der p 2	Yes	Australian	Unknown	296
			Specicfi IgE to Der p 1	Yes	Spanish Gypsy		243
AACT	14q32	Thr(−15)Ala	Atopic asthma, total IgE, BHR	Yes	Italian	Unknown	297
IL4RA	16p12	Ile50Val	Atopic asthma, total IgE	Yes	Japanese	Yes 120	298
			Atopic asthma	No	Japanese		299
			Atopy	No	Singapore		300
			Atopic asthma	Yes	Japanese		121
			AD	No	Japanese		301
			Atopy	No	Danish		302
			AD	No	Japanese		114
			Atopic asthma	Yes	Japanese		112
			Atopic asthma	No	Mexican		303
		Glu375Ala	AD	No	Japanese	Unknown	301
			AD	No	Japanese		114
			Atopic asthma	No	Mexican		303
			Total IgE	Yes	Dutch		12
		Cys406Arg	AD	No	Japanese	Unknown	301
			Atopic asthma	No	Mexican		303
		Ser478Pro	Total IgE	Yes	Dutch		12
			Total IgE	Yes	German	Yes	122
			Total IgE, SPT, asthma, BHR	Yes	Dutch		12
		Gln551Arg	AD, hyper-IgE syndrome	Yes	American	Yes 118; No 304	118
			Total IgE	Yes	German		122
			Asthma, atopy	No	Japanese		305
			Asthma, asthma severity	Yes	American		306
			Atopic asthma	No	Italian		307
			FEV$_1$	Yes	Canadian		108
			AD	Yes	Japanese		301

Table 8.3 (continued) Genes Associated with Asthma- or Atopy-Related Traits in at Least One Study

Gene	Chromosomal Location	Locus	Phenotype	Association?	Population	Influence on Function?§	Ref.
			Atopy	No	Danish		302
			AD	No	Japanese		114
			Atopic asthma	No	Japanese		112
		Ser786Pro	Asthma	No	American	No	308
		Haplotypes	Total IgE	Yes	German		309
			Total IgE	Yes	Finnish		310
			Asthma, atopy	Yes	Hutterite		28
			Asthma, atopy	Yes	CSGA (American)		28
			Atopic asthma	Yes	American	Yes	29
			Total IgE	Yes	British		124
CARD15	16q12	2104C/T	Allergic rhinitis	Yes	German	Unknown	311
		2722G/C	Allergic rhinitis, AD	Yes	German	Unknown	311
		3020insC	Atopy, total IgE	Yes	German	Yes 312	311
NOS2A	17cen-q11	(CCTTT)ₙ	Atopy	Yes	Japanese	Yes 313	314
RANTES	17q11-q12	−403A/G	AD	Yes	German	Yes	315
			Asthma, atopy	Yes	Caucasian		316
			AD	No	Hungarian		317
			Asthma, atopy	No	Hungarian		318
			Asthma onset	No	Japanese		319
		−28C/G	Late-onset asthma	Yes	Japanese	Yes 320	319
			AD	No	Hungarian		317
			Asthma, atopy	No	Hungarian		318
MCP1	17q11-q12	−2518A/G	Asthma, eosinophil level	Yes	Hungarian	Yes 321	318
			Atopic asthma	No	Icelandic		103
			AD	No	Hungarian		317

Gene	Location	Polymorphism	Phenotype		Population		Ref
EOTAXIN1	17q21	Ala23Thr	Eosinophil level, lung function	Yes	American	Yes	322
			Asthma	No	Japanese		323
			Atopic asthma	No	Icelandic		103
			AD	No	Japanese		324
		−426C/T, −384A/G	Total IgE	Yes	Korean		257
			Total IgE in AD	Yes	Japanese		324
ACE	17q23	In/Del	Asthma	Yes	French	Yes 325	326
			Atopic diseases	Yes	Czech		327
			Asthma	No	Japanese		328
			Asthma, atopy	No	British, Japanese		329
			Asthma	No	Japanese		330
			Asthma	No	South Korean		265
			Asthma, asthma severity	No	Caucasian		73
			Childhood asthma	No	British, South Asian		74
TBXA2R	19p13	924T/C	Asthma	Yes	Japanese		197
			Childhood asthma, FEV₁, specific IgE	Yes	Japanese		331
TGFB1	19q13.1	−509C/T	Total IgE	Yes	American	Yes 332	196
			Asthma severity	Yes	British		333
			Asthma, atopy	No	Czech		334
			Atopic asthma	No	Icelandic		103
		Arg25Pro	AD	Yes	British	Yes	335
			Asthma severity	No	British		333
			Asthma, atopy	No	Czech		334
		Leu10Pro	AD	No	British	Yes	335
			Asthma severity	No	British		333
			Asthma, atopy	No	Czech		334

Table 8.3 (continued) Genes Associated with Asthma- or Atopy-Related Traits in at Least One Study

Gene	Chromosomal Location	Locus	Phenotype	Association?	Population	Influence on Function?§	Ref.
IFNGR2	21q22	Gln64Arg	Total IgE	Yes	British	Unknown	256
			Atopic asthma	No	Japanese		222
IL13RA1	Xq13	1398A/G	Total IgE	Yes	British	Unknown	100
		−1050C/T	Atopic asthma	No	Japanese	Unknown	336

HNMT = histamine N-methyltransferase. IL10 = interleukin 10. CHRM3 = cholinergic receptor, muscarinic 3. CTLA4 = cytytoxic T lymphocyte-associated 4. CCR3 (5) = chemokine receptor 3 (5). TLR9 = toll-like receptor 9. EDNRA = endothelin receptor A. IRF2(1) = interferon regulatory factor 2(1). CSF2 = colony stimulating factor 2. IL4 (13) = interleukin 4 (13). CD14 = monocyte differentiation antigen 14. UGRP1 = uteroglobin-related protein 1. IL12B = interleukin 12B. ADRB2 = beta-2 adrenergic receptor. SPINK5 = serine protease inhibitor, kazal type 5. LTC4S = leukotriene C4 synthase. HLA = human leukocyte antigen. TNF = tumor necrosis factor. LTA = lymphotoxin-alpha. TAP1 = transporter, ATP-binding cassette 1. PAFAH = platelet activating factor acetylhydrolase. EDN1 = endothelin 1. IFNGR1 = interferon gamma receptor 1. CFTR = cystic fibrosis transmembrane conductance regulator. NOS3 = nitric oxide synthase 3. NAT2 = N-acetyltransferase 2. ALOX5 = arachidonate 5-lipoxygenase. CC16 (10) = Clara cell-specific 16-kD protein (10). FCER1B = high affinity IgE receptor beta chain. GSTP1 = glutathione S-transferase P1. IL18 = interleukin 18. AICDA = activation-induced cytidine deaminase. STAT6 = signal transducer and activator of transcription 6. IFNG = interferon gamma. NOS1 = nitric oxide synthase 1. TCRA/D = T cell antigen receptor alpha/delta. AACT = alpha-1-antichymotrypsin (serpin A3). IL4RA = interleukin 4 receptor alpha chain. CARD15 = caspase recruitment domain-containing protein 15. NOS2A = nitric oxide synthase 2A. RANTES = regulated upon activation, normally T-expressed and secreted. MCP1 = monocyte chemotactic protein 1. ACE = angiotensin 1-converting enzyme. TBXA2R = thromboxane A2 receptor. TGFB1 = transforming growth factor 1. IFNGR2 = interferon gamma receptor 2. IL13RA1 = interleukin 13 receptor alpha-1.

§ Has this variant been shown to influence gene function or expression *in vivo* or *in vitro*? Numbers represent references.

with respect to design and specific phenotypes, overall sample sizes are small (<100 cases in most studies), few studies examined more than a single SNP within each gene, and relatively few positive findings have been replicated. However, some genes have shown associations with an asthma or atopy-related phenotype in multiple studies. These include *HLA-DRB1, IL13, IL4, IL4RA, FCER1B, CD14,* and *ADRB2,* described in more detail below. In addition, the few studies that investigated gene–gene and gene–environment interactions in asthma suscepti- bility are discussed.

A. *HLA-DRB1:* From the Early Studies to Today

The first genetic association studies of atopy focused on the role of the human leukocyte antigen (HLA) genes on chromosome 6p21 in specific IgE responses.[45–47] The HLA class II genes, HLA-DR and HLA DQ, are intriguing candidate genes because their main function is to present antigen to the T cell receptor. As early as 1972, an association of a class II locus with ragweed hay fever was reported.[45] That group and others subsequently identified associations between the HLA-DR antigens (and more recently DRB1 alleles) and specific IgE responses to short ragweed pollen (*Amb a* 6),[48,49] rye grass (*Lol p* 1 and 2),[50] birch pollen (*Bet v* 1),[51] cat (*Fel d* 1),[52,53] mold (*Alt a* 1),[52] olive pollen (*Ole e* 1),[54] *Parietaria* (*Par o* 1),[55] cockroach,[56,57] and house dust mites (*Der p* 1, 2 and 5).[53,58,59]

In addition to specific IgE, associations with *HLA-DRB1,* alleles were reported for total IgE,[53,60,61] atopy,[62] and asthma.[63–65] A few studies failed to replicate some of these associations.[66–68] It is noteworthy that even though the *HLA-DRB1* locus has been associated consistently with atopy-related phenotypes in many populations, the associations and phenotypes vary among studies. This is not unexpected because the polymorphic amino acid sequences in the *DRB1* gene contribute to differential binding of peptides derived from a variety of allergens. Therefore, different HLA-DRB1 alleles may specify IgE responses to different allergens.

On the other hand, many excellent candidate genes other than the HLA genes per se are found in the HLA region. These include the genes encoding tumor necrosis factor (TNF)-α (*TNF*) and lymphotoxin-α (*LTA*). TNF-α is a potent pro-inflammatory cytokine shown to be elevated in asthmatic lungs and bronchoalveolar fluid.[69] A functional polymorphism in the promoter region of the *TNF* gene (C-308T)[70] was associated with asthma,[71–75] BHR,[76] and atopy,[77] although associations of this polymorphism with asthma-related phenotypes were not replicated in other studies.[78–83] Similarly, a variant in intron 1 of the *LTA* gene was associated with asthma phenotypes in some studies[72,75,78,81] and not in oth- ers.[76,77,83,84] Interestingly, the extended haplotype including the *LTA* NcoI*1/*TNF*-308*2/*HLA-DRB1**02 alleles was strongly associated with asthma and BHR in an Australian population sample.[85] Curiously, however, the many linkages to this region on 6p21 (Table 8.2) are not obviously attributable to variations in *HLA-DRB1*, *TNF* or *LTA*, suggesting that additional variation in HLA region genes may contribute to asthma susceptibility.

B. Genes in the IL-4/IL-13 Pathway

IL-4 and IL-13 are T helper (Th)-2 cytokines that play an important role in asthma pathophysiology.[86,87] The genes encoding both cytokines are located adjacent to each other in the cytokine cluster on chromosome 5q31 which has been linked to asthma or atopic phenotypes in five genome screens and in several linkage studies that focused solely on this region.[88–93]

Two variants in the *IL13* gene are among the most consistently replicated associations, although no study has demonstrated that variation in this (or any other) gene explains the evidence for linkage in this region. A C/T SNP in the promoter region at position –1112 and a coding SNP in exon 4 (G4464A) resulting in an amino acid exchange from arginine to glutamine at position 110 (Arg110Gln) have been associated with asthma-related phenotypes in eight studies. Further, these SNPs may directly affect the function of the gene.

The –1112T allele was associated with increased IL-13 production and increased binding of nuclear proteins to this region[94] and with asthma,[94,95] and BHR, and SPT[95] in two different Dutch populations. Curiously, associations of this promoter SNP have not been replicated in other populations yet. However, the 110Gln allele was associated with total IgE levels,[16,96–98] atopic dermatitis,[96,99] asthma,[100] and atopy.[101] This SNP was shown to influence function, with the Gln allele having a lower affinity to the IL-13 receptor alpha-2 chain, leading to slower clearance and enhanced stability in plasma.[102] Overall, however, most studies did not find an association of this variant with asthma per se,[32,98,101,103] suggesting that variation in the *IL13* gene may instead influence susceptibility to atopy. Only studies in Icelandic[103] and Costa Rican[104] populations were unable to detect any association between variants in this gene and asthma- or atopy-related phenotypes.

Compared with *IL13*, association studies with variants of the *IL4* gene have been more contradictory. A functional SNP in the promoter region –509C/T has been associated with total and specific IgE,[105,106] childhood asthma,[79,107] asthma severity,[108] AD,[109,110] and FEV$_1$.[111] However, negative results were reported for childhood asthma,[112] asthma,[32,103] and AD.[113,114] The –509C/T variant did not account for the evidence of linkage to the 5q cytokine cluster.[32,115] A second promoter SNP (+33C/T) was associated with total IgE levels in one study[116] but not AD in another.[113]

The common α chain shared by the IL-4 and IL-13 receptors is encoded by the *IL4RA* gene on chromosome 16p12. To date, 14 SNPs in coding regions have been described,[28,117–119] 10 of which result in amino acid substitutions. Three have been reported to influence function: Ile50Val, the only variant in the extracellular domain,[120,121] and Gln551Arg[118] and Ser478Pro[122] in the intracellular domain. Association studies taking into account only single SNPs were contradictory[123] (Table 8.3). As a result, subsequent studies examined haplotypes rather than single SNPs. In a large study of the Hutterites, a founder population, individual alleles were only modestly associated with asthma, but haplotypes composed of combinations of alleles in the intracellular domain were highly associated with asthma.[28]

Similarly, in other samples, haplotypes but not single SNPs showed associations with both asthma and SPT.[28,29,124] Functional synergisms between alleles were demonstrated for Ser478 and Arg551 alleles[122] and for Val50 and Arg551 alleles,[29] further emphasizing the importance of evaluating more than one SNP simultaneously. Recently, a promoter SNP in *IL4RA* was identified (−3223C/T).[125] The −3223T allele was associated with lower levels of soluble IL4R, but association studies of disease susceptibility with this new variant have not yet been reported. However, associations between coding region variation and asthma or atopic phenotypes in at least 11 independent studies indicate that the *IL4RA* gene is indeed an asthma susceptibility locus.

The first evidence for a gene–gene interaction in the IL-4–Il-13 pathway was reported by Howard et al. in a study of Dutch asthma cases and controls.[12] In this population, the *IL13* −1112T allele was significantly associated with BHR[95] and the *IL4RA* Ser478 variant with elevated serum IgE levels.[12] When the interaction effects of these two SNPs in the same sample were examined, individuals who were homozygous for the *IL4RA* Ser478 allele and carried the *IL13* −1112T allele had almost a five times greater risk for developing asthma than individuals with other genotypes.[12] This intriguing example of a gene–gene interaction must be confirmed by other studies, but it highlights the importance of considering multiple genes simultaneously.

C. *FCER1B*

The first linkage to asthma was reported for a region on chromosome 11q13.[126] The same region is also one of the five that met genome-wide criteria of significance (Table 8.2) and has been linked to asthma or related phenotypes in multiple studies.[35,43,92,126–131] The 11q13 region has attracted much attention because it houses the gene encoding the beta chain of the high affinity IgE receptor (*FCER1B*) that plays an important role in IgE-mediated inflammation. The receptor is composed of three subunits — alpha, beta, and gamma; the alpha chain is responsible for ligand binding and the gamma chain for signal transduction. The beta chain serves as an amplifier for signal strength.[132] Unlike the region on 11q13, the chromosomal region encoding the alpha and gamma chains (1q) provided little evidence for linkage to asthma in genome screens.

Several polymorphisms in the *FCER1B* gene have been identified, including three amino acid substitutions (Ile181Leu, Val183Leu, and Glu237Gly). However, detection of the 181Leu and 183Leu variants has been technically difficult. They were identified in only a few populations[133–135] and were not detectable in many European populations.[136–138] Thus, these variants are unlikely to be important atopy-susceptibility alleles.

The 237Gly allele, on the other hand, has been associated with allergic sensitization and BHR,[139] childhood atopic asthma and elevated IgE,[140] allergic rhinitis,[141] and atopy[142] although some studies failed to replicate these associations.[79,108,112] Further, additional polymorphisms that do not alter the amino acid sequence (*Rsa*I_in2 and *Rsa*I_ex7) were associated with asthma and total IgE,[143] AD,[144] and specific IgE response.[145] A promoter polymorphism (–109C/T) associated with total IgE levels was identified recently in a Japanese population.[146] These studies indicate that *FCER1B* may be a susceptibility gene on 11q13, although no one has shown that variation in this gene accounts for the evidence of linkage in this region. Further, the associated variants may be in linkage disequilibrium with other susceptibility loci in close proximity. In fact, many other candidate genes in the region have been studied, including *CC16*, the Clara cell protein (CC10),[147,148] and *GSTP1*, encoding glutathione S-transferase.[149–151] Further studies of these genes and of the *FCER1B* gene are needed to identify the true susceptibility variation in this region.

D. *CD14* and the "Hygiene Hypothesis"

Association studies with the *CD14* gene on chromosome 5q31 have provided an exciting new perspective on the role of gene–environment interactions in asthma susceptibility. CD14 is the primary receptor for lipopolysaccharide (LPS or endotoxin).[152] Growing evidence indicates that exposure to LPS in the first years of life may prevent allergic sensitization by stimulating the early development of a Th1-like immune response[153] or suppress cytokine production.[154] Thus, the rising incidence of allergic diseases in industrialized countries may be due in part to the lack of microbial stimuli, especially LPS, in our modern, rather sterile environment (the so-called hygiene hypothesis).[155,156]

A functional SNP in the promoter region of the *CD14* gene (–159C/T) was identified.[157,158] The –159T allele was associated with higher levels of soluble CD14 (sCD14) and reduced levels of serum IgE levels in the Tucson Respiratory Study.[157] This same allele was also associated with low IgE levels in a Dutch population.[159] However, in the Hutterites, a farming population, the –159T allele was associated with atopy (defined by 1 positive SPT).[32] Neither allele was associated with asthma or atopic phenotypes in the German Multicenter Allergy Study (MAS)[160] or in the Icelandic population.[103]

These seemingly contradictory results may be due to gene–environment interactions. In particular, Vercelli recently proposed an intriguing explanation for these discrepant findings.[161] She hypothesized that the level of endotoxin exposure influences the "switch" from the Th2-biased cytokine profile at birth to a Th1-biased cytokine profile in early life, and that endotoxin exposure levels interact with *CD14* genotype to confer either risk to or protection from atopic phenotypes later in life.[161] According to this model, children with very low levels of exposure to endotoxin, such as those in the German MAS and Icelandic studies, would remain primarily Th2-skewed and be at highest risk for developing atopic phenotypes. However, this risk would be independent of their genotypes at the *CD14* loci. Children in the Tucson Respiratory Study, and presumably in the Dutch study, had intermediate levels of endotoxin exposure. In these populations, the −159T allele facilitates this "switch" and protects against the subsequent development of atopic disease. However, in farming populations with exposures to very high levels of endotoxin, for example, the Hutterites, the "switch" occurs earlier in children with the −159C allele. Thus, in populations with very high levels of endotoxin exposure, the −159C allele would be protective against the development of atopic phenotypes, as it is in the Hutterites. In populations with moderate exposure levels, the −159T allele would be protective, as shown in the Tucson and Dutch studies.

Finally, in populations with very low exposure levels, neither allele would be associated with risk, as in the German MAS and Icelandic studies. This model is supported by a recent study of the development of atopic phenotypes in the first year of life in a cohort of high-risk children.[162] Dogs lived in the homes of 36.8% of the children in this cohort and this is consistent with moderate levels of endotoxin exposure.[163] A significant interaction of the *CD14* genotype and the presence of a dog in the home with the development of AD in the first year of life was reported. The −159TT genotype was protective against developing AD in children with dogs, whereas no such protection was evident in the children without dogs in their homes.[163]

These combined studies demonstrate that it is important to consider gene–environment interactions related to asthma risk. Studies of *CD14* polymorphism indicate that the lack of replication in association studies may be due in some instances to the failure to account for environmental risk factors that may modulate the effect of genotype on disease susceptibility. How generalizable this is to other susceptibility loci remains to be determined, but again it illustrates the complexity of susceptibility to asthma and related phenotypes.

E. *ADRB2* and Drug Response

Variation in the β_2 adrenoceptor (*ADRB2*) gene provides another example of a gene–environment interaction, but in this case genetic variation is associated with response to β_2 agonists. In fact, *ADRB2* is the most examined gene with regard to pharmacogenetics in asthma and provides one of the best examples overall of genotype–drug interactions.

β_2 adrenoceptor agonists are the most widely used bronchodilator drugs in asthma management. They activate β_2 adrenoceptors on the bronchial smooth muscle cells, leading to relaxation of airway tone and thus bronchodilation.[164] However, long-term use of these drugs induces both desensitization and down-regulation of the receptors in some, but not all, asthmatic patients. Thus, it was proposed that genetic variation in the ADRB2 gene might influence responses to β_2 agonists.[165]

ADRB2, a single-exon gene, is located on chromosome 5q32-34. Four amino acid substitutions have been reported, of which Arg16Gly and Gln27Glu are the most common. Functional studies have shown that the Gly16 allele leads to increased agonist-promoted down-regulation of the receptor, whereas the Glu27 allele is relatively resistant to such down-regulation.[166] Additionally, an SNP in the 5′ leader cistron regulates protein translation.[167] Most case-control studies to date have not found an association between any of these variants and asthma per se, but rather implicate ADRB2 as a disease-modifying gene. For example, the Gly16 allele was associated with steroid-dependent asthma,[168] nocturnal asthma,[169] asthma severity,[170] and lung function[171] but did not show different frequencies between asthmatics and controls in many studies.[170–172] The Glu27 allele was associated with lower airway reactivity in asthma patients,[173] and the Gln27 allele with elevated IgE and self-reported childhood asthma.[172,174] However, both polymorphisms are in tight LD so that distinguishing the effects of a single SNP in this gene is difficult.

Both Arg16Gly and Gln27Glu have been studied for their roles in response to bronchodilator treatment in several clinical trials, but the results to date are conflicting. Some investigators found reduced responses to inhaled β_2 agonists and greater amounts of receptor desensitization in Gly16/Gly16 homozygotes,[175–177] whereas others reported declines in morning peak flows in Arg16/Arg16 subjects who used bronchodilators regularly[178] or increases in asthma exacerbations during long-term treatment in Arg16/Arg16 homozygotes.[179]

Other studies failed to replicate associations with drug responses entirely.[179,180] Drysdale et al. recently examined haplotypes composed of 13 SNPs in promoter and coding regions of *ADRB2* and reported associations between certain haplotypes and *in vivo* bronchodilator responses and *in vitro* expression levels.[30] This study suggests that haplotypes may have greater predictive powers than individual SNPs as loci involved in drug responses and may account for some of the contradictory results discussed above. Evidence indicates that variation at the *ADRB2* locus may indeed influence drug response, but the relative importance of this effect on treatment outcomes and the specific SNPs and haplotypes that influence responses remains to be determined.

V. Conclusion

Despite the methodologic problems in mapping and identifying genes for complex diseases, considerable progress has been made over the past 10 years. Twelve genome-wide screens for asthma-related phenotypes identified at least 20 regions in the genome that likely house asthma or atopy genes. The first "asthma gene" was positionally cloned in 2002. However, it is evident that many different genes contribute to asthma susceptibility, each producing only minor individual effects. The results of candidate gene studies further highlight this hypothesis: variants in 52 genes have been associated with asthma or related phenotypes in at least one study; however, many of these studies are methodologically limited and must be replicated. Developing more sophisticated analytical tools that incorporate gene–gene and gene–environment interactions on a genome-wide level may provide a better understanding of the complex genetic background that underlies asthma and atopic diseases.

References

1. Asher MI, Keil U, Anderson HR, Beasley R, Crane J, Martinez F, Mitchell EA, Pearce N, Sibbald B, Stewart AW Strachen D, Weiland SK, and Williams HC. International Study of Asthma and Allergies in Childhood (ISAAC): rationale and methods. *Eur Respir J* 1995; 8: 483–491.
2. Beasley R. The burden of asthma with specific reference to the United States. *J Allergy Clin Immunol* 2002; 109: S482–S489.
3. Edfors-Lubs ML. Allergy in 7000 twin pairs. *Acta Allergol* 1971; 26: 249–285.
4. Hopp RJ, Bewtra AK, Watt GD, Nair NM, and Townley RG. Genetic analysis of allergic disease in twins. *J Allergy Clin Immunol* 1984; 73: 265–270.
5. Hopper JL, Hannah MC, Macaskill GT, and Mathews JD. Twin concordance for a binary trait III. A bivariate analysis of hay fever and asthma. *Genet Epidemiol* 1990; 7: 277–289.
6. Duffy DL, Martin NG, Battistutta D, Hopper JL, and Mathews JD. Genetics of asthma and hay fever in Australian twins. *Am Rev Respir Dis* 1990; 142: 1351–1358.
7. Nieminen MM, Kaprio J, and Koskenvuo M. A population-based study of bronchial asthma in adult twin pairs. *Chest* 1991; 100: 70–75.
8. Strachan DP. Family size, infection and atopy: the first decade of the "hygiene hypothesis." *Thorax* 2000; 55: S2–S10.
9. von Hertzen LC. Puzzling associations between childhood infections and the later occurrence of asthma and atopy. *Ann Med* 2000; 32: 397–400.
10. Varner AE. The increase in allergic respiratory diseases: survival of the fittest? *Chest* 2002; 121: 1308–1316.
11. Weiss ST. Eat dirt — the hygiene hypothesis and allergic diseases. *New Engl J Med* 2002; 347: 930–931.

12. Howard TD, Koppelman GH, Xu J, Zheng SL, Postma DS, Meyers DA, and Bleecker ER. Gene–gene interaction in asthma: IL4RA and IL13 in a Dutch population with asthma. *Am J Hum Genet* 2002; 70: 230–236.
13. Wang Z, Chen C, Niu T, Wu D, Yang J, Wang B, Fang Z, Yandava CN, Drazen JM, Weiss ST, and Xu X. Association of asthma with beta-(2)-adrenergic receptor gene polymorphism and cigarette smoking. *Am J Respir Crit Care Med* 2001; 163: 1404–1409.
14. Baldini M, Vercelli D, and Martinez FD. CD14: an example of gene by environment interaction in allergic disease. *Allergy* 2002; 57: 188–192.
15. Colilla S, Nicolae D, Pluzhnikov A, Blumenthal MN, Beaty TH, Bleecker ER, Lange EM, Rich SS, Meyers DA, Ober C, and Cox NJ. Evidence for gene–environment interactions in a linkage study of asthma and smoking exposure. *J Allergy Clin Immunol* 2003; 111: 840–846.
16. Ober C, Hoffjan S, Newman DL, Nicolae D, Ostrovnaja I, Colilla S, Parry R, Meyers DA, Rich SS, Gangnon R, Solway J, Beaty TH, Blumenthal MN, Bleecker ER, Cox NJ, Mirel DB, Gern JE, and Lemanske RF, Jr. Exposure to environmental tobacco smoke in the first year of life interacts with IL13 genotype to confer risk for asthma. Submitted.
17. Botstein D, White RL, Skolnick M, and Davis RW. Construction of a genetic linkage map in man using restriction fragment length polymorphisms. *Am J Hum Genet* 1980; 32: 314–331.
18. Lander E and Kruglyak L. Genetic dissection of complex traits: guidelines for interpreting and reporting linkage results. *Nat Genet* 1995; 11: 241–247.
19. Curtis D. Genetic dissection of complex traits. *Nat Genet* 1996; 12: 356–358.
20. Witte JS, Elston RC, and Schork NJ. Genetic dissection of complex traits. *Nat Genet* 1996; 12: 355–358.
21. Botstein D and Risch N. Discovering genotypes underlying human phenotypes: past successes for mendelian disease, future approaches for complex disease. *Nat Genet* 2003; 33: S228–S237.
22. Risch N and Merikangas K. The future of genetic studies of complex human diseases. *Science* 1996; 273: 1516–1517.
23. Altmuller J, Palmer LJ, Fischer G, Scherb H, and Wjst M. Genome-wide scans of complex human diseases: true linkage is hard to find. *Am J Hum Genet* 2001; 69: 936–950.
24. Kruglyak L. Prospects for whole-genome linkage disequilibrium mapping of common disease genes. *Nat Genet* 1999; 22: 139–144.
25. Jorde LB. Linkage disequilibrium and the search for complex disease genes. *Genome Res 2000*; 10: 1435–1444.
26. Shifman S, Kuypers J, Kokoris M, Yakir B, and Darvasi A. Linkage disequilibrium patterns of the human genome across populations. *Hum Mol Genet* 2003; 12: 771–776.
27. Spielman RS and Ewens WJ. The TDT and other family-based tests for linkage disequilibrium and association. *Am J Hum Genet* 1996; 59: 983–989.

28. Ober C, Leavitt SA, Tsalenko A, Howard TD, Hoki DM, Daniel R, Newman DL, Wu X, Parry R, Lester LA, Solway J, Blumenthal M, King RA, Xu J, Meyers DA, Bleecker ER, and Cox NJ. Variation in the interleukin 4-receptor alpha gene confers susceptibility to asthma and atopy in ethnically diverse populations. *Am J Hum Genet* 2000; 66: 517–526.

29. Risma KA, Wang N, Andrews RP, Cunningham CM, Ericksen MB, Bernstein JA, Chakraborty R, and Hershey GK. V75R576 IL-4 receptor alpha is associated with allergic asthma and enhanced IL-4 receptor function. *J Immunol* 2002; 169: 1604–1610.

30. Drysdale CM, McGraw DW, Stack CB, Stephens JC, Judson RS, Nandabalan K, Arnold K, Ruano G, and Liggett SB. Complex promoter and coding region beta 2-adrenergic receptor haplotypes alter receptor expression and predict *in vivo* responsiveness. *Proc Natl Acad Sci USA* 2000; 97: 10483–10488.

31. Xu X, Fang Z, Wang B, Chen C, Guang W, Jin Y, Yang J, Lewitzky S, Aelony A, Parker A, Meyer J, and Weiss ST. A genomewide search for quantitative trait loci underlying asthma. *Am J Hum Genet* 2001; 69: 1271–1277.

32. Ober C, Tsalenko A, Parry R, and Cox NJ. A second-generation genomewide screen for asthma susceptibility alleles in a founder population. *Am J Hum Genet* 2000; 67: 1154–1162.

33. Yokouchi Y, Nukaga Y, Shibasaki M, Noguchi E, Kimura K, Ito S, Nishihara M, Yamakawa-Kobayashi K, Takeda K, Imoto N, Ichikawa K, Matsui A, Hamaguchi H, and Arinami T. Significant evidence for linkage of mite-sensitive childhood asthma to chromosome 5q31-q33 near the interleukin 12B locus by a genome-wide search in Japanese families. *Genomics* 2000; 66: 152–160.

34. Xu J, Postma DS, Howard TD, Koppelman GH, Zheng SL, Stine OC, Bleecker ER, and Meyers DA. Major genes regulating total serum immunoglobulin E levels in families with asthma. *Am J Hum Genet* 2000; 67: 1163–1173.

35. Daniels SE, Bhattacharrya S, James A, Leaves NI, Young A, Hill MR, Faux JA, Ryan GF, Le Souef PN, Lathrop GM, Musk AW, and Cookson WO. A genome-wide search for quantitative trait loci underlying asthma. *Nature* 1996; 383: 247–250.

36. Hakonarson H, Bjornsdottir US, Halapi E, Palsson S, Adalsteinsdottir E, Gislason D, Finnbogason G, Gislason T, Kristjansson K, Arnason T, Birkisson I, Frigge ML, Kong A, Gulcher JR, and Stefansson K. A major susceptibility gene for asthma maps to chromosome 14q24. *Am J Hum Genet* 2002; 71: 483–491.

37. De Sanctis GT, Merchant M, Beier DR, Dredge RD, Grobholz JK, Martin TR, Lander ES, and Drazen JM. Quantitative locus analysis of airway hyperresponsiveness in A/J and C57BL/6J mice. *Nat Genet* 1995; 11: 150–154.

38. De Sanctis GT, Singer JB, Jiao A, Yandava CN, Lee YH, Haynes TC, Lander ES, Beier DR, and Drazen JM. Quantitative trait locus mapping of airway responsiveness to chromosomes 6 and 7 in inbred mice. *Am J Physiol* 1999; 277: L1118–L1123.

39. Ewart SL, Kuperman D, Schadt E, Tankersley C, Grupe A, Shubitowski DM, Peltz G, and Wills-Karp M. Quantitative trait loci controlling allergen-induced airway hyperresponsiveness in inbred mice. *Am J Respir Cell Mol Biol* 2000; 23: 537–545.

40. Zhang Y, Lefort J, Kearsey V, Lapa e Silva JR, Cookson WO, and Vargaftig BB. A genome-wide screen for asthma-associated quantitative trait loci in a mouse model of allergic asthma. *Hum Mol Genet* 1999; 8: 601–605.

41. Van Eerdewegh P, Little RD, Dupuis J, Del Mastro RG, Falls K, Simon J, Torrey D, Pandit S, McKenny J, Braunschweiger K, Walsh A, Liu Z, Hayward B, Folz C, Manning SP, Bawa A, Saracino L, Thackston M, Benchekroun Y, Capparell N, Wang M, Adair R, Feng Y, Dubois J, FitzGerald MG, Huang H, Gibson R, Allen KM, Pedan A, Danzig MR, Umland SP, Egan RW, Cuss FM, Rorke S, Clough JB, Holloway JW, Holgate ST, and Keith TP. Association of the ADAM33 gene with asthma and bronchial hyperresponsiveness. *Nature* 2002; 418: 426–430.

42. Garlisi CG, Zou J, Devito KE, Tian F, Zhu FX, Liu J, Shah H, Wan Y, Motasim Billah M, Egan RW, and Umland SP. Human ADAM33: protein maturation and localization. *Biochem Biophys Res Commun* 2003; 301: 35–43.

43. Xu J, Meyers DA, Ober C, Blumenthal MN, Mellen B, Barnes KC, King RA, Lester LA, Howard TD, Solway J, Langefeld CD, Beaty TH, Rich SS, Bleecker ER, and Cox NJ. Genomewide screen and identification of gene-gene interactions for asthma-susceptibility loci in three U.S. populations: collaborative study on the genetics of asthma. *Am J Hum Genet* 2001; 68: 1437–1446.

44. Horikawa Y, Oda N, Cox NJ, Li X, Orho-Melander M, Hara M, Hinokio Y, Lindner TH, Mashima H, Schwarz PE, del Bosque-Plata L, Oda Y, Yoshiuchi I, Colilla S, Polonsky KS, Wei S, Concannon P, Iwasaki N, Schulze J, Baier LJ, Bogardus C, Groop L, Boerwinkle E, Hanis CL, and Bell GI. Genetic variation in the gene encoding calpain-10 is associated with type 2 diabetes mellitus. *Nat Genet* 2000; 26: 163–175.

45. Levine BB, Stember RH, and Fotino M. Ragweed hay fever: genetic control and linkage to HL-A haplotypes. *Science* 1972; 178: 1201–1203.

46. Blumenthal MN, Amos DB, and Noreen H. Genetic mapping of Ir locus in man: linkage to second locus of HL-A. *Science* 1974; 184: 1301–1303.

47. Bias WB and Marsh DG. HL-A linked antigen E immune response genes: an unproved hypothesis. *Science* 1975; 188: 375–377.

48. Marsh DG, Hsu SH, Roebber M, Ehrlich-Kautzky E, Freidhoff LR, Meyers DA, Pollard MK, and Bias WB. HLA-Dw2: a genetic marker for human immune response to short ragweed pollen allergen Ra5. I. Response resulting primarily from natural antigenic exposure. *J Exp Med* 1982; 155: 1439–1451.

49. Marsh DG, Freidhoff LR, Ehrlich-Kautzky E, Bias WB, and Roebber M. Immune responsiveness to *Ambrosia artemisiifolia* (short ragweed) pollen allergen Amb a-VI (Ra6) is associated with HLA-DR5 in allergic humans. *Immunogenetics* 1987; 26: 230–236.

50. Freidhoff LR, Ehrlich-Kautzky E, Meyers DA, Ansari AA, Bias WB, and Marsh DG. Association of HLA-DR3 with human immune response to Lol p I and Lol p II allergens in allergic subjects. *Tissue Antigens* 1988; 31: 211–219.

51. Fischer GF, Pickl WF, Fae I, Ebner C, Ferreira F, Breiteneder H, Vikoukal E, Scheiner O, and Kraft D. Association between IgE response against Bet v-I, the major allergen of birch pollen, and HLA-DRB alleles. *Hum Immunol* 1992; 33: 259–265.

52. Young RP, Dekker JW, Wordsworth BP, Schou C, Pile KD, Matthiesen F, Rosenberg WM, Bell JI, Hopkin JM, and Cookson WO. HLA-DR and HLA-DP genotypes and immunoglobulin E responses to common major allergens. *Clin Exp Allergy* 1994; 24: 431–439.

53. Moffatt MF, Schou C, Faux JA, Abecasis GR, James A, Musk AW, and Cookson WO. Association between quantitative traits underlying asthma and the HLA- DRB1 locus in a family-based population sample. *Eur J Hum Genet* 2001; 9: 341–346.

54. Cardaba B, Vilches C, Martin E, de Andres B, del Pozo V, Hernandez D, Gallardo S, Fernandez JC, Villalba M, Rodriguez R, Bogomba A, Kreisler M, Palomino P, and Lahoz C. DR7 and DQ2 are positively associated with immunoglobulin-E response to the main antigen of olive pollen (Ole e I) in allergic patients. *Hum Immunol* 1993; 38: 293–299.

55. D'Amato M, Scotto d'Abusco A, Maggi E, Menna T, Sacerdoti G, Maurizio SM, Iozzino S, De Santo C, Oreste U, Tosi R, D'Amato G, Baltadijeva D, Bjorksten B, Freidhoff LR, Lahoz C, Marsh DG, Rashef A, and Ruffilli A. Association of responsiveness to the major pollen allergen of *Parietaria officinalis* with HLA-DRB1* alleles: a multicenter study. *Hum Immunol* 1996; 46: 100–106.

56. Donfack J, Tsalenko A, Hoki DM, Parry R, Solway J, Lester LA, and Ober C. HLA-DRB1*01 alleles are associated with sensitization to cockroach allergens. *J Allergy Clin Immunol* 2000; 105: 960–966.

57. Kalpaklioglu AF and Turan M. Possible association between cockroach allergy and HLA class II antigens. *Ann Allergy Asthma Immunol* 2002; 89: 155–158.

58. Hu C, Hsu PN, Lin RH, Hsieh KH, and Chua KY. HLA DPB1*0201 allele is negatively associated with immunoglobulin E responsiveness specific for house dust mite allergens in Taiwan. *Clin Exp Allergy* 2000; 30: 538–545.

59. Kim YK, Oh SY, Oh HB, Lee BJ, Son JW, Cho SH, Kim YY, and Min KU. Positive association between HLA-DRB1*07 and specific IgE responses to purified major allergens of *D. pteronyssinus* (Der p 1 and Der p 2). *Ann Allergy Asthma Immunol* 2002; 88: 170–174.

60. Woszczek G, Kowalski ML, and Borowiec M. Association of asthma and total IgE levels with human leucocyte antigen-DR in patients with grass allergy. *Eur Respir J* 2002; 20: 79–85.

61. Moffatt MF, Faux JA, Lester S, Pare P, McCluskey J, Spargo R, James A, Musk AW, and Cookson WO. Atopy, respiratory function and HLA-DR in Aboriginal Australians. *Hum Mol Genet* 2003; 12: 625–630.

62. Aron Y, Desmazes-Dufeu N, Matran R, Polla BS, Dusser D, Lockhart A, and Swierczewski E. Evidence of a strong, positive association between atopy and the HLA class II alleles DR4 and DR7. *Clin Exp Allergy* 1996; 26: 821–828.

63. Soriano JB, Ercilla G, Sunyer J, Real FX, Lazaro C, Rodrigo MJ, Estivill X, Roca J, Rodriguez-Roisin R, Morell F, and Anto JM. HLA class II genes in soybean epidemic asthma patients. *Am J Respir Crit Care Med* 1997; 156: 1394–1398.

64. Howell WM, Standring P, Warner JA, and Warner JO. HLA class II genotype, HLA-DR B cell surface expression and allergen specific IgE production in atopic and non-atopic members of asthmatic family pedigrees. *Clin Exp Allergy* 1999; 29: S35–S38.

65. Cho SH, Kim YK, Oh HB, Jung JW, Son JW, Lee MH, Jee HS, Kim YY, and Min KU. Association of HLA-DRB1(*)07 and DRB1(*)04 to citrus red mite (*Panonychus citri*) and house dust mite-sensitive asthma. *Clin Exp Allergy* 2000; 30: 1568–1575.

66. Holloway JW, Doull I, Begishvili B, Beasley R, Holgate ST, and Howell WM. Lack of evidence of a significant association between HLA-DR, DQ and DP genotypes and atopy in families with HDM allergy. *Clin Exp Allergy* 1996; 26: 1142–1149.

67. Rihs HP, Barbalho-Krolls T, Huber H, and Baur X. No evidence for the influence of HLA class II in alleles in isocyanate-induced asthma. *Am J Ind Med* 1997; 32: 522–527.

68. Dekker JW, Nizankowska E, Schmitz-Schumann M, Pile K, Bochenek G, Dyczek A, Cookson WO, and Szczeklik A. Aspirin-induced asthma and HLA-DRB1 and HLA-DPB1 genotypes. *Clin Exp Allergy* 1997; 27: 574–577.

69. Thomas PS. Tumour necrosis factor-alpha: the role of this multifunctional cytokine in asthma. *Immunol Cell Biol* 2001; 79: 132–140.

70. Wilson AG, Symons JA, McDowell TL, McDevitt HO, and Duff GW. Effects of a polymorphism in the human tumor necrosis factor alpha promoter on transcriptional activation. *Proc Natl Acad Sci USA* 1997; 94: 3195–3199.

71. Moffatt MF and Cookson WO. Tumour necrosis factor haplotypes and asthma. *Hum Mol Genet* 1997; 6: 551–554.

72. Albuquerque RV, Hayden CM, Palmer LJ, Laing IA, Rye PJ, Gibson NA, Burton PR, Goldblatt J, and Lesouef PN. Association of polymorphisms within the tumour necrosis factor (TNF) genes and childhood asthma. *Clin Exp Allergy* 1998; 28: 578–584.

73. Chagani T, Pare PD, Zhu S, Weir TD, Bai TR, Behbehani NA, Fitzgerald JM, and Sandford AJ. Prevalence of tumor necrosis factor-alpha and angiotensin converting enzyme polymorphisms in mild/moderate and fatal/near-fatal asthma. *Am J Respir Crit Care Med* 1999; 160: 278–282.

74. Winchester EC, Millwood IY, Rand L, Penny MA, and Kessling AM. Association of the TNF-alpha-308 (G→A) polymorphism with self- reported history of childhood asthma. *Hum Genet* 2000; 107: 591–596.

75. Witte JS, Palmer LJ, O'Connor RD, Hopkins PJ, and Hall JM. Relation between tumour necrosis factor polymorphism TNF-alpha-308 and risk of asthma. *Eur J Hum Genet* 2002; 10: 82–85.

76. Li Kam Wa TC, Mansur AH, Britton J, Williams G, Pavord I, Richards K, Campbell DA, Morton N, Holgate ST, and Morrison JF. Association between −308 tumour necrosis factor promoter polymorphism and bronchial hyperreactivity in asthma. *Clin Exp Allergy* 1999; 29: 1204–1208.

77. Castro J, Telleria JJ, Linares P, and Blanco-Quiros A. Increased TNFA*2, but not TNFB*1, allele frequency in Spanish atopic patients. *J Invest Allergol Clin Immunol* 2000; 10: 149–154.

78. Trabetti E, Patuzzo C, Malerba G, Galavotti R, Martinati LC, Boner AL, and Pignatti PF. Association of a lymphotoxin alpha gene polymorphism and atopy in Italian families. *J Med Genet* 1999; 36: 323–325.

79. Zhu S, Chan-Yeung M, Becker AB, Dimich-Ward H, Ferguson AC, Manfreda J, Watson WT, Pare PD, and Sandford AJ. Polymorphisms of the IL-4, TNF-alpha, and Fc-epsilon RI-beta genes and the risk of allergic disorders in at-risk infants. *Am J Respir Crit Care Med* 2000; 161: 1655–1659.

80. Louis R, Leyder E, Malaise M, Bartsch P, and Louis E. Lack of association between adult asthma and the tumour necrosis factor alpha-308 polymorphism gene. *Eur Respir J* 2000; 16: 604–608.

81. Malerba G, Trabetti E, Patuzzo C, Lauciello MC, Galavotti R, Pescollderungg L, Boner AL, and Pignatti PF. Candidate genes and a genome-wide search in Italian families with atopic asthmatic children. *Clin Exp Allergy* 1999; 29: S27–S30.

82. Lin YC, Lu CC, Su HJ, Shen CY, Lei HY, and Guo YL. The association between tumor necrosis factor, HLA-DR alleles, and IgE-mediated asthma in Taiwanese adolescents. *Allergy* 2002; 57: 831–834.

83. Buckova D, Holla LI, Vasku A, Znojil V, and Vacha J. Lack of association between atopic asthma and the tumor necrosis factor alpha-308 gene polymorphism in a Czech population. *J Invest Allergol Clin Immunol* 2002; 12: 192–197.

84. Izakovicova Holla L, Vasku A, Izakovic V, and Znojil V. The interaction of the polymorphisms in transporter of antigen peptides (TAP) and lymphotoxin alpha (LT-alpha) genes and atopic diseases in the Czech population. *Clin Exp Allergy* 2001; 31: 1418–1423.

85. Moffatt MF, James A, Ryan G, Musk AW, and Cookson WO. Extended tumour necrosis factor/HLA-DR haplotypes and asthma in an Australian population sample. *Thorax* 1999; 54: 757–761.

86. Punnonen J, Yssel H, and de Vries JE. The relative contribution of IL-4 and IL-13 to human IgE synthesis induced by activated CD4+ or CD8+ T cells. *J Allergy Clin Immunol* 1997; 100: 792–801.

87. Wills-Karp M, Luyimbazi J, Xu X, Schofield B, Neben TY, Karp CL, and Donaldson DD. Interleukin-13: central mediator of allergic asthma. *Science* 1998; 282: 2258–2261.

88. Marsh DG, Neely JD, Breazeale DR, Ghosh B, Freidhoff LR, Ehrlich-Kautzky E, Schou C, Krishnaswamy G, and Beaty TH. Linkage analysis of IL4 and other chromosome 5q31.1 markers and total serum immunoglobulin E concentrations. *Science* 1994; 264: 1152–1156.

89. Meyers DA, Postma DS, Panhuysen CI, Xu J, Amelung PJ, Levitt RC, and Bleecker ER. Evidence for a locus regulating total serum IgE levels mapping to chromosome 5. *Genomics* 1994; 23: 464–470.

90. Postma DS, Bleecker ER, Amelung PJ, Holroyd KJ, Xu J, Panhuysen CI, Meyers DA, and Levitt RC. Genetic susceptibility to asthma: bronchial hyperresponsiveness coinherited with a major gene for atopy. *New Engl J Med* 1995; 333: 894–900.

91. Martinez FD, Solomon S, Holberg CJ, Graves PE, Baldini M, and Erickson RP. Linkage of circulating eosinophils to markers on chromosome 5q. *Am J Respir Crit Care Med* 1998; 158: 1739–1744.

92. Palmer LJ, Daniels SE, Rye PJ, Gibson NA, Tay GK, Cookson WO, Goldblatt J, Burton PR, and LeSouef PN. Linkage of chromosome 5q and 11q gene markers to asthma-associated quantitative traits in Australian children. *Am J Respir Crit Care Med* 1998; 158: 1825–1830.

93. Holberg CJ, Halonen M, Solomon S, Graves PE, Baldini M, Erickson RP, and Martinez FD. Factor analysis of asthma and atopy traits shows two major components, one of which is linked to markers on chromosome 5q. *J Allergy Clin Immunol* 2001; 108: 772–780.

94. van der Pouw Kraan TC, van Veen A, Boeije LC, van Tuyl SA, de Groot ER, Stapel SO, Bakker A, Verweij CL, Aarden LA, and van der Zee JS. An IL-13 promoter polymorphism associated with increased risk of allergic asthma. *Genes Immunol* 1999; 1: 61–65.

95. Howard TD, Whittaker PA, Zaiman AL, Koppelman GH, Xu J, Hanley MT, Meyers DA, Postma DS, and Bleecker ER. Identification and association of polymorphisms in the interleukin-13 gene with asthma and atopy in a Dutch population. *Am J Respir Cell Mol Biol* 2001; 25: 377–384.

96. Liu X, Nickel R, Beyer K, Wahn U, Ehrlich E, Freidhoff LR, Bjorksten B, Beaty TH, and Huang SK. An IL13 coding region variant is associated with a high total serum IgE level and atopic dermatitis in the German multicenter atopy study (MAS-90). *J Allergy Clin Immunol* 2000; 106: 167–170.

97. Graves PE, Kabesch M, Halonen M, Holberg CJ, Baldini M, Fritzsch C, Weiland SK, Erickson RP, von Mutius E, and Martinez FD. A cluster of seven tightly linked polymorphisms in the IL-13 gene is associated with total serum IgE levels in three populations of white children. *J Allergy Clin Immunol* 2000; 105: 506–513.

98. Leung TF, Tang NL, Chan IH, Li AM, Ha G, and Lam CW. A polymorphism in the coding region of interleukin-13 gene is associated with atopy but not asthma in Chinese children. *Clin Exp Allergy* 2001; 31: 1515–1521.

99. Tsunemi Y, Saeki H, Nakamura K, Sekiya T, Hirai K, Kakinuma T, Fujita H, Asano N, Tanida Y, Wakugawa M, Torii H, and Tamaki K. Interleukin-13 gene polymorphism G4257A is associated with atopic dermatitis in Japanese patients. *J Dermatol Sci* 2002; 30: 100–107.

100. Heinzmann A, Mao XQ, Akaiwa M, Kreomer RT, Gao PS, Ohshima K, Umeshita R, Abe Y, Braun S, Yamashita T, Roberts MH, Sugimoto R, Arima K, Arinobu Y, Yu B, Kruse S, Enomoto T, Dake Y, Kawai M, Shimazu S, Sasaki S, Adra CN, Kitaichi M, Inoue H, Yamauchi K, Tomichi N, Kurimoto F, Hamasaki N, Hopkin JM, Izuhara K, Shirakawa T, and Deichmann KA. Genetic variants of IL-13 signalling and human asthma and atopy. *Hum Mol Genet* 2000; 9: 549–559.

101. DeMeo DL, Lange C, Silverman EK, Senter JM, Drazen JM, Barth MJ, Laird N, and Weiss ST. Univariate and multivariate family-based association analysis of the IL-13 ARG130GLN polymorphism in the Childhood Asthma Management program. *Genet Epidemiol* 2002; 23: 335–348.

102. Arima K, Umeshita-Suyama R, Sakata Y, Akaiwa M, Mao XQ, Enomoto T, Dake Y, Shimazu S, Yamashita T, Sugawara N, Brodeur S, Geha R, Puri RK, Sayegh MH, Adra CN, Hamasaki N, Hopkin JM, Shirakawa T, and Izuhara K. Upregulation of IL-13 concentration *in vivo* by the IL13 variant associated with bronchial asthma. *J Allergy Clin Immunol* 2002; 109: 980–987.

103. Hakonarson H, Bjornsdottir US, Ostermann E, Arnason T, Adalsteinsdottir AE, Halapi E, Shkolny D, Kristjansson K, Gudnadottir SA, Frigge ML, Gislason D, Gislason T, Kong A, Gulcher J, and Stefansson K. Allelic frequencies and patterns

of single-nucleotide polymorphisms in candidate genes for asthma and atopy in Iceland. *Am J Respir Crit Care Med* 2001; 164: 2036–2044.

104. Celedon JC, Soto-Quiros ME, Palmer LJ, Senter J, Mosley J, Silverman EK, and Weiss ST. Lack of association between a polymorphism in the interleukin-13 gene and total serum immunoglobulin E level among nuclear families in Costa Rica. *Clin Exp Allergy* 2002; 32: 387–390.

105. Rosenwasser LJ, Klemm DJ, Dresback JK, Inamura H, Mascali JJ, Klinnert M, and Borish L. Promoter polymorphisms in the chromosome 5 gene cluster in asthma and atopy. *Clin Exp Allergy* 1995; 25: S74–S78.

106. Walley AJ and Cookson WO. Investigation of an interleukin-4 promoter polymorphism for associations with asthma and atopy. *J Med Genet* 1996; 33: 689–692.

107. Noguchi E, Shibasaki M, Arinami T, Takeda K, Yokouchi Y, Kawashima T, Yanagi H, Matsui A, and Hamaguchi H. Association of asthma and the interleukin-4 promoter gene in Japanese. *Clin Exp Allergy* 1998; 28: 449–453.

108. Sandford AJ, Chagani T, Zhu S, Weir TD, Bai TR, Spinelli JJ, Fitzgerald JM, Behbehani NA, Tan WC, and Pare PD. Polymorphisms in the IL4, IL4RA, and FCERIB genes and asthma severity. *J Allergy Clin Immunol* 2000; 106: 135–140.

109. Kawashima T, Noguchi E, Arinami T, Yamakawa-Kobayashi K, Nakagawa H, Otsuka F, and Hamaguchi H. Linkage and association of an interleukin 4 gene polymorphism with atopic dermatitis in Japanese families. *J Med Genet* 1998; 35: 502–504.

110. Novak N, Kruse S, Kraft S, Geiger E, Kluken H, Fimmers R, Deichmann KA, and Bieber T. Dichotomic nature of atopic dermatitis reflected by combined analysis of monocyte immunophenotyping and single nucleotide polymorphisms of the interleukin-4/interleukin-13 receptor gene: the dichotomy of extrinsic and intrinsic atopic dermatitis. *J Invest Dermatol* 2002; 119: 870–875.

111. Burchard EG, Silverman EK, Rosenwasser LJ, Borish L, Yandava C, Pillari A, Weiss ST, Hasday J, Lilly CM, Ford JG, and Drazen JM. Association between a sequence variant in the IL-4 gene promoter and FEV(1) in asthma. *Am J Respir Crit Care Med* 1999; 160: 919–922.

112. Takabayashi A, Ihara K, Sasaki Y, Suzuki Y, Nishima S, Izuhara K, Hamasaki N, and Hara T. Childhood atopic asthma: positive association with a polymorphism of IL-4 receptor alpha gene but not with that of IL-4 promoter or Fc epsilon receptor I beta gene. *Exp Clin Immunogenet* 2000; 17: 63–70.

113. Elliott K, Fitzpatrick E, Hill D, Brown J, Adams S, Chee P, Stewart G, Fulcher D, Tang M, Kemp A, King E, Varigos G, Bahlo M, and Forrest S. The –590C/T and –34C/T interleukin-4 promoter polymorphisms are not associated with atopic eczema in childhood. *J Allergy Clin Immunol* 2001; 108: 285–287.

114. Tanaka K, Sugiura H, Uehara M, Hashimoto Y, Donnelly C, and Montgomery DS. Lack of association between atopic eczema and the genetic variants of interleukin-4 and the interleukin-4 receptor alpha chain gene: heterogeneity of genetic backgrounds on immunoglobulin E production in atopic eczema patients. *Clin Exp Allergy* 2001; 31: 1522–1527.

115. Dizier MH, Sandford A, Walley A, Philippi A, Cookson W, and Demenais F. Indication of linkage of serum IgE levels to the interleukin-4 gene and exclusion

of the contribution of the (–590 C to T) interleukin-4 promoter polymorphism to IgE variation. *Genet Epidemiol* 1999; 16: 84–94.

116. Suzuki I, Hizawa N, Yamaguchi E, and Kawakami Y. Association between a C+33T polymorphism in the IL-4 promoter region and total serum IgE levels. *Clin Exp Allergy* 2000; 30: 1746–1749.

117. Deichmann K, Bardutzky J, Forster J, Heinzmann A, and Kuehr J. Common polymorphisms in the coding part of the IL4-receptor gene. *Biochem Biophys Res Commun* 1997; 231: 696–697.

118. Hershey GK, Friedrich MF, Esswein LA, Thomas ML, and Chatila TA. The association of atopy with a gain-of-function mutation in the alpha subunit of the interleukin-4 receptor. *New Engl J Med* 1997; 337: 1720–1725.

119. Wu X, Di Rienzo A, and Ober C. A population genetics study of single nucleotide polymorphisms in the interleukin 4 receptor alpha (IL4RA) gene. *Genes Immunol* 2001; 2: 128–134.

120. Mitsuyasu H, Yanagihara Y, Mao XQ, Gao PS, Arinobu Y, Ihara K, Takabayashi A, Hara T, Enomoto T, Sasaki S, Kawai M, Hamasaki N, Shirakawa T, Hopkin JM, and Izuhara K. Cutting edge: dominant effect of Ile50Val variant of the human IL-4 receptor alpha-chain in IgE synthesis. *J Immunol* 1999; 162: 1227–1231.

121. Izuhara K, Yanagihara Y, Hamasaki N, Shirakawa T, and Hopkin JM. Atopy and the human IL-4 receptor alpha chain. *J Allergy Clin Immunol* 2000; 106: S65–S71.

122. Kruse S, Japha T, Tedner M, Sparholt SH, Forster J, Kuehr J, and Deichmann KA. The polymorphisms S503P and Q576R in the interleukin-4 receptor alpha gene are associated with atopy and influence the signal transduction. *Immunology* 1999; 96: 365–371.

123. Hoffjan S and Ober C. Present status on the genetic studies of asthma. *Curr Opin Immunol* 2002; 14: 709–717.

124. Bottini N, Borgiani P, Otsu A, Saccucci P, Stefanini L, Greco E, Fontana L, Hopkin JM, Mao XQ, and Shirakawa T. IL-4 receptor alpha chain genetic polymorphism and total IgE levels in the English population: two-locus haplotypes are more informative than individual SNPs. *Clin Genet* 2002; 61: 288–292.

125. Hackstein H, Hecker M, Kruse S, Bohnert A, Ober C, Deichmann KA, and Bein G. A novel polymorphism in the 5' promoter region of the human interleukin-4 receptor alpha-chain gene is associated with decreased soluble interleukin-4 receptor protein levels. *Immunogenetics* 2001; 53: 264–269.

126. Cookson WO, Sharp PA, Faux JA, and Hopkin JM. Linkage between immunoglobulin E responses underlying asthma and rhinitis and chromosome 11q. *Lancet* 1989; 1: 1292–1295.

127. Huang SK, Mathias RA, Ehrlich E, Plunkett B, Liu X, Cutting GR, Wang XJ, Li XD, Togias A, Barnes KC, Malveaux F, Rich S, Mellen B, Lange E, and Beaty TH. Evidence for asthma susceptibility genes on chromosome 11 in an African-American population. *Hum Genet* 2003; 27: 27.

128. Rigoli L, Salpietro DC, Lavalle R, Cafiero G, Zuccarello D, and Barberi I. Allelic association of gene markers on chromosome 11q in Italian families with atopy. *Acta Paediatr* 2000; 89: 1056–1061.

129. Shirakawa T, Hashimoto T, Furuyama J, Takeshita T, and Morimoto K. Linkage between severe atopy and chromosome 11q13 in Japanese families. *Clin Genet* 1994; 46: 228–232.
130. Sandford AJ, Shirakawa T, Moffatt MF, Daniels SE, Ra C, Faux JA, Young RP, Nakamura Y, Lathrop GM, Cookson WO, and Hopkin JM, Localisation of atopy and beta subunit of high-affinity IgE receptor (Fc epsilon RI) on chromosome 11q. *Lancet* 1993; 341: 332–334.
131. Cookson WO, Young RP, Sandford AJ, Moffatt MF, Shirakawa T, Sharp PA, Faux JA, Julier C, LeSonef PN, Nakumuura Y, Lathrop GM, and Hopkin JM. Maternal inheritance of atopic IgE responsiveness on chromosome 11q. *Lancet* 1992; 340: 381–384.
132. Kinet JP. The high-affinity IgE receptor (Fc epsilon RI): from physiology to pathology. *Annu Rev Immunol* 1999; 17: 931–972.
133. Shirakawa T, Li A, Dubowitz M, Dekker JW, Shaw AE, Faux JA, Ra C, Cookson WO, and Hopkin JM. Association between atopy and variants of the beta subunit of the high-affinity immunoglobulin E receptor. *Nat Genet* 1994; 7: 125–129.
134. Li A and Hopkin JM. Atopy phenotype in subjects with variants of the beta subunit of the high affinity IgE receptor. *Thorax* 1997; 52: 654–655.
135. Green SL, Gaillard MC, Song E, Dewar JB, and Halkas A. Polymorphisms of the beta chain of the high-affinity immunoglobulin E receptor (F cepsilon RI-beta) in South African black and white asthmatic and nonasthmatic individuals. *Am J Respir Crit Care Med* 1998; 158: 1487–1492.
136. Deichmann KA, Hildebrandt F, Heinzmann A, Schlenther S, Forster J, and Kuehr J. Absence of mutations in the sixth exon of Fc epsilon RI-beta. *Adv Exp Med Biol* 1996; 409: 355–358.
137. Kofler H, Aichberger S, Ott G, Casari A, and Kofler R. Lack of association between atopy and the Ile181Leu variant of the beta subunit of the high-affinity immunoglobulin E receptor. *Int Arch Allergy Immunol* 1996; 111: 44–47.
138. Dickson PW, Wong ZY, Harrap SB, Abramson MJ, and Walters EH. Mutational analysis of the high affinity immunoglobulin E receptor beta subunit gene in asthma. *Thorax* 1999; 54: 409–412.
139. Hill MR and Cookson WO. A new variant of the beta subunit of the high-affinity receptor for immunoglobulin E (Fc epsilon RI-beta E237G): associations with measures of atopy and bronchial hyper-responsiveness. *Hum Mol Genet* 1996; 5: 959–962.
140. Shirakawa T, Mao XQ, Sasaki S, Enomoto T, Kawai M, Morimoto K, and Hopkin J. Association between atopic asthma and a coding variant of Fc epsilon RI beta in a Japanese population. *Hum Mol Genet* 1996; 5: 1129–1130.
141. Nagata H, Mutoh H, Kumahara K, Arimoto Y, Tomemori T, Sakurai D, Arase K, Ohno K, Yamakoshi T, Nakano K, Okawa T, Numata T, and Konno A. Association between nasal allergy and a coding variant of the Fc epsilon RI beta gene Glu237Gly in a Japanese population. *Hum Genet* 2001; 109: 262–266.
142. Laprise C, Boulet LP, Morissette J, Winstall E, and Raymond V. Evidence for association and linkage between atopy, airway hyper-responsiveness, and the beta subunit Glu237Gly variant of the high-affinity receptor for immunoglobulin E in the French-Canadian population. *Immunogenetics* 2000; 51: 695–702.

143. Palmer LJ, Rye PJ, Gibson NA, Moffatt MF, Goldblatt J, Burton PR, Cookson WO, and Lesouef PN. Association of Fc-epsilon R1-beta polymorphisms with asthma and associated traits in Australian asthmatic families. *Clin Exp Allergy* 1999; 29: 1555–1562.

144. Cox HE, Moffatt MF, Faux JA, Walley AJ, Coleman R, Trembath RC, Cookson WO, and Harper JI. Association of atopic dermatitis to the beta subunit of the high affinity immunoglobulin E receptor. *Br J Dermatol* 1998; 138: 182–187.

145. van Hage-Hamsten M, Johansson E, Kronqvist M, Loughry A, Cookson WO, and Moffatt MF. Associations of Fc epsilon R1-beta polymorphisms with immunoglobin E antibody responses to common inhalant allergens in a rural population. *Clin Exp Allergy* 2002; 32: 838–842.

146. Hizawa N, Yamaguchi E, Jinushi E, and Kawakami Y. A common FCER1B gene promoter polymorphism influences total serum IgE levels in a Japanese population. *Am J Respir Crit Care Med* 2000; 161: 906–909.

147. Laing IA, Hermans C, Bernard A, Burton PR, Goldblatt J, and Le Souef PN. Association between plasma CC16 levels, the A38G polymorphism, and asthma. *Am J Respir Crit Care Med* 2000; 161: 124–127.

148. Sengler C, Heinzmann A, Jerkic SP, Haider A, Sommerfeld C, Niggemann B, Lau S, Forster J, Schuster A, Kamin W, Bauer C, Laing I, LeSouef P, Wahn U, Deichmann K, and Nickel R. Clara cell protein 16 (CC16) gene polymorphism influences the degree of airway responsiveness in asthmatic children. *J Allergy Clin Immunol* 2003; 111: 515–519.

149. Fryer AA, Bianco A, Hepple M, Jones PW, Strange RC, and Spiteri MA. Polymorphism at the glutathione S-transferase GSTP1 locus: a new marker for bronchial hyperresponsiveness and asthma. *Am J Respir Crit Care Med* 2000; 161: 1437–1442.

150. Gilliland FD, Gauderman WJ, Vora H, Rappaport E, and Dubeau L. Effects of glutathione-S-transferase M1, T1, and P1 on childhood lung function growth. *Am J Respir Crit Care Med* 2002; 166: 710–716.

151. Mapp CE, Fryer AA, De Marzo N, Pozzato V, Padoan M, Boschetto P, Strange RC, Hemmingsen A, and Spiteri MA. Glutathione S-transferase GSTP1 is a susceptibility gene for occupational asthma induced by isocyanates. *J Allergy Clin Immunol* 2002; 109: 867–872.

152. Aderem A and Ulevitch RJ. Toll-like receptors in the induction of the innate immune response. *Nature* 2000; 406: 782–787.

153. Gereda JE, Leung DY, Thatayatikom A, Streib JE, Price MR, Klinnert MD, and Liu AH. Relation between house-dust endotoxin exposure, type 1 T-cell development, and allergen sensitisation in infants at high risk of asthma. *Lancet* 2000; 355: 1680–1683.

154. Braun-Fahrlander C, Riedler J, Herz U, Eder W, Waser M, Grize L, Maisch S, Carr D, Gerlach F, Bufe A, Lauener RP, Schierl R, Renz H, Nowak D, and von Mutius E. Environmental exposure to endotoxin and its relation to asthma in school-age children. *New Engl J Med* 2002; 347: 869–877.

155. Martinez FD. The coming-of-age of the hygiene hypothesis. *Respir Res* 2001; 2: 129–132.

156. Liu AH and Murphy JR. Hygiene hypothesis: fact or fiction? *J Allergy Clin Immunol* 2003; 111: 471–478.

157. Baldini M, Lohman IC, Halonen M, Erickson RP, Holt PG, and Martinez FD. A Polymorphism in the 5′ flanking region of the CD14 gene is associated with circulating soluble CD14 levels and with total serum immunoglobulin E. *Am J Respir Cell Mol Biol* 1999; 20: 976–983.

158. LeVan TD, Bloom JW, Bailey TJ, Karp CL, Halonen M, Martinez FD, and Vercelli D. A common single nucleotide polymorphism in the CD14 promoter decreases the affinity of Sp protein binding and enhances transcriptional activity. *J Immunol* 2001; 167: 5838–5844.

159. Koppelman GH, Reijmerink NE, Colin Stine O, Howard TD, Whittaker PA, Meyers DA, Postma DS, and Bleecker ER. Association of a promoter polymorphism of the CD14 gene and atopy. *Am J Respir Crit Care Med* 2001; 163: 965–969.

160. Sengler C, Haider A, Sommerfeld C, Lau S, Baldini M, Martinez F, Wahn U, and Nickel R. Evaluation of the CD14 C-159 T polymorphism in the German Multicenter Allergy Study cohort. *Clin Exp Allergy* 2003; 33: 166–169.

161. Vercelli D. Learning from discrepancies: CD14 polymorphisms, atopy and the endotoxin switch. *Clin Exp Allergy* 2003; 33: 153–155.

162. Lemanske RF, Jr. The Childhood Origins of Asthma (COAST) study. *Pediatr Allergy Immunol* 2002; 15: 1–6.

163. Gern JE, Rock C, Hoffjan S, Nicolae D, Zhanhai L, Roberg KA, Carlson-Dakes K, Adler K, R. H, Anderson E, Gilbertson-White S, Tisler C, DaSilva D, Anklam K, Mikus LD, Rosenthal LA, Ober C, Gangnon R, and Lemanske RF, Jr. Effect of dog ownership and genotype on immune development and atopy in infancy. *J Allergy Clin Immunol* 2004; 113: 307–314.

164. Johnson M. The beta adrenoceptor. *Am J Respir Crit Care Med* 1998; 158: S146–S153.

165. Drazen JM, Silverman EK, and Lee TH. Heterogeneity of therapeutic responses in asthma. *Br Med Bull* 2000; 56: 1054–1070.

166. Green SA, Turki J, Bejarano P, Hall IP, and Liggett SB. Influence of beta 2-adrenergic receptor genotypes on signal transduction in human airway smooth muscle cells. *Am J Respir Cell Mol Biol* 1995; 13: 25–33.

167. McGraw DW, Forbes SL, Kramer LA, and Liggett SB. Polymorphisms of the 5′ leader cistron of the human beta-2-adrenergic receptor regulate receptor expression. *J Clin Invest* 1998; 102: 1927–1932.

168. Reihsaus E, Innis M, MacIntyre N, and Liggett SB. Mutations in the gene encoding for the beta 2-adrenergic receptor in normal and asthmatic subjects. *Am J Respir Cell Mol Biol* 1993; 8: 334–339.

169. Turki J, Pak J, Green SA, Martin RJ, and Liggett SB. Genetic polymorphisms of the beta 2-adrenergic receptor in nocturnal and nonnocturnal asthma: evidence that Gly16 correlates with the nocturnal phenotype. *J Clin Invest* 1995; 95: 1635–1641.

170. Holloway JW, Dunbar PR, Riley GA, Sawyer GM, Fitzharris PF, Pearce N, Le Gros GS, and Beasley R. Association of beta 2-adrenergic receptor polymorphisms with severe asthma. *Clin Exp Allergy* 2000; 30: 1097–1103.

171. Summerhill E, Leavitt SA, Gidley H, Parry R, Solway J, and Ober C. Beta(2)-adrenergic receptor Arg16/Arg16 genotype is associated with reduced lung function, but not with asthma, in the Hutterites. *Am J Respir Crit Care Med* 2000; 162: 599–602.

172. Dewar JC, Wilkinson J, Wheatley A, Thomas NS, Doull I, Morton N, Lio P, Harvey JF, Liggett SB, Holgate ST, and Hall IP. The glutamine 27 beta 2-adrenoceptor polymorphism is associated with elevated IgE levels in asthmatic families. *J Allergy Clin Immunol* 1997; 100: 261–265.

173. Hall IP, Wheatley A, Wilding P, and Liggett SB. Association of Glu 27 beta 2-adrenoceptor polymorphism with lower airway reactivity in asthmatic subjects. *Lancet* 1995; 345: 1213–1214.

174. Hopes E, McDougall C, Christie G, Dewar J, Wheatley A, Hall IP, and Helms PJ. Association of glutamine 27 polymorphism of beta 2 adrenoceptor with reported childhood asthma: population based study. *Br Med J* 1998; 316: 664.

175. Martinez FD, Graves PE, Baldini M, Solomon S, and Erickson R. Association between genetic polymorphisms of the beta 2-adrenoceptor and response to albuterol in children with and without a history of wheezing. *J Clin Invest* 1997; 100: 3184–3188.

176. Kotani Y, Nishimura Y, Maeda H, and Yokoyama M. Beta 2-adrenergic receptor polymorphisms affect airway responsiveness to salbutamol in asthmatics. *J Asthma* 1999; 36: 583–590.

177. Tan S, Hall IP, Dewar J, Dow E, and Lipworth B. Association between beta 2-adrenoceptor polymorphism and susceptibility to bronchodilator desensitisation in moderately severe stable asthmatics. *Lancet* 1997; 350: 995–999.

178. Israel E, Drazen JM, Liggett SB, Boushey HA, Cherniack RM, Chinchilli VM, Cooper DM, Fahy JV, Fish JE, Ford JG, Kraft M, Kunselman S, Lazarus SC, Lemanske RF, Jr., Martin RJ, McLean DE, Peters SP, Silverman EK, Sorkness CA, Szefler SJ, Weiss ST, and Yandava CN. Effect of polymorphism of the beta(2)-adrenergic receptor on response to regular use of albuterol in asthma. *Int Arch Allergy Immunol* 2001; 124: 183–186.

179. Taylor DR, Hancox RJ, McRae W, Cowan JO, Flannery EM, McLachlan CR, and Herbison GP. The influence of polymorphism at position 16 of the beta 2-adreno-ceptor on the development of tolerance to beta agonists. *J Asthma* 2000; 37: 691–700.

180. Lipworth BJ, Hall IP, Aziz I, Tan KS, and Wheatley A. Beta 2-adrenoceptor poly-morphism and bronchoprotective sensitivity with regular short- and long-acting beta 2-agonist therapy. *Clin Sci (Lond)* 1999; 96: 253–259.

181. A genome-wide search for asthma susceptibility loci in ethnically diverse popula-tions: the Collaborative Study on the Genetics of Asthma (CSGA). *Nat Genet* 1997; 15: 389–392.

182. Mathias RA, Freidhoff LR, Blumenthal MN, Meyers DA, Lester L, King R, Xu JF, Solway J, Barnes KC, Pierce J, Stine OC, Togias A, Oetting W, Marshik PL, Hetmanski JB, Huang SK, Ehrlich E, Dunston GM, Malveaux F, Banks-Schlegel S, Cox NJ, Bleecker E, Ober C, Beaty TH, and Rich SS. Genome-wide linkage analyses of total serum IgE using variance components analysis in asthmatic fam-ilies. *Genet Epidemiol* 2001; 20: 340–355.

183. Ober C, Cox NJ, Abney M, Di Rienzo A, Lander ES, Changyaleket B, Gidley H, Kurtz B, Lee J, Nance M, Pettersson A, Prescott J, Richardson A, Schlenker E, Summerhill E, Willadsen S, and Parry R. Genome-wide search for asthma susceptibility

loci in a founder population: the Collaborative Study on the Genetics of Asthma. *Hum Mol Genet* 1998; 7: 1393–1398.

184. Ober C, Tsalenko A, Willadsen S, Newman D, Daniel R, Wu X, Andal J, Hoki D, Schneider D, True K, Schou C, Parry R, and Cox N. Genome-wide screen for atopy susceptibility alleles in the Hutterites. *Clin Exp Allergy* 1999; 29: S11–S15.

185. Wjst M. Specific IgE: one gene fits all? *Clin Exp Allergy* 1999; 29: S5–S10.

186. Alcais A, Plancoulaine S, and Abel L. An autosome-wide search for loci underlying wheezing age of onset in German asthmatic children identifies a new region of interest on 6q24–q25. *Genet Epidemiol* 2001; 21: S168–S173.

187. Dizier MH, Besse-Schmittler C, Guilloud-Bataille M, Annesi-Maesano I, Boussaha M, Bousquet J, Charpin D, Degioanni A, Gormand F, Grimfeld A, Hochez J, Hyne G, Lockhart A, Luillier-Lacombe M, Matran R, Meunier F, Neukirch F, Pacheco Y, Parent V, Paty E, Pin I, Pison C, Scheinmann P, Thobie N, Vervloet D, Kauffmann F, Feingold J, Lathrop M, and Demenais F. Genome screen for asthma and related phenotypes in the French EGEA study. *Am J Respir Crit Care Med* 2000; 162: 1812–1818.

188. Koppelman GH, Stine OC, Xu J, Howard TD, Zheng SL, Kauffman HF, Bleecker ER, Meyers DA, and Postma DS. Genome-wide search for atopy susceptibility genes in Dutch families with asthma. *J Allergy Clin Immunol* 2002; 109: 498–506.

189. Laitinen T, Daly MJ, Rioux JD, Kauppi P, Laprise C, Petays T, Green T, Cargill M, Haahtela T, Lander ES, Laitinen LA, Hudson TJ, and Kere J. A susceptibility locus for asthma-related traits on chromosome 7 revealed by genome-wide scan in a founder population. *Nat Genet* 2001; 28: 87–91.

190. Haagerup A, Bjerke T, Schoitz PO, Binderup HG, Dahl R, and Kruse TA. Allergic rhinitis: a total genome scan for susceptibility genes suggests a locus on chromosome 4q24–q27. *Eur J Hum Genet* 2001; 9: 945–952.

191. Haagerup A, Bjerke T, Schiotz PO, Binderup HG, Dahl R, and Kruse TA. Asthma and atopy: a total genome scan for susceptibility genes. *Allergy* 2002; 57: 680–686.

192. Yokouchi Y, Shibasaki M, Noguchi E, Nakayama J, Ohtsuki T, Kamioka M, Yamakawa-Kobayashi K, Ito S, Takeda K, Ichikawa K, Nukaga Y, Matsui A, Hamaguchi H, and Arinami T. A genome-wide linkage analysis of orchard grass-sensitive childhood seasonal allergic rhinitis in Japanese families. *Genes Immun* 2002; 3: 9–13.

193. Yan L, Galinsky RE, Bernstein JA, Liggett SB, and Weinshilboum RM. Histamine N-methyltransferase pharmacogenetics: association of a common functional polymorphism with asthma. *Pharmacogenetics* 2000; 10: 261–266.

194. Sasaki Y, Ihara K, Ahmed S, Yamawaki K, Kusuhara K, Nakayama H, Nishima S, and Hara T. Lack of association between atopic asthma and polymorphisms of the histamine H1 receptor, histamine H2 receptor, and histamine N-methyltransferase genes. *Immunogenetics* 2000; 51: 238–240.

195. Rosenwasser LJ. Promoter polymorphism in the candidate genes, IL-4, IL-9, TGF-beta 1, for atopy and asthma. *Int Arch Allergy Immunol* 1999; 118: 268–270.

196. Hobbs K, Negri J, Klinnert M, Rosenwasser LJ, and Borish L. Interleukin-10 and transforming growth factor-beta promoter polymorphisms in allergies and asthma. *Am J Respir Crit Care Med* 1998; 158: 1958–1962.

197. Unoki M, Furuta S, Onouchi Y, Watanabe O, Doi S, Fujiwara H, Miyatake A, Fujita K, Tamari M, and Nakamura Y. Association studies of 33 single nucleotide polymorphisms (SNPs) in 29 candidate genes for bronchial asthma: positive association a T924C polymorphism in the thromboxane A2 receptor gene. *Hum Genet* 2000; 106: 440–446.

198. Immervoll T, Loesgen S, Dutsch G, Gohlke H, Herbon N, Klugbauer S, Dempfle A, Bickeboller H, Becker-Follmann J, Ruschendorf F, Saar K, Reis A, Wichmann HE, and Wjst M. Fine mapping and single nucleotide polymorphism association results of candidate genes for asthma and related phenotypes. *Hum Mutat* 2001; 18: 327–336.

199. Karjalainen J, Hulkkonen J, Nieminen MM, Huhtala H, Aromaa A, Klaukka T, and Hurme M. Interleukin-10 gene promoter region polymorphism is associated with eosinophil count and circulating immunoglobulin E in adult asthma. *Clin Exp Allergy* 2003; 33: 78–83.

200. Donfack J, Kogut P, Forsythe S, Solway J, and Ober C. Sequence variation in the promoter region of the cholinergic receptor muscarinic 3 gene and asthma and atopy. *J Allergy Clin Immunol* 2003; 111: 527–532.

201. Ligers A, Teleshova N, Masterman T, Huang WX, and Hillert J. CTLA-4 gene expression is influenced by promoter and exon 1 polymorphisms. *Genes Immunol* 2001; 2: 145–152.

202. Heinzmann A, Plesnar C, Kuehr J, Forster J, and Deichmann KA. Common polymorphisms in the CTLA-4 and CD28 genes at 2q33 are not associated with asthma or atopy. *Eur J Immunogenet* 2000; 27: 57–61.

203. Nakao F, Ihara K, Ahmed S, Sasaki Y, Kusuhara K, Takabayashi A, Nishima S, and Hara T. Lack of association between CD28/CTLA-4 gene polymorphisms and atopic asthma in the Japanese population. *Exp Clin Immunogenet* 2000; 17: 179–184.

204. Hizawa N, Yamaguchi E, Jinushi E, Konno S, Kawakami Y, and Nishimura M. Increased total serum IgE levels in patients with asthma and promoter polymorphisms at CTLA4 and FCER1B. *J Allergy Clin Immunol* 2001; 108: 74–79.

205. Lee SY, Lee YH, Shin C, Shim JJ, Kang KH, Yoo SH, and In KH. Association of asthma severity and bronchial hyperresponsiveness with a polymorphism in the cytotoxic T-lymphocyte antigen-4 gene. *Chest* 2002; 122: 171–176.

206. Maurer M, Loserth S, Kolb-Maurer A, Ponath A, Wiese S, Kruse N, and Rieckmann P. A polymorphism in the human cytotoxic T-lymphocyte antigen 4 (CTLA4) gene (exon 1 + 49) alters T-cell activation. *Immunogenetics* 2002; 54: 1–8.

207. Howard TD, Postma DS, Koppelman GA, Koppelman GH, Zheng SL, Wysong AK, Xu J, Meyers DA, and Bleecker ER. Fine mapping of an IgE-controlling gene on chromosome 2q: analysis of CTLA4 and CD28. *J Allergy Clin Immunol* 2002; 110: 743–751.

208. Fukunaga K, Asano K, Mao XQ, Gao PS, Roberts MH, Oguma T, Shiomi T, Kanazawa M, Adra CN, Shirakawa T, Hopkin JM, and Yamaguchi K. Genetic polymorphisms of CC chemokine receptor 3 in Japanese and British asthmatics. *Eur Respir J* 2001; 17: 59–63.

209. Liu R, Paxton WA, Choe S, Ceradini D, Martin SR, Horuk R, MacDonald ME, Stuhlmann H, Koup RA, and Landau NR. Homozygous defect in HIV-1 coreceptor accounts for resistance of some multiply exposed individuals to HIV-1 infection. *Cell* 1996; 86: 367–377.

210. Hall IP, Wheatley A, Christie G, McDougall C, Hubbard R, and Helms PJ. Association of CCR5 delta32 with reduced risk of asthma. *Lancet* 1999; 354: 1264–1265.
211. Mitchell TJ, Walley AJ, Pease JE, Venables PJ, Wiltshire S, Williams TJ, and Cookson WO. Delta 32 deletion of CCR5 gene and association with asthma or atopy. *Lancet* 2000; 356: 1491–1492.
212. Szalai C, Bojszko A, Beko G, and Falus A. Prevalence of CCR5 delta 32 in allergic diseases. *Lancet* 2000; 355: 66.
213. Sandford AJ, Zhu S, Bai TR, Fitzgerald JM, and Pare PD. The role of the CC chemokine receptor-5 delta 32 polymorphism in asthma and in the production of regulated on activation: normal T cells expressed and secreted. *J Allergy Clin Immunol* 2001; 108: 69–73.
214. Nagy A, Kozma GT, Bojszko A, Krikovszky D, Falus A, and Szalai C. No association between asthma or allergy and the CCR5 delta 32 mutation. *Arch Dis Child* 2002; 86: 426.
215. McGinnis R, Child F, Clayton S, Davies S, Lenney W, Illig T, Wjst M, Spurr N, Debouck C, Hajeer AH, Ollier WE, Strange R, and Fryer AA. Further support for the association of CCR5 allelic variants with asthma susceptibility. *Eur J Immunogenet* 2002; 29: 525–528.
216. Srivastava P, Helms PJ, Stewart D, Main M, and Russell G. Association of CCR5 delta 32 with reduced risk of childhood but not adult asthma. *Thorax* 2003; 58: 222–226.
217. Lazarus R, Klimecki WT, Raby BA, Vercelli D, Palmer LJ, Kwiatkowski DJ, Silverman EK, Martinez F, and Weiss ST. Single-nucleotide polymorphisms in the Toll-like receptor 9 gene (TLR9): frequencies, pairwise linkage disequilibrium, and haplotypes in three U.S. ethnic groups and exploratory case-control disease association studies. *Genomics* 2003; 81: 85–91.
218. Mao XQ, Gao PS, Roberts MH, Enomoto T, Kawai M, Sasaki S, Shaldon SR, Coull P, Dake Y, Adra CN, Hagihara A, Shirakawa T, and Hopkin JM. Variants of endothelin-1 and its receptors in atopic asthma. *Biochem Biophys Res Commun* 1999; 262: 259–262.
219. Nishio Y, Noguchi E, Ito S, Ichikawa E, Umebayashi Y, Otsuka F, and Arinami T. Mutation and association analysis of the interferon regulatory factor 2 gene (IRF2) with atopic dermatitis. *J Hum Genet* 2001; 46: 664–667.
220. Rohrbach M, Frey U, Kraemer R, and Liechti-Gallati S. A variant in the gene for GM-CSF, I117T, is associated with atopic asthma in a Swiss population of asthmatic children. *J Allergy Clin Immunol* 1999; 104: 247–248.
221. He JQ, Ruan J, Chan-Yeung M, Becker AB, Dimich-Ward H, Pare PD, and Sandford AJ. Polymorphisms of the GM-CSF genes and the development of atopic diseases in at-risk children. *Chest* 2003; 123: 438S.
222. Nakao F, Ihara K, Kusuhara K, Sasaki Y, Kinukawa N, Takabayashi A, Nishima S, and Hara T. Association of IFN-gamma and IFN regulatory factor 1 polymorphisms with childhood atopic asthma. *J Allergy Clin Immunol* 2001; 107: 499–504.
223. Noguchi E, Nukaga-Nishio Y, Jian Z, Yokouchi Y, Kamioka M, Yamakawa-Kobayashi K, Hamaguchi H, Matsui A, Shibasaki M, and Arinami T. Haplotypes of the 5′ region of the IL-4 gene and SNPs in the intergene sequence between the IL-4 and IL-13 genes are associated with atopic asthma. *Hum Immunol* 2001; 62: 1251–1257.

224. Gao PS, Mao XQ, Baldini M, Roberts MH, Adra CN, Shirakawa T, Holt PG, Martinez FD, and Hopkin JM. Serum total IgE levels and CD14 on chromosome 5q31. *Clin Genet* 1999; 56: 164–165.

225. Niimi T, Munakata M, Keck-Waggoner CL, Popescu NC, Levitt RC, Hisada M, and Kimura S. A polymorphism in the human UGRP1 gene promoter that regulates transcription is associated with an increased risk of asthma. *Am J Hum Genet* 2002; 70: 718–725.

226. Morahan G, Huang D, Wu M, Holt BJ, White GP, Kendall GE, Sly PD, and Holt PG. Association of IL12B promoter polymorphism with severity of atopic and non-atopic asthma in children. *Lancet* 2002; 360: 455–459.

227. Morahan G, Huang D, Ymer SI, Cancilla MR, Stephen K, Dabadghao P, Werther G, Tait BD, Harrison LC, and Colman PG. Linkage disequilibrium of a type 1 diabetes susceptibility locus with a regulatory IL12B allele. *Nat Genet* 2001; 27: 218–221.

228. Tsunemi Y, Saeki H, Nakamura K, Sekiya T, Hirai K, Fujita H, Asano N, Kishimoto M, Tanida Y, Kakinuma T, Mitsui H, Tada Y, Wakugawa M, Torii H, Komine M, Asahina A, and Tamaki K. Interleukin-12 p40 gene (IL12B) 3′ untranslated region polymorphism is associated with susceptibility to atopic dermatitis and psoriasis vulgaris. *J Dermatol Sci* 2002; 30: 161–166.

229. Noguchi E, Yokouchi Y, Shibasaki M, Kamioka M, Yamakawa-Kobayashi K, Matsui A, and Arinami T. Identification of missense mutation in the IL12B gene: lack of association between IL12B polymorphisms and asthma and allergic rhinitis in the Japanese population. *Genes Immunol* 2001; 2: 401–403.

230. Deichmann KA, Schmidt A, Heinzmann A, Kruse S, Forster J, and Kuehr J. Association studies on beta 2-adrenoceptor polymorphisms and enhanced IgE responsiveness in an atopic population. *Clin Exp Allergy* 1999; 29: 794–799.

231. Kim SH, Oh SY, Oh HB, Kim YK, Cho SH, Kim YY, and Min KU. Association of beta 2-adrenoreceptor polymorphisms with nocturnal cough among atopic subjects but not with atopy and nonspecific bronchial hyperresponsiveness. *J Allergy Clin Immunol* 2002; 109: 630–635.

232. Binaei S, Christensen M, Murphy C, Zhang Q, and Quasney M. Beta 2-adrenergic receptor polymorphisms in children with status asthmaticus. *Chest* 2003; 123: 375S.

233. D'Amato M, Vitiani LR, Petrelli G, Ferrigno L, di Pietro A, Trezza R, and Matricardi PM. Association of persistent bronchial hyperresponsiveness with beta 2-adrenoceptor (ADRB2) haplotypes. A population study. *Am J Respir Crit Care Med* 1998; 158: 1968–1973.

234. Ulbrecht M, Hergeth MT, Wjst M, Heinrich J, Bickeboller H, Wichmann HE, and Weiss EH. Association of beta(2)-adrenoreceptor variants with bronchial hyperresponsiveness. *Am J Respir Crit Care Med* 2000; 161: 469–474.

235. Walley AJ, Chavanas S, Moffatt MF, Esnouf RM, Ubhi B, Lawrence R, Wong K, Abecasis GR, Jones EY, Harper JI, Hovnanian A, and Cookson WO. Gene polymorphism in Netherton and common atopic disease. *Nat Genet* 2001; 29: 175–178.

236. Sanak M, Pierzchalska M, Bazan-Socha S, and Szczeklik A. Enhanced expression of the leukotriene C(4) synthase due to overactive transcription of an allelic variant associated with aspirin-intolerant asthma. *Am J Respir Cell Mol Biol* 2000; 23: 290–296.

237. Van Sambeek R, Stevenson DD, Baldasaro M, Lam BK, Zhao J, Yoshida S, Yandora C, Drazen JM, and Penrose JF. 5' flanking region polymorphism of the gene encoding leukotriene C4 synthase does not correlate with the aspirin-intolerant asthma phenotype in the United States. *J Allergy Clin Immunol* 2000; 106: 72–76.

238. Kawagishi Y, Mita H, Taniguchi M, Maruyama M, Oosaki R, Higashi N, Kashii T, Kobayashi M, and Akiyama K. Leukotriene C4 synthase promoter polymorphism in Japanese patients with aspirin-induced asthma. *J Allergy Clin Immunol* 2002; 109: 936–942.

239. Sayers I, Barton S, Rorke S, Beghe B, Hayward B, Van Eerdewegh P, Keith T, Clough JB, Ye S, Holloway JW, Sampson AP, and Holgate ST. Allelic association and functional studies of promoter polymorphism in the leukotriene C4 synthase gene (LTC4S) in asthma. *Thorax* 2003; 58: 417–424.

240. Huang SK, Zwollo P, and Marsh DG. Class II major histocompatibility complex restriction of human T cell responses to short ragweed allergen, Amb aV. *Eur J Immunol* 1991; 21: 1469–1473.

241. Ansari AA, Freidhoff LR, Meyers DA, Bias WB, and Marsh DG. Human immune responsiveness to *Lolium perenne* pollen allergen Lol p III (rye III) is associated with HLA-DR3 and DR5. *Hum Immunol* 1989; 25: 59–71.

242. Stephan V, Kuehr J, Seibt A, Saueressig H, Zingsem S, Dinh TD, Moseler M, Wahn V, and Deichmann KA. Genetic linkage of HLA-class II locus to mite-specific IgE immune responsiveness. *Clin Exp Allergy* 1999; 29: 1049–1054.

243. Cardaba B, Moffatt MF, Fernandez E, Jurado A, Rojo M, Garcia M, Ansotegui IJ, Cortegano I, Arrieta I, Etxenagusia MA, del Pozo V, Urraca J, Aceituno E, Gallardo S, Palomino P, Cookson W, and Lahoz C. Allergy to dermatophagoides in a group of Spanish gypsies: genetic restrictions. *Int Arch Allergy Immunol* 2001; 125: 297–306.

244. Di Somma C, Charron D, Deichmann K, Buono C, and Ruffilli A. Atopic asthma and TNF-308 alleles: linkage disequilibrium and association analyses. *Hum Immunol* 2003; 64: 359–365.

245. Jeal H, Draper A, Jones M, Harris J, Welsh K, Taylor AN, and Cullinan P. HLA associations with occupational sensitization to rat lipocalin allergens: a model for other animal allergies? *J Allergy Clin Immunol* 2003; 111: 795–799.

246. Lara-Marquez ML, Yunis JJ, Layrisse Z, Ortega F, Carvallo-Gil E, Montagnani S, Makhatadze NJ, Pocino M, Granja C, and Yunis E. Immunogenetics of atopic asthma: association of DRB1*1101 DQA1*0501 DQB1*0301 haplotype with dermatophagoides species: sensitive asthma in a sample of the Venezuelan population. *Clin Exp Allergy* 1999; 29: 60–71.

247. Tan EC, Lee BW, Tay AW, Chew FT, and Tay AH. Asthma and TNF variants in Chinese and Malays. *Allergy* 1999; 54: 402–403.

248. El Bahlawan L, Christensen M, Binaei S, Murphy C, Zhang Q, and Quasney M. Lack of association between the tumor necrosis factor-alpha regulatory region genetic polymorphisms associated with elevated tumor necrosis factor-alpha levels and children with asthma. *Chest* 2003; 123: 374S–375S.

249. Noguchi E, Yokouchi Y, Shibasaki M, Inudou M, Nakahara S, Nogami T, Kamioka M, Yamakawa-Kobayashi K, Ichikawa K, Matsui A, and Arinami T. Association between TNFA polymorphism and the development of asthma in the Japanese population. *Am J Respir Crit Care Med* 2002; 166: 43–46.

250. Ismail A, Bousaffara R, Kaziz J, Zili J, el Kamel A, Tahar Sfar M, Remadi S, and Chouchane L. Polymorphism in transporter antigen peptides gene (TAP1) associated with atopy in Tunisians. *J Allergy Clin Immunol* 1997; 99: 216–223.

251. Hang LW, Hsia TC, Chen WC, Chen HY, and Tsai FJ. TAP1 gene AccI polymorphism is associated with atopic bronchial asthma. *J Clin Lab Anal* 2003; 17: 57–60.

252. Stafforini DM, Numao T, Tsodikov A, Vaitkus D, Fukuda T, Watanabe N, Fueki N, McIntyre TM, Zimmerman GA, Makino S, and Prescott SM. Deficiency of platelet-activating factor acetylhydrolase is a severity factor for asthma. *J Clin Invest* 1999; 103: 989–997.

253. Satoh N, Asano K, Naoki K, Fukunaga K, Iwata M, Kanazawa M, and Yamaguchi K. Plasma platelet-activating factor acetylhydrolase deficiency in Japanese patients with asthma. *Am J Respir Crit Care Med* 1999; 159: 974–979.

254. Ito S, Noguchi E, Shibasaki M, Yamakawa-Kobayashi K, Watanabe H, and Arinami T. Evidence for an association between plasma platelet-activating factor acetylhydrolase deficiency and increased risk of childhood atopic asthma. *J Hum Genet* 2002; 47: 99–101.

255. Kruse S, Mao XQ, Heinzmann A, Blattmann S, Roberts MH, Braun S, Gao PS, Forster J, Kuehr J, Hopkin JM, Shirakawa T, and Deichmann KA. The Ile198Thr and Ala379Val variants of plasmatic PAF-acetylhydrolase impair catalytical activities and are associated with atopy and asthma. *Am J Hum Genet* 2000; 66: 1522–1530.

256. Gao PS, Mao XQ, Jouanguy E, Pallier A, Doffinger R, Tanaka Y, Nakashima H, Otsuka T, Roberts MH, Enomoto T, Dake Y, Kawai M, Sasaki S, Shaldon SR, Coull P, Adra CN, Niho Y, Casanova JL, Shirakawa T, and Hopkin JM. Nonpathogenic common variants of IFNGR1 and IFNGR2 in association with total serum IgE levels. *Biochem Biophys Res Commun* 1999; 263: 425–429.

257. Shin HD, Kim LH, Park BL, Jung JH, Kim JY, Chung IY, Kim JS, Lee JH, Chung SH, Kim YH, Park HS, Choi JH, Lee YM, Park SW, Choi BW, Hong SJ, and Park CS. Association of eotaxin gene family with asthma and serum total IgE. *Hum Mol Genet* 2003; 12: 1279–1285.

258. Schroeder SA, Gaughan DM, and Swift M. Protection against bronchial asthma by CFTR delta F508 mutation: a heterozygote advantage in cystic fibrosis. *Nat Med* 1995; 1: 703–705.

259. Mennie M, Gilfillan A, Brock DJ, and Liston WA. Heterozygotes for the delta F508 cystic fibrosis allele are not protected against bronchial asthma. *Nat Med* 1995; 1: 978–979.

260. Dahl M, Tybjaerg-Hansen A, Lange P, and Nordestgaard BG. Delta F508 heterozygosity in cystic fibrosis and susceptibility to asthma. *Lancet* 1998; 351: 1911–1913.

261. Castellani C, Quinzii C, Altieri S, Mastella G, and Assael BM. A pilot survey of cystic fibrosis clinical manifestations in CFTR mutation heterozygotes. *Genet Test* 2001; 5: 249–254.

262. de Cid R, Chomel JC, Lazaro C, Sunyer J, Baudis M, Casals T, Le Moual N, Kitzis A, Feingold J, Anto J, Estivill X, and Kauffmann F. CFTR and asthma in the French EGEA study. *Eur J Hum Genet* 2001; 9: 67–69.

263. Lazaro C, de Cid R, Sunyer J, Soriano J, Gimenez J, Alvarez M, Casals T, Anto JM, and Estivill X. Missense mutations in the cystic fibrosis gene in adult patients with asthma. *Hum Mutat* 1999; 14: 510–519.

264. Tzetis M, Efthymiadou A, Strofalis S, Psychou P, Dimakou A, Pouliou E, Doudounakis S, and Kanavakis E. CFTR gene mutations including three novel nucleotide substitutions and haplotype background in patients with asthma, disseminated bronchiectasis and chronic obstructive pulmonary disease. *Hum Genet* 2001; 108: 216–221.

265. Lee YC, Cheon KT, Lee HB, Kim W, Rhee YK, and Kim DS. Gene polymorphisms of endothelial nitric oxide synthase and angiotensin-converting enzyme in patients with asthma. *Allergy* 2000; 55: 959–963.

266. Holla LI, Buckova D, Kuhrova V, Stejskalova A, Francova H, Znojil V, and Vacha J. Prevalence of endothelial nitric oxide synthase gene polymorphisms in patients with atopic asthma. *Clin Exp Allergy* 2002; 32: 1193–1198.

267. Gao PS, Kawada H, Kasamatsu T, Mao XQ, Roberts MH, Miyamoto Y, Yoshimura M, Saitoh Y, Yasue H, Nakao K, Adra CN, Kun JF, Moro-oka S, Inoko H, Ho LP, Shirakawa T, and Hopkin JM. Variants of NOS1, NOS2, and NOS3 genes in asthmatics. *Biochem Biophys Res Commun* 2000; 267: 761–763.

268. Zielinska E, Niewiarowski W, Bodalski J, Stanczyk A, Bolanowski W, and Rebowski G. Arylamine N-acetyltransferase (NAT2) gene mutations in children with allergic diseases. *Clin Pharmacol Ther* 1997; 62: 635–642.

269. Gawronska-Szklarz B, Luszawska-Kutrzeba T, Czaja-Bulsa G, and Kurzawski G. Relationship between acetylation polymorphism and risk of atopic diseases. *Clin Pharmacol Ther* 1999; 65: 562–569.

270. Nacak M, Aynacioglu AS, Filiz A, Cascorbi I, Erdal ME, Yilmaz N, Ekinci E, and Roots I. Association between the N-acetylation genetic polymorphism and bronchial asthma. *Br J Clin Pharmacol* 2002; 54: 671–674.

271. Makarova SI, Vavilin VA, Lyakhovich VV, and Gavalov SM. Allele NAT2*5 determines resistance to bronchial asthma in children. *Bull Exp Biol Med* 2000; 129: 575–577.

272. In KH, Asano K, Beier D, Grobholz J, Finn PW, Silverman EK, Silverman ES, Collins T, Fischer AR, Keith TP, Serino K, Kim SW, De Sanctis GT, Yandava C, Pillari A, Rubin P, Kemp J, Israel E, Busse W, Ledford D, Murray JJ, Segal A, Tinkleman D, and Drazen JM. Naturally occurring mutations in the human 5-lipoxygenase gene promoter that modify transcription factor binding and reporter gene transcription. *J Clin Invest* 1997; 99: 1130–1137.

273. Drazen JM, Yandava CN, Dube L, Szczerback N, Hippensteel R, Pillari A, Israel E, Schork N, Silverman ES, Katz DA, and Drajesk J. Pharmacogenetic association between ALOX5 promoter genotype and the response to anti-asthma treatment. *Nat Genet* 1999; 22: 168–170.

274. Fowler SJ, Hall IP, Wilson AM, Wheatley AP, and Lipworth BJ. 5-Lipoxygenase polymorphism and *in vivo* response to leukotriene receptor antagonists. *Eur J Clin Pharmacol* 2002; 58: 187–190.

275. Laing IA, Goldblatt J, Eber E, Hayden CM, Rye PJ, Gibson NA, Palmer LJ, Burton PR, and Le Souef PN. A polymorphism of the CC16 gene is associated with an increased risk of asthma. *J Med Genet* 1998; 35: 463–467.

276. Gao PS, Mao XQ, Kawai M, Enomoto T, Sasaki S, Tanabe O, Yoshimura K, Shaldon SR, Dake Y, Kitano H, Coull P, Shirakawa T, and Hopkin JM. Negative association between asthma and variants of CC16 (CC10) on chromosome 11q13 in British and Japanese populations. *Hum Genet* 1998; 103: 57–59.

277. Choi M, Zhang Z, Ten Kate LP, Collee JM, Gerritsen J, and Mukherjee AB. Human uteroglobin gene polymorphisms and genetic susceptibility to asthma. *Ann NY Acad Sci* 2000; 923: 303–306.
278. Mansur AH, Fryer AA, Hepple M, Strange RC, and Spiteri MA. An association study between the Clara cell secretory protein CC16 A38G polymorphism and asthma phenotypes. *Clin Exp Allergy* 2002; 32: 994–999.
279. Mao XQ, Shirakawa T, Kawai M, Enomoto T, Sasaki S, Dake Y, Kitano H, Hagihara A, Hopkin JM, and Morimoto K. Association between asthma and an intragenic variant of CC16 on chromosome 11q13. *Clin Genet* 1998; 53: 54–56.
280. Donnadieu E, Cookson WO, Jouvin MH, and Kinet JP. Allergy-associated polymorphisms of the Fc epsilon RI beta subunit do not impact its two amplification functions. *J Immunol* 2000; 165: 3917–3922.
281. Furumoto Y, Hiraoka S, Kawamoto K, Masaki S, Kitamura T, Okumura K, and Ra C. Polymorphisms in Fc epsilon RI beta chain do not affect IgE-mediated mast cell activation. *Biochem Biophys Res Commun* 2000; 273: 765–771.
282. Hill MR, James AL, Faux JA, Ryan G, Hopkin JM, Le Souef P, Musk AW, and Cookson WO. Fc epsilon RI beta polymorphism and risk of atopy in a general population sample. *Br Med J* 1995; 311: 776–779.
283. Hijazi Z, Haider MZ, Khan MR, and Al-Dowaisan AA. High frequency of IgE receptor Fc epsilon RI beta variant (Leu181/Leu183) in Kuwaiti Arabs and its association with asthma. *Clin Genet* 1998; 53: 149–152.
284. Rohrbach M, Kraemer R, and Liechti-Gallati S. Screening of the Fc epsilon RI-beta gene in a Swiss population of asthmatic children: no association with E237G and identification of new sequence variations. *Dis Markers* 1998; 14: 177–186.
285. Ishizawa M, Shibasaki M, Yokouchi Y, Noguchi E, Arinami T, Yamakawa-Kobayashi K, Matsui A, and Hamaguchi H. No association between atopic asthma and a coding variant of Fc epsilon R1 beta in a Japanese population. *J Hum Genet* 1999; 44: 308–311.
286. Castro J, Telleria JJ, Blanco-Quiros A, Linares P, and Andion R. Lack of association between atopy and RsaI polymorphism within intron 2 of the Fc (epsilon) RI-beta gene in a Spanish population sample. *Allergy* 1998; 53: 1083–1086.
287. Watson MA, Stewart RK, Smith GB, Massey TE, and Bell DA. Human glutathione S-transferase P1 polymorphisms: relationship to lung tissue enzyme activity and population frequency distribution. *Carcinogenesis* 1998; 19: 275–280.
288. Kruse S, Kuehr J, Moseler M, Kopp MV, Kurz T, Deichmann KA, Foster PS, and Mattes J. Polymorphisms in the IL 18 gene are associated with specific sensitization to common allergens and allergic rhinitis. *J Allergy Clin Immunol* 2003; 111: 117–122.
289. Noguchi E, Shibasaki M, Inudou M, Kamioka M, Yokouchi Y, Yamakawa-Kobayashi K, Hamaguchi H, Matsui A, and Arinami T. Association between a new polymorphism in the activation-induced cytidine deaminase gene and atopic asthma and the regulation of total serum IgE levels. *J Allergy Clin Immunol* 2001; 108: 382–386.
290. Gao PS, Mao XQ, Roberts MH, Arinobu Y, Akaiwa M, Enomoto T, Dake Y, Kawai M, Sasaki S, Hamasaki N, Izuhara K, Shirakawa T, and Hopkin JM. Variants of STAT6 (signal transducer and activator of transcription 6) in atopic asthma. *J Med Genet* 2000; 37: 380–382.

291. Amoli MM, Hand S, Hajeer AH, Jones KP, Rolf S, Sting C, Davies BH, and Ollier WE. Polymorphism in the STAT6 gene encodes risk for nut allergy. *Genes Immunol* 2002; 3: 220–224.
292. Tamura K, Arakawa H, Suzuki M, Kobayashi Y, Mochizuki H, Kato M, Tokuyama K, and Morikawa A. Novel dinucleotide repeat polymorphism in the first exon of the STAT-6 gene is associated with allergic diseases. *Clin Exp Allergy* 2001; 31: 1509–1514.
293. Duetsch G, Illig T, Loesgen S, Rohde K, Klopp N, Herbon N, Gohlke H, Altmueller J, and Wjst M. STAT6 as an asthma candidate gene: polymorphism-screening, association and haplotype analysis in a Caucasian sib-pair study. *Hum Mol Genet* 2002; 11: 613–621.
294. Nagarkatti R, Rao CB, Rishi JP, Chetiwal R, Shandilya V, Vijayan V, Kumar R, Pemde HK, Sharma SK, Sharma S, Singh AB, Gangal SV, and Ghosh B. Association of IFNG gene polymorphism with asthma in the Indian population. *J Allergy Clin Immunol* 2002; 110: 410–412.
295. Grasemann H, Yandava CN, Storm van's Gravesande K, Deykin A, Pillari A, Ma J, Sonna LA, Lilly C, Stampfer MJ, Israel E, Silverman EK, and Drazen JM. A neuronal NO synthase (NOS1) gene polymorphism is associated with asthma. *Biochem Biophys Res Commun* 2000; 272: 391–394.
296. Moffatt MF, Schou C, Faux JA, and Cookson WO. Germline TCR-A restriction of immunoglobulin E responses to allergen. *Immunogenetics* 1997; 46: 226–230.
297. Malerba G, Patuzzo C, Trabetti E, Lauciello MC, Galavotti R, Pescollderungg L, Whalen MB, Zanoni G, Martinati LC, Boner AL, and Pignatti PF. Chromosome 14 linkage analysis and mutation study of two serpin genes in allergic asthmatic families. *J Allergy Clin Immunol* 2001; 107: 654–658.
298. Mitsuyasu H, Izuhara K, Mao XQ, Gao PS, Arinobu Y, Enomoto T, Kawai M, Sasaki S, Dake Y, Hamasaki N, Shirakawa T, and Hopkin JM. Ile50Val variant of IL4R alpha upregulates IgE synthesis and associates with atopic asthma. *Nat Genet* 1998; 19: 119–120.
299. Noguchi E, Shibasaki M, Arinami T, Takeda K, Yokouchi Y, Kobayashi K, Imoto N, Nakahara S, Matsui A, and Hamaguchi H. No association between atopy/asthma and the ILe50Val polymorphism of IL-4 receptor. *Am J Respir Crit Care Med* 1999; 160: 342–345.
300. Tan EC, Lee BW, Chew FT, Shek L, Tay AW, and Tay AH. IL-4R alpha gene Ile50Val polymorphism. *Allergy* 1999; 54: 1005–1007.
301. Oiso N, Fukai K, and Ishii M. Interleukin 4 receptor alpha chain polymorphism Gln551Arg is associated with adult atopic dermatitis in Japan. *Br J Dermatol* 2000; 142: 1003–1006.
302. Haagerup A, Bjerke T, Schiotz PO, Dahl R, Binderup HG, and Kruse TA. No linkage and association of atopy to chromosome 16 including the interleukin-4 receptor gene. *Allergy* 2001; 56: 775–779.
303. Mujica-Lopez KI, Flores-Martinez SE, Ramos-Zepeda R, Castaneda-Ramos SA, Gazca-Aguilar A, Garcia-Perez J, and Sanchez-Corona J. Association analysis of polymorphisms in the interleukin-4 receptor (alpha) gene with atopic asthma in patients from western Mexico. *Eur J Immunogenet* 2002; 29: 375–378.

304. Wang HY, Shelburne CP, Zamorano J, Kelly AE, Ryan JJ, and Keegan AD. Cutting edge: effects of an allergy-associated mutation in the human IL-4R alpha (Q576R) on human IL-4-induced signal transduction. *J Immunol* 1999; 162: 4385–4389.

305. Noguchi E, Shibasaki M, Arinami T, Takeda K, Yokouchi Y, Kobayashi K, Imoto N, Nakahara S, Matsui A, and Hamaguchi H. Lack of association of atopy/asthma and the interleukin-4 receptor alpha gene in Japanese. *Clin Exp Allergy* 1999; 29: 228–233.

306. Rosa-Rosa L, Zimmermann N, Bernstein JA, Rothenberg ME, and Khurana-Hershey GK. The R576 IL-4 receptor alpha allele correlates with asthma severity. *J Allergy Clin Immunol* 1999; 104: 1008–1014.

307. Patuzzo C, Trabetti E, Malerba G, Martinati LC, Boner AL, Pescollderungg L, Zanoni G, and Pignatti PF. No linkage or association of the IL-4R alpha gene Q576R mutation with atopic asthma in Italian families. *J Med Genet* 2000; 37: 382–384.

308. Andrews RP, Burrell L, Rosa-Rosa L, Cunningham CM, Brzezinski JL, Bernstein JA, and Khurana-Hershey GK. Analysis of the Ser786Pro interleukin-4 receptor alpha allelic variant in allergic and nonallergic asthma and its functional consequences. *Clin Immunol* 2001; 100: 298–304.

309. Hackstein H, Hofmann H, Bohnert A, and Bein G. Definition of human interleukin-4 receptor alpha chain haplotypes and allelic association with atopy markers. *Hum Immunol* 1999; 60: 1119–1127.

310. Kauppi P, Lindblad-Toh K, Sevon P, Toivonen HT, Rioux JD, Villapakkam A, Laitinen LA, Hudson TJ, Kere J, and Laitinen T. A second-generation association study of the 5q31 cytokine gene cluster and the interleukin-4 receptor in asthma. *Genomics* 2001; 77: 35–42.

311. Kabesch M, Peters W, Carr D, Leupold W, Weiland SK, and Von Mutius E. Association between polymorphisms in caspase recruitment domain containing protein 15 and allergy in two German populations. *J Allergy Clin Immunol* 2003; 111: 813–817.

312. Ogura Y, Bonen DK, Inohara N, Nicolae DL, Chen FF, Ramos R, Britton H, Moran T, Karaliuskas R, Duerr RH, Achkar JP, Brant SR, Bayless TM, Kirschner BS, Hanauer SB, Nunez G, and Cho JH. A frameshift mutation in NOD2 associated with susceptibility to Crohn's disease. *Nature* 2001; 411: 603–606.

313. Warpeha KM, Xu W, Liu L, Charles IG, Patterson CC, Ah-Fat F, Harding S, Hart PM, Chakravarthy U, and Hughes AE. Genotyping and functional analysis of a polymorphic (CCTTT)(n) repeat of NOS2A in diabetic retinopathy. *FASEB J* 1999; 13: 1825–1832.

314. Konno S, Hizawa N, Yamaguchi E, Jinushi E, and Nishimura M. (CCTTT)n repeat polymorphism in the NOS2 gene promoter is associated with atopy. *J Allergy Clin Immunol* 2001; 108: 810–814.

315. Nickel RG, Casolaro V, Wahn U, Beyer K, Barnes KC, Plunkett BS, Freidhoff LR, Sengler C, Plitt JR, Schleimer RP, Caraballo L, Naidu RP, Levett PN, Beaty TH, and Huang SK. Atopic dermatitis is associated with a functional mutation in the promoter of the C-C chemokine RANTES. *J Immunol* 2000; 164: 1612–1616.

316. Fryer AA, Spiteri MA, Bianco A, Hepple M, Jones PW, Strange RC, Makki R, Tavernier G, Smilie FI, Custovic A, Woodcock AA, Ollier WE, and Hajeer AH. The -403 G→A promoter polymorphism in the RANTES gene is associated with atopy and asthma. *Genes Immunol* 2000; 1: 509–514.

317. Kozma GT, Falus A, Bojszko A, Krikovszky D, Szabo T, Nagy A, and Szalai C. Lack of association between atopic eczema/dermatitis syndrome and polymorphisms in the promoter region of RANTES and regulatory region of MCP-1. *Allergy* 2002; 57: 160–163.

318. Szalai C, Kozma GT, Nagy A, Bojszko A, Krikovszky D, Szabo T, and Falus A. Polymorphism in the gene regulatory region of MCP-1 is associated with asthma susceptibility and severity. *J Allergy Clin Immunol* 2001; 108: 375–381.

319. Hizawa N, Yamaguchi E, Konno S, Tanino Y, Jinushi E, and Nishimura M. A functional polymorphism in the RANTES gene promoter is associated with the development of late-onset asthma. *Am J Respir Crit Care Med* 2002; 166: 686–690.

320. Liu H, Chao D, Nakayama EE, Taguchi H, Goto M, Xin X, Takamatsu JK, Saito H, Ishikawa Y, Akaza T, Juji T, Takebe Y, Ohishi T, Fukutake K, Maruyama Y, Yashiki S, Sonoda S, Nakamura T, Nagai Y, Iwamoto A, and Shioda T. Polymorphism in RANTES chemokine promoter affects HIV-1 disease progression. *Proc Natl Acad Sci USA* 1999; 96: 4581–4585.

321. Rovin BH, Lu L, and Saxena R. A novel polymorphism in the MCP-1 gene regulatory region that influences MCP-1 expression. *Biochem Biophys Res Commun* 1999; 259: 344–348.

322. Nakamura H, Luster AD, Nakamura T, In KH, Sonna LA, Deykin A, Israel E, Drazen JM, and Lilly CM. Variant eotaxin: its effects on the asthma phenotype. *J Allergy Clin Immunol* 2001; 108: 946–953.

323. Miyamasu M, Sekiya T, Ohta K, Ra C, Yoshie O, Yamamoto K, Tsuchiya N, Tokunaga K, and Hirai K. Variations in the human CC chemokine eotaxin gene. *Genes Immunol* 2001; 2: 461–463.

324. Tsunemi Y, Saeki H, Nakamura K, Sekiya T, Hirai K, Fujita H, Asano N, Tanida Y, Kakinuma T, Wakugawa M, Torii H, and Tamaki K. Eotaxin gene single nucleotide polymorphisms in the promoter and exon regions are not associated with susceptibility to atopic dermatitis, but two of them in the promoter region are associated with serum IgE levels in patients with atopic dermatitis. *J Dermatol Sci* 2002; 29: 222–228.

325. Rigat B, Hubert C, Alhenc-Gelas F, Cambien F, Corvol P, and Soubrier F. An insertion/deletion polymorphism in the angiotensin I-converting enzyme gene accounting for half the variance of serum enzyme levels. *J Clin Invest* 1990; 86: 1343–1346.

326. Benessiano J, Crestani B, Mestari F, Klouche W, Neukirch F, Hacein-Bey S, Durand G, and Aubier M. High frequency of a deletion polymorphism of the angiotensin-converting enzyme gene in asthma. *J Allergy Clin Immunol* 1997; 99: 53–57.

327. Holla L, Vasku A, Znojil V, Siskova L, and Vacha J. Association of three gene polymorphisms with atopic diseases. *J Allergy Clin Immunol* 1999; 103: 702–708.

328. Tomita H, Sato S, Matsuda R, Ogisu N, Mori T, Niimi T, and Shimizu S. Genetic polymorphism of the angiotensin-converting enzyme (ACE) in asthmatic patients. *Respir Med* 1998; 92: 1305–1310.

329. Gao PS, Mao XQ, Kawai M, Enomoto T, Sasaki S, Shaldon SR, Dake Y, Kitano H, Coull P, Hagihara A, Shirakawa T, and Hopkin JM. Lack of association between ACE gene polymorphisms and atopy and asthma in British and Japanese populations. *Clin Genet* 1998; 54: 245–247.

330. Nakahama H, Obata K, Nakajima T, Nakamura H, Kitada O, Sugita M, Fujita Y, Kawada N, and Moriyama T. Renin–angiotensin system component gene polymorphism in Japanese bronchial asthma patients. *J Asthma* 1999; 36: 187–193.

331. Leung TF, Tang NL, Lam CW, Li AM, Chan IH, and Ha G. Thromboxane A2 receptor gene polymorphism is associated with the serum concentration of cat-specific immunoglobulin E as well as the development and severity of asthma in Chinese children. *Pediatr Allergy Immunol* 2002; 13: 10–17.

332. Grainger DJ, Heathcote K, Chiano M, Snieder H, Kemp PR, Metcalfe JC, Carter ND, and Spector TD. Genetic control of the circulating concentration of transforming growth factor type beta1. *Hum Mol Genet* 1999; 8: 93–97.

333. Pulleyn LJ, Newton R, Adcock IM, and Barnes PJ. TGF beta 1 allele association with asthma severity. *Hum Genet* 2001; 109: 623–627.

334. Buckova D, Izakovicova Holla L, Benes P, Znojil V, and Vacha J. TGF-beta 1 gene polymorphisms. *Allergy* 2001; 56: 1236–1237.

335. Arkwright PD, Chase JM, Babbage S, Pravica V, David TJ, and Hutchinson IV. Atopic dermatitis is associated with a low-producer transforming growth factor beta(1) cytokine genotype. *J Allergy Clin Immunol* 2001; 108: 281–284.

336. Ahmed S, Ihara K, Sasaki Y, Nakao F, Nishima S, Fujino T, and Hara T. Novel polymorphism in the coding region of the IL-13 receptor alpha' gene: association study with atopic asthma in the Japanese population. *Exp Clin Immunogenet* 2000; 17: 18–22.

9

Birth Order

**TRICIA MCKEEVER, RICHARD HUBBARD, SARAH LEWIS,
and JOHN BRITTON**

University of Nottingham
Nottingham, U.K.

I. Introduction

One finding that has emerged consistently from epidemiological studies as a potentially important risk factor for allergic disease is birth order; the more older siblings a child has, the lower the risk of allergic disease. This finding was first reported by David Strachan in an analysis of a 1958 British birth cohort in which he observed that the risks of hay fever at age 11 and at age 23 and the risk of eczema in the first year of life were reduced in relation to the number of older siblings in the family. He suggested that "allergic diseases were prevented by infection in early childhood, transmitted by unhygienic contact with older siblings." He went on to propose, "Over the past century, declining family size, improvements in household amenities, and higher standards of personal cleanliness have reduced the opportunity for cross-infection in young families."[1]

This hypothesis, widely termed the "hygiene hypothesis," opened up new areas of research into the etiology of allergic disease and many studies addressed the clinical manifestations of allergic diseases including asthma, eczema, hay fever, bronchial hyperresponsiveness, and the presence of allergic sensitization determined through positive skin prick testing (SPT) to specific allergens or elevated IgE levels. Since Strachan's initial report appeared, several studies have demonstrated a reduced risk of eczema and hay fever in relation to birth order and this has now become one of the most consistent findings in the epidemiological studies of these diseases. However, in contrast, the evidence for asthma had been inconsistent and in this chapter the evidence for asthma is discussed separately.

II. Hay Fever, Eczema, and Allergic Sensitization in Relation to Birth Order

The protective effects of older siblings on the risk of hay fever present in the 1958 British birth cohort were also present (at age 16) in a 1970 British birth cohort. In this dataset, having five or more older siblings was protective for the development of hay fever by an odds ratio of 0.35 (95% confidence interval [CI], 0.27–0.44).[2] Data from 150,000 male conscripts born between 1973 and 1975 collected as part of the Swedish Military Enrollment Register were analyzed and represents one of the largest studies.[3] Braback et al. found a strong birth order effect for allergic rhinitis such that having four or more older siblings reduced the risk of developing disease by an odds ratio of 0.63 (95% CI, 0.55–0.72).

A number of other studies support the protective effect of larger family size or increased numbers of older siblings on the risk of having hay fever.[1,3–14] Although eczema has not been as extensively researched as hay fever, the evidence overall supports a protective effect of family size and birth order.[1,5–7,11,14–17] Results from our own study using primary care records indicate that having three or more older siblings reduced the risk of developing eczema with a hazard ratio of 0.70 (95%, 0.64–0.76).[17]

The first research paper report linking birth order and an objective marker of allergic disease was a cross-sectional study of 6,786 children in Germany.[18] This study demonstrated a decreased risk of a positive SPT as the number of siblings in a family increased (Figure 9.1). Further evidence to support the protective effect of siblings on objective markers of allergic disease comes from a European Community Heath Survey of 13,932 adults that showed that having three siblings (compared with no siblings) reduced the risk of having increased IgE levels to specific allergens by an odds ratio of 0.75 (95% CI, 0.65–0.87).[19] A reduced prevalence of objective markers of allergic disease has also been demonstrated in relation to both family size and also, more specifically, the number of older siblings.[20,21]

A recent systematic review article by Karmaus and Botezan summarizes research on the relationship between having three or more siblings and the risk of having eczema, hay fever, and positive skin prick or IgE tests (Figures 9.2 through Figure 9.4).[22] The authors calculated the average odds ratio, weighted

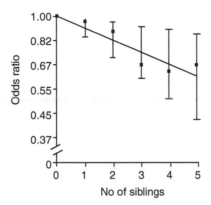

Figure 9.1   Odds ratios (95% confidence intervals) of being atopic by number of siblings after correction for other risk factors in a multivariate logistic regression analysis (logarithmic scale). (From *Br Med J* 1994; 308: 604. With permission from BMJ Publishing Group.)

for sample size, and found that overall three or more siblings reduced the risk of eczema by an odds ratio of 0.66, hay fever by an odds ratio of 0.56, and positive SPT or increased IgE by an odds ratio of 0.62. In summary, current evidence suggests very strongly that an increased number of siblings decreases the risk of developing allergic disease.

III. Asthma and Birth Order

One of the first studies to report the impact of family size on the prevalence of asthma was conducted before David Strachan's initial paper on the hygiene hypothesis and suggested that children from larger families had higher asthma prevalence rates.[23] A number of years later, a study by Crane et al. found that increasing number of older siblings protected against wheezing illness and that having two or more older siblings reduced the risk of wheezing in children aged 8 to 13 by an odds ratio of 0.5 (95% CI, 0.2–1.0).[24] The inconsistency between birth order and asthma or wheezing illness has been a recurring theme over the years and is at odds with the evidence for hay fever, eczema, and SPT.

A number of studies found no association between birth order or family size and asthma.[3,6,13,23,25–35] In addition, studies that found protective impacts of birth order on asthma[4,12,14,25,26,33,36–39] demonstrated effects of a smaller size than those reported for hay fever, eczema, and objective markers of atopy. This inconsistency in the evidence for asthma sets it aside from the other allergic diseases and may reflect the more complex etiologies of asthma and wheezing illness in

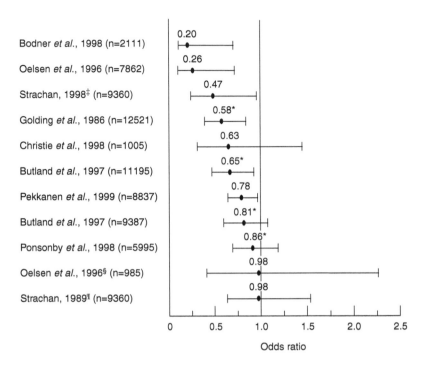

Figure 9.2 Summary of studies of the relationship between eczema and number of siblings (three or more versus none). Odds ratios and 95% confidence intervals for large number of siblings. Odds ratios are adjusted for other risk factors except for those marked with asterisks. † = Specialist diagnosis of atopic dermatitis, older siblings only. ‡ = Older siblings only. § = Parent's report of diagnosis of atopic dermatitis, older siblings only; ¶ = younger siblings only. (With permission from BMJ Publishing Group.)

children. In their systematic review, Karmaus and Botezan also demonstrated a birth order influence on the prevalence of asthma (Figure 9.5).[22]

Some of these inconsistencies may arise from the difficulties of standardizing the asthma diagnosis in population studies and because asthma appears to include at least two distinct phenotypes. This is evident from the fact that wheezing illness in the first two years of life tends to be relatively transient and risk factors include environmental tobacco smoke, exposure to viral infections, and small airways. Allergy, bronchial hyperresponsiveness, and other environmental factors become more important risk factors in the onset of wheezing in later childhood.[41] Consistent with this evidence are indications of a cross-over effect in the relationship between number of older siblings and development of asthma, such that having older siblings increases the risk of early transient wheezing and is a protective factor for development of wheeze later in life.

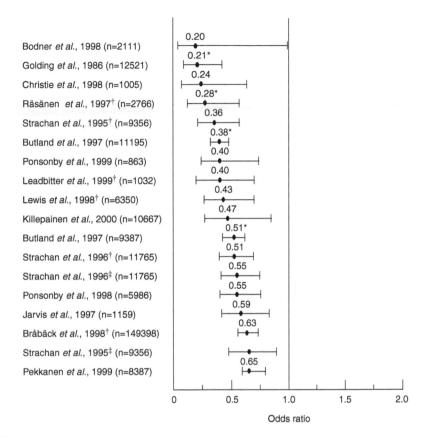

Figure 9.3 Summary of studies of the relationship between hay fever and number of siblings (three or more versus none). Odds ratios and 95% confidence intervals for large number of siblings. Odds ratios are adjusted for other risk factors except for those marked with asterisks. † = Older siblings only; ‡ = younger siblings only. (With permission from BMJ Publishing Group.)

For example, in the Tucson Children's Respiratory Study in which 1,035 children were followed from birth, those who had one or more older siblings or attended day care were more likely to exhibit early wheezing but were protected from later onset of asthma.[38] Similarly, another study found that the presence of siblings increased the risk of transient early wheezing but was protective for late onset wheezing.[27] Our own studies of a cohort of 29,238 children demonstrated that increased numbers of older siblings were risk factors for asthma diagnosed before the age of 2 years, but were protective for asthma diagnosed after the age of 2 (Figure 9.6). This cross-over in risk could occur as early as 1 year of age.[17] The likely explanation is that asthma-like symptoms with a later onset are more

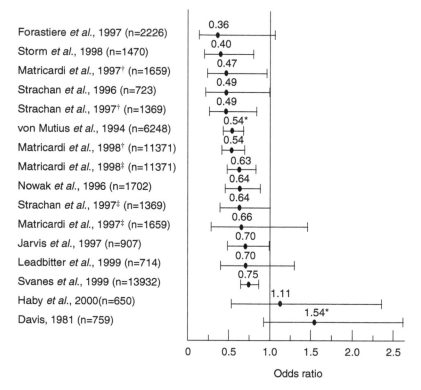

Figure 9.4 Summary of studies of the relationship between SPT/IgE reactivity to at least one allergen and number of siblings. Odds ratios and 95% confidence intervals for large number of siblings. Odds ratios are adjusted for other risk factors except for those marked with asterisks. † = Older siblings only; ‡ = younger siblings only. (With permission from BMJ Publishing Group.)

frequently driven by allergy than by symptoms that develop very early in life[41] and that siblings protect against the former but not the latter.

IV. Infections

Exposure to infection is one of the more plausible explanations for the birth order effect, although consistent evidence of a protective effect of infection on the development of allergic disease has not emerged to date. Data have demonstrated protective effects of measles,[10,42,43] hepatitis A,[44–46] mycobacterial infections,[47,48] and repeated episodes of runny nose[49] in relation to a variety of allergic outcomes. Despite evidence for a protective effect, few of these studies explored their data further to determine whether the infections could explain the birth order effect.

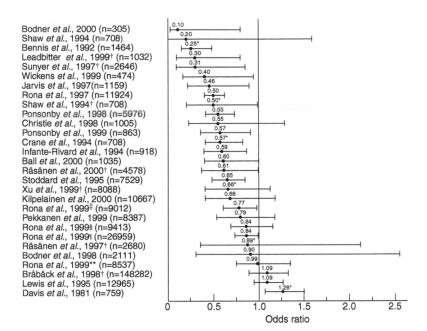

Figure 9.5 Summary of studies of the relationship between asthma and number of siblings. Odds ratios and 95% confidence intervals for large number of siblings. Odds ratios are adjusted for other risk factors except for those marked with asterisks. † = Older siblings only. ‡ = 1994 survey. § = 1986 survey. ¶ = All surveys. ** = 1977 survey. (With permission from BMJ Publishing Group.)

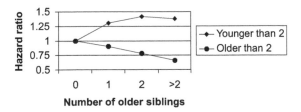

Figure 9.6 Birth order and asthma by age of diagnosis. (Constructed from data in *Thorax* 2002; 56: 761. With permission.)

In a study of hepatitis A, a birth order effect was noted in subjects who were seronegative, but no birth order effect was seen in seropositive subjects.[20] Our own study of the 1970 British birth cohort suggests that a protective effect from exposure to measles was limited to children who had greater numbers of older siblings,[10] although this finding was not confirmed by analyses of the 1958

British birth cohort.[50] A few studies examined the effects of early infection on birth order and found that exposure to infection had no impact on the strong birth order effects noted in their data.[8,34,51] No convincing evidence that exposure to infections explains the birth order effects on allergic outcomes has appeared to date.

V. Immune System

Enthusiasm for the hygiene hypothesis has fueled the emergence of the TH1–TH2 hypothesis that exposure to viral and bacterial infections stimulates the production of TH1 lymphocyte subsets that in turn inhibit the production of pro-allergic TH2 cells.[52] It has been suggested that babies are born with their immune systems skewed toward TH2 responses that help maintain successful pregnancies, and then after birth, exposure to pathogens switches the immune system to a TH1 profile.[52] Recent evidence in humans suggests that the system is more complex and doubts have been expressed about the usefulness of the TH1–TH2 model in humans.[53]

VI. Day Care

A logical extension to birth order is to examine exposures to other children outside the family unit. Thus, some studies have examined whether exposure to other children through attendance at day care also reduces the risk of developing allergic disease. The data from current studies are rather inconsistent, however, and are summarized in Table 9.1. Most studies found no protective effect between day care attendance and development of allergic diseases although one study has shown that use of day care facilities reduced the risk of PST (odds ratio [OR] 0.26, 95% CI, 0.14–0.50).[54]

Another study revealed that a younger age of entry into day care reduced the risk of asthma at age 13[38] and also that children from small families who had a later entries into day nurseries were at increased risk of having positive SPTs although this association was present only in a subset analysis of small families.[55] No consistent evidence currently suggests that attending day care early in life protects against the development of allergic disease.

VII. Multiple Births

As a unique extension to the birth order effect, evidence suggests that being part of a multiple birth may reduce the risk for asthma and other allergic diseases. The first study to show an effect of multiple gestation was conducted in Swedish conscripts and found a reduction in allergic rhinitis by an odds ratio of 0.74 (95% CI, 0.64–0.85) and a reduction in asthma by an odds ratio of 0.80 (95% CI,

Table 9.1 Summary of Studies Examining Effect of Day Care Use on Asthma and Allergic Disease

Lead Author, Year, Ref. Number	Study Design and Population	Outcome	Exposure	Size of Effect
Nafstad, 1993 (85)	Cross-sectional survey; children aged 4–5; N = 3749	Asthma	Age of entry into day care	Adj. OR
			Never in day care	1.00
			3 years or more	1.01 (0.68–1.49)
			2–3 years	1.16 (0.76–1.77)
			0–2 years	1.59 (1.07–2.36)
		Hay fever	Never in day care	1.00
			3 years or more	0.78 (0.49–12.3)
			2–3 years	0.95 (0.57–1.58)
			0–2 years	0.83 (0.51–1.37)
Forastiere, 1997 (86)	Cross-sectional survey; children aged 7–11; N = 2226	Positive skin prick test	Day care attendance	OR
			No	1.00
			Yes	1.23 (0.86–1.75)
Strachan, 1997 (87)	Nested case-control within birth cohort; follow-up data until age 34–35; N = 1369	Positive SPT	Nursery preschool attendance	Prevalence of positive SPT
			Yes	35.5%
			No	32.3% NS
Celedon, 1999 (88)	Birth cohort, selected by requiring at least one atopic parent; follow-up of children at age 2–4; N = 498	Two or more wheezing episodes	Day care in first 2 years of life	Adj. OR
			No	1.0
			Yes	1.4 (0.8–2.3)

Table 9.1 (continued) Summary of Studies Examining Effect of Day Care Use on Asthma and Allergic Disease

Lead Author, Year, Ref. Number	Study Design and Population	Outcome	Exposure	Size of Effect
Kramer, 1999 (55)	Cross-sectional survey; ages 5–7, 8–10, and 11–14; N = 2250	Doctor-diagnosed asthma	Age of entry into day nursery	
			Small families:	P = 0.03 for positive trend
			6–11 months	
			12–23 months	
			24 months	
			Large families:	Adj. OR
			6–11 months	1.00
			12–23 months	1.76 (0.38–8.22)
			24 months	2.77 (0.54–14.14)
		Positive SPT	Age of entry into day nursery	
			Small families:	
			6–11 months	1.00
			12–23 months	1.99 (1.08–3.66)
			24 months	2.72 (1.37–5.40)
			Large families:	
			6–11 months	1.00
			12–23 months	0.98 (0.67–1.42)
			24 months	1.16 (0.75–1.77)
Nystad, 1999 (26)	Cross-sectional survey; ages 6–16; N = 1447	Asthma	Full-time day care	OR
			No	1.0
			Yes	1.2 (0.8–1.9)
Wickens, 1999 (39)	Case-control study; ages 7–9; case N = 233; control N = 241	Doctor-diagnosed asthma and asthma medications used in previous 12 months	Day care in first year of life	OR
			No	1.00
			Yes	1.81 (0.93–3.51)

Study	Description	Outcome	Exposure	RR / OR
Ball, 2000 (38)	Birth cohort; follow-up data to age 13; N = 996	Doctor-diagnosed asthma	Age of entry into day care 0–6 months 7–12 months >12 months	RR 0.4 (0.2–1.0) 0.9 (0.4–2.1) 1.0
Haby, 2000 (54)	Cross-sectional survey; ages 3–5; N = 650	Positive SPT	No day care Family day care Day care center	Adj. OR (95% CI) 1.00 0.66 (0.41–1.04) 0.26 (0.14–0.50)
Infante-Rivard, 2001 (33)	Case-control study; ages 3–4; case N = 457; control N = 457	Doctor-diagnosed asthma	Day care attendance before age 1 No Yes	OR 1.00 0.65 (0.47–0.89)
Svanes, 2002 (35)	Cross-sectional study; ages 20–44; N = 18,530	Various phenotypes of wheeze, hay fever, eczema	Day care attendance any time before age 5	In subgroup analyses in subjects with no siblings: Hay fever 0.76 (0.60–0.98) Wheeze 1.48 (1.12–1.95) No other significant associations

Adj. OR = adjusted odds ratio. NS = not significant risk. RR = relative risk.

0.65–0.97).[56] In a cohort study of Scottish children up to the age of 10, a reduction in asthma admissions to hospital was found in multiple birth children as compared with singletons, a rate ratio of 0.47 (95% CI, 0.39–0.57).[40] Our own research demonstrated a protective effect of multiple birth with an inverse relation between number of multiple birth siblings and the risk of developing asthma and eczema and a broadly similar relationship for hay fever.[17] Thus, a protective effect seems to result from being born in a multiple birth. These findings may be helpful when determining the underlying cause of the protective effect from older siblings.

VIII.   Is the Birth Order Effect Already Present at Birth?

The fact that the birth order effects have proven surprisingly difficult to explain in terms of early infection[8,57,58] has prompted a search for alternative explanations. One such explanation is that the birth order effects are mediated by changes in the mother arising from successive pregnancies. For example, a cross-sectional study found that women who had greater numbers of children were less likely to be SPT-positive with adjusted odds ratios for increasing numbers of offspring being 0.71, 0.79, and 0.26.[59] This suggests that successive pregnancies may reduce the risk of atopy or that atopic women are less fertile. One cohort study also demonstrated that cord blood IgE levels were lower in children with more older siblings and that cord blood IgE level was a better predictor of atopic sensitization than number of older siblings at age 4, implying that the birth order effect is established *in utero*.[60]

Research has also shown that cord blood mononuclear cells in children from a first pregnancy have increased proliferative responses after stimulation with house dust mite extract as compared with children from subsequent pregnancies.[61] We have addressed this question by looking at the effects of previous pregnancies terminated through abortions, miscarriages, or stillbirths and found no evidence that termination reduced the risk of developing allergic disease.[62] It therefore remains unclear whether the birth order effect is a result of changes of *in utero* exposures or changes in environmental exposures surrounding subsequent births or both influences.

IX.   Birth Order and Other Diseases

If the simple TH1–TH2 hypothesis is true, it potentially has importance for other diseases and suggests that diseases associated with TH1 responses rather than TH2 responses should be more common in children with more older siblings. This association has been mainly researched in type I diabetes, a TH1 disease. Some studies demonstrated increased risk of disease with increasing birth order,[63–65] and others found no association.[66,67] Evidence has emerged that TH1 and TH2 diseases may not be mutually exclusive. One study revealed an increase in prevalence of allergic disease in TH1-mediated disorders.[53] This evidence argues against a simple TH1–TH2 model.

The birth order effect has been investigated in multiple sclerosis, another TH1-immune disease. The evidence generally points to low birth order increasing the risk of multiple sclerosis,[68–70] and again this result runs counter to the simple TH1–TH2 hypothesis. In Crohn's disease, another TH1-immune condition, a case–control study of over 300 patients demonstrated increased prevalence of eczema in cases as compared with controls.[71] This represents further evidence that TH1–TH2 diseases are not exclusive. This study found no relationship between Crohn's disease or ulcerative colitis and birth order.

Birth order effects have been investigated in relation to other diseases including various cancers,[72–80] congenital defects,[81] epilepsy,[82] and cardiovascular disease.[83,84] The greatest amount of work was conducted in the area of cancer research. In a large matched case–control study of 10,162 childhood cancers, the authors found an increase in birth order related to a decrease in the risk of cancer such that having five or more older siblings halved the risk of developing disease (adjusted odds ratio of 0.5, 95% CI, 0.3–0.8).[75] A significant birth order effect showing increased risk in lower birth orders was also noted for breast[73,77] and testicular cancer[72,76] in adults. These studies show that the birth order effect is not limited to immune-related diseases and may, in fact, be a phenomenon of producing "healthier" children with each pregnancy.

X. Summary

Evidence suggests strongly that allergic disorders are less common in children with several older siblings. For asthma and wheezing, however, the relationship is more complex. There appears to be a cross-over effect under which a greater number of older siblings increases the risk of early wheezing, but decreases the risk diagnosis of asthma after the age of 2. The mechanism of these associations is not clear, and we have strong reasons to doubt the original suggestions that these associations are due to patterns of exposure to infection. Because a consistency exists in the relationship between birth order and other diseases, further investigation is needed to determine how birth order exerts its effects on health.

References

1. Strachan DP. Hay fever, hygiene, and household size. *Br Med J* 1989; 299: 1259–1260.
2. Butland B.K, Strachan DP, Lewis S, Bynner J, Butler N, and Britton J. Investigation into the increase in hay fever and eczema at age 16 observed between the 1958 and 1970 British birth cohorts. *Br Med J* 1997; 315: 717–721.

3. Braback L and Hedberg A. Perinatal risk factors for atopic disease in conscripts. *Clin Exp Allergy* 1998; 28: 936–942.

4. Ponsonby AL, Couper D, Dwyer T, and Carmichael A. Cross-sectional study of the relation between sibling number and asthma, hay fever, and eczema. *Arch Dis Child* 1998; 79: 328–333.

5. Butland B.K, Strachan DP, Lewis S, Bynner J, Butler N, and Britton J. Investigation into the increase in hay fever and eczema at age 16 observed between the 1958 and 1970 British birth cohorts. *Br Med J* 1997; 315: 717–721.

6. Bodner C, Godden D, and Seaton A. Family size, childhood infections and atopic diseases. *Thorax* 1998; 53: 28–32.

7. Xu B, Jarvelin MR, and Pekkanen J. Prenatal factors and occurrence of rhinitis and eczema among offspring. *Allergy* 1999; 54: 829–836.

8. Strachan DP, Taylor EM, and Carpenter RG. Family structure, neonatal infection, and hay fever in adolescence. *Arch Dis Child* 1996; 74: 422–426.

9. Kulig M, Klettke U, Wahn V, Forster J, Bauer CP, and Wahn U. Development of seasonal allergic rhinitis during the first seven years of life. *J Allergy Clin Immunol* 2000; 106: 832–839.

10. Lewis SA and Britton JR. Measles infection, measles vaccination and the effect of birth order in the aetiology of hay fever. *Clin Exp Allergy* 1998; 28: 1493–1500.

11. Butler NR and Golding J. *From Birth to Five*. Oxford: Pergamon Press, 1986.

12. Leadbitter P, Pearce N, Cheng S, Sears MR, Holdaway MD, Flannery EM, Herbison GP, and Beasley R. Relationship between fetal growth and the development of asthma and atopy in childhood. *Thorax* 1999; 54: 905–910.

13. Kilpelainen M, Terho EO, Helenius H, and Koskenvuo M. Farm environment in childhood prevents the development of allergies. *Clin Exp Allergy* 2000; 30: 201–208.

14. Pekkanen J, Remes S, Kajosaari M, Husman T, and Soininen L. Infections in early childhood and risk of atopic disease. *Acta Paediatr* 1999; 88: 710–714.

15. Golding J and Peters TJ. The epidemiology of childhood eczema I. A population-based study of associations. *Paediatr Perinatal Epidemiol* 1987; 1: 67–79.

16. Olesen AB, Ellingsen AR, Olesen H, Juul S, and Thestrup-Pedersen K. Atopic dermatitis and birth factors: historical follow-up by record linkage. *Br Med J* 1997; 314: 1003–1008.

17. McKeever TM, Lewis SA, Smith C, Collins J, Heatlie H, Frischer M et al. Siblings, multiple births, and the incidence of allergic disease: a birth cohort study using the West Midlands general practice research database. *Thorax* 2001; 56: 758–762.

18. von Mutius E, Martinez FD, Fritzsch C, Nicolai T, Reitmeir P, and Thiemann HH. Skin test reactivity and number of siblings. *Br Med J* 1994; 308: 692–695.

19. Svanes C, Jarvis D, Chinn S, and Burney P. Childhood environment and adult atopy: results from the European Community Respiratory Health Survey. *J Allerg Clin Immunol* 1999; 103: 415–420.

20. Matricardi PM, Rosmini F, Ferrigno L, Nisini R, Rapicetta M, Chionne P et al. Cross-sectional retrospective study of prevalence of atopy among Italian military students with antibodies against hepatitis A virus. *Br Med J* 1997; 314: 999–1003.

21. Strachan DP, Harkins LS, Johnston IDA, and Anderson HR. Childhood antecedents of allergic sensitization in young British adults. *J Allerg Clin Immunol* 1997; 99: 6–12.

22. Karmaus W and Botezan C. Does a higher number of siblings protect against the development of allergy and asthma? A review. *J Epidemiol Commun Health* 2002; 56: 209–217.

23. Davis JB and Bulpitt CJ. Atopy and wheeze in children according to parental atopy and family size. *Thorax* 1981; 36: 185–189.

24. Crane J, Pearce N, Shaw R, Fitzharris P, and Mayes C. Asthma and having siblings. *Br Med J* 1994; 309: 272.

25. Rona RJ, Hughes JM, and Chinn S. Association between asthma and family size between 1977 and 1994. *J Epidemiol Commun Health* 1999; 53: 15–19.

26. Nystad W, Skrondal A, and Magnus P. Day care attendance, recurrent respiratory tract infections and asthma. *Int J Epidemiol* 1999; 28: 882–887.

27. Rusconi F, Galassi C, Corbo GM, Forastiere F, Biggeri A, Ciccone G et al. Risk factors for early, persistent, and late-onset wheezing in young children: SIDRIA Collaborative Group. *Am J Respir Crit Care Med* 1999; 1605: 161–1622.

28. Lewis S, Butland B, Strachan D, Bynner J, Richards D, Butler N et al. Study of the aetiology of wheezing illness at age 16 in two national British birth cohorts. *Thorax* 1996; 51: 670–676

29. Lewis S, Richards D, Bynner J, Butler N, and Britton J. Prospective study of risk factors for early and persistent wheezing in childhood. *Eur Resp J* 1995; 8: 349–356.

30. Horwood LJ, Fergusson DM, and Shannon FT. Social and familial factors in the development of early childhood asthma. *Pediatrics* 1985; 75: 859–868.

31. Haby MM, Peat JK, Marks GB, Woolcock AJ, and Leeder SR. Asthma in preschool children: prevalence and risk factors. *Thorax* 2001; 56: 589–595.

32. Wickens K, Crane J, Pearce N, and Beasley R. The magnitude of the effect of smaller family sizes on the increase in the prevalence of asthma and hay fever in the United Kingdom and New Zealand. *J Allerg Clin Immunol* 1999; 104: 55–558.

33. Infante-Rivard C, Amre D, Gautrin D, and Malo JL. Family size, day-care attendance, and breastfeeding in relation to the incidence of childhood asthma. *Am J Epidemiol* 2001; 153: 653–658.

34. Bodner C, Anderson WJ, Reid TS, and Godden DJ. Childhood exposure to infection and risk of adult onset wheeze and atopy. *Thorax* 2000; 55: 383–387.

35. Svanes C, Jarvis D, Chinn S, Omenaas E, Gulsvik A, and Burney P. Early exposure to children in family and day care as related to adult asthma and hay fever: results from the European Community Respiratory Health Survey. *Thorax* 2002; 57: 945–950.

36. Rona RJ, Duran-Tauleria E, and Chinn S. Family size, atopic disorders in parents, asthma in children, and ethnicity. *J Allerg Clin Immunol* 1997; 99: 454–460.

37. Rasanen M, Kaprio J, Laitinen T, Winter T, Koskenvuo M, and Laitinen LA. Perinatal risk factors for asthma in Finnish adolescent twins. *Thorax* 2000; 55: 25–31.

38. Ball TM, Castro-Rodriguez JA, Griffith KA, Holberg CJ, Martinez FD, and Wright AL. Siblings, day-care attendance, and the risk of asthma and wheezing during childhood. *New Engl J Med* 2000; 343: 538–543.

39. Wickens KL, Crane J, Kemp TJ, Lewis SJ, D'Souza WJ, Sawyer GM et al. Family size, infections, and asthma prevalence in New Zealand children. *Epidemiology* 1999; 10: 699–705.

40. Strachan DP, Moran SE, McInneny K, and Smalls M. Reduced risk of hospital admission for childhood asthma among Scottish twins: record linkage study. *Br Med J* 2000; 321: 732–733.
41. Silverman M and Wilson N. Wheezing phenotypes in childhood. *Thorax* 1997; 52: 936–937.
42. Shaheen SO, Aaby P, Hall AJ, Barker DJP, Heyes CB, Shiell AW et al. Measles and atopy in Guinea–Bissau. *Lancet* 1996; 347: 1792–1796.
43. Shaheen SO, Aaby P, Hall AJ, Barker DJP, Heyes CB, Shiell AW et al. Cell-mediated immunity after measles in Guinea–Bissau: historical cohort study. *Br Med J* 1996; 313: 969–974.
44. Matricardi PM, Rosmini F, Riondino S, Fortini M, Ferrigno L, Rapicetta M et al. Exposure to foodborne and orofecal microbes versus airborne viruses in relation to atopy and allergic asthma: epidemiological study. *Br Med J* 2000; 320: 412–417.
45. Matricardi PM, Rosmini F, Ferrigno L, Nisini R, Rapicetta M, Chionne P et al. Cross sectional retrospective study of prevalence of atopy among Italian military students with antibodies against hepatitis A virus. *Br Med J* 1997; 314: 999–1003.
46. Matricardi PM, Rosmini F, Panetta V, Ferrigno L, and Bonini S. Hay fever and asthma in relation to markers of infection in the United States. *J Allergy Clin Immunol* 2002; 110: 381–387.
47. Shirakawa T, Enomoto T, Shimazu S, and Hopkin JM. The inverse association between tuberculin responses and atopic disorder. *Science* 1997; 275: 77–79.
48. von Hertzen L, Klaukka T, Mattila H, and Haahtela T. *Mycobacterium tuberculosis* infection and the subsequent development of asthma and allergic conditions. *J Allergy Clin Immunol* 1999; 104: 1211–1214.
49. Illi S, von Mutius E, Lau S, Bergmann R, Niggemann B, Sommerfeld C et al. Early childhood infectious diseases and the development of asthma up to school age: a birth cohort study. *Br Med J* 2001; 322: 390–395.
50. Strachan DP. Family size, infection and atopy: the first decade of the "hygiene hypothesis." *Thorax* 2000; 55: S2–10.
51. McKeever TM, Lewis SA, Smith C, Collins J, Heatlie H, Frischer M et al. Early exposure to infections and antibiotics and the incidence of allergic disease: a birth cohort study with the West Midlands General Practice Research Database. *J Allergy Clin Immunol* 2002; 109: 43–50.
52. Donovan CE and Finn PW. Immune mechanisms of childhood asthma. *Thorax* 1999; 54: 938–946.
53. Skeikh A, Smeeth L, and Hubbard R. What is the relationship between atopic allergic conditions and autoimmune disorders? *Am J Resp Crit Care Med* 2002; 165: A313.
54. Haby MM, Marks GB, Peat JK, and Leeder SR. Daycare attendance before the age of two protects against atopy in preschool age children. *Pediatr Pulmonol* 2000; 30: 377–384.
55. Kramer U, Heinrich J, Wjst M, and Wichmann HE. Age of entry to day nursery and allergy in later childhood. *Lancet* 1999; 353: 450–454.
56. Braback L and Hedberg A. Perinatal risk factors for atopic disease in conscripts. *Clin Exp Allergy* 1998; 28: 936–942.

57. Alm JS, Swartz J, Lilja G, Scheynius A, and Pershagen G. Atopy in children of families with an anthroposophic lifestyle. *Lancet* 1999; 353: 1485–1488.
58. Bodner C, Godden D, Seaton A. Family size, childhood infections and atopic diseases. *Thorax* 1998; 53: 28–32.
59. Sunyer J, Anto JM, Harris J, Torrent M, Vall O, Cullinan P et al. Maternal atopy and parity. *Clin Exp Allergy* 2001; 31: 1352–1355.
60. Karmaus W, Arshad H, and Mattes J. Does the sibling effect have its origin *in utero*? Investigating birth order, cord blood immunoglobulin E concentration, and allergic sensitization at age four years. *Am J Epidemiol* 2001; 154: 909–915.
61. Devereux G, Barker RN, and Seaton A. Antenatal determinants of neonatal immune responses to allergens. *Clin Exp Allergy* 2002; 32: 43–50.
62. McKeever TM, Lewis SA, Smith C, and Hubbard R. The importance of prenatal exposures on the development of allergic disease: a birth cohort study using the west midlands general practice database. *Am J Respir Crit Care Med* 2002; 166: 827–832.
63. Tuomilehto J, Podar T, Tuomilehto-Wolf E, and Virtala E. Evidence for importance of gender and birth cohort for risk of IDDM in offspring of IDDM parents. *Diabetologia* 1995; 38: 975–982.
64. Soltesz G. IDDM in Hungarian children: population-based clinical characteristic and their possible implication for diabetic health care. *Padiatr Padol* 1992; 27: 63–66.
65. Ramachandran A, Snehalatha C, Joseph A, Viswanathan V, and Viswanathan M. Maternal age and birth order of young IDDM patients: a study from southern India. *Diabetes Care* 1993; 16: 636–637.
66. Warram JH, Martin BC, and Krolewski AS. Risk of IDDM in children of diabetic mothers decreases with increasing maternal age at pregnancy. *Diabetes* 1991; 40: 1679–1684.
67. Wagener DK, LaPorte RE, Orchard TJ, Cavender D, Kuller LH, and Drash AL. The Pittsburgh diabetes mellitus study 3: increased prevalence with older maternal age. *Diabetologia* 1983; 25: 82–85.
68. James WH. Multiple sclerosis and birth order. *J Epidemiol Commun Health* 1984; 38: 21–22.
69. Zilber N, Kutai-Berman M, Kahana E, and Korczyn AD. Multiple sclerosis and birth order. *Acta Neurol Scand* 1988; 78: 313–317.
70. Isager H, Andersen E, and Hyllested K. Risk of multiple sclerosis inversely associated with birth order position. *Acta Neurol Scand* 1980; 61: 393–396.
71. Gilat T, Hacohen D, Lilos P, and Langman MJ. Childhood factors in ulcerative colitis and Crohn's disease: an international cooperative study. *Scand J Gastroenterol* 1987; 22: 1009–1024.
72. Prener A, Hsieh CC, Engholm G, Trichopoulos D, and Jensen OM. Birth order and risk of testicular cancer. *Cancer Causes Control* 1992; 33: 265–272.
73. Hsieh CC, Tzonou A, and Trichopoulos D. Birth order and breast cancer risk. *Cancer Causes Control* 1991; 2: 95–98.
74. Gold E, Gordis L, Tonascia J, and Szklo M. Risk factors for brain tumors in children. *Am J Epidemiol* 1979; 109: 309–319.

75. Dockerty JD, Draper G, Vincent T, Rowan SD, and Bunch KJ. Case-control study of parental age, parity and socioeconomic level in relation to childhood cancers. *Int J Epidemiol* 2001; 30: 1428–1437.
76. Swerdlow AJ, Huttly SR, and Smith PG. Prenatal and familial associations of testicular cancer. *Br J Cancer* 1987; 55: 571–577.
77. Hemminki K and Mutanen P. Birth order, family size, and the risk of cancer in young and middle-aged adults. *Br J Cancer* 2001; 84: 1466–1471.
78. Westergaard T, Andersen PK, Pedersen JB, Olsen JH, Frisch M, Sorensen HT et al. Birth characteristics, sibling patterns, and acute leukemia risk in childhood: a population-based cohort study. *J Natl Cancer Inst* 1997; 89: 939–947.
79. Gutensohn N and Cole P. Childhood social environment and Hodgkin's disease. *New Engl J Med* 1981; 304: 135–140.
80. Vianna NJ and Polan AK. Immunity in Hodgkin's disease: importance of age at exposure. *Ann Intern Med* 1978; 89: 550–556.
81. Choudhury AR, Mukherjee M, Sharma A, Talukder G, and Ghosh PK. Study of 126,266 consecutive births for major congenital defects. *Indian J Pediatr* 1989; 56: 493–499.
82. Tay JS, Yip WC, Joseph R, and Wong HB. Parental age and birth order effects in children with febrile convulsions. *Eur J Pediatr* 1985; 144:88–89.
83. Yasuda N, Nara Y, Kojima S, Mikami H, Hiwada K, Tsuda K et al. Family history study on hypertension in Japan. *Clin Exp Pharmacol Physiol Suppl* 1992; 20: 7–9.
84. Whincup PH, Cook DG, and Shaper AG. Early influences on blood pressure: a study of children aged 5–7 years. *Br Med J* 1989; 299: 587–591.
85. Nafstad P, Hagen JA, Oie L, Magnus P, and Jaakkola JJ. Day care centers and respiratory health. *Pediatrics* 1999; 103: 753–758.
86. Forastiere F, Agabiti N, Corbo GM, Dell'Orco V, Porta D, Pistelli R et al. Socio-economic status, number of siblings, and respiratory infections in early life as determinants of atopy in children. *Epidemiology* 1997; 8: 566–570.
87. Strachan DP, Harkins LS, Johnston IDA, and Anderson HR. Childhood antecedents of allergic sensitization in young British adults. *J Allergy Clin Immunol* 1997; 99: 6–12.
88. Celedon JC, Litonjua AA, Weiss ST, and Gold DR. Day care attendance in the first year of life and illnesses of the upper and lower respiratory tract in children with a familial history of atopy. *Pediatrics* 1999; 104: 495-500.

10

Infections: Causative

G. DANIEL BROOKS and ROBERT F. LEMANSKE, JR.

University of Wisconsin–Madison
Madison, Wisconsin, U.S.A.

I. Introduction

Respiratory viruses typically cause self-limited upper respiratory symptoms that produce discomfort and inconvenience in most people. However, for people with asthma, respiratory viruses can cause severe exacerbations. Childhood infection with respiratory viruses may even contribute to the initiation of asthma. This review addresses the epidemiologic evidence that respiratory viruses contribute to asthma inception or asthma exacerbation, possible mechanisms by which viruses may initiate or aggravate asthma, and potential therapeutic approaches to prevent the effects of viruses on asthma.

II. Asthma Inception

A. Association between Bronchiolitis and Asthma

Seventy percent of emergency room visits for wheezing in children under the age of 2 years are associated with a respiratory syncytial virus (RSV) infection.[1] RSV is usually the cause of an infant's first wheezing episode, and many infants go on to develop a post-bronchiolitic syndrome that includes more prolonged wheezing and response to inhaled steroids, similar to asthma. Prospective trials have been performed in Nottingham, Sweden, and Tucson to determine whether RSV bronchiolitis is associated with asthma later in life.

In Nottingham, Noble and colleagues conducted a prospective case–control study in which they followed 101 infants admitted to the hospital for bronchiolitis.[2] After 5 years, age- and gender-matched controls with no histories of bronchiolitis were recruited. At 9 to 10 years of age, 61 subjects with histories of bronchiolitis and 47 controls were tested for pulmonary function. Children with histories of bronchiolitis were significantly more likely to have coughing (odds ratio [OR] 4.02), wheezing (OR 3.59), or a diagnosis of asthma (39 versus 13%). They also showed decreases in peak expiratory flow rate (PEFR) and forced expiratory volume in 1 second (FEV_1). The index cases were not more likely to demonstrate positive skin tests or family histories of atopy. Although RSV is the virus most commonly implicated in bronchiolitis, this study did not include viral testing and some episodes of bronchiolitis may have been caused by other viruses.

In Sweden, Sigurs and colleagues prospectively followed 47 infants with RSV bronchiolitis and 93 age- and gender-matched controls to age 7.5 years.[3] Children with histories of bronchiolitis were more likely to have had three or more physician-diagnosed episodes of bronchial obstruction (30 versus 3%), allergic rhinoconjunctivitis (15 versus 2%), and skin prick tests positive to inhalant allergens (20 versus 6%). A family history of atopy in both parents appeared to be a more significant risk factor than RSV bronchiolitis for positive skin tests (ORs 5.7 versus 2.4) but less important for asthma (ORs 3.1 versus 12.7).

In Tucson, Martinez and colleagues followed 888 children in a prospective birth cohort.[4] During the first 3 years, all children with symptoms of lower respiratory illness were assessed by their pediatricians and nasopharyngeal swabs were collected and tested for RSV and parainfluenza. Five hundred nineteen children had at least one lower respiratory tract infection; RSV was detected in 207 children, parainfluenza in 68 children, and other respiratory pathogens in 68 children. Children who had RSV lower respiratory tract infections during the first 3 years of life were significantly more likely to have parent-reported wheezing at ages 6, 8, and 11 years.

The risk of wheezing in the children with RSV decreased over time and was no longer significant by age 13 years. Parainfluenza was not associated with an increased risk of wheezing; however, children with negative cultures or with other respiratory pathogens identified were more likely to have wheezing at age 13. Children with RSV infections also had lower FEV_1 values at age 11 (not measured at age 13). In contrast to the findings of Sigurs et al., Martinez found no relationship between RSV infection and allergen skin prick tests or total serum IgE levels.

When considered together, these three studies indicate that bronchiolitis and RSV lower respiratory tract infections are risk factors for childhood asthma, but the Tucson study indicates that the risk declines over time and is no longer present by adolescence — a finding that was noted earlier with less powerful study designs.[5,6] The importance of bronchiolitis and RSV infections as risk factors for asthma beyond 10 years of age still remains controversial.[7]

B. Importance of Host Response

The epidemiologic association of RSV lower respiratory tract infections and childhood asthma led to the hypothesis that RSV can cause asthma; however, the causal linkage between RSV and asthma is not clear. Most children who had wheezing in the first 3 years of life did not go on to develop asthma by 6 years of age.[7] Only a subset of children had lower respiratory symptoms during RSV infections. The majority of children showed serologic evidence of previous RSV infection by 1 year of age and 75% had had RSV infections by the age of 2.[9,10] However, only a small fraction of these children had had severe lower respiratory tract infections. Of those who developed lower respiratory infections with RSV, studies indicate that 30% or fewer would go on to have asthma.[3,11] For this reason, it is necessary to consider that the host response of bronchiolitis or wheezing and not the specific virus is the marker for asthma later in childhood.

In Finland, Kotaniemi-Syrjanen and colleagues evaluated 81 infants for wheezing at the time of hospital admission and reevaluated them 6 years later.[12] During the initial hospitalization, nasopharyngeal aspirates were collected for identification of pathogenic viruses using an immunoassay and polymerase chain reaction (PCR). The incorporation of PCR allowed accurate detection of rhinovirus (RV), which is usually missed by the conventional virology techniques used in previous studies. RV was detected in 27 infants and RSV was identified in 21 infants, 67% of whom were under 6 months of age. At follow-up, children were categorized as having asthma if they were on maintenance medications for asthma or had symptoms suggestive of asthma and positive exercise challenges. Children who had previous episodes of RV-associated wheezing were more likely to develop asthma than children with wheezing due to other viruses. In contrast to previous studies,[3,11] RSV was not associated with asthma, but fewer subjects with RSV were included. One interpretation is that RSV can induce wheezing even in children with little risk of asthma, but RV affects only children with significant risk for asthma (Figure 10.1).

In Germany, Illi and colleagues[13] compared the effects of lower respiratory tract infections with upper respiratory tract infections in 1314 children recruited at birth. During the first 3 years, parents were asked to keep a diary of all illnesses, including upper and lower respiratory infections. Until the children reached age 7, parents were asked whether a physician had diagnosed asthma. When the children reached age 7, histamine challenges were performed. This study was limited by the lack of specific laboratory viral identification, but comparisons of

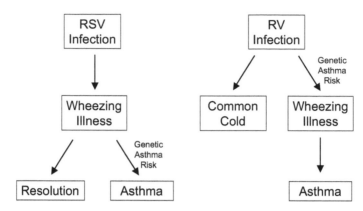

Figure 10.1 Model demonstrating the observation that a wheezing infection with rhinovirus (RV) is a greater risk factor for developing asthma than a wheezing infection with respiratory syncytial virus (RSV). RSV infection causes wheezing illness in many children. Only children with genetic risks will develop asthma. In contrast, RV infection is unlikely to cause wheezing in children without genetic risk for asthma.

upper and lower respiratory tract infections were still possible. Children with two or more upper respiratory infections during the first year of life were less likely to have asthma or bronchial hyperreactivity by age 7. In contrast, children with four or more lower respiratory infections were more likely to develop asthma by age 7; the trend was similar for bronchial hyperreactivity.

The findings of Kotaniemi-Syrjanen and Illi reaffirm the concept that a specific virus may not be a primary risk factor for developing asthma. Instead, the host response of bronchiolitis or lower respiratory symptoms appears to be a risk factor for asthma.

C. Host Factors Contributing to Wheezing or Asthma

Several factors that predispose children to develop wheezing during viral infections have been discovered. One risk factor is lung size, as measured by length-adjusted functional residual capacity. Children with reduced pulmonary function are more likely to have wheezing with infections in the first year of life.[8] Maternal smoking is also associated with wheezing during infections early in life, partially due to reduced pulmonary function.[8] However, children with these "physiologic" risk factors often have wheezing that does not persist beyond the age of 3.[8]

Immunologic factors appear to exert a greater influence on the persistence of wheezing later in life. Three studies indicate that infants with reduced production of interferon gamma (IFN), an important antiviral cytokine, during RSV infections appear to be at greater risk for wheezing after infection.

Renzi and colleagues[14] studied 32 infants admitted to the hospital for bronchiolitis. During the hospitalization, peripheral blood mononuclear cells (PBMCs) from the infants were incubated with interleukin (IL)-2 and supernatants were analyzed for IFN. After 4.9 months, histamine challenges were performed, and at 2 years, the infants were assessed for the presence of asthma-like symptoms. Infants with reduced production of IFNγ during infection showed greater histamine responsiveness 4.9 months later and a greater incidence of asthma-like symptoms 2 years later.

Aberle and colleagues[15] studied 20 infants hospitalized for acute lower respiratory illness due to RSV. IFN messenger RNA (mRNA) was measured in PBMCs from all of the children. The children with more severe RSV disease had lower amounts of IFN mRNA production than children with milder disease, although both groups showed increases in IFN compared with levels during convalescence.

Legg and colleagues[16] examined cytokine protein secretion in nasopharyngeal aspirates and PBMC cultures from 28 infants with documented RSV illness. Infants with upper respiratory tract infections secreted more IFN than infants with bronchiolitis, again suggesting a relative deficit in IFN production. However, this finding does not agree with a previous study by Van Schaik and colleagues,[17] who compared 82 infants with virus-induced wheezing with 47 infants with upper respiratory symptoms and 18 healthy controls. Nasal secretions from infants with upper respiratory tract symptoms contained less IFN mRNA than secretions from children with lower respiratory symptoms. Thus, there is a discrepancy between the two studies, and the role of IFN in nasal secretions during an RSV infection requires further study.

A rat model also supports the hypothesis that host immune responses to the virus affect the development of post-bronchiolitic syndromes. After weanling Brown–Norway rats were infected with Sendai virus, they developed episodic, reversible airway obstruction, airway hyperresponsiveness to methacholine, chronic airway inflammation, and airway wall remodeling.[18,19] Fischer 344 rats did not develop the post-bronchiolitic syndrome. During the Sendai virus infection, Brown–Norway weanlings exhibited decreased production of IFNγ compared with Fischer 344 weanlings. Administering aerosolized IFNγ to Brown–Norway weanlings prevented the post-viral sequelae.[20] Thus, abnormal host immune response to respiratory viruses (specifically, low IFNγ production) appears to be a risk factor for persistent asthma-like symptoms.

D. Effects of RSV Bronchiolitis May Contribute to Asthma

Although the host immune response to RSV is a critical risk factor for the development of wheezing, effects of RSV on the host immune system or lungs may also be necessary to cause asthma. RSV is an enveloped paramyxovirus that expresses two antigenic proteins to which neutralizing antibodies can be directed. The attachment glycoprotein (G) mediates attachment to host epithelial cells, and the fusion (F) protein is necessary for fusion between the viral envelope and cell membranes.

RSV type A and type B are distinguished by variations in the structure of the G protein. Experiments have been performed in BALB/c mice to determine whether the F and G proteins stimulate different types of immune responses.[21,22] The G protein generated a T helper (Th) type 2 response and animals later exposed to RSV developed severe lung disease with eosinophilia. In contrast, the F protein generated a Th1 response and animals later exposed to RSV had much milder lung diseases without eosinophilia. These findings have raised the question of whether children who have more severe reactions to RSV infection (bronchiolitis) also have reduced Th1 responses or exaggerated Th2 responses to the G protein in the virus that may be a risk factor for asthma later in life.

Because the G protein can generate an increase in Th2 cytokine production,[21,22] it is theoretically possible that RSV infection can cause a deviation in the host immune system toward a more Th2 phenotype.

Some evidence indicates that RSV infection may promote allergic sensitization in humans. In the Swedish cohort,[3] children with histories of RSV bronchiolitis were more likely to show positive skin tests to environmental allergens. In addition, a subset of 37 children with histories of bronchiolitis and 69 matched controls had PBMCs cultured with RSV at the time of their follow-ups at age 7.[23] More IL-4 producing cells were found in the group with histories of RSV bronchiolitis. However, both groups had more IFN-producing T cells than IL-4-producing T-cells. In the Tucson cohort, no greater incidence of allergen sensitization in the children with a history of RSV was found,[11] and the hypothesis that a natural RSV infection can induce a Th2 response in humans is still controversial. In mouse studies of RSV infection and allergic sensitization, RSV infection may promote or inhibit allergic sensitization, depending on the specific timing of infection and sensitization.[24] Because of the varying effects of protocol on the outcome of infection, it is difficult to extrapolate these results to humans.

It is important to keep in mind that human subjects infected with RSV produce significant amounts of IFNγ but minimal IL-4, suggesting that the primary response to RSV is a Th1 response, although this may be deficient in some individuals.[16,17,25] In addition, the inflammation that occurs in the lower airway does not contain cells that are associated with an allergic response. Bronchoalveolar lavage (BAL) fluid from children with RSV bronchiolitis contained more neutrophils than any other cell type.[26] Although this response is neutrophilic, it still may be pathogenic. Neutrophils are the primary cell types found in children with recurrent wheezing.[27] In summary, RSV may exert possible allergic and nonallergic effects on the lower airway and more study is required to elucidate possible cause-and-effect relationships.

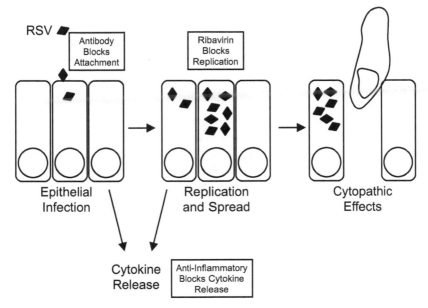

Figure 10.2 Respiratory syncytial virus (RSV) infects bronchial epithelial cells, replicates, spreads, induces inflammatory cytokine release, and eventually kills infected cells. Four treatment approaches have been proposed to interrupt this process. AntiRSV antibody may prevent infection by blocking attachment. Ribavirin may limit replication and spread. Anti-inflammatory treatments may alter the cytokines released during infection. Vaccination (not shown) has the potential to prevent infection through antibody production, prevent spread by eliminating infected cells, and alter the cytokine response to infection.

III. Strategies for Preventing RSV

Strategies that may prevent the effects of RSV on the airway include vaccination, prophylaxis with RSV immune globulin, antiviral therapies, and treatment of inflammation during infection (Figure 10.2).

A. RSV Vaccination

A formalin-inactivated intramuscular RSV vaccine was tested in the 1960s. Unfortunately, vaccinated children under the age of 2 years had increased respiratory disease in response to natural infection compared with unvaccinated children.[28–31] A mouse model has been used to determine the mechanism of this adverse reaction. Mice immunized with formalin-inactivated RSV vaccine had poor immune responses to subsequent RSV infection and lung histology was consistent with a Th2 response.[32] This suggests that the formalin-inactivated vaccine promoted Th2 inflammation during subsequent RSV infections, possibly because of a Th2 response to the G subunit of the vaccine.

Live attenuated, temperature-sensitive RSV vaccines did not produce the increased pulmonary inflammation seen with the formalin-inactivated vaccines. However, the strains used were not attenuated sufficiently. Vaccine recipients typically developed upper respiratory infections from the vaccine and shed virus for up to 3 weeks. Some nonrecipients also were infected.[33,34]

A subunit vaccine using the F protein that stimulates neutralizing antibodies and is conserved between serotypes has been developed.[35] It is unlikely that a subunit vaccine will be tested on infants any time soon because of the problems with the formalin-inactivated vaccine.[36] However, a subunit vaccine has been proposed for maternal immunization. It is administered during the second or third trimester to increase maternal production of RSV-neutralizing antibodies that are transported across the placenta to the fetus.[37,38]

Infants born prior to or during RSV season should have protection because of increased levels of RSV-neutralizing antibodies during the first 6 months of life — a particularly vulnerable period for RSV bronchiolitis.[39] When an F protein subunit vaccine was given to 35 women at 30 to 34 weeks of gestation, only a small increase in maternal antibody was noted, but the antibody was transported across the placenta effectively, suggesting that a more immunogenic vaccine may be successful.[36]

B. Antiviral Medications

Ribavirin is a virustatic nucleoside analog with activity against RSV that has been approved by the U.S. Food and Drug Administration (FDA). Ribavirin demonstrated efficacy in several early clinical trials, but these trials included small numbers of infants who were given the medication in the first 72 hours of symptoms.[40,41] A large prospective study has suggested that ribavirin is not effective, but this study was not randomized, and ribavirin was sometimes administered late in the infection.[42] Because of these conflicting results, it is not clear whether the benefits of ribavirin for bronchiolitis outweigh the costs. In addition, ribavirin should be used in the first 72 hours after onset of symptoms and this limits its practical usage.[40]

Two studies have examined whether administering ribavirin during an episode of RSV bronchiolitis can prevent the development of asthma later in life. Rodriguez and colleagues[43] randomized 35 infants with RSV bronchiolitis to ribavirin or placebo and followed them to age 7. Significantly more children from the placebo group had two or more wheezing episodes in the next 6 years; however, lung volumes and methacholine sensitivity were not statistically different between groups. Long and colleagues[44] studied 28 children treated with ribavirin and 26 controls 9 years after episodes of RSV-induced bronchiolitis.

They noted no significant difference between groups in the incidence of wheezing or in lung volumes. Thus, ribavirin appears to have little effect on the chances of developing asthma later in childhood.

C. Passive Immunization

Passive immunization is accomplished by administering antibodies against an organism to a susceptible host. Two preparations of antiRSV antibodies have been studied as preventive therapy for RSV bronchiolitis: RSV immunoglobulin and palivizumab. RSV immunoglobulin is an intravenous preparation isolated from blood donors with high levels of serum antibodies to RSV. Prophylaxis with human RSV intravenous immunoglobulin has been demonstrated to decrease the rate of acute RSV lower respiratory infection symptoms and RSV-associated hospitalization.[45,46] Palivizumab is a humanized monoclonal antibody against RSV, which is also effective in the prevention of lower respiratory infection due to RSV.[47]

There is some evidence that the preventive use of antiRSV antibodies may decrease the risk of asthma later in life. Wenzel and colleagues[48] evaluated 13 children at high risk for respiratory disease 7 to 10 years after prophylaxis with RSV immune globulin and 26 high risk controls. Control subjects were of similar age and gestational age, but had significantly higher incidence of RSV lower respiratory tract infection during infancy. At 7 to 10 years, children treated with RSV immune globulin had higher FEV_1/FVC ratios and were less likely to have asthma exacerbations or positive skin tests to common allergens. The children in this study all had bronchopulmonary dysplasia or another chronic lung disease, so the results may not apply to a broader population. However, the effect of passive immunization to RSV on subsequent development of asthma warrants further study.

D. Anti-Inflammatory Therapy

While cytopathic effects of RSV on airways may contribute to postbronchiolitic wheezing, the inflammatory response to RSV almost certainly plays a role as well. Because they exert broad anti-inflammatory effects, corticosteroids have been used to treat inflammation during RSV infections. Several studies have examined the effects of inhaled and systemic corticosteroids during RSV infection on pulmonary function or the incidence of wheezing in children aged 6 months to 1 year with mixed results.[49–54]

One study examined the effect of corticosteroid use during RSV infection on asthma later in childhood. Van Woensel and colleagues[55] followed 47 infants under 2 years of age who were treated with oral prednisolone or placebo. At age 5 years, no significant difference between treatment and placebo groups was noted. Thus, little evidence indicates that administering corticosteroids during RSV bronchiolitis protects a child from wheezing later in life.

Because RSV bronchiolitis has been associated with elevated levels of leukotrienes,[17] leukotriene receptor antagonists have been evaluated for RSV bronchiolitis. Bisgaard and colleagues[56] gave either montelukast or placebos for 28 days to infants admitted to the hospital for bronchiolitis. The treatment group showed significantly fewer lower respiratory tract symptoms, but the follow-up in this study was limited to 3 months.

IV. Asthma Exacerbations

A. Presence of Respiratory Viruses during Exacerbations

Epidemiology studies have detected a seasonal pattern of asthma admissions that coincides with seasonal increases in RV infections.[57,58] Three prospective studies of asthma exacerbations revealed viral respiratory infections in the majority of cases. Nicholson and colleagues[59] performed a longitudinal study of 138 asthmatic adults 19 to 46 years of age. Nasal swabs were collected for 61 asthma exacerbations; 27 subjects showed evidence of respiratory pathogens, with RV most commonly detected.

Johnston and colleagues[60] used symptom diaries and peak flow monitoring to follow 108 children aged 9 to 11 years who had histories of wheezing or persistent cough. If an episode of upper or lower respiratory symptoms was reported, a nasal aspirate was obtained for viral culture, immunofluorescence, and RV PCR studies. During the 13 months of the study, respiratory viruses were detected in 161 of 200 episodes of lower respiratory tract infection and 125 of 153 episodes of peak flow reduction (>50 liters/min). More than half the viruses detected were rhinoviruses.

Rakes and colleagues[1] performed a cross-sectional analysis of 48 children aged 2 to 16 years who presented to emergency departments with wheezing. Forty children had detectable respiratory virus infections, including 34 with RV identified by PCR. In summary, viral respiratory infections are present in about half of adult asthma exacerbations and 75 to 80% of childhood asthma exacerbations.

B. Host Risk Factors for Virus-Induced Exacerbations

Although a very high prevalence of RV was detected during asthma exacerbations, not all RV infections lead to exacerbations. Sometimes asthmatic patients have only upper respiratory infections or even asymptomatic infections. Corne and colleagues[61] followed 76 adult atopic asthmatic subjects for 3 months during the peak RV cold season. Subjects maintained symptom diaries and nasal aspirates were taken every 2 weeks regardless of symptoms. Twenty-eight RV infections were detected via PCR. Of these, only 16 had upper respiratory symptoms and

12 had lower respiratory symptoms. Thus, many of the infections were asymptomatic and most of the infections did not cause worsening of asthma. These results suggest that some RV strains may be more asthmogenic or that some asthmatic patients are more likely to develop lower respiratory symptoms with the same infection.

To better understand why some RV infections generate lower respiratory symptoms while others do not, experimental inoculations were performed with RV16. Despite infection with standardized inocula of RV, significant individual variability was noted among subjects in viral shedding, symptom scores, and inflammatory infiltrate.[62,63] This further suggests that individual variability in the clinical response to RV infections is due to host-related factors rather than the virus. The experimental inoculations also provided a method to study specific host responses that contribute to RV-induced asthma exacerbations.

Before discussing RV inoculations further, it is necessary to address certain limitations of experimental infections. Because of safety concerns, patients with severe asthma or histories of virus-induced asthma exacerbations are usually excluded. Also, some attenuation of the virus in culture media may occur over time. As a result of these factors, experimental RV16 infections rarely led to asthma exacerbations, causing only minimal lower respiratory obstruction, if any.[62–65] However, using experimental inoculations produced some distinct benefits. The same quantity and strain of virus can be administered to all subjects, and the timing of infection and subsequent studies of viral shedding, symptoms, and inflammation can be determined more precisely than in natural infections.

Virus-specific host immune factors that predispose to more severe infections have been identified. Parry and colleagues[63] experimentally infected 22 asthmatic or allergic subjects with RV16. Prior to inoculation with the virus, PBMCs from the subjects were incubated with RV16 for 6 days and IFN production was measured. Subjects with increased IFN production or increased RV-induced cell proliferation at baseline demonstrated less viral shedding during infection. Similarly, Gern and colleagues[62] found that subjects with higher sputum IFN mRNA-to-IL-5 mRNA ratios prior to RV16 infection had fewer peak cold symptoms and more rapid clearance of virus during infection. These findings in experimental infection suggest that host immune responses, specifically the capacity to produce IFN in response to virus, may affect the outcomes of RV infections and theoretically may contribute to the wide variety of symptomatic responses seen in asthmatic subjects during infection.

C. Effects of RV on Airway Inflammation

Although RV is typically thought of as an upper airway virus, results of experimental infections have demonstrated that RV can also induce inflammation in the lower airways. During an RV infection, neutrophilic inflammation can be found

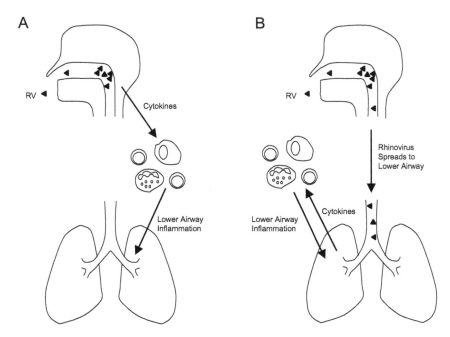

Figure 10.3 Two general mechanisms have been proposed to explain how rhinovirus (RV) infection generates lower airway inflammation. A: RV infection of the nasal mucosa indirectly causes lower airway inflammation. B: The spread of RV to the lower airway directly stimulates lower airway inflammation.

in both sputum and BAL fluid,[66,67] while eosinophils have been found to increase in bronchial biopsy specimens.[68] Eosinophilic cationic protein increases during experimental infection and correlates with histamine responsiveness.[69] In addition, asthma infections caused by natural colds are associated with increases in sputum neutrophils and eosinophil cationic protein (ECP).[1,70]

The mechanism by which RV attracts these cells to the airways is still not fully understood, but at least two possible models have been proposed (Figure 10.3). First, RV infection in the upper airway may stimulate cytokine release, which could increase baseline or allergen-induced inflammation in the lungs. Second, RV may infect the lower airway and directly induce inflammation as a result of the immune response to virus. These two mechanisms are not mutually exclusive and both probably occur to some extent.

Although many immune mechanisms are activated during RV infection, the relation between IL-8 and granulocyte colony stimulating factor (G-CSF) secretion and the subsequent recruitment of neutrophils to the airway has been particularly well described by three observations:

1. Nasal G-CSF levels correlate with peripheral blood neutrophilia on the second day of infection.[62,67]
2. Serum and nasal G-CSF levels correlate with nasal lavage neutrophils on the second day of infection and bronchial lavage neutrophils on the fourth day of infection.[67]
3. Increases in G-CSF and IL-8 during experimental infection correlate with histamine-induced airway responsiveness.[71]

Based on these three observations, it can be concluded that RV infection causes the secretion of IL-8 and G-CSF from the nose. The secretion attracts neutrophils to the blood on day 2 and into the lungs by day 4. The relationship of these cytokines to histamine responsiveness suggests that they may be important in the pathogenesis of lower airway symptoms, although the exact signal that attracts neutrophils to the lung has yet to be described.

RV may also up-regulate existing allergic inflammation. Allergen challenge can be used in conjunction with experimental RV infection to examine this relationship. After an asthmatic subject is administered an allergen challenge, the immediate response is an initial drop in lung function followed by a slow return to baseline. In some subjects, a second drop in lung function (late response) will occur approximately 4 to 6 hours later. Significantly more subjects exhibit late responses to allergen challenge during experimental RV infections that can still be elicited by allergen challenge weeks after infection.[72] The increased incidence of late responses to allergens may be due to increases in pulmonary eosinophils or ECP that occur during both allergen challenges and RV infections.[68,69] Regardless of the mechanism, the presence of an altered late response to allergen weeks after infection suggests that natural exposures to RVs may significantly alter the inflammatory responses induced by low level allergen exposure in the environment.

Although RV is traditionally thought of as strictly an upper airway virus, evidence now indicates that it can extend into the lower airways as well. Bronchial epithelial cells express the primary RV receptor ICAM-1, and expression of this receptor appears to be greater in the bronchial epithelia of asthmatic patients.[73] RV can also replicate effectively at the temperatures found in the lower airways.[74] Furthermore, RV RNA has been detected in bronchial lavage cells from eight of eight subjects experimentally inoculated with RV16 and has been cultured from bronchial brushings from other subjects.[66,75] One criticism of these findings is that introduction of a bronchoscope through the nasopharynx could transfer RV to the lower airway. However, experiments using *in situ* hybridization to minimize chances of contamination detected RV RNA in bronchial epithelial cells from five of ten subjects experimentally infected with RV.[76]

It is likely that RV infection of the lower airway exacerbates asthma by effects other than direct toxicity to the bronchial epithelial cells. Only a small fraction of epithelial cells were infected — with little cytopathic effect observed; cilia function was preserved.[76–78] However, RV can induce pulmonary epithelial cell cultures to increase expression of IL-6, IL-8, IL-11, RANTES, eotaxin, and ICAM-1, which can lead to the migration of inflammatory cells.[79] Together, these mediators may synergize with existing asthmatic inflammation or work to redirect inflammation from the upper airway.

IV. Preventive Strategies

A. Immunization

Because RV is implicated in such a large percentage of asthma exacerbations, an RV vaccine has the potential to affect asthma morbidity significantly. Although a vaccine that prevented RV infection would be ideal, a vaccine could prevent lower airway spread of the virus or decrease virus-induced airway inflammation to produce positive effects for asthmatic patients. Decades ago, RV vaccines were developed but were not successful for treating natural infections.[80,81]

One of the primary goals of antiviral vaccines is to produce neutralizing antibodies to prevent viruses from infecting cells. Because more than 100 serotypes of RVs exist and each requires separate neutralizing antibodies, any future RV vaccine would likely have to express proteins from many different RV strains to be effective against natural infections.[82,83]

B. Interferon Alpha (IFN)

Although RV vaccine development has not yet been successful, other immune-stimulating treatments have shown some promise. IFN is an antiviral cytokine released during RV infections that is known to inhibit RV growth in epithelial cells.[84,85] When recombinant IFN is delivered intranasally prior to an experimental RV infection, reductions in illness severity, nasal secretions, and virus isolation occur.[86] In addition, household contacts of people with natural RV infection are less likely to develop RV infections if given intranasal IFN prophylaxis.[87] However, the widespread use of IFN prophylaxis has been prevented because it has been associated with increased incidence of nasal mucosal bleeding.[86,87] It was tested as a therapy for established RV infections but was not effective.[88] While IFN appears to reduce upper respiratory symptoms during RV colds, its effect on asthmatic exacerbations remains unknown.

C. Antiviral Medications

Antiviral medications serve as nonimmunologic methods of limiting RV infections. Theoretically, these medications could help an asthmatic patient with RV infection by limiting the spread of RV to the lower airway or by reducing the viral load that stimulates the immune system. Pleconaril is a promising antiviral medication that inhibits the capsid function of RV and thereby blocks RV entry into the cells.[89,90] Hayden and colleagues[91] conducted two placebo-controlled trials of pleconaril with a total of 1363 picornavirus-infected subjects who presented within 24 hours of the onset of symptoms. Subjects receiving pleconaril had significantly fewer upper respiratory symptoms, less viral shedding, and less time until symptom resolution. Although pleconaril was effective in reducing upper airway symptoms from RV, this study excluded patients who had received asthma medications within the previous 2 months. Determining whether pleconaril will truly reduce the severity of RV-associated asthma exacerbations requires further study.

D. Anti-Inflammatory Therapy

Many of the adverse symptoms caused by RV infection have been attributed to the inflammatory response of the host against the virus, so another approach to treating RV infections has been the use of anti-inflammatory therapy. The effects of prophylaxis with nasal steroids on nasal symptoms during an experimental cold have been studied. Administering prednisone prior to RV inoculation caused viral shedding to increase without improvement in symptoms.[92] Prophylaxis with intranasal beclomethasone and prednisone led to a decrease in symptoms during the first 2 days but not afterward.[93]

One study has examined the effects of inhaled corticosteroids (ICS) on lower airways during experimental RV infection. Grunberg and colleagues[94] experimentally infected 25 atopic asthmatic adults with RV16 after treatment with inhaled budesonide (800 µg twice a day) or a placebo. The budesonide-treated group exhibited no change in RV-induced airway inflammation or ICAM-1 expression, but showed significant reductions in airway responsiveness, suggesting a possible role for ICS in preventing RV-induced lower airway hyperresponsiveness.[77,94]

Two treatment strategies have been pursued to prevent natural colds from causing asthma exacerbations: long-term treatment with ICS at low doses or short-term treatment with ICS at high doses. Doull and colleagues[95] investigated the effects of long-term treatment with low doses of ICS in 104 children aged 7 to 9 years with a history of wheezing during upper respiratory infections. The children received 200 µg of beclomethasone or placebo for 6 months and were followed for upper and lower respiratory symptoms but not with cultures for virus. The beclomethasone-treated children had fewer days with upper or lower respiratory symptoms compared with placebo, but the difference was not quite statistically significant. Thus, long-term treatment with low doses of ICS does not appear to alter the course of RV-induced asthma exacerbation greatly. Administering higher doses of ICS for this duration was avoided because of concerns about side effects, particularly in children. Using ICS in combination with long-acting beta-agonists or leukotriene modifiers can significantly reduce asthma exacerbations, but studies have not reported data relating specifically to infection-related exacerbations.[96–100]

A short-term approach, administering high doses of ICS at the first sign of a cold, has been effective in preventing lower respiratory symptoms in two studies involving different ages of children. Svedmyr and colleagues[101] studied 31 children aged 3 to 10 years with histories of asthma deterioration during upper respiratory tract infections. The children inhaled budesonide or a placebo at the first sign of an upper respiratory tract infection. Those receiving budesonide required fewer emergency room visits and had significantly higher peak flow rates, but did not exhibit significantly fewer symptoms than children treated with placebos. Connett and colleagues[102] found that preschool children treated with high doses of budesonide (>800 µg/day) at the first sign of upper respiratory tract infections had decreased asthmatic symptoms. Thus, administering ICS at the first sign of this type of infection appeared promising and warrants further investigation.

V. Conclusions

Respiratory viruses are major sources of asthma exacerbations and may contribute to asthma inception as well. The risk factors that make a host susceptible to viruses and the mechanisms by which these viruses worsen asthmatic responses still require study. Immunizations, antiviral therapies, and anti-inflammatory medications demonstrate some promise in protecting susceptible individuals from the effects of virus; however, the beneficial effects of these treatments have generally been mild. Increased knowledge of the mechanisms of interaction of viruses and asthma can potentially provide direction for the development of safe and effective treatment modalities.

References

1. Rakes GP, Arruda E, Ingram JM, Hoover GE, Zambrano JC, Hayden FG, Platts-Mills TA, and Heymann PW, Rhinovirus and respiratory syncytial virus in wheezing children requiring emergency care: IgE and eosinophil analyses. *Am J Respir Crit Care Med* 1999; 159: 785–790.
2. Noble V, Murray M, Webb MS, Alexander J, Swarbrick AS, and Milner AD. Respiratory status and allergy nine to ten years after acute bronchiolitis. *Arch Dis Child* 1997; 76: 315–319.
3. Sigurs N, Bjarnason R, Sigurbergsson F, and Kjellman B. Respiratory syncytial virus bronchiolitis in infancy is an important risk factor for asthma and allergy at age 7. *Am J Respir Crit Care Med* 2000; 161: 1501–1507.

4. Hsia J, Goldstein AL, Simon GL, Sztein M, and Hayden FG. Peripheral blood mononuclear cell interleukin-2 and interferon-gamma production, cytotoxicity, and antigen-stimulated blastogenesis during experimental rhinovirus infection. *J Infect Dis* 1990; 162: 591–597.

5. Kneyber MCJ, Steyerberg EW, de Groot R, and Moll HA. Long-term effects of respiratory syncytial virus (RSV) bronchiolitis in infants and young children: a quantitative review. *Acta Paediatr* 2000; 89: 654–660.

6. McConnochie KM and Roghmann KJ. Wheezing at 8 and 13 years: changing importance of bronchiolitis and passive smoking. *Pediatr Pulmonol* 1989; 6: 138–146.

7. Wennergren G and Kristjansson S. Relationship between respiratory syncytial virus bronchiolitis and future obstructive airway diseases. *Eur Respir J* 2001; 18: 1044–1058.

8. Martinez FD, Wright AL, Taussig LM, Holberg CJ, Halonen M, and Morgan WJ. Asthma and wheezing in the first six years of life. *New Engl J Med* 1995; 332: 133–138.

9. Openshaw PJ. Immunopathological mechanisms in respiratory syncytial virus disease. *Springer Semin Immunopathol* 1995; 17-173: 187–201.

10. Harsten G, Prellner K, Lofgren B, Heldrup J, Kalm O, and Kornfalt R. Serum antibodies against respiratory tract viruses: a prospective three-year follow-up from birth. *J Laryngol Otol* 1989; 103: 904–908.

11. Stein RT, Sherrill D, Morgan WJ, Holberg CJ, Halonen M, Taussig LM, Wright AL, and Martinez FD, Respiratory syncytial virus in early life and risk of wheeze and allergy by age 13 years. *Lancet* 1999; 354: 541–545.

12. Kotaniemi-Syrjanen A, Vainionpaa R, Reijonen TM, Waris M, Korhonen K, and Korppi M. Rhinovirus-induced wheezing in infancy: the first sign of childhood asthma? *J Allergy Clin Immunol* 2003; 111: 66–71.

13. Illi S, von Mutius E, Lau S, Bergmann R, Niggemann B, Sommerfeld C, and Wahn U. Early childhood infectious diseases and the development of asthma up to school age: a birth cohort study. *Br Med J* 2001; 322: 390–395.

14. Renzi PM, Turgeon JP, Marcotte JE, Drblik SP, Berube D, Gagnon MF, and Spier S. Reduced interferon-gamma production in infants with bronchiolitis and asthma. *Am J Respir Crit Care Med* 1999; 159: 1417–1422.

15. Aberle JH, Aberle SW, Dworzak MN, Mandl CW, Rebhandl W, Vollnhofer G, Kundi M, and Popow-Kraupp T. Reduced interferon-gamma expression in peripheral blood mononuclear cells of infants with severe respiratory syncytial virus disease. *Am J Respir Crit Care Med* 1999; 160: 1263–1268.

16. Legg JP, Hussain IR, Warner JA, Johnston SL, and Warner JO. Type 1 and type 2 cytokine imbalance in acute respiratory syncytial virus bronchiolitis. *Am J Respir Crit Care Med* 2003; 168: 633–639.

17. van Schaik SM, Tristram DA, Nagpal IS, Hintz KM, and Welliver RC. Increased production of IFN-gamma and cysteinyl leukotrienes in virus-induced wheezing. *J Allergy Clin Immunol* 1999; 103: 630–636.

18. Kumar A, Sorkness RL, Kaplan MR, and Lemanske RF, Jr. Chronic, episodic, reversible airway obstruction after viral bronchiolitis in rats. *Am J Respir Crit Care Med* 1997; 155: 130–134.

19. Uhl EW, Castleman WL, Sorkness RL, Busse WW, Lemanske RF, Jr., and McAllister PK. Parainfluenza virus-induced persistence of airway inflammation, fibrosis, and dysfunction associated with TGF-beta 1 expression in brown Norway rats. *Am J Respir Crit Care Med* 1996; 154: 1834–1842.

20. Sorkness RL, Castleman WL, Kumar A, Kaplan MR, and Lemanske RF, Jr. Prevention of chronic postbronchiolitis airway sequelae with IFN-gamma treatment in rats. *Am J Respir Crit Care Med* 1999; 160: 705–710.

21. Alwan WH, Record FM, and Openshaw PJ. Phenotypic and functional characterization of T cell lines specific for individual respiratory syncytial virus proteins. *J Immunol* 1993; 150: 5211–5218.

22. Alwan WH, Kozlowska WJ, and Openshaw PJ. Distinct types of lung disease caused by functional subsets of antiviral T cells. *J Exp Med* 1994; 179: 81–89.

23. Pala P, Bjarnason R, Sigurbergsson F, Metcalfe C, Sigurs N, and Openshaw PJ. Enhanced IL-4 responses in children with a history of respiratory syncytial virus bronchiolitis in infancy. *Eur Respir J* 2002; 20: 376–382.

24. Schwarze J and Gelfand EW. Respiratory viral infections as promoters of allergic sensitization and asthma in animal models. *Eur Respir J* 2002; 19: 341–349.

25. Roman M, Calhoun WJ, Hinton KL, Avendano LF, Simon V, Escobar AM, Gaggero A, and Diaz PV. Respiratory syncytial virus infection in infants is associated with predominant Th-2-like response. *Am J Respir Crit Care Med* 1997; 156: 190–195.

26. Everard ML, Swarbrick A, Wrightham M, McIntyre J, Dunkley C, James PD, Sewell HF, and Milner AD. Analysis of cells obtained by bronchial lavage of infants with respiratory syncytial virus infection. *Arch Dis Child* 1994; 71: 428–432.

27. Krawiec ME, Westcott JY, Chu HW, Balzar S, Trudeau JB, Schwartz LB, and Wenzel SE. Persistent wheezing in very young children is associated with lower respiratory inflammation. *Am J Respir Crit Care Med* 2001; 163: 1338–1343.

28. Chin J, Magoffin RL, Shearer LA, Schieble JH, and Lennette EH. Field evaluation of a respiratory syncytial virus vaccine and a trivalent parainfluenza virus vaccine in a pediatric population. *Am J Epidemiol* 196; 894: 449–463.

29. Fulginiti VA, Eller JJ, Sieber OF, Joyner JW, Minamitani M, and Meiklejohn G. Respiratory virus immunization. I. A field trial of two inactivated respiratory virus vaccines; an aqueous trivalent parainfluenza virus vaccine and an alum-precipitated respiratory syncytial virus vaccine. *Am J Epidemiol* 1969; 89: 435–448.

30. Kim HW, Canchola JG, Brandt CD, Pyles G, Chanock RM, Jensen K, and Parrott RH. Respiratory syncytial virus disease in infants despite prior administration of antigenic inactivated vaccine. *Am J Epidemiol* 1969; 89: 422–434.

31. Kapikian AZ, Mitchell RH, Chanock RM, Shvedoff RA, and Stewart CE. An epidemiologic study of altered clinical reactivity to respiratory syncytial RS virus infection in children previously vaccinated with an inactivated RS virus vaccine. *Am J Epidemiol* 1969; 89: 405–421.

32. Domachowske JB and Rosenberg HF. Respiratory syncytial virus infection: immune response, immunopathogenesis, and treatment. *Clin Microbiol Rev* 1999; 12: 298–309.

33. Wright PF, Karron RA, Belshe RB, Thompson J, Crowe JE, Jr., Boyce TG, Halburnt LL, Reed GW, Whitehead SS, Anderson EL, Wittek AE, Casey R, Eichelberger M, Thumar B, Randolph VB, Udem SA, Chanok RM, and Murphy BR. Evaluation of

a live, cold-passaged, temperature-sensitive, respiratory syncytial virus vaccine candidate in infancy. *J Infect Dis* 2000; 182: 1331–1342.

34. Karron RA, Wright PF, Crowe JE, Jr., Clements-Mann ML, Thompson J, Makhene M, Casey R, and Murphy BR. Evaluation of two live, cold-passaged, temperature-sensitive respiratory syncytial virus vaccines in chimpanzees and in human adults, infants, and children. *J Infect Dis* 1997; 176: 1428–1436.

35. Walsh EE, Brandriss MW, and Schlesinger JJ. Purification and characterization of the respiratory syncytial virus fusion protein. *J Gen Virol* 1985; 66: 409–415.

36. Piedra PA. Clinical experience with respiratory syncytial virus vaccines. *Pediatr Infect Dis J* 2003; 22: S94–S99.

37. Glezen WP and Alpers M. Maternal immunization. *Clin Infect Dis* 1999; 28: 219–224.

38. Suara RO, Piedra PA, Glezen WP, Adegbola RA, Weber M, Mulholland EK, and Smith J. Prevalence of neutralizing antibody to respiratory syncytial virus in sera from mothers and newborns residing in the Gambia and in the United States. *Clin Diagn Lab Immunol* 1996; 3: 477–479.

39. Glezen WP, Paredes A, Allison JE, Taber LH, and Frank AL. Risk of respiratory syncytial virus infection for infants from low-income families in relationship to age, sex, ethnic group, and maternal antibody level. *J Pediatr* 1981; 98: 708–715.

40. Jafri HS. Treatment of respiratory syncytial virus: antiviral therapies. *Pediatr Infect Dis J* 2003; 22: S89–S92.

41. Groothuis JR, Woodin KA, Katz R, Robertson AD, McBride JT, Hall CB, McWilliams BC, and Lauer BA. Early ribavirin treatment of respiratory syncytial viral infection in high-risk children. *J Pediatr* 1990; 117: 792–798.

42. Law BJ, Wang EE, MacDonald N, McDonald J, Dobson S, Boucher F, Langley J, Robinson, J, Mitchell I, and Stephens D. Does ribavirin impact on the hospital course of children with respiratory syncytial virus RSV infection? An analysis using the pediatric investigators collaborative network on infections in Canada PICNIC RSV database. *Pediatrics* 1997; 99: E7.

43. Rodriguez WJ, Arrobio J, Fink R, Kim HW, and Milburn C. Prospective follow-up and pulmonary functions from a placebo-controlled randomized trial of ribavirin therapy in respiratory syncytial virus bronchiolitis. *Arch Pediatr Adolesc Med* 1999; 153: 469–474.

44. Long CE, Voter KZ, Barker WH, and Hall CB. Long-term follow-up of children hospitalized with respiratory syncytial virus lower respiratory tract infection and randomly treated with ribavirin or placebo. *Pediatr Infect Dis J* 1997; 161: 1023–1028.

45. Groothuis JR, Simoes EA, Levin MJ, Hall CB, Long CE, Rodriguez WJ, Arrobio J, Meissner HE, Fulton DR, and Welliver RC. Prophylactic administration of respiratory syncytial virus immune globulin to high-risk infants and young children. *New Engl J Med* 1993; 329: 1524–1530.

46. PREVENT Study Group. Reduction of respiratory syncytial virus hospitalization among premature infants and infants with bronchopulmonary dysplasia using respiratory syncytial virus immune globulin prophylaxis. *Pediatrics* 1997; 99: 93–99.

47. Romero JR. Palivizumab prophylaxis of respiratory syncytial virus disease from 1998 to 2002: results from four years of palivizumab usage. *Pediatr Infect Dis J* 2003; 22: S46–S54.

48. Wenzel SE, Gibbs RL, Lehr MV, and Simoes EA. Respiratory outcomes in high-risk children 7 to 10 years after prophylaxis with respiratory syncytial virus immune globulin. *Am J Med* 2002; 112: 627–633.
49. Carlsen KH, Leegaard J, Larsen S, and Orstavik I. Nebulised beclomethasone dipropionate in recurrent obstructive episodes after acute bronchiolitis. *Arch Dis Child* 1988; 63: 1428–1433.
50. Reijonen T, Korppi M, Kuikka L, and Remes K. Anti-inflammatory therapy reduces wheezing after bronchiolitis. *Arch Pediatr Adolesc Med* 1996; 150: 512–517.
51. Richter H and Seddon P. Early nebulized budesonide in the treatment of bronchiolitis and the prevention of postbronchiolitic wheezing. *J Pediatr* 1998; 132: 849–853.
52. Fox GF, Everard ML, Marsh MJ, and Milner AD. Randomised controlled trial of budesonide for the prevention of post-bronchiolitis wheezing. *Arch Dis Child* 1999; 80: 343–347.
53. Kajosaari M, Syvanen P, Forars M, and Juntunen-Backman K. Inhaled corticosteroids during and after respiratory syncytial virus bronchiolitis may decrease subsequent asthma. *Pediatr Allergy Immunol* 2000; 11: 198–202.
54. Cade A, Brownlee KG, Conway SP, Haigh D, Short A, Brown J, Dassa D, Mason SA, Phillips A, Eglin R, Graham M, Chetcuti A, Chatrath M, Hudson N, Thomas A, and Chetcuti, PA. Randomised placebo controlled trial of nebulised corticosteroids in acute respiratory syncytial viral bronchiolitis. *Arch Dis Child* 2000; 82: 126–130.
55. van Woensel JB, Kimpen JL, Sprikkelman AB, Ouwehand A, and van Aalderen WM. Long-term effects of prednisolone in the acute phase of bronchiolitis caused by respiratory syncytial virus. *Pediatr Pulmonol* 2000; 30: 92–96.
56. Bisgaard H. A randomized trial of montelukast in respiratory syncytial virus post-bronchiolitis. *Am J Respir Crit Care Med* 2003; 167: 379–383.
57. Dales RE, Schweitzer I, Toogood JH, Drouin M, Yang W, Dolovich J, and Boulet J. Respiratory infections and the autumn increase in asthma morbidity. *Eur Respir J* 1996; 9: 72–77.
58. Johnston SL, Pattemore PK, Sanderson G, Smith S, Campbell MJ, Josephs LK et al. The relationship between upper respiratory infections and hospital admissions for asthma: a time-trend analysis. *Am J Respir Crit Care Med* 1996; 154: 654–660.
59. Nicholson KG, Kent J, and Ireland DC. Respiratory viruses and exacerbations of asthma in adults. *Br Med J* 1993; 30: 982–986.
60. Johnston SL, Pattemore PK, Sanderson G, Smith S, Lampe F, Josephs L, Symington P, O'Toole S, Myint SH, and Tyrrell DA. Community study of role of viral infections in exacerbations of asthma in 9- to 11-year-old children. *Br Med J* 1995; 310: 1225–1229.
61. Corne JM, Marshall C, Smith S, Schreiber J, Sanderson G, Holgate ST, and Johnston SL. Frequency, severity, and duration of rhinovirus infections in asthmatic and non-asthmatic individuals: a longitudinal cohort study. *Lancet* 2002; 359: 831–834.
62. Gern JE, Vrtis R, Grindle KA, Swenson C, and Busse WW. Relationship of upper and lower airway cytokines to outcome of experimental rhinovirus infection. *Am J Respir Crit Care Med* 2000; 162: 2226–2231.
63. Parry DE, Busse WW, Sukow KA, Dick CR, Swenson C, and Gern JE. Rhinovirus-induced PBMC responses and outcome of experimental infection in allergic subjects. *J Allergy Clin Immunol* 2000; 105: 692–698.

64. Grunberg K, Timmers MC, de Klerk EP, Dick EC, and Sterk PJ. Experimental rhinovirus 16 infection causes variable airway obstruction in subjects with atopic asthma. *Am J Respir Crit Care Med* 1999; 160: 1375–1380.

65. Bardin PG, Fraenkel DJ, Sanderson G, van Schalkwyk EM, Holgate ST, and Johnston SL. Peak expiratory flow changes during experimental rhinovirus infection. *Eur Respir J* 2000; 16: 980–985.

66. Gern JE, Galagan DM, Jarjour NN, Dick EC, and Busse WW. Detection of rhinovirus RNA in lower airway cells during experimentally induced infection. *Am J Respir Crit Care Med* 1997; 155: 1159–1161.

67. Jarjour NN, Gern JE, Kelly EA, Swenson CA, Dick CR, and Busse WW. The effect of an experimental rhinovirus 16 infection on bronchial lavage neutrophils. *J Allergy Clin Immunol* 2000; 105: 1169–1177.

68. Fraenkel DJ, Bardin PG, Sanderson G, Lampe F, Johnston SL, and Holgate ST. Lower airways inflammation during rhinovirus colds in normal and in asthmatic subjects. *Am J Respir Crit Care Med* 1995; 151: 879–886.

69. Grunberg K, Smits HH, Timmers MC, de Klerk EP, Dolhain RJ, Dick EC et al. Experimental rhinovirus 16 infection: effects on cell differentials and soluble markers in sputum in asthmatic subjects. *Am J Respir Crit Care Med* 1997; 156: 609–616.

70. Pizzichini MM, Pizzichini E, Efthimiadis A, Chauhan AJ, Johnston SL, Hussack P et al. Asthma and natural colds. Inflammatory indices in induced sputum: a feasibility study. *Am J Respir Crit Care Med* 1998; 158: 1178–1184.

71. Grunberg K, Timmers MC, Smits HH, de Klerk EP, Dick EC, Spaan WJ et al. Effect of experimental rhinovirus 16 colds on airway hyperresponsiveness to histamine and interleukin-8 in nasal lavage in asthmatic subjects *in vivo*. *Clin Exp Allergy* 1997; 27: 36–45.

72. Lemanske RF, Jr., Dick EC, Swenson CA, Vrtis RF, and Busse WW. Rhinovirus upper respiratory infection increases airway hyperreactivity and late asthmatic reactions. *J Clin Invest* 1989; 83: 1–10.

73. Bentley AM, Durham SR, Robinson DS, Menz G, Storz C, Cromwell O et al. Expression of endothelial and leukocyte adhesion molecules intercellular adhesion molecule-1, E-selectin, and vascular cell adhesion molecule-1 in the bronchial mucosa in steady-state and allergen-induced asthma. *J Allergy Clin Immunol* 1993; 92: 857–868.

74. Papadopoulos NG, Sanderson G, Hunter J, and Johnston SL. Rhinoviruses replicate effectively at lower airway temperatures. *J Med Virol* 1999; 58: 100–104.

75. Halperin SA, Eggleston PA, Hendley JO, Suratt PM, Groschel DH, and Gwaltney JM, Jr. Pathogenesis of lower respiratory tract symptoms in experimental rhinovirus infection. *Am Rev Respir Dis* 1983; 128: 806–810.

76. Papadopoulos NG, Bates PJ, Bardin PG, Papi A, Leir SH, Fraenkel DJ et al. Rhinoviruses infect the lower airways. *J Infect Dis* 2000; 181: 1875–1884.

77. Grunberg K, Sharon RF, Hiltermann TJ, Brahim JJ, Dick EC, Sterk PJ et al. Experimental rhinovirus 16 infection increases intercellular adhesion molecule-1 expression in bronchial epithelium of asthmatics regardless of inhaled steroid treatment. *Clin Exp Allergy* 2000; 30: 1015–1023.

78. Gerrard CS, Levandowski RA, Gerrity TR, Yeates DB, and Klein E. The effects of acute respiratory virus infection upon tracheal mucous transport. *Arch Environ Health* 1985; 40: 322–325.

79. Gern JE and Busse WW. The role of viral infections in the natural history of asthma. *J Allergy Clin Immunol* 2000; 106: 201–212.
80. Douglas RG, Jr. and Couch RB. Parenteral inactivated rhinovirus vaccine: minimal protective effect. *Proc Soc Exp Biol Med* 1972; 139: 899–902.
81. Perkins JC, Tucker DN, Knope HL, Wenzel RP, Hornick RB, Kapikian AZ, and Chanock RM, Evidence for protective effect of an inactivated rhinovirus vaccine administered by the nasal route. *Am J Epidemiol* 1969; 90: 319–326.
82. Monto AS, Bryan ER, and Ohmit S. Rhinovirus infections in Tecumseh, Michigan: frequency of illness and number of serotypes. *J Infect Dis* 1987; 156: 43–49.
83. Savolainen C, Blomqvist S, Mulders MN, and Hovi T. Genetic clustering of all 102 human rhinovirus prototype strains: serotype 87 is close to human enterovirus 70. *J Gen Virol* 2002; 83: 333–340.
84. Levandowski RA and Horohov DW. Rhinovirus induces natural killer-like cytotoxic cells and interferon alpha in mononuclear leukocytes. *J Med Virol* 1991; 35: 116–120.
85. Sperber SJ, Hunger SB, Schwartz B, and Pestka S. Anti-rhinoviral activity of recombinant and hybrid species of interferon alpha. *Antiviral Res* 1993; 22: 121–129.
86. Samo TC, Greenberg SB, Couch RB, Quarles J, Johnson PE, Hook S, and Harmon MW. Efficacy and tolerance of intranasally applied recombinant leukocyte A interferon in normal volunteers. *J Infect Dis* 1983; 148: 535–542.
87. Hayden FG, Albrecht JK, Kaiser DL, and Gwaltney JM, Jr. Prevention of natural colds by contact prophylaxis with intranasal alpha 2-interferon. *New Engl J Med* 1986; 314: 71–75.
88. Hayden FG, Kaiser DL, and Albrecht JK. Intranasal recombinant alfa-2b interferon treatment of naturally occurring common colds. *Antimicrob Agents Chemother* 1988; 32: 224–230.
89. McKinlay MA, Pevear DC, and Rossmann MG. Treatment of the picornavirus common cold by inhibitors of viral uncoating and attachment. *Annu Rev Microbiol* 1992; 46: 635–654.
90. Pevear DC, Tull TM, Seipel ME, and Groarke JM. Activity of pleconaril against enteroviruses. *Antimicrob Agents Chemother* 1999; 43: 2109–2115.
91. Hayden FG, Herrington DT, Coats TL, Kim K, Cooper EC, Villano SA, Liu S, Hudson S, Pevear DC, Collett M, and McKinlay M, Efficacy and safety of oral pleconaril for treatment of colds due to picornaviruses in adults: results of 2 double-blind, randomized, placebo-controlled trials. *Clin Infect Dis* 2003; 36: 1523–1532.
92. Gustafson LM, Proud D, Hendley JO, Hayden FG, and Gwaltney JM, Jr. Oral prednisone therapy in experimental rhinovirus infections. *J Allergy Clin Immunol* 1996; 97: 1009–1014.
93. Farr BM, Gwaltney JM, Jr., Hendley JO, Hayden FG, Naclerio RM, McBride T, Doyle WJ, Sorrentino JV, Riker DK, and Proud D. A randomized controlled trial of glucocorticoid prophylaxis against experimental rhinovirus infection. *J Infect Dis* 1990; 162: 1173–1177.
94. Grunberg K, Sharon RF, Sont JK, In V, van Schadewijk WA, de Klerk EP, Dick CR, Van Krieker JH, and Sterk PJ. Rhinovirus-induced airway inflammation in asthma: effect of treatment with inhaled corticosteroids before and during experimental infection. *Am J Respir Crit Care Med* 2001; 164: 1816–1822.

95. Doull IJ, Lampe FC, Smith S, Schreiber J, Freezer NJ, and Holgate ST. Effect of inhaled corticosteroids on episodes of wheezing associated with viral infection in school age children: randomised double blind placebo controlled trial. *Br Med J* 1997; 315: 858–862.

96. Lalloo UG, Malolepszy J, Kozma D, Krofta K, Ankerst J, Johansen B, and Thomson NC. Budesonide and formoterol in a single inhaler improves asthma control compared with increasing the dose of corticosteroid in adults with mild-to-moderate asthma. *Chest* 2003; 123: 1480–1487.

97. Pauwels RA, Lofdahl CG, Postma DS, Tattersfield AE, O'Byrne P, Barnes PJ, and Ulman A. Effect of inhaled formoterol and budesonide on exacerbations of asthma. *New Engl J Med* 1997; 337: 1405–1411.

98. Tattersfield AE, Postma DS, Barnes PJ, Svensson K, Bauer CA, O'Byrne PM, Lofdahl CG, Pawvels RA, and Ullman A. Exacerbations of asthma: a descriptive study of 425 severe exacerbations. *Am J Respir Crit Care Med* 1999; 160: 594–599.

99. O'Byrne PM, Barnes PJ, Rodriguez-Roisin R, Runnerstrom E, Sandstrom T, Svensson K, and Tattersfiled AE. Low dose inhaled budesonide and formoterol in mild persistent asthma: the OPTIMA randomized trial. *Am J Respir Crit Care Med* 2001; 164: 1392–1397.

100. Matz J, Emmett A, Rickard K, and Kalberg C. Addition of salmeterol to low-dose fluticasone versus higher-dose fluticasone: an analysis of asthma exacerbations. *J Allergy Clin Immunol* 2001; 107: 783–789.

101. Svedmyr J, Nyberg E, Asbrink-Nilsson E, and Hedlin G. Intermittent treatment with inhaled steroids for deterioration of asthma due to upper respiratory tract infections. *Acta Paediatr* 1995; 84: 884–888.

102. Connett G and Lenney W. Prevention of viral-induced asthma attacks using inhaled budesonide. *Arch Dis Child* 1993; 68: 85–87.

11

Allergens

ELIZABETH A. ERWIN, JUDITH A. WOODFOLK, PETER W. HEYMANN, and THOMAS A.E. PLATTS-MILLS

University of Virginia
Charlottesville, Virginia, U.S.A.

I. Introduction

It has long been believed that inhalant allergens play a role in the etiology of asthma. Initially this view was supported by the results of bronchial challenge tests.[1] However, it is clear that inhalation tests do not reflect natural exposure. On the other hand, the evidence for causality is supported by a combination of association of sensitization with disease, exposure studies, avoidance studies, and the biological plausibility that allergens induce inflammation in the lungs of allergic subjects.[2–5]

As the disease has become more common and studies grow in number and sophistication, the evidence for a relationship between allergic sensitivity and asthma has persisted. However, several caveats have become apparent. First, sensitivities to certain allergens such as those from dust mites, animal dander, fungi, and cockroaches are more strongly related to asthma than sensitivities to pollens. Second, the overlap of etiologies for early wheezing involving viral infections and allergens is confusing. Furthermore, it has been difficult to prove a direct link between allergen *exposure* and asthma in part because many homes in specific areas contain similar allergen levels.

The relationship of allergens and asthma is studied to reveal causation and alleviate the disease. The prevalence and severity of asthma increased steadily over 40 years to reach epidemic proportions in the late 1990s. Primary prevention of disease has proven impossible in these days of a mobile society in which both parents may work outside the home and children spend time in several different environments, e.g., home and daycare, from a very early age. Despite increased exposures to allergens, an appropriate avoidance regimen can result in symptomatic improvement among patients with established disease. Also, it is vital for patients to perceive that they have some control over their disease and that factors specific to their problem are being addressed.

It has been shown that the connection between exposure and sensitization is not a simple dose–response relationship for all allergens. Exposure to dust mite allergens is directly related to allergic sensitivity and appears to be more important during early years of childhood when an individual's atopic predisposition is still unknown. In contrast, high exposure to cat allergens at levels found in homes of children who live with cats has paradoxically been associated with decreased sensitization to cats. In areas like northern Sweden where cats and dogs are the sources of predominant allergens, this paradoxical relationship to pet ownership may have a major impact on the prevalence and severity of asthma.

This chapter will focus on the allergens that represent significant risk factors for asthma, i.e., those from dust mites, animals, fungi, and cockroaches. The clinical relevance, dose response, characteristics, and outcomes of avoidance studies are discussed for each allergen.

II. Dust Mites

The importance of house dust as a source of allergens was first recognized early in the 20th century when several authors speculated that house dust had to contain more than animal dander and molds. In 1967, Spieksma and Voorhorst established that dust mites were the single most important sources of indoor allergens in Holland.[6] They also developed techniques for growing mites to produce skin test extracts, so that their results were rapidly confirmed in humid climates around the world. The significance of dust mites has been confirmed via prospective studies, cross-sectional population-based studies, emergency room data, and avoidance studies.[1,3,4,5] The conclusions are that dust mite exposure increases the risk of IgE ab production, and that in a community with high levels of dust mites, this can lead to sensitization of a large proportion of the population, i.e., up to 35%.[7]

Recent data indicate that the titer of IgE ab to dust mites increases progressively with higher exposure. Although plenty of prospective studies show the onset of sensitization over the first 5 years of life, it is not clear whether an early window for exposure exists. Certainly many children do not develop positive skin tests or IgE ab in the first 2 years of life. However, it is difficult to exclude or prove early priming of T cells. Our prospective data suggested that exposure in the first 2 years of life was more important than exposure to mite allergens at age 10.[3] That study did not provide information about exposure between the ages of 3 and 5 years. Indeed, few studies provide sequential exposure measurements and the measurements (i.e., floor or bedding dust allergen concentrations) are not sufficiently accurate to produce the kinds of conclusions about timing of exposure that many authors imply.[8]

Avoidance experiments have provided consistent evidence about the effects of moving mite-allergic patients out of their houses.[9] Indeed the results show progressive improvement in symptoms with highly significant decreases in bronchial hyperreactivity (BHR).[10,11] The degree of clinical improvement in these studies is greater than those reported for most asthma medications. Although the results of controlled trials of dust mite allergen avoidance in patients' houses have been less consistent, a series of studies reported *both* prolonged decreases in mite allergens and decreased BHR.[12–14] Two recent controlled trials of mattress covers reported negative results, [15,16] But both these studies had major problems in that they only tested one element of the protocol shown to be effective.[17]

Our conclusion is that a full regime of dust mite control in the bedroom is an important part of the treatment of asthma in mite-allergic patients. By contrast, most studies on primary avoidance have been unsuccessful. This initially appeared confusing because we were certain that sensitization required exposure and also that the concentration found in a patient's home correlated with sensitization.[18] Thus it seemed irrational that decreasing exposure in a patient's home did not decrease sensitization. However, primary avoidance studies are based on the assumption that exposure only takes place at home.

In northern Sweden, very few children (~3%) become sensitized to mites, but there are no mites in any houses so that 2 weeks spent at Granny's house would not expose a child to mite allergens. By contrast, in Manchester, United Kingdom, Atlanta, Georgia, Sydney, Australia, and Vancouver, British Columbia, most houses contain high concentrations of mite allergens. As a result, children get transient exposure in other houses or in day care facilities in spite of careful avoidance measures carried out in their own homes.

Taking all the data about dust mites and applying the criteria for causality proposed by Bradford Hill, it is possible to make a strong case for causality.[19] We consider that sufficient criteria have been met to imply that dust mite exposure is a cause of asthma although several problems have arisen. First, it is clear that many children have bronchiolitis that includes wheezing in the first 2 years of life, before sensitization to mites or other inhaled allergens develops. Second, several authors have stressed that a simple dose response relationship is more difficult to show for asthma than for sensitization.[20] We believe that early wheezing is unrelated to allergy; is extremely common, up to 40% in some studies; and

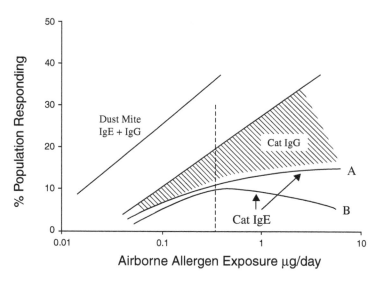

Figure 11.1 Exposure to high levels of dust mite allergen is associated with a high prevalence of allergy to mite. High exposure to cat allergen is associated with a plateau (A) or a decrease (B) in allergy to cat.

is equally common among children who will become allergic and those who will not.[3,21] Thus, up to 40% of children who develop chronic allergic asthma would have histories of early wheezing by chance.

The dose response issue is complicated. It may simply reflect the inadequacy of our exposure measurements. However it is important to recognize that the relationship between dust mite (or other allergen) exposure and asthma requires at least one intervening step: production of IgE and/or inflammation (Figure 11.1). If the association between sensitization and asthma is very strong (e.g., odds ratio >6) and the quantity of allergen necessary to cause disease is *less* than the quantity necessary to cause sensitization, the relationship between allergen exposure and asthma will be obscured.

The reasons mite allergens are such important risk factors for asthma are not immediately obvious. Although exposure which is primarily in bedding, may be concentrated close to the head where it could be inhaled, it is unlikely that exposure is greater than that to other important allergens. Some features of mite allergens may be relevant (Table 11.1). First, mite allergens accumulate in dust *and* become airborne as fecal pellets.[22] These particles are ~20 µm in diameter and contain very high concentrations of allergens — by some estimates as high as 10 mg/ml. Furthermore, despite the chitinous peritrophic membrane of fecal pellets, the allergens elute rapidly in salt water. Thus, the impaction of a fecal particle in the nose or lungs gives rise to high local concentrations of allergens.

The second important issue is the nature of the proteins that are allergens. Der p 1 demonstrates both sequence homology with proteinases and *in vitro* enzymatic activity. Excellent studies have shown that this protein can cleave CD23 and CD25 and also open epithelial junctions.[23-25] These studies led to the argument that the enzymatic activity of Der p 1 is an important consideration in its "allergenicity." However, it is important to remember that Der p 2, which has neither homology with any known enzymes nor enzymatic activity *in vitro,* is also a major allergen.

III. Animal Dander Allergens

The importance of cats, dogs, rodents, and other small mammals as causes of allergic diseases has been obvious since the first studies using skin testing. The recent NHANES, ISAAC, and ECRHS investigations indicate that skin tests of 4 to 10% of the population are positive for cat dander.[7,26] Furthermore, the fact that exposure to cats can cause sneezing, conjunctivitis, and wheezing is obvious to most patients who are specifically allergic.

The immediacy of symptoms following exposure is a common feature of animal allergy. It is also important to recognize that similar immediate responses are unusual with dust mite, cockroach, or fungal sensitivity. Thus, it is unusual to find mite- or cockroach-allergic individuals who report the onset of wheezing within a few hours of entering a house with high concentrations of mite allergen in the floor dust.

Animal allergens such as Fel d 1, Can f 1, Equ c 1, and Mus m 1, are a diverse group of proteins. Many are derived from the skin but the rodent allergens are primarily present in urine (Table 11.1). These animal proteins have no obvious common characteristics, but one striking feature is common to particles that become airborne. For all the dander allergens and also for rodent urinary allergens, the aerodynamic sizes of particles that become airborne are smaller than the average sizes of mite feces, pollen grains, and cockroach debris.[27] In keeping with this allergens from animals remain airborne with only moderate disturbance. Thus, the most likely explanation for the rapid onset of symptoms with cat or rat exposure is that these allergens are airborne continuously.[28]

In addition, the particle size suggests that a larger proportion of these particles would reach the lungs. However, particle size is a complex issue. With increasing size, a smaller *proportion* of the inhaled particles will enter the lungs, but even with particles as large as 20 µm diameter, ~5% will enter the lungs. On the other hand, the volume of particles increases as the cube of the diameter. Thus 5% of 100 fecal particles or pollen grains may represent the same quantity of allergen entering the lungs as 50% of 10,000 particles of 2 µm diameter (i.e. rat allergen or the spores of Aspergillus or Penicillium).

Table 11.1 Major Allergens from Dust Mite, Mammals, Cockroach, and Alternaria
(See www.allergen.org)

Source	Allergen	MW (kD)	Function (Homology)	Mode of Exposure
Dust mite				
Dermatophagoides spp.	Der p 1	25	Cysteine protease	Fecal particles
Mammals	Der p 2		(Epididymal protein)	
Felis domesticus	Fel d 1	36	(Uteroglobin)[a]	Sebaceous secretions
Canis familiaris	Can f 1	25	Lipocalin	Saliva, dander
Equus caballus	Equ c 1	25	Lipocalin	
Mus musculus	Mus m 1	19	Lipocalin-MUPs[b]	Urine
Rattus norvegicus	Rat n 1	17	RUPs[b]	Urine
Cockroach				
Blattella germanica	Bla g 1		(Mosquito protein precursor)	Saliva
	Bla g 2	36	Inactive aspartic protease	Fecal particles
	Bla g 4	21	Lipocalin-calycin	
	Bla g 5	22	Glutathione transferase	
Periplaneta americana	Per a 1		(Mosquito protein precursor)	
	Per a 3	72	Insect storage protein	
	Per a 7	37	Tropomyosin	
Alternaria				
Alternaria alternata	Alt a 1	31	Unknown	Mycelia

[a] uteroglobin is also called Clara Cell Secretory Protein (or CCSP)
[b] mouse and rat urinary proteins respectively

In population-based studies, sensitization to cat allergens is consistently an important risk factor for wheezing and/or bronchial hyperresponsiveness (BHR). In some countries, e.g. Sweden and Finland, and certain geographic areas, e.g. the mountain states and southwestern region of the United States, sensitization to animal dander is the strongest risk factor for asthma. However, in countries where dust mites are present in larger numbers (≥ 200/g dust), animal dander is generally less significant than dust mite.[29] Furthermore, in areas where cats are not kept as pets e.g., the inner cities of Atlanta or Chicago, cat sensitization is less common.[30] The implication is that although cat sensitization is a significant cause of asthma, it is less "important" than mite or cockroach allergens. The question is whether cat dander is as good as an allergen as these others *or* whether the dose response is the same.

A. Paradoxical Effects of Animal Ownership

Although cats release large quantities of dander into the environment and one of the proteins in dander, Fel d 1, appears to be a potent allergen, data about the effects of cat ownership are not simple. On a population basis, the countries studied as part of ECRHS, which had the highest prevalences of cat ownership (~50% in Australia and New Zealand) did not have the highest prevalence of cat sensitization (see Roost et al.[26]). Indeed, consistently in New Zealand, the prevalence of sensitization to cat allergens was one half to one third of that for dust mites.[7,26,29] Furthermore, in several Scandinavian studies, children raised in houses with cats showed *decreased* prevalence of IgE antibodies (ab) to cats compared to those who had never lived in houses with cats.[31,32]

Initially it appeared possible that this effect was attributable to choice, i.e., that allergic families chose not to keep cats. The assumption was that families who kept cats would then be less allergic in general. However, the effect of cat ownership has now been seen in the United States, United Kingdom, and New Zealand in communities where cat ownership is common and choice is not a major factor.[33,34] Choice may be relevant in Scandinavia and the Netherlands, but still only explains a small part of the observations.

In some studies, the effect of cat ownership appears to be nonspecific, i.e., animal ownership decreases the prevalence of IgE ab to all allergens.[35] Obviously, a general lack of response to allergens might reflect choice, but could also reflect a nonspecific suppressive effect related to the animal(s). A nonspecific effect may result either because of endotoxins produced by the animals *or* because the immune response to the animal proteins creates a cytokine milieu that is suppressive to the IgE ab responses. The results from the cohort in Sweden suggest that the presence of a cat in a home can inhibit responses to dog and birch allergens. On the other hand, the data on endotoxins do not provide clear evidence because the differences in houses with animals are not sufficient to explain the effect.[33]

In environments with high concentrations of dust mite allergens in houses, sensitization to mites is very common regardless of the number of cats.[3,5,29] In New Zealand, we have recently shown that children who *ever* lived with cats had decreased prevalence of sensitization to cats with slightly higher prevalence of IgE ab to dust mites.[33] Indeed, among children living with cats, only 26% of the allergic children had IgE ab to cat. The results established that sensitization to dust mites is *not* influenced by the presence of a cat. Thus there is no doubt that the two allergens have different effects and different dose response relationships. However, the results can be seen in two ways. Cat allergens can induce tolerance or control, which reflects a special property of cat allergen, or the response to dust mites is very resistant to suppression or control *and* this reflects a special property of the mite allergen (Table 11.2).

Table 11.2 Characteristics of the Major Allergens of Dust Mite (Der p 1) and cat (Fel d 1)

	Der p 1	Fel d 1
Source	Fecal particles	Sebacious secretions, saliva
Size (median)	~20 μm	~5 μm
Quantity airborne	Undetectable without disturbance	0.2–20 ng/m³
Structure	Non glycosylated	Glycosylated
Homology	Cysteine protease	Uteroglobin
Enzymatic activity	Can cleave CD23 and CD25	None
Tolerance	No evidence; increased exposure associated with increased IgE ab	Increased exposure associated with decreased IgE ab

B. Mechanisms of Control: Are All Allergens Created Equal?

Although some simple versions of the hygiene hypothesis argue that the effect of exposure to dirt or more specifically mycobacteria is to induce a Th1 response, the evidence for this remains unclear.[36] In particular, the common inhalant allergens (dust mite, cat, and pollen) do not induce delayed hypersensitivity on skin testing. In addition, although human T cell responses *in vitro* almost always include interferon-gamma (IFN-γ), the quantity is not comparable to responses to tuberculin. Our results with cat allergens show that many children with high exposure have developed IgG and IgG$_4$ ab responses to Fel d 1.[37] Since IgG$_4$ production is interleukin (IL)-4 dependent, this form of immunity is better seen as a "modified Th2 response" than as a Th1 response.

The mechanism for the difference between mite and cat responses is not clear. However, recent studies on overlapping peptides of Fel d 1 identified two peptides of the n-terminal end of the second chain that selectively induce IL-10 and IFN-γ.[38] These results strongly suggest that it is the response to Fel d 1 that explains why this allergen is associated with "control" at high doses. Furthermore, the results strongly suggest that this control also occurs in allergic patients, which could explain why the *titer* of IgE ab to cat is much lower than that to mite.[33]

Although T cell responses may provide a mechanism, other striking differences between mite and cat exposure may explain the differences (Table 11.2). The measurements of airborne cat allergens in houses with cats imply that the inhaled dose could be as much as 1 μg/day. Since most of the allergen impacts the nose or pharynx, it would be swallowed, and it is possible that the response to cat allergens occurs in the gut. Finally, the enzymatic activity of mite allergen may be relevant to its *allergenicity* and equally to the lack of a control mechanism.

IV. Allergens Derived from Fungi

The relevance of fungal allergens to asthma is undoubted, but establishing dose response relationships or indeed simply measuring exposure remains difficult.

Unlike other allergens, certain fungi (e.g., Aspergillus) can grow in the lungs or elsewhere in the body (Trichophyton or Candida).[39] There are several possible mechanisms by which fungi can contribute to asthma and the differences have profound implications for prevention and treatment.

The strongest data about asthma and inhaled fungal allergens relates to fungi of the genus Alternaria. Sensitivity to this fungus has been related to asthma in prospective and cross-sectional studies on children and in relation to the severity of asthma in adults. Interestingly, the spores of Alternaria are larger than most other fungal spores, often as large as 10×14 μm. By contrast the spores of Penicillium or Aspergillus are generally 2 μm in diameter. Thus, an Alternaria spore may be 200 times larger in volume than other spores, and the very high counts for fungal spores in the outdoor air may be misleading if their volume is not taken into account. However, comparison of spore sizes makes two assumptions: (1) that fungal allergens become airborne as spores rather than as "mycelia fragments" and (2) that spores release proteins in the same way that pollen grains, mite feces, and cat dander particles do.

Fungal spores are generally designed to be resistant to desiccation and consequently have an outside layer that resists rapid release of the contents. In some cases, the situation is more extreme because the relevant allergens are not expressed in the spores until after they germinate.[40] A good example is the *Aspergillus fumigatus* allergen Asp f 1 that is expressed rapidly after germination. The obvious conclusion is that fungal spores are not directly comparable to other airborne particles.

The epidemiology of sensitization to Alternaria allergens correlates in general with the known presence of outdoor spores even if it does not correlate well with the quantitative spore count and reports have come from the upper midwest, Tucson, Arizona, and Los Alamos, New Mexico.[41,42] A report from the Mayo Clinic suggested that Alternaria sensitization was associated with severe asthma.[43] More importantly, the attacks occurred during the "Alternaria season." While it is easy to argue that the prolonged season of Alternaria exposure explains the severity of symptoms, it is difficult to explain why this should be more severe than asthma associated with the major indoor allergens.

Aspergillus is well recognized as an inhalant allergen; exposure predominantly occurs outdoors. Among children, sensitization to this fungus is not common (<5%), but the association with asthma may be very strong [odds ratio $\geq$6).[29] Clearly, very few of these children have the fungi growing in their lungs. On the other hand, allergic bronchopulmonary aspergillosis (ABPA) is a well recognized complication of allergic asthma in adults. The reasons some patients develop this complication are not clear. Many of them are reported to have relatively mild asthma prior to developing this syndrome, which includes specific IgE ab to Aspergillus, productive sputum, transient lung infiltrates, eosinophilia, and steroid dependence.

Some studies suggest that exposure too high levels of viable fungi, for example, from chicken or turkey farms, contributes to the risk, but this can only be part of the explanation. Fungal growth in the lungs is certain and production of sputum with viable Aspergillus can persist for many years. Although single sputum cultures may be negative, repeated cultures will usually produce positive results.

The fungus may also be identified from bronchoalveolar lavage (BAL). Cultures must be obtained for several reasons. First, occasionally other fungi (i.e. Candida or Curvularia) may cause a similar syndrome, and second, the *in vitro* sensitivity of Aspergillus may help predict response to oral antifungal treatment.[44] A cardinal feature of ABPA or ABPX (where X denotes another fungal etiology) is that the serum IgE is elevated (usually >400 IU/ml). This appears to be a characteristic feature of fungal colonization of the respiratory tract because it has not been reported in relation to bacteria in the lungs, for example, in traditional bronchiectasis.

The early descriptions of "intrinsic asthma" recognized a severe disease with generally late onset associated with infection. Sulzberger recognized a role for local fungal infection, particularly with Trichophyton species.[45] Although not common, extensive onychomycosis combined with immediate hypersensitivity to Trichophyton species is found in a proportion of men with late onset and severe asthma. These cases are worth identifying because they respond to antifungal treatment with fluconazole.[39,46] In addition, the syndrome is of considerable theoretical interest because Trichophyton species are strict dermatophytes and cannot grow in the respiratory tract.

The implication is that antigens absorbed from sites of fungal growth in the skin or nailbeds can induce an inflammatory response elsewhere in the body. Obviously, this poses several questions because T cells primed in the periphery would not be expected to localize to the lungs. However, almost all these cases involve extensive sinus disease and it seems possible that T cells are primed secondarily in the sinus and can then localize to the lungs. Whatever the mechanism, these patients do not get better when admitted to hospitals (an early criterion for intrinsic asthma) but do improve with antifungal treatment.[46]

V. Cockroach Exposure

In 1964, Bernton and Brown first suggested a relationship between cockroach exposure and allergic sensitization in atopic individuals.[47] They initially studied 367 individuals and found that among their 114 allergic patients, the prevalence of sensitivity by skin test was 28%. In subsequent studies, the prevalence has varied from 10 to 40%, depending on the geographic area and group of patients studied. Poor individuals, particularly African Americans living in inner cities, are at greatest risk.[48–50] The cockroach has been shown to be a significant allergen, not only in the United States, but also in Brazil, France, and eastern Asia where the temperatures also support cockroach survival.

The potential for cockroach exposure to cause asthma was initially observed in an occupational setting.[51] Two entomologists reported asthma and dermatitis upon exposure to cockroaches. A third patient who worked in a laboratory for breeding cockroaches also experienced asthma when exposed. Bronchial challenge studies supported the relationship to asthma. Bernton et al. reported positive challenges consisting of decreased FEV_1 and symptoms in 10 of 10 sensitized patients with asthma.[51] Kang et al. observed similar immediate reactions in their patients.[52] Furthermore, the majority of their patients experienced late asthmatic responses 6 to 10 hours after challenge and increased peripheral blood eosinophilia at 24 hours.

Studies of patients presenting to emergency rooms and living in inner cities associated cockroach sensitivity with acute asthma. Gelber et al. found that among adults presenting to an emergency room in Delaware, sensitization and exposure to cockroaches were associated with a six times greater risk for asthma.[50] Call et al. found a correlation between asthma and high cockroach exposure in sensitized children presenting to an emergency room in Atlanta.[49] Rosenstreich et al. studied eight inner city areas and reported higher rates of hospitalization and unscheduled clinic visits for sensitized children exposed to high levels of cockroach (>8 units Bla g 1/g dust).[48] Common to all these studies was the observation that exposure alone was not a sufficient risk factor for asthma; sensitization was a necessary intermediate step.[47–50]

In Boston, lower levels of exposure were associated with incident asthma and recurrent wheeze in a dose response fashion.[53] In a birth cohort study, the presence of cockroach allergen in the home predicted recurrent episodes of wheezing during the first year of life with a higher relative risk at higher levels of exposure.[54] Furthermore, in a study of the siblings of the birth cohort, cockroach allergen levels were found to be significant predictors of incident asthma.[53] In fact, levels ranging from 0.05 to 2 U/g were associated with an 8- to 9-fold risk and levels ≥ 2 U/g were associated with a 20-fold risk of developing asthma.

Airborne exposures are believed to be more clinically relevant for aeroallergens; thus several studies were undertaken with the purpose of characterizing exposures to cockroach allergens. In Strasbourg, France, although very high levels of cockroach allergen were measured in dust from mattresses, airborne allergens were undetectable either without disturbance or with natural disturbance alone.[55] With vigorous disturbance, particles >10 μm in size were collected. In contrast, using polyvinylidene difluoride membranes for collection, DeLucca et al. measured cockroach allergen with (normal movement) and without disturbance (at night) with a greater proportion of smaller particles airborne without disturbance.[56] The particles were amorphous and flake-like or fibrous, and described as having "many similarities to dust mite."

The two primary species of cockroaches in the United States are *Blattella germanica* (German cockroach) and *Periplaneta americana* (American cockroach). A number of allergens have been described for both species (Table 11.1). The only two allergens that have shown evidence of cross-reactivity are Bla g 1 and Per a 1.[57] They are unique in that they contain tandem amino acid repeats and thus can occur in multiple molecular forms, depending on the number of repeats present.[58] These allergens are found primarily in the digestive tract and are homologous to a mosquito precursor protein.

Bla g 2 is also found in highest content in the digestive tract.[59] It is a 36-kD protein with three possible glycosylation sites although it does not appear to be glycosylated. Although Bla g 2 has extensive sequence homology with aspartic proteases, it does not exert *in vitro* enzymatic activity. The structure of Per a 7 has recently been elucidated as a 33-kD protein without glycosylation that is homologous to invertebrate tropomyosin and similar to that found in dust mites and shrimp.[60]

VI. Relationship of Specific IgE Antibody Responses and Total IgE in Asthma Patients

The total IgE elevations found in many patients with asthma were recognized soon after the techniques for measuring this isotype became available. It was also clear that, on average, children and young adults with more severe disease had higher total IgE levels. Although specific IgE antibody responses can be large enough to contribute to total IgE, it is by no means clear whether total IgE is elevated in patients with asthma *because* of specific responses. Burrows and his colleagues argued in an influential paper that allergen-specific IgE correlated with allergic rhinitis but not with asthma even though total IgE correlated with asthma.[61]

The implication was that total IgE was elevated nonspecifically in patients with asthma. However, the data were difficult to interpret because the researchers did not perform skin tests with mite, cockroach, or cat allergens. It subsequently became clear that Alternaria was the most important factor in relation to asthma in Arizona.[41] Although RAST is a quantitative technique, the units originally were arbitrary, and it was difficult to compare units among allergens.[5,62]

The development of the ImmunoCAP (Pharmacia, Uppsala, Sweden), a high capacity immunosorbent, has provided much greater confidence about the absolute values. It is now possible to compare units of IgE ab with the same units used to measure total serum IgE. The fact that many sera contain as many as 100 to 300 IU of IgE ab to mite allergen means that this ab alone makes a significant contribution to total IgE.[33] In contrast, IgE ab to cat allergens is generally less than 10 IU/ml; this represents less than 3% of circulating IgE if the total is 400 IU/ml.

The correlation between total IgE and wheezing is widely accepted. Less well accepted is the fact that total IgE is on average much higher (300 to 400 IU/ml) among children and young adults who present to the hospital with acute episodes.[63] Many of these children aged 3 to 18 (~45%) have recently had rhinovirus infections.[63,64] The implication is that rhinovirus can cause acute episodes of asthma in "highly allergic" subjects. In keeping with this, it is well recognized that experimental human rhinovirus (HRV) infection can up-regulate the responses of the lungs to allergen challenges.[65,66] We recently demonstrated that responses to HRV challenges in asthmatics are much greater in subjects with total IgE values above 300 IU/ml compared to those with levels of ~100 IU/ml.[67]

The interaction of total and specific IgE can also be seen in population-based studies.[68] Total IgE has been associated consistently with asthma, but surprisingly many studies show little relationship between total IgE and allergic rhinitis.[69] However, seasonal rhinitis is consistently and strongly associated with IgE ab to relevant seasonal pollen allergens such as grass, ragweed, trees, and weeds. The implication is that the IgE ab response to pollen does not make a significant contribution to total serum IgE. Although we would argue that immediate hypersensitivity to some allergens is associated with elevated total serum IgE because the IgE ab response makes a contribution to the total, other explanations are possible. Perhaps the response creates a milieu that nonspecifically enhances IgE ab responses. It is also possible that most of these patients are *highly allergic* and that the increase in total IgE results from multiple IgE ab responses. It is increasingly probable that some allergens "push" total IgE more than others. Based on the striking correlation between total serum IgE and severity of asthma, it is likely that some allergens inherently predispose children to more severe asthma.

VII. Conclusions

The environment in which we live is also inhabited by a wide range of plants, fungi, insects, acarids, and mammals. All these organisms produce proteins that are antigenically foreign and can become airborne. The characteristics that lead to IgE antibody formation are still not well defined, but they have some striking characteristics. Almost all the important allergens are soluble glycoproteins with molecular weights between 10,000 and 60,000 (Table 11.1). The allergens that have been studied become airborne on particles ranging in size from 30 μm to less than 1 μm in diameter. Thus the properties of the allergens include the properties of the particles, the quantities of allergens inhaled, and the solubilities of the proteins. In addition, whether an allergen is an outdoor (generally seasonal) type or indoor and in most cases perennial type may be an important factor.

Because populations are diverse and responses to allergens are complex (Figure 11.1), it is no surprise that many different genes influence the relationship to asthma. We would now add that the ability to become tolerant with high dose exposure may be genetically controlled.[38]

The rise in asthma prevalence has occurred in all countries with Western lifestyles and the rise is now appearing in developing countries. The important fact is that the increases have occurred in countries that have completely different patterns of allergic sensitization so it is most unlikely that the increases can be attributed solely to increased exposure. It is now clear that increased exposure to cat allergens does not increase the risk of sensitization or asthma. The fact that asthma has also increased in areas where cats are the most important sources of allergens associated with asthma also argues against increased exposure as the cause of the increase.

Although asthma has increased in many countries and the increases in some countries have been ten-fold or greater, the prevalence of disease is not the same.[70] Recent analyses of ISAAC and other data show that the absolute prevalence may be much higher in some areas. In addition, the disease appears to be more severe in areas with higher prevalence rates. Thus, the increase in Finland has been recorded as 0.2 to 4%, or twenty-fold.[71] In contrast, figures for New Zealand and the United Kingdom appear to have increased from 4 to 20%.[70,72] Recent data from New York City suggest that up to 20% of the children have objective evidence of asthma. Over the same period (1960 through 2000) an increase in hospitalizations among African Americans living in poverty in the United States has been documented.[73]

The correct question is whether the natures of the allergens can influence the prevalence or severity of disease. If, as now seems clear, increasing exposure to certain allergens does not increase either the prevalence or titer of IgE ab, would these allergens be associated with less disease and less severe disease? In this respect, a select handful of allergens have been associated with *severity* of asthma. They include dust mite, cockroach, and Alternaria.[41,48–50,74] Interestingly, both dust mite and Alternaria have been found to give rise to high titer IgE ab.[33,75] There is a real possibility that allergens that do not induce *control* of the IgE ab response can give rise to more severe disease.

The total IgE ab data may also argue that some allergens can increase total IgE while others have little effect. Given the strong relationship between total IgE and asthma hospitalization, this again suggests that those allergens that give rise to high titer IgE ab may be relevant to increased hospitalization. These facts together provide very good evidence that the combination of allergen exposure and sensitization is a major risk factor for asthma. However, it appears that a hierarchy in allergens related to their biological and physical properties may be relevant to the overall prevalence and severity of disease.

References

1. Platts-Mills TAE, Vervloet D, Thomas WR, Aalberse RC, and Chapman MD. Indoor allergens and asthma: Third International Workshop, Cuenca Spain. *J Allergy Clin Immunol* 1997; 100: S1–S24.
2. Burrows B, Sears MR, Flannery EM, Herbison GP, and Holdaway MD. Relations of bronchial responsiveness to allergy skin test reactivity, lung function, respiratory symptoms and diagnoses in thirteen-year-old New Zealand children. *J Allergy Clin Immunol* 1995; 95: 548–556.
3. Sporik R, Holgate ST, Platts-Mills TAE, and Cogswell JJ. Exposure to house-dust mite allergen (Der p 1) and the development of asthma in childhood: a prospective study. *New Engl J Med* 1990; 323: 502–507.
4. Peat JK, Tovey E, Toelle BG, Haby MM, Xuan W, and Woolcock AJ. House dust mite allergens: a major risk factor for childhhod asthma in Australia. *Am J Respir Crit Care Med* 1996; 153: 141–146.
5. Pollart SM, Chapman MD, Fiocco GP, Rose G, and Platts-Mills TAE. Epidemiology of acute asthma: IgE antibodies to common inhalant allergen as a risk factor for emergency room visits. *J Allergy Clin Immunol* 1989; 83: 875–882.
6. Spieksma F. and Voorhorst R. Comparison of skin reactions to extracts of house dust, mites and human skin scales. *Acta Allergol* 1969; 24: 124.
7. Asher MI, Barry D, Clayton T et al. The burden of symptoms of asthma, allergic rhinoconjunctivitis and atopic eczema in children and adolescents in six New Zealand centers: ISAAC Phase One. *N Z Med J* 2001; 114: 114–120.
8. Prescott SL, Macaubas C, Holt BJ et al. Transplacental priming of the human immune system to environmental allergens: universal skewing of initial T cell responses toward the Th2 cytokine profile. *J Immunol* 1998; 160: 4730–4737.
9. Platts-Mills TAE, Tovey ER, Mitchell EB et al. Reduction of bronchial hyperreactivity during prolonged allergen avoidance. *Lancet* 1982; ii: 675–678.
10. Boner AL, Niero E, Antolini I et al. Pulmonary function and bronchial hyperreactivity in asthmatic children with house dust mite allergy during prolonged stay in the Italian Alps (Misurina, 1756 m). *Ann Allergy* 1985; 54: 42–45.
11. Kerrebijn KF. Endogenous factors in childhood CNSLD: methodological aspects in population studies, in Orie NGM and van de Lende R, Eds., *Bronchitis III*. Netherlands: Royal Vangorcum Assen; 1970; 38–48.
12. van der Heide S, Kauffman HF, Dubois AEJ, and deMonchy JGR. Allergen avoidance measures in homes of house dust mite allergic asthmatic patients: effects of acaricides and mattress encasing. *Allergy* 1997; 52: 921–927.
13. Htut T, Higenbottam TW, Gill GW et al. Eradication of house dust mite from homes of atopic asthmatic subjects: a double-blind trial. *J Allergy Clin Immunol* 2001; 107: 55–60.
14. Ehnert B, Lau-Schadendorf S, Weber A et al. Reducing domestic exposure to dust mite allergen reduces bronchial hyperreactivity in sensitive children with asthma. *J Allergy Clin Immunol* 1992; 90: 135–138.
15. Terreehorst I, Hak E, Oosting AJ, Tempels-Pavlica, MD et al. Evaluation of impermeable covers for bedding in patients with allergic rhinitis. *New Engl J Med* 2003; 349: 237–246.

16. Woodcock A, Forster L, Matthews E et al. Control of exposure to mite allergen and allergen-impermeable bed covers for adults with asthma. *New Engl J Med* 2003; 349: 225–236.

17. Platts-Mills TAE, Vaughan JW, Carter MC, and Woodfolk, JA. The role of intervention in established allergy: avoidance of indoor allergens in the treatment of chronic allergic disease. *J Allergy Clin Immunol* 2000; 106: 787–804.

18. Arshad SH, Matthews S, Gant C, and Hide DW. Effect of allergen avoidance on development of allergic disorders in infancy. *Lancet* 1992; 339: 1493–1497.

19. Sporik R, Chapman MD, and Platts-Mills TAE. House dust mite exposure as a cause of asthma. *Clin Exp Allergy* 1992; 22: 897–906.

20. Lau S and Sommerfeld C et al. Early exposure to house-dust mite and cat allergens and development of childhood asthma: a cohort study. *Lancet* 2000; 356: 1392–1397.

21. Martinez FD, Wright AL, Taussig LM, Holberg CJ, and Halonen M. Asthma and wheezing in the first six years of life. *New Engl J Med* 1995; 332: 133–138.

22. Tovey ER, Chapman MD, and Platts-Mills TAE. Mite faeces are a major source of house dust allergens. *Nature* 1981; 289: 592–593.

23. Schulz O, Sewell HF, and Shakib F. Proteolytic cleavage of CD25, the α subunit of the human T cell Interleukin 2 receptor, by Der p 1, a major mite allergen with cysteine protease activity. *J Exp Med* 1998; 187: 271–275.

24. Wan H, Winton HL, Soeller C et al. Der p 1 facilitates transepithelial allergen delivery by disruption of tight junctions. *J Clin Invest* 1999; 104: 3–4.

25. Hewitt CRA, Brown AP, Hart BD, and Pritchard DI. A major house dust mite allergen disrupts the IgE network by selectively cleaving CD23. *J Exp Med* 1995; 182: 1537–1544.

26. Roost HP, Hunzli N, Schindler C et al. Role of current and childhood exposure to cat and atopic sensitization. *J Allergy Clin Immunol* 1999; 104: 941–947.

27. Luczynska CM, Li Y, Chapman MD, and Platts-Mills TAE. Airborne concentrations and particle size distribution of allergen derived from domestic cats (*Felis domesticus*): measurements using cascade impactor, liquid impinger, and a two-site monoclonal antibody assay for Fel d 1. *Amer Rev Respir Dis* 1990; 141: 361–367.

28. De Blay F, Heymann PW, Chapman MD, and Platts-Mills TAE. Airborne dust mite allergens: comparison of group II allergens with group I mite allergen and cat allergen Fel d 1. *J Allergy Clin Immunol* 1991; 88: 919–926.

29. Sears MR, Herbison GP, Holdaway MD, Hewitt CJ et al. The relative risks of sensitivity to grass pollen, house dust mite, and cat dander in the development of childhood asthma. *Clin Exp Allergy* 1989; 19: 419–424.

30. Carter MC, Perzanowski MS. Raymond A, and Platts-Mills TAE. Home intervention in the treatment of asthma among inner-city children. *J Allergy Clin Immunol* 2001; 108: 732–737.

31. Hesselmar B, Aberg N, Aberg B, Eriksson, and Bjorksten B. Does early exposure to cat or dog protect against later allergy development? *Clin Exp Allergy* 1999; 29: 611–617.

32. Perzanowski MS, Ronmark E, Platts-Mills TAE, and Lundback B. Effect of cat and dog ownership on sensitization and development of asthma among preteenage children. *Am J Respir Crit Care Med* 2002; 166: 696–702.

33. Erwin EA, Wickens K, Custis NJ, Siebers R, Woodfolk J, Barry D, Crane J, and Platts-Mills TAE. Cat and dust mite sensitivity and tolerance in relation to wheezing among children raised with high exposure to both allergens. *Journal of Allergy and Clin Immunol.* In press.

34. Custovic A, Hallam CL, Simpson BM, Craven M, Simpson A, and Woodcock A. Decreased prevalence of sensitization to cats with high exposure to cat allergen. *J Allergy Clin Immunol* 2001; 108: 537–539.

35. Ownby DD, Johnson CC, and Peterson EL. Exposure to dogs and cats in the first year of life and risk of allergic sensitization at 6 to 7 years of age. *JAMA* 2002; 288: 963–972.

36. Busse WW and Lemanske RF, Jr. Asthma. *New Engl J Med* 2001; 344: 350–362.

37. Platts-Mills TAE, Vaughan J, Squillace S, Woodfolk J, and Sporik R. Sensitisation, asthma, and a modified Th2 response in children exposed to cat allergen: a population-based cross-sectional study. *Lancet* 2001; 357; 752–756.

38. Reefer AJ, Carneiro RM, Custus NJ, Platts-Mills, TAE, Sung, SSJ, Hammer J, and Woodfolk JA. Evidence of a role for IL-10-mediated HLA-DR7-restricted T-cell dependant events in development of the modified Th2 response to cat allergens. *J Immunol* 2004 (in press).

39. Ward GWJ, Karlsson G, Rose G, and Platts-Mills TAE. Trichophyton asthma: sensitization of bronchi and upper airways to dermatophyte antigen. *Lancet* 1989; 1: 859–862.

40. Sporik RB, Arruda LK, Woodfolk J et al. Environmental exposure to *Asperigillus fumigatus* allergen (Asp f 1). *Clin Exp Allergy* 1993; 23: 326–331.

41. Halonen M, Stern DA, Wright AL, Taussig LM, and Martinez FD. Alternaria as a major allergen for asthma in children raised in a desert environment. *Amer J Respir Crit Care Med* 1997; 155: 1356–1361.

42. Perzanowski MS, Sporik R, Squillace SP, Gelber LE et al. Association of sensitization to Alternaria allergens with asthma among school-age children. *J Allergy Clin Immunol* 1998; 101: 626–632.

43. O'Hallaren MT, Yunginger J, Offord KP et al. Exposure to an aeroallergen as a possible precipitating factor in respiratory arrest in young patients with asthma. *New Engl J Med* 1991; 324: 359–363.

44. Stevens DA, Schwartz HJ, Lee JY, Moskovitz BL, Jerome DC, Catanzaro A, Bamberger DM, Weinmann AJ, Tuazon CU, Judson MA, Platts-Mills TAE, and DeGraff AC. A randomized trial of itraconazole in allergic bronchopulmonary aspergillosis. *New Engl J Med* 2000; 342: 756–762.

45. Wise F and Sulzberger MD. Urticaria and hay fever due to Trichophyton *(Epidermophyton interdigital). JAMA* 1930; 95: 1504–1508.

46. Ward GW, Woodfolk JA, Hayden ML, Jackson S, and Platts-Mills TAE. Asthma, rhinitis, other respiratory diseases: treatment of late-onset asthma with fluconazole. *J Allergy Clin Immunol* 1998; 104: 541–546.

47. Bernton HS and Brown H. Insect allergy: preliminary studies of the cockroach. *J Allergy* 1964; 35: 506–513.

48. Rosenstreich DL, Eggleston P, Kattan M, Baker D et al. The role of cockroach allergy and exposure to cockroach allergen in causing mordibity among inner-city children with asthma. *New Engl J Med* 1997; 336: 1356–1363.

49. Call RS, Smith TF, Morris E, Chapman MD, and Platts-Mills TAE. Risk factors for asthma in inner city children. *J Pediatr* 1992; 121: 862–866.
50. Gelber LE, Seltzer LH, Bouzoukis JK, Pollart SM et al. Sensitization and exposure to indoor allergens as risk factors for asthma among patients presenting to hospital. *Am Rev Respir Dis* 1993; 147: 573–578.
51. Bernton HS, McMahon TF, and Brown H. Cockroach asthma. *Brit J Dis Chest* 1972; 66: 61–66.
52. Kang B. Study on cockroach antigen as a probable causative agent in bronchial asthma. *J Allergy Clin Immunol* 1976; 58: 357–365.
53. Litonjua AA, Carey VJ, Burge HA, Weiss ST et al. Exposure to cockroach allergen in the home is associated with incident doctor-diagnosed asthma and recurrent wheezing. J *Allergy Clin Immunol* 2001; 107: 41–47.
54. Gold DR, Burge HA, Carey V, Milton DK et al. Predictors of repeated wheeze in the first year of life. The relative roles of cockroach, birth weight, acute lower respiratory illness, and maternal smoking. *Am J Respir Crit Care Med* 1999; 160: 227–236.
55. deBlay F, Sanchez J, Hedelin G, Perez-Infante A et al. Dust and airborne exposure to allergens derived from cockroach (*Blattella germanica*) in low-cost public housing in Strasbourg (France). *J Allergy Clin Immunol* 1997; 99: 107–112.
56. DeLucca SD, Taylor DJM, O'Meara TJ, Jones AS, and Tovey ER. Measurement and characterization of cockroach allergens detected during normal domestic activity. *J Allergy Clin Immunol* 1999; 104: 672–680.
57. Melen E, Pomes A, Vailes LD, Arruda LK, and Chapman MD. Molecular cloning of Per a 1 and definition of the cross-reactive Group 1 cockroach allergens. *J Allergy Clin Immunol* 1999; 103: 859–864.
58. Pomes A, Melen E, Vailes LD, Retief JD et al. Novel allergen structures with tandem amino acid repeats derived from German and American cockroach. *J Biol Chem* 1998; 273: 30801–30807.
59. Arruda LK, Vailes LD, Platts-Mills TAE, Hayden ML, and Chapman MD. Induction of IgE antibody responses by glutathione S-transferase from the german cockroach (*Blattella gerrmanica*). *J Biol Chem* 1997; 272: 20907–20912.
60. Santos AR, Chapman MD, Aalberse RC, Vailes LD et al. Cockroach allergen and asthma in Brazil: Identification of tropomyosin as a major allergen with potential cross-reactivity with mite and shrimp allergens. *J Allergy Clin Immunol* 1999; 104: 329–337.
61. Burrows B, Martinez FD, Halonen M, Barbee RA, and Cline MG. Association of asthma with serum IgE levels and skin-test reactivity to allergens. *New Engl J Med* 1989; 320: 271–277.
62. Dolen, WK. IgE antibody in the serum: detection and diagnostic significance. *Allergy* 2003; 58: 717–723.
63. Rakes GP, Arruda E, Ingram JM et al. Rhinovirus and respiratory syncytial virus in wheezing children requiring emergency care: IgE and eosinophil analyses. *Am J Respir Crit Care Med* 1999; 159: 785–790.
64. Green RM, Custovic A, Sanderson G, Hunter J, Johnston SL, and Woodcock A. Synergism between allergens and viruses and risk of hospital admission with asthma: case-control study. *Br Med J* 2002; 324: 763 and 1131.

65. Lemanske RF, Dick EC, Swenson CA, Vrtis RF, and Busse WW. Rhinovirus upper respiratory tract infection increases airway hyperreactivity and late asthmatic reactions. *J Clin Invest* 1989; 83: 1–10.

66. Calhoun WJ, Dick EC, Schwartz LB, and Busse WW. A common cold virus, rhinovirus 16, potentiates airway inflammation after segmental antigen bronchoprovocation in allergic subjects. *J Clin Invest* 1994; 94: 2220–2228.

67. Zambrano JC, Carper HT, Rakes GP, Patrie J, Murphy DD, Platts-Mills TAE, Hayden FG, Gwaltney JM, Hatley TK, Owens AM, and Heymann, PW. Experimental rhinovirus challenges in adults with mild asthma: response to infection in relation to IgE. *J Allergy Clin Immunol* 2003; 111: 1006–1016.

68. Sporik R, Ingram JM, Price W, Sussman JH, Honsinger RW, and Platts-Mills TAE. Association of asthma with serum IgE and skin test reactivity to allergens among children living at high altitude: tickling the dragon's breath. *Am J Respir Crit Care Med* 1995; 151: 1388–1392.

69. Platts-Mills TA, Erwin EA, Allison AB, Blumenthal K, Barr M, Sredl D, Burge H, and Gold D. The relevance of maternal immune responses to inhalant allergens to maternal symptoms, passive transfer to the infant, and development of antibodies in the first two years of life. *J Allergy Clin Immunol* 2003; 111: 123–130.

70. Beasley R, Ellwood P, and Asher I. International patterns of the prevalence of pediatric asthma: the ISAAC program. *Pediatr Clin North Am* 2003; 50: 539–553.

71. Haahtela T, Lindholm H, Bjorkstein F, Koshenvuo K, and Laitinen LA. Prevalence of asthma in Finnish young men. *NMJ* 1990; 301: 226–268.

72. Seaton A, Godden DJ, and Brown K. Increase in asthma: a more toxic environment or a more susceptible population? *Thorax* 1994; 49: 171–174.

73. Crater DD, Heise S, Perzanowski M et al. Asthma hospitalization trends in Charleston, South Carolina, from 1956–1997: twenty-fold increase among African-American children over a thirty-year period. *Pediatrics* 2001; 108: E97.

74. Sporik R, Platts-Mills TA, and Cogswell JJ. Exposure to house dust mite allergen of children admitted to hospital with asthma. *Clin Exp Allergy* 1993; 23: 740–746.

75. Mari A, Schneider P, Wally V. Bretenbach M, and Simon-Nobbe B. Sensitization to fungi: epidemiology, comparative skin tests, and IgE reactivity of fungal extracts. *Clin Exp Allergy* 2003; 33L: 1429–1438.

12

Asthma and Nonrespiratory Infections

PAOLO MARIA MATRICARDI

Bambino Gesù Pediatric Hospital, Research Institute
Rome, Italy

I. Odd Influence on Asthma of Certain Nonrespiratory Infections (NRIs)

While overwhelming evidence links asthma to respiratory infections, it seems strange based on superficial evaluation that both the inception and the natural history of asthma may be affected by infections not directly involving the respiratory tract. Umberto Serafini pioneered this concept in 1950. He described five patients with asthma whose clinical manifestations disappeared with the onset of hepatitis and were absent for the duration of the disease; in one patient, a decrease in blood eosinophils was also recorded.[1] Serafini hypothesized that biological activities stimulated by infection were able to suppress those factors causing eosinophilic inflammation and asthmatic symptoms. He also described a therapeutic effect of provoked fever on asthma and observed both remission of symptomatology, marked decreases of blood eosinophils and lymphocytes, and an increase in neutrophils.[2] He also reported that provoked fever could prevent an asthma crisis induced by the injection of histamine (1 mg).[2] Fifty years later, he revisited his early observations in the light of modern knowledge about the role of cytokines and their balance in the regulation of eosinophilia and bronchial inflammation.[3-4]

Serafini's concept was extended from individual patients to populations as soon as the rising trend of asthma reached epidemic proportions in westernized countries. In the 1970s, Gerrard observed that the Saskatchewan Metis, a Cree Indian community living a very traditional lifestyle, exhibited higher total IgE levels but less atopic diseases than white Caucasians living a hygienic way of life. Gerrard anticipated that declining exposure to helminths and the fight against infectious diseases would have caused a rising trend in allergic asthma and other atopic diseases among populations living a western lifestyle.[5]

These predictions re-emerged as a comprehensive theory only in the 1990s when the "hygiene hypothesis" of Strachan,[6-7] originally based on epidemiological observations only, acquired biological plausibility through the TH1–TH2 paradigm[8-10] (stimulation of TH1 immunity by certain infections would suppress TH2 responses against allergens) and later through expanding knowledge of the so-called anti-inflammatory network[12,13] (certain infections will trigger and ensure strong immunoregulation that will prevent or suppress allergic and other immune-mediated inflammations).

II. Testing Hygiene Hypothesis in Europe

The hygiene hypothesis is indirectly supported by the evidence that in the course of westernization, atopy displays a characteristic distribution, as it is less frequent in children raised in large and poor families,[6,14] on farms,[15] in communities living traditional-type lifestyles,[16] and in children attending day care centers.[16-18] Thus, hygiene that reduces exposure to infections facilitates atopic responses and their inflammatory consequences at mucosal and skin surfaces, namely allergic asthma, rhinitis, and atopic eczema.[6-12]

Less indirect information was obtained by studies based on the assumption that individuals reared in poor hygiene conditions in countries undergoing westernization could be identified roughly from the presence of certain infectious agents in their sera, for example, hepatitis A virus (HAV). Under this strategy, poor hygiene was associated inversely with hay fever and allergic asthma in a group of Italian military cadets.[19] Atopy was also inversely related to other orofecal and foodborne infections [*Toxoplasma gondii* (TG) and *Helicobacter pylori* (HP)] but not to a series of airborne viruses.[20] Of note, allergic asthma was rare (1 of 245 or 0.4%) among subjects exposed to at least two orofecal and foodborne infections (TG, HP, HAV).

The inverse association of atopy and HAV antibodies was confirmed in an Italian adult population.[21] In Albania, the European country with the lowest prevalence of asthma,[22] the prevalence of positive serology for HAV among adults was well over 80% (A. Priftanji, personal communication).

III. Testing Hygiene Hypothesis in the United States

The hygiene hypothesis was questioned in the United States, where allergic asthma since the 1970s has reached minorities living in poverty under less-than-optimal hygienic conditions. The condition is known as "inner city asthma."[23] However, comparing criteria that discriminate between rural poverty in Europe and inner city poverty in North America can be instructive in finding what kind of NRI can affect the inception and natural history of asthma. In Europe, protection from atopy is mainly the hallmark of a "rugged" rural lifestyle, with daily exposure to animals and their waste, and thus to a high turnover of orofecal and foodborne infections. Low socioeconomic conditions in the American inner cities, on the other hand, entail living in an urban environment where exposure to indoor allergens such as cockroaches and rodent urine is chronic and foodborne and orofecal infections are less prevalent.

Recently, the same approach based on HAV serology used to test the hygiene hypothesis in Europe was applied also to a large general population sample of the United States.[24] The data of 33,994 residents recorded in a public database of a nationally representative cross-sectional survey [Third National Health and Nutrition Examination Survey (NHANES-III) 1988–1994] were analyzed. The variables examined were sociodemographic information, lifetime diagnosis and age at first diagnosis of hay fever or asthma, current skin sensitization to nine airborne allergens and peanuts, and current serology for hepatitis A, B, and C viruses, TG, and herpes simplex viruses type 1 and 2.

Hay fever [adjusted odds ratio (OR) 0.27; 95% confidence interval (CI) 0.18–0.41; p <0.001] and asthma (adjusted OR 0.45; 95% CI 0.31–0.66; p <0.001) were less frequent in subjects seropositive for hepatitis A virus, TG, and herpes simplex virus 1 versus seronegative subjects, after adjusting for age, sex, race, urban residence, census region, family size, income, and education. Skin sensitization to peanuts and to all airborne allergens examined (except cockroach) was less frequent among HAV-seropositive versus -seronegative subjects under the age of 40 years.

It was very interesting to note that the prevalences of hay fever and asthma diagnosed at or before 18 years of age in HAV-seronegative subjects increased progressively from 2.7% (95% CI 0.7–4.7%) and 0.4% (95% CI 0.1–1.6%), respectively, in cohorts born before 1920 to 8.5% (95% CI 7.3–9.7%) and 5.8% (95% CI 4.8–6.8%) in cohorts born in the 1960s. The prevalences remained constant, around 2%, in all cohorts of HAV-seropositive subjects (Figure 12.1).

To evaluate whether a positive HAV serology was simply a surrogate of poverty, the same associations were tested in a subgroup of participants (n = 2,711) aged 6 through 59 and living with annual incomes lower than $10,000 U.S. HAV seropositivity in this subgroup was inversely associated with hay fever

A)

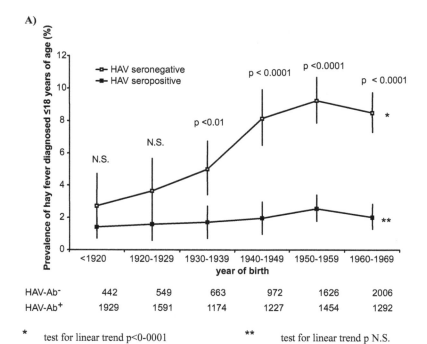

| HAV-Ab⁻ | 442 | 549 | 663 | 972 | 1626 | 2006 |
| HAV-Ab⁺ | 1929 | 1591 | 1174 | 1227 | 1454 | 1292 |

*   test for linear trend p<0-0001   **   test for linear trend p N.S.

B)

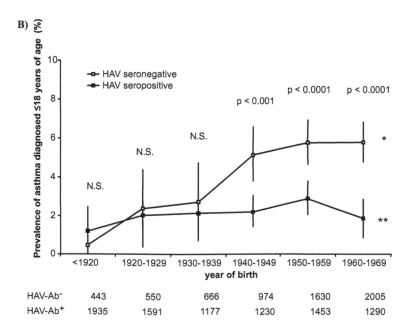

| HAV-Ab⁻ | 443 | 550 | 666 | 974 | 1630 | 2005 |
| HAV-Ab⁺ | 1935 | 1591 | 1177 | 1230 | 1453 | 1290 |

Figure 12.1 (See caption on opposite page)

(OR 0.47; 95% CI 0.32–0.68; p <0.0001) or asthma (OR 0.66; 95% CI 0.47–0.91; p <0.02) after adjusting for age, race, and sex. An interesting finding was the association of one food allergen, peanut — an emerging trigger of fatal allergic reactions in the United States. This study showed that serologic evidence of acquisition of certain infections, mainly foodborne and orofecal, in the United States is associated with a lower probability of developing atopic sensitizations not only to inhalants, but also to food allergens, and it supported the hypothesis that hygiene is a major factor contributing to the rise of hay fever and asthma in westernized countries.[25]

IV. Does the Hygiene Hypothesis Explain Inner City Asthma?

The results of the NHANES-III study suggest that a primary cause of the asthma epidemic in the United States is the reduction of those infections that may confer protection from atopy and allergic airway inflammation. It has been speculated that this reduction did not occur simultaneously in all socioeconomic strata. It started among the wealthiest in the nineteenth century, then extended to the middle class and involved the poorest classes only after the 1970s. The poorest group is now suffering from the most severe consequence of atopic susceptibility — a greater severity of allergic asthma — because of the concurrent exposure to secondary risk factors typical of poor urban environments, for example, exposure to cockroaches, smoking, dampness, and inadequate access to health care. Inner city asthma may thus be explained in the framework of the hygiene hypothesis as the final stage of a class-driven urbanization and westernization process that in the United States started two centuries ago and that it is only now coming to an end (Figure 12.2).[24]

A relevant consequence of these concepts is that if this hypothesis remains true, the recent increase in allergic asthma in the inner cities would be only partially overcome by preventive strategies aimed at reducing exposure to known, but secondary, risk factors. By contrast, the identification of primary protective factors, namely those linked to infections today and typical of a "traditional" rural European lifestyle, may lead to future strategies for primary prevention tentatively linked to infections today and still associated with a European "traditional" rural lifestyle, may inspire future strategies for primary prevention[26]

Figure 12.1 (Opposite) Prevalences of participants with histories of hay fever (a) and asthma (b) diagnosed before 18 years of age in relation to serology for hepatitis A virus by decade of birth (NHANES-III, 1988–1994). The bars represent the 95% confidence intervals. The p values reflect comparisons of prevalences of hay fever (a) and asthma (b) among participants seropositive or seronegative for HAV at examination. (From Matricardi, P.M. et al., *J Allergy Clin Immunol* 2002; 110: 381–387. With permission from Elsevier.)

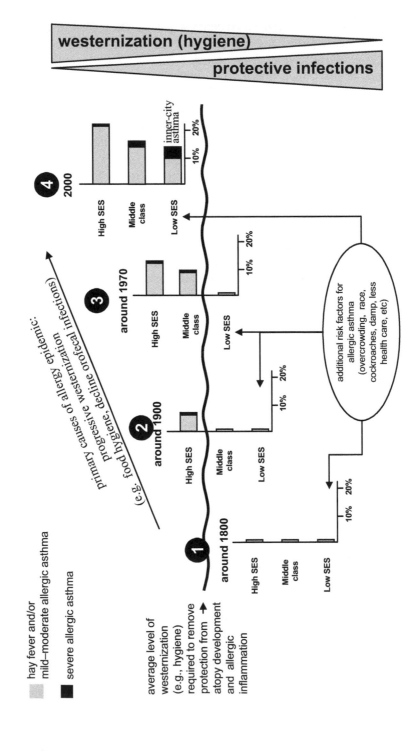

Figure 12.2 Hypothetical model (not to scale) of the spread of hay fever and allergic asthma in the U.S. according to socioeconomic status (y axis), westernization level, and exposure to relevant infections protecting from allergy. Before the industrial revolution, lifestyle factors that protected from allergy (persistent exposure to foodborne and orofecal pathogens under the hygiene hypothesis) were so common throughout society that allergy was rare. The slow progress of westernization meant these factors were gradually lost starting with the highest income groups downward during the 19th century. This correlated to the emergence of hay fever among the more affluent classes. Further progress toward westernization and more hygienic conditions led to the decline of the same protective factors among the more numerous middle income groups during the first seven decades of the 20th century; this reinforced the epidemic trend of hay fever and allergic asthma that spared the lowest socioeconomic classes, still exposed then to sufficient levels of protective factors. Indeed, although unsanitary environmental conditions always plagued inner cities (overcrowding, dampnesss, cockroaches, suboptimal health care, etc.), allergic asthma prevalence was low in the inner cities until the 1970s. As a result of further westernization (hygiene improvement and further decline of infections, mainly foodborne and orofecal), protective factors disappeared even from the inner cities. Exposure to overcrowding, and other unsanitary conditions worsened the primary effects of increasing atopy susceptibility and made new asthma cases more severe in this population. (From Matricardi, P.M. et al., *Ann Allergy Asthma Immunol* 2002; 89 Suppl.: 69–74. With permission.)

V. Protection Provided by Nonrespiratory Infections

The issue whether the asthma-protective roles of certain NRIs are lung-specific and targeted to any kind of wheezing or whether NRIs act primarily on the propensity of the immune system to develop allergic inflammation has been debated. In the first case, a decline of NRI should cause an increase of any kind of wheezing; in the second case, the epidemic of asthma should be limited to the allergic type.

It is becoming clear that the increase in asthma cases observed in developed countries is only an indicator of a more complex phenomenon. This is suggested, for example, by ISAAC phase I studies that demonstrated a significant correlation between the prevalence of asthma and that of allergic rhinoconjunctivitis and atopic eczema in the 155 centers examined.[22] On the other hand, studies examining cohorts at least 10 years apart showed parallel increases in the prevalence of asthma and also of allergic rhinitis and atopic eczema. For example, in school children aged 8 to 13 years in Aberdeen, Scotland who were administered the same questionnaires in 1964, 1989, and 1994, the prevalence of asthma increased from 4.1% (1964) to 10.2% (1989) and to 19.6% (1994).[27–28] Similarly, hay fever increased from 3.2% to 11.9% and to 12.7%; atopic eczema increased from 5.3% to 12.0% and to 17.7%, indicative of an underlying increase in susceptibility to atopy.[27–28]

The increased prevalence of asthma in westernized countries is almost totally accounted for by an excess in atopic sensitization. Asthma was more frequent in children from West Germany with respect to East Germany in 1992, but the difference was almost totally due to a marked difference in the prevalence of atopic sensitization.[29] Among Scottish adults, the prevalence of asthma increased more than two-fold in 20 years, but subjects "responsible" for excess rates were also affected by hay fever.[30]

Objective increases in atopic sensitization were demonstrated in several studies (reviewed by Woolcock and Peat).[31] Perhaps the most striking is a study of 13- to 14-year old female students in Akita, Japan. Serum IgE against airborne allergens (mites and grass and tree pollens) occurred in 21.4% in 1978, 25% in 1981, 35.5% in 1985, and 39.4% in 1991.[32] These data strongly suggest that the asthma epidemic is primarily an epidemic of "bronchial allergy" which in turn is only one aspect of a rising trend of the propensity to produce atopic responses toward allergens and mucosal or cutaneous eosinophilic inflammation leading to organ-specific symptoms (involving bronchial and/or nasal mucosae and/or skin). This rising trend of allergic inflammation is now considered only one component of an even more complex epidemiological phenomenon characterized by the simultaneous increases with westernization of both TH1- and TH2-like immune disorders.[12,33]

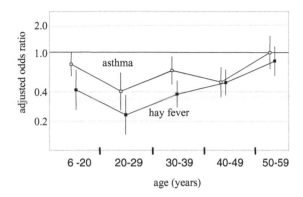

Figure 12.3 Asthma and hay fever in relation to serology for hepatitis A virus and age in the U.S. (NHANES-III, 1988–1994) after adjusting for age, sex, education, income, and residence (see Matricardi, P.M. et al., *Ann Allergy Asthma Immunol* 2002; 89 Suppl.: 69–74 for definitions).

The NHANES-III provides an opportunity to answer the question whether the asthma-protective roles of some NRIs are lung-specific and target any kind of wheezing or they act primarily on the propensity of the immune system to develop allergic inflammation. In the NHANES-III, an inverse relationship between serum antibodies to certain infectious agents and respiratory disease was stronger for hay fever than for asthma.[24] In addition, the protective effect on asthma was much stronger in the age range between 20 and 39 years, when asthma is mainly associated with allergy. Conversely, the inverse association of asthma with positive HAV serology was weaker both among children (whose wheezing is often due to infection in the absence of allergic sensitization) and in subjects 40 years of age or older (whose diagnoses of asthma are less frequently associated with allergy). See Figure 12.3.

The observation that a positive HAV serology was inversely associated also to food allergens, such as peanuts, is of interest. Indeed, this suggested that "protection" from hay fever and asthma by certain NRI is not a lung-specific phenomenon but involves atopic responses at the level of other mucosal surfaces, including those of the gastrointestinal tract.[10,20,34]

VI. Ability of HAV to Protect against Asthma

The exact nature (viral, bacterial, or parasitic) of nonrespiratory infectious agents that may prevent allergic asthma and other atopic diseases remains uncertain.

Among those examined, HAV is perhaps the one most consistently found to be inversely associated with allergic asthma and hay fever. Although a positive HAV serology was used as a marker of exposure to more infection in general and of orofecal and/or foodborne transmission in particular, a causal role of HAV in protection from allergic asthma has been proposed on the basis of clinical observations[1,4] and potential molecular mechanisms identified.[35]

In congenic mice that differed at the homologous chromosomal segment 5q23–35, a Mendelian trait was recently identified that encodes by a T cell and airway phenotype regulator (Tapr). Tapr is genetically distinct from known cytokine genes and controls the development of airway hyperreactivity and T cell production of interleukin 4 (IL-4) and IL-13.[35] Positional cloning identified a gene family that encodes T cell membrane proteins (TIMs); major sequence variants of this gene family completely cosegregated with Tapr. Since the human homolog of TIM-1 is the HAV receptor, the authors made the hypothesis that the interaction of HAV with its receptor may protect from atopy by reducing TH2 differentiation and also reducing the likelihood of developing airway hyperreactivity.[35] This explanation for the inverse relationship between HAV infection and the development of allergic asthma was considered rather weak.[36]

VII. Bacteria: Do Exogenous Endotoxins Protect from Asthma?

The most relevant evidence suggesting that bacteria may play a role in protection from allergy relies upon the consistent inverse association between exposure to endotoxins in early life and the risk of developing allergy later in childhood.[37] In Bavarian farming families, where allergies are less frequent,[38] endotoxin concentrations were highest in stables and were also significantly higher in dust from kitchen floors and children's mattresses in households where children had regular contacts with farm animals as compared to control subjects who had no such contacts. It was concluded that environmental exposure to endotoxins and other bacterial wall components is an important protective determinant for the development of atopic diseases in childhood.[40]

In addition, ingestion of unpasteurized milk and exposure to stables accounted for most of the protection against the development of asthma and atopy linked to the farming environment.[40] This is supported by recent data on the inverse association of the concentration of endotoxin in mattresses with atopy, hay fever, allergic asthma, and the production of type 2 cytokines by peripheral blood lymphocytes (PBL) stimulated by staphylococcal enterotoxin β (SEB).[41] Interestingly, nonatopic wheezing was not significantly associated with endotoxin level, further suggesting that a protective effect is exerted on the development of atopy, rather than on the development of bronchial hyperreactivity per se.[41]

Similarly, in Denver, Colorado, low levels of endotoxin in the dust of houses of children with asthma were associated with peripheral blood CD4 T lymphocytes producing IFN and with skin sensitization to common allergens.[42]

VIII. Bacteria: Gut Microflora and Allergy

Exposure to endotoxin should serve as a proxy of exposure to Gram-negative bacteria. However, the gut microflora is by far the most relevant source of Gram-negative bacteria; moreover, it is also conceivable that endotoxins stimulating our immune systems are derived from both endogenous and exogenous bacterial sources.

The first studies in this field suggested a relation of the composition of gut microflora with allergy by describing differences in intestinal microflora composition of infants raised in Estonia, a country with a low prevalence of atopy, compared to microflora of infants raised in Sweden where atopy is much more prevalent.[43] It was then proposed that a persistent "pressure" on the human immune system by bacteria colonizing the gastrointestinal tract may prevent atopic sensitization to airborne allergens.[44]

Indeed, gut microflora enhance host resistance to infections both by limiting intestinal colonization with potential pathogens (bacterial competition) and by priming the immunological defense mechanisms against invading pathogens. The presence of normal microflora in the gut seems to be required for the development of a fully functional immune system.

It was reasoned that the gastrointestinal flora of westernized children may predispose to atopy through one or more of three distinct potential mechanisms: (1) absence of bacteria that suppress atopy; (2) stable predominance of bacteria stimulating atopy; or (3) lower turnover of bacterial species and strains.[45]

A. Absence of Bacteria Suppressing Atopy

Data supporting the first hypothesis derive from studies reporting that allergic 2-year old children were colonized less often by Lactobacilli than non allergic children.[44] In a follow-up study, however, the same group reported that the prevalence of infants with Lactobacilli in the feces during the first year of life was even significantly higher at 1 week of age in children who developed atopic dermatitis and/or positive skin tests in the first 2 years of life,[46] suggesting a lack of protection by Lactobacillus spp. under physiologic conditions.

This inconsistency may put in question the use of Lactobacilli in prevention of allergy. However, daily administration of *Lactobacillus rhamnosus* GG in early life to bottle-fed children or breast-feeding mothers was reported to reduce by 50% the incidence of atopic eczema in the first 2 years of life;[47] some of the limitations of this study are discussed elsewhere.[48]

Studies showing that early exposure to endotoxin is inversely associated with the development of atopy later in life may guide future studies on the role of gut microflora, a major endogenous source of endotoxin. Interestingly, during the 1980s, colonization with *Escherichia coli* in the first week of life occurred in more than 80% of children in Pakistan and only in 40% of children in Sweden.[49] Similarly, over 40% of Italian infants were still not colonized by *E.coli* at 2 months of age (P.M. Matricardi et al., unpublished data).

B. Stable Predominance of Bacteria Stimulating Atopy

The second hypothesis that excessive allergy in westernized populations is determined by a stable predominance of bacteria stimulating atopy may find support from data showing that allergic 2-year old Swedish and Estonian children harbored higher counts of aerobic bacteria, including *Staphylococcus aureus*, than nonallergic controls.[44] Staphylococcal enterotoxins exert a profound immunostimulatory influence and a key role for them in allergy has been proposed.[50] *S. aureus* colonization of skin lesions aggravates atopic eczema. A putative role for the development of allergy by early gut colonization with *S. aureus* is still to be evaluated.

Clostridia have also been found more frequently in allergic children than in nonallergic children.[44] In a subsequent study, the fecal compositions of short chain fatty acids (indicators of colon microflora composition) in allergic and nonallergic 13-month-old infants were evaluated.[51] Allergic subjects had higher levels of i-caproic acid, a marker of colonization by *Clostridium difficile*, and lower levels of propionic, i-butyric, butyric, i-valeric, and valeric acids.[51]

According to the first two hypotheses, atopy may be prevented simply by substituting one colonizing species with another. However, it is evolutionistically unlikely that one single bacterial species has the important task of protecting mammals from atopic diseases. Moreover, translocation through the epithelial barrier and subsequent potent stimulation of the local immune system by a bacterium are only transient and limited to initial colonization phases, and they are soon prevented by an IgA response[52]; otherwise, we probably could not tolerate our own microflora.

C. Lower Turnover of Bacterial Species and Strains

The third hypothesis proposing that a high turnover of bacterial species and strains at the gut level[45] would guarantee that "continuous pressure"[44] on the immune system, essential to prevent atopy, may be considered stronger. Indeed, this hypothesis would have evolutionistic plausibility (attributing an atopy-preventing effect to many different bacterial species) and in principle could explain the "effects" of sibship size and birth order on atopy.[6]

Indeed, cross-infections with new bacterial strains, rather than a specific and stable colonization, are facilitated in large families living a traditional lifestyle. An interesting observation derived from longitudinal studies on the ontogenesis of gut microflora of Swedish and Pakistani infants.[53] After colonization with *E. coli,* Swedish children harbored the same strain for months or years, while Pakistani children underwent high turnover of *E.coli* and other enterobacteria during the first 6 months of life.[53] To test this "turnover" hypothesis, longitudinal studies on the strain turnover rates of several different bacterial species colonizing the gut mucosa in birth cohorts are in progress.

IX. Parasites and Asthma

The relationship of helminths and asthma has been debated since the 1970s and epidemiological studies have led to opposite conclusions on the asthma-protective or -causative role of helminthic infections.[54]

Epidemiologic studies on populations living in temperate areas of developed countries where helminths are not endemic have shown that helminth infection is associated with a higher risk of allergic asthma. For example, occurrences of asthma/recurrent bronchitis and hospitalization due to asthma/recurrent bronchitis were significantly associated with seroprevalence for *Toxocara canis* in Dutch children.[55] German children who were Ascaris–IgE seropositive had higher levels of total IgE, higher prevalence rates of allergen-specific IgE seropositivity, allergic rhinitis, and asthma when compared to Ascaris–IgE seronegative children.[56]

By contrast, epidemiologic studies of populations living in tropical areas of developing countries where helminths are still highly endemic have shown that helminth infection is associated with a low risk of allergic asthma.[57] For example, the prevalence of physician-diagnosed asthma and allergic rhinitis was lower in pinworm-positive compared to uninfested children in Taipei.[58] Specific IgE antibodies to Ascaris and Necator species were less frequent among adult asthmatics compared with a control group of nonasthmatics in Gondar, Ethiopia.[59] The risk of wheeze was reduced by hookworm infection in a population of adults living in Jimma, Ethiopia.[60]

A unifying explanation of this contrasting data proposes that acute, sporadic, and mild helminthic infection typical of temperate areas of developed countries can enhance atopic responses in predisposed individuals, thus facilitating asthma exacerbations. By contrast, chronic and heavy helminth infection typical of poor rural areas of tropical countries would stimulate polyclonal IgE production and also prevent allergic inflammation and allergic asthma by several mechanisms including mast cell saturation and enhanced production of IgG4 blocking antibodies and anti-inflammatory cytokines such as IL-10 and transforming growth factor beta (TGF).[12,61]

The latter mechanism was suggested by the observation that Gabonese school children with urinary schistosomiasis had similar levels of dust mite specific IgE and lower prevalences of positive skin reactions to dust mites than schistosome-free children. The production of IL-10 obtained by incubating peripheral blood mononuclear cells with schistosoma antigens was inversely associated with skin reactivity to mite allergens, suggesting that helminth-induced IL-10 can play a part in counteracting inflammation-mediated allergic diseases.

This study provided insights to the mechanisms by which helminths may sustain IgE responses while preventing damage from the bystander induction of specific IgE responses against common allergens.[62] Interestingly, this model would also explain the apparently conflicting data showing that deworming of asthmatic patients with mild helminth infections is associated with an improvement of asthma,[63] while deworming of patients heavily infected by helminths is associated with enhanced skin reactivity to common allergens and exacerbation of asthmatic symptoms.[64]

The issue of the interaction of helminth infections, allergies, and asthma remains extremely complex. It will be interesting to learn more about the role played by acquisition of helminth infections in protection against allergic asthma conferred by exposure to foodborne and/or orofecal infection and to a traditional farming environment.

X. The Role of NRIs in Preventing and Treating Asthma

The role of bacteria as potential modulators of the immune response against allergens and regulators of allergic inflammation has been investigated frequently. At least five kinds of bacteria or bacterial substances are currently under investigation for their potential atopy-preventing effects (Table 12.1).[65] However, the hygiene hypothesis also remains a subject for further research. We cannot attribute the hypothesis with immediate implications related to prevention and treatment of allergic diseases until most of the questions it originated[66] are answered.

Table 12.1 Categories of Bacterial Products Used against Allergies

1,	Bacterial vaccines
2.	ISS-ODN
3.	Probiotics
4.	LPS derivatives
5.	*Mycobacterium vaccae*

From Matricardi, P.M. et al., Allergy 2003; 58: 461–471. With permission.

XI. Conclusions

Although we continue to learn more about the influence of nonrespiratory infections on asthma, their role in the inception and natural history of this disease must be seen within the framework of airway–respiratory infection interactions, environmental risk factors, and the genetic backgrounds of affected individuals. This framework elicits the complexity of the system we are trying to investigate. Nevertheless, we hope that future studies of the interactions of NRIs and asthma may ultimately open new avenues for preventive and therapeutic strategies based on the safe use of molecules derived from nonrespiratory infectious agents.

References

1. Serafini U and Di Nardo U. Sulla remissione dei sintomi asmatici nel corso di sindromi itteriche. *Gaz Intern Med Chir* 1950; 54: 338–344.
2. Serafini U, De Sanctis C, and Fabiani F. Alcune modificazioni ematiche ed ematochimiche negli asmatici nel corso della febbre provocata. *Clin Nuova* 1964; 2: 43–48.
3. Serafini U. Long-term asthma remission. *Eur J Int Med* 1996; 7: 5–12.
4. Serafini U. Do infections have a protective effect on asthma and atopy? *Allergy* 1997; 52: 955–957.
5. Gerrard JW, Geddes CA, Reggin PL, Gerrard CD, and Horne S. Serum IgE levels in white and Metis communities in Saskatchewan. *Ann Allergy* 1976; 37: 91–100.
6. Strachan DP. Hay fever, hygiene and household size. *Br Med J* 1989; 299: 1259–1260.
7. Strachan DP. Family size, infection and atopy: the first decade of the "hygiene hypothesis." *Thorax* 2000; 55: S2–S10.
8. Romagnani, S. Regulation of the development of type 2 T-helper cells in allergy. *Curr Opin Immunol* 1994; 6: 838–846.
9. Cookson WO and Moffatt MF. Asthma: an epidemic in the absence of infection? *Science* 1997; 275: 41–42.
10. Martinez FD and Holt PG. Role of microbial burden in aetiology of allergy and asthma. *Lancet* 1999; 354: 12–15.
11. Wills-Karp M, Santeliz J, and Karp CL. The germless theory of allergic disease: revisiting the hygiene hypothesis. *Nature Rev Immunol* 2001; 1: 69–75.
12. Yazdanbakhsh M, Kremsner PG, and van Ree R. Allergy, parasites and the hygiene hypothesis. *Science* 2002; 296: 490–494.
13. Matricardi PM and Bonini S. Why is the incidence of asthma increasing? In Johnston SL and Holgate ST, Eds., *Asthma: Critical Debates*. Blackwell Science, Oxford, 2002, pp 3–17.
14. Matricardi PM, Franzinelli F, Franco A, Caprio G, Murru F, Cioffi D, Ferrigno L, Palermo A, Ciccarelli N, and Rosmini F. Sibship size, birth order, and atopy in 11,371 Italian young men. *J Allergy Clin Immunol* 1998; 101: 439–444.

15. Braun-Fahrlander C, Gassner M, Grize L, Neu U, Sennhauser FH, Varonier HS, Vuille JC, and Wuthrich B. Prevalence of hay fever and allergic sensitization in farmers' children and their peers living in the same rural community. *Clin Exp Allergy* 1999; 29: 28–34.
16. Alm JS, Swartz J, Lilja G, Scheynius A, and Pershagen G. Atopy in children with an anthroposophic lifestyle. *Lancet* 1999; 353: 1485–1488.
17. Kramer U, Heinrich J, Wjst M, and Wichmann HE. Age of entry to day nursery and allergy in later childhood. *Lancet* 1999; 353: 450–454.
18. Ball TM, Castro-Rodriguez JA, Griffith KA, Holberg CJ, Martinez FD, and Wright AL. Siblings, day-care attendance, and the risk of asthma and wheezing during childhood. *New Eng J Med* 2000; 343: 538–543.
19. Matricardi PM, Rosmini F, Ferrigno L, Nisini R, Rapicetta M, Chionne P, Stroffolini T, Pasquini P, and D'Amelio R. Cross-sectional retrospective study of prevalence of atopy among Italian military students with antibodies against hepatitis A virus. *Br Med J* 1997; 314: 999–1003.
20. Matricardi PM, Rosmini F, Riondino S, Fortini M, Ferrigno L, Rapicetta M, and Bonini S. Exposure to foodborne and orofecal microbes versus airborne viruses in relation to atopy and allergic asthma: epidemiological study. *Br Med J* 2000; 320: 412–417.
21. Matricardi PM, Rosmini F, Rapicetta M, Gasbarrini G, and Stroffolini T. Atopy, hygiene and anthroposophic lifestyle. *Lancet* 1999; 354: 430.
22. The International Study of Asthma and Allergies in Childhood (ISAAC) Steering Committee. Worldwide variation in prevalence of symptoms of asthma, allergic rhinoconjunctivitis, and atopic eczema. *Lancet* 1998; 351: 1225–1232.
23. Platts-Mills TAE, Woodfolk JA, and Sporik RB. The increase in asthma cannot be ascribed to cleanliness. *Am J Resp Crit Care Med* 2001; 164: 1107–1108.
24. Matricardi PM, Bouygue GR, and Tripodi S. Inner-city asthma and the hygiene hypothesis. *Ann Allergy Asthma Immunol* 2002; 89: 69–74.
25. Matricardi PM and Bonini S. Mimicking microbial "education" of the immune system: a strategy to revert the epidemic trend of atopy and allergic asthma? *Respir Res* 2001; 1: 129–132.
26. Matricardi PM, Rosmini F, Panetta V, Ferrigno L, Bonini S. Hay fever and asthma in relation to markers of infection in the United States. *J Allergy Clin Immunol* 2002; 110: 381–387.
27. Ninan TK and Russell G. Respiratory symptoms and atopy in Aberdeen schoolchildren: evidence from two surveys 25 years apart. *Br Med J* 1992; 304: 873–875.
28. Omran M and Russel G. Continuing increase in respiratory symptoms and atopy in Aberdeen schoolchildren. *Br Med J* 1996; 312: 334.
29. Von Mutius E, Martinez FD, Fritzsch C, Nicolai T, Roell G, and Thiemann HH. Prevalence of asthma and atopy in two areas of West and East Germany. *Am J Respir Crit Care Med* 1994; 149: 358–364.
30. Upton MN, McConnachie A, McSharry C, Hart CL, Davey Smith G, Gillis CR, and Watt GC. Intergenerational 20 year trends in the prevalence of asthma and hay fever in adults: the Midspan family study surveys of parents and offspring. *Br Med J* 2000; 321: 88–92.

31. Woolcock AJ and Peat JK. Evidence for the increase of asthma worldwide. *Ciba Found Symp* 1997; 206: 122–139.
32. Nakagomi T, Itaya H, Tominaga T, Yamaki M, Hisamatsu S, and Nakagomi O. Is atopy increasing? *Lancet* 1994; 343: 121–122.
33. Bach JF. The effect of infections on susceptibility to autoimmune and allergic diseases. *New Eng J Med* 2002; 347: 911–920.
34. Holgate ST. Science, medicine, and the future: allergic disorders. *Br Med J* 2000; 320: 231–234.
35. McIntire JJ, Umetsu SE, Akbari O, Potter M, Kuchroo VK, Barsh GS, Freeman GJ, Umetsu DT, and DeKruyff RH. Identification of Tapr (an airway hyperreactivity regulatory locus) and the linked TIM gene family. *Nature Immunol* 2001; 2: 1109–1116.
36. Wills-Karp M. Asthma genetics: not for the TIMid? *Nature Immunol* 2001; 2: 1095–1096.
37. Von Mutius E. Environmental factors influencing the development and progression of pediatric asthma. *J Allergy Clin Immunol* 2002; 109: S525–S532.
38. Von Ehrenstein OS, von Mutius E, Illi S, Baumann L, Bohm O, and von Kries R. Reduced risk of hay fever and asthma among children of farmers. *Clin Exp Allergy* 2000; 30: 187–193.
39. Von Mutius E, Braun-Fahrlander C, Schierl R, Riedler J, Ehlermann S, Maisch S, Waser M, and Nowak D. Exposure to endotoxin or other bacterial components might protect against the development of atopy. *Clin Exp Allergy* 2000; 30: 1230–1234.
40. Riedler J, Braun-Fahrländer C, Eder W, Schreuer M, Waser M, Maisch S, Carr D, Schierl R, Nowak D, and von Mutius E. Exposure to farming in early life and development of asthma and allergy: a cross-sectional survey. *Lancet* 2001; 358: 1129–1132.
41. Braun-Fahrlander C, Riedler J, Herz U, Eder W, Waser M, Grize L, Maisch S, Carr D, Gerlach F, Bufe A, Lauener RP, Schierl R, Renz H, Nowak D, and von Mutius E. Environmental exposure to endotoxin and its relation to asthma in school-age children. *New Engl J Med* 2002; 347: 869–877.
42. Gereda JE, Leung DYM, Thatayatikom A, Streib JE, Price MR, Klinnert MD, and Liu AH. Relation between house-dust endotoxin exposure, type 1 T-cell development, and allergen sensitisation in infants at high risk of asthma. *Lancet* 2000; 355: 1680–1683.
43. Sepp E, Julge K, Vasar M, Naaber P, Bjorksten B, and Mikelsaar M. Intestinal microflora of Estonian and Swedish infants. *Acta Pediatr* 1997; 86: 956–961.
44. Bjorksten B, Naaber P, Sepp E, and Mikelsaar M. The intestinal microflora in allergic Estonian and Swedish 2-year-old children. *Clin Exp Allergy* 1999; 29: 342–346.
45. Wold AE. The hygiene hypothesis revised: is the rising frequency of allergy due to changes in the intestinal flora? *Allergy* 1998; 53S46: 20–25.
46. Bjorksten B, Sepp E, Julge K, Voor T, and Mikelsaar M. Allergy development and the intestinal microflora during the first year of life. *J Allergy Clin Immunol* 2001; 108: 516–520.

47. Kalliomaki M, Salminen S, Arvilommi H, Kero P, Koskinen P, and Isolauri E. Probiotics in primary prevention of atopic disease: a randomised placebo-controlled trial. *Lancet* 2001; 357: 1076–1079.

48. Matricardi PM. Probiotics against allergy: data, doubts, and perspectives. *Allergy* 2002; 57: 185–187.

49. Adlerberth I, Carlsson B, De Man P, Jalil F, Khan SR, Larsson P, Mellander L, Svanborg C, Wold AE, and Hanson LA. Intestinal colonization with enterobacteriaceae in Pakistani and Swedish hospital-delivered infants. *Acta Paediatr Scand* 1991; 80: 602–610.

50. Bachert C, Gevaert P, and Van Cauwenberge P. *Staphylococcus aureus* enterotoxins: a key in allergic diseases? *Allergy* 2002; 57: 480–487.

51. Bottcher MF, Nordin EK, Sandin A, Midtvedt T, and Bjorksten B. Microflora-associated characteristics in faeces from allergic and nonallergic infants. *Clin Exp Allergy* 2000; 30: 1590–1596.

52. Shroff KE, Meslin K, and Cebra JJ. Commensal enteric bacteria engender a self-limiting humoral mucosal immune response while permanently colonizing the gut. *Infect Immun* 1995; 63: 3904–3913.

53. Adlerberth I, Jalil F, Carlsson B, Mellander L, Hanson LA, Jalil F, Khalil K, and Wold AE. High turnover rate of *Escherichia coli* strains in the intestinal flora of infants in Pakistan. *Epidemiol Infect* 1998; 121: 587–598.

54. Weiss ST. Parasites and asthma/allergy: what is the relationship? *J Allergy Clin Immunol* 2000; 105: 205–210.

55. Buijs J, Borsboom G, van Gemund JJ, Hazebroek A, van Dongen PA, van Knapen F, and Neijens HJ. Toxocara seroprevalence in 5-year-old elementary schoolchildren: relation with allergic asthma. *Am J Epidemiol* 1994; 140: 839–847.

56. Dold S, Heinrich J, Wichmann HE, and Wjst M. Ascaris-specific IgE and allergic sensitization in a cohort of school children in the former East Germany. *J Allergy Clin Immunol* 1998; 102: 414–420.

57. Masters S and Barrett-Connor E. Parasites and asthma: predictive or protective? *Epidemiol Rev* 1985; 7: 49–58.

58. Huang SL, Tsai PF, and Yeh YF. Negative association of Enterobius infestation with asthma and rhinitis in primary school children in Taipei. *Clin Exp Allergy* 2002; 32: 1029–1032.

59. Selassie FG, Stevens RH, Cullinan P, Pritchard D, Jones M, Harris J, Ayres JG, and Newman-Taylor AJ. Total and specific IgE (house dust mite and intestinal helminths) in asthmatics and controls from Gondar, Ethiopia. *Clin Exp Allergy* 2000; 30: 356–358.

60. Scrivener S, Yemaneberhan H, Zebenigus M, Tilahun D, Girma S, Ali S, McElroy P, Custovic A, Woodcock A, Pritchard D, Venn A, and Britton J. Independent effects of intestinal parasite infection and domestic allergen exposure on risk of wheeze in Ethiopia: a nested case-control study. *Lancet* 2001; 358: 1493–1499.

61. Cooper PJ. Can intestinal helminth infections (geohelminths) affect the development and expression of asthma and allergic disease? *Clin Exp Immunol* 2002; 128: 398–404.

62. van den Biggelaar AH, van Ree R, Rodrigues LC, Lell B, Deelder AM, Kremsner PG, and Yazdanbakhsh M. Decreased atopy in children infected with *Schistosoma haematobium*: a role for parasite-induced interleukin-10. *Lancet* 2000; 356: 1723–1727.
63. Lynch NR, Hagel I, Perez M, Di Prisco M, Lopez R, and Alvarez N. Effect of antihelminthic treatment on the allergic reactivity of children in a tropical slum. *J Allergy Clin Immunol* 1993; 92: 404–411.
64. Lynch NR, Palenque M, Hagel I, and Di Prisco MC. Clinical improvement of asthma after anthelminthic treatment in a tropical situation. *Am J Respir Crit Care Med* 1997; 156: 50–54.
65. Matricardi PM, Bjorksten B, Bonini S, Bousquet J, Djukanovic R, Dreborg S, Gereda J, Malling HJ, Popov T, Raz E, and Wold A. Microbial products in allergy prevention and therapy: EAACI position paper. *Allergy* 2003; 58; 461–471.

13

Antibiotics as Risk Factors in the Development of Asthma

BENGT BJÖRKSTÉN

Karolinska Institutet
Stockholm, Sweden

I. Introduction

The normal ontogeny of the immune responses to allergens depends on appropriate antigenic stimulation early in life. Microbes in our environment, particularly the gut microflora, play a pivotal role in this process and may thus affect the development of allergic asthma. Furthermore, infections may serve as both causative and protective factors with regard to the development of asthma, depending on the circumstances and type of asthma, i.e., atopic and nonatopic asthma. The fact that host–microbe interactions apparently are important for the development of asthma has raised interest in the potential influence of antibiotics in this process. In this chapter, the possible role of antibiotics early in life as risk factors for the development of asthma and other allergic diseases will be discussed. The use of antibiotics in the treatment of asthma lies beyond the scope of the review.

II. Epidemiological Studies

A. Antibiotics in Infancy

In 1998, Farooqi and Hopkin, in a retrospective analysis, investigated the putative relationship between childhood infections and atopic diseases in over 1900 children and young adults, aged 12 to 21 years.[1] Treatment with antibiotics in the first 2 years of life was found to be significantly associated with subsequent atopic disease with an odds ratio (OR) of 2.07 [95% confidence interval (CI) 1.64–2.60]. The association was even stronger for asthma (OR 3.19; 95% CI 2.43–4.18). The authors cautioned for possible confounders and reverse causation because the study was retrospective and the outcome was based on clinical diagnosis only in a single general practice comprising ten family doctors.

The study is important, however, as the authors analyzed the effects of different types of antibiotics given during the first years of life and the indications for treatment. They found a statistically significant association between antibiotic treatment of a range of infections in the first year of life and subsequent atopic disorders. The relationship was not limited to treatment of upper and lower respiratory infections, but was also noted for urinary tract infections, for example. Importantly, the association was more marked for treatment with broad-spectrum antibiotics, i.e., cephalosporins and macrolides, while no such trend was observed for infections treated with penicillin.

The findings were similar for other outcomes, such as the use of antiasthmatic compounds at age 5, including β2 agonists, bronchial disodium cromoglycate, and corticosteroid preparations. Furthermore, heredity for allergy did not affect the results. The association between treatment with antibiotics and subsequent development of asthma or other atopic disorders was limited to treatment with broad-spectrum antibiotics in the first and second years of life, and increased with the number of antibiotic courses received in the first 2 years of life. Thus, treatment with broad-spectrum antibiotics after age 2 did not seem to be associated with any particularly increased risk for atopic disease.

Several authors subsequently assessed the possibility that antibiotics may be risk factors for the development of asthma and other allergies and the results are slightly conflicting (Table 13.1). In a study from New Zealand, antibiotic use during the first year of life was significantly associated with histories of asthma in 5- to 10-year-old children (OR 4.05; 95% CI 1.55–10.59).[2]

In contrast, the use of antibiotics after the first year was only associated with a slightly increased risk for asthma that did not reach statistical significance (OR 1.64; 95% CI 0.60–4.46). Although unknown lifestyle factors and other biases may have influenced the findings, a greater than seven-fold risk of symptoms was observed when antibiotic use in the first year of life preceded the development of symptoms. This would argue against attributing the increased risk to antibiotics prescribed in response to episodes of wheezy bronchitis that

Table 13.1 Studies of Antibiotic (ab) Treatment Early in Life as a Putative Risk Factor for Asthma and Other Allergy

Study	Design	Increased Risk for Disease
Infancy		
Farooqi and Hopkin[1]	Retrospective	Yes, broad-spectrum ab
Wickens et al.[2]	Retrospective	Yes
Droste et al.[3]	Retrospective	Yes
McKeever et al.[4]	Retrospective	Yes, broad-spectrum ab
Ponsonby et al.[6]	Prospective	No
Celedon et al.[7]	Prospective	No
Pregnancy		
Benn et al.[9]	Prospective	Yes
McKeever et al.[5]	Prospective	Yes, if more than once

could be forerunners of asthma. The study also supported the initial observation that the first year or two of life may be particularly important.

Droste et al. investigated the association between the use of antibiotics in the first year of life and subsequent development of asthma and other allergic diseases in a population-based sample of 1200 7- and 8-year-old children.[3] Antibiotic treatment was associated with asthma (OR 1.7; 95% CI 1.0–3.1) and hay fever (OR 2.3; 95% CI 1.3–3.8) and weakly with eczema; no significant relationship with skin test positivity was noted. The associations with asthma and hay fever were particularly obvious in children with parental hay fever, i.e., with family histories of allergy.

In a large retrospective study comprising 24,700 children, McKeever et al. analyzed exposure to antibiotics both early in life[4] and prenatally.[5] All infections and antibiotic usage after birth were recorded at 6-month intervals and the results were related to incident diagnoses of asthma and wheeze, eczema, and hay fever up to a mean follow-up time of 2.9 years (range 2 to 11 years). Usage of penicillin was not associated with any increased risk for disease. An association was noted between asthma and previous treatment with amoxicillin, macrolides, and cephalosporins, with statistically significant odds ratios of 1.25 to 1.44 and a slightly increasing odds ratio with increasing numbers of prescriptions of antibiotics.

The authors concluded that exposure to antibiotics during infancy was associated with an increased risk of developing allergic disease, but the effects were small and could be explained to a large extent by frequency of consulting physicians.

The relationship of antibiotic use in the first year of life with asthma, allergic rhinitis, and eczema has also been assessed in two prospective studies. Ponsonby et al. followed 863 children from birth.[6] Data were collected through parental interviews when the infants were 1 and 3 months old and then at 7 years.

Antibiotic use during the first 3 months of life was not associated with subsequent development of either asthma or hay fever.

The second prospective study comprised 488 children. Telephone interviews were conducted every 2 months during the first year of their lives, and then every 6 months until they reached 5 years of age.[7] No significant association between antibiotic use in the first year of life and having one or more atopic diseases at age 5 years was noted. In this carefully conducted study, a number of potential confounding factors were considered and several analytic models were tested. No objective markers of allergy were employed, however, and the type of antibiotic given was not considered. Furthermore, the statistical power of the study was limited, as only 90 children developed at least one of the three atopic diseases and of these only 30 had not received any antibiotics.

Epidemiological studies could in a more indirect way suggest that antibiotic treatment may be a risk factor for asthma. In a Swedish study, a low prevalence of allergic diseases was observed among children living in an anthroposophic community.[8] Since the use of antibiotics in the community was very restricted, the findings were suggested to indicate antibiotics as risk factors for allergy development. However, there are many other differences in environmental exposures that are characteristic for anthroposophic communities, e.g., fewer vaccinations and, particularly important, as noted below, high intakes of fermented foods.

B. Antibiotic Treatment during Pregnancy

Exposure to antibiotic treatment before birth has been suggested in two studies as a risk factor for the development of asthma and other allergic diseases. In a population-based cohort comprising 3000 children and their mothers, the use of antibiotics in pregnancy was associated with a modest increase in asthma, as defined by usage of antiasthmatic medication during the fifth year of life in the children (OR 1.7; 95% CI 1.1–2.6).[9]

A similar independent association between usage of antiasthmatic medication by the children and the presence of Staphylococci in the maternal vaginal flora during pregnancy was noted (OR, 2.2; 95% CI 1.4–3.4). These bacteria are not part of the normal vaginal flora normally dominated by lactic acid bacteria. The findings are interesting, as the vaginal flora is the first microbial environment with which an infant comes into contact during the birth process and thus has an impact on postnatal colonization.

In the large British study of 24,700 children discussed in the previous section,[4] a number of perinatal exposures were also related to the incidence of asthma, eczema, and hay fever.[5] More than two courses of antibiotics during pregnancy were associated with increased risks for asthma in the children (OR 1.68; 95% CI 1.51–1.87) and similar significant associations were present for eczema and hay fever. Although a range of intrauterine infections was also associated with increased risk of developing allergic disease, the association was smaller than for antibiotic treatment alone.

C. Lessons from Epidemiological Studies

None of the epidemiological studies of a possible relationship between antibiotic treatment and subsequent development of asthma and other allergies was conclusive and the results may appear conflicting. Most of the postnatal studies were designed to analyze the putative role of infections early in life and were not particularly focused on antibiotic usage. Thus, antibiotic use was treated more as a marker and modifier of infection than as a risk factor. In recent years, however, interest has focused more on the possible modifying role of microbial products on the developing immune system than on respiratory infections per se.[10,11]

Antibiotics vary with regard to the effects on microbial ecology in the gut. While penicillin does not affect gut microbiota, nor does it inhibit endotoxin-producing microorganisms, antibiotics with broader antimicrobial spectra may profoundly affect the gut flora and are often deadly to Gram-negative bacteria.

As discussed in the following section, the establishment of a microbial gut flora in the neonatal period and infancy is a dynamic process that may have long-term consequences also for the development of immune regulation and tolerance.[12,13] In order to study any relationship between antibiotic treatment early in life and subsequently developing asthma and other allergies, the effects of broad-spectrum antibiotics should be separated from those of regular penicillin and other antibiotics with narrow antimicrobial spectra. This was done in only two of the published studies.[1,4] In both studies, the use of broad-spectrum antibiotics was associated with development of asthma and allergy, while penicillin was not.

It is reasonable to suspect that atopic individuals, particularly those who develop asthma, may be more likely to have suffered from wheezing early in life and as a consequence be more likely to have used antibiotics. Recall bias is another possible confounder in that parents of an asthmatic child may be more likely to remember infections that required antibiotics. For these reasons, retrospective studies are problematic, particularly since any observed relationships between previous antibiotics usage and current asthma are rather weak, with odds ratios around or below two. Unfortunately, several studies reported have been retrospective and only two were prospective. Furthermore, the diagnoses were mostly based on questionnaires or telephone interviews. In the only study in which allergy was verified, no association between antibiotic usage and skin prick test positivity was noted.[3]

A third area of concern when interpreting the results of published epidemiological studies is the fact that any effect of antibiotics on subsequently developing disease would be expected to be more related to IgE-mediated allergy than to symptoms such as wheeze or rhinitis that can also be triggered by nonallergic mechanisms. According to the hypothesis that microbial pressure stimulates the maturation of the immune system and enhances tolerance induction,[11,14] any negative effects of antibiotics would be expected to be particularly obvious for IgE-mediated symptoms. On the other hand, it is common knowledge that wheezing and asthma attacks may be triggered by infections, which could confound any inverse relationship between antibiotic treatment and asthma development. Thus, any effect on allergy may be obscured on questionnaire surveys that ask only about symptoms.

III. Aspects of Microbial Ecology

The biological and medical communities increasingly realize that the microflora of the large gut may play important roles in human health and disease. The perspective of the human colon in health and disease is by no means a new concept. Elie Metchnikoff, a Russian scientist, indicated the clinical importance of host colonic microflora a century ago. He also suggested that certain live microorganisms might promote health.

Despite this, only modest interest in this concept was exhibited among researchers for many years, and only during the past 10 years has microbial ecology again become a major research area. It is now generally accepted that the bacterial microflora of the human gut is an integral component of the host defense system and may provide a primary signal for driving the postnatal maturation of the immune system and the induction of a balanced immunity.[13]

Because microorganisms have been present throughout the evolution of humans, evolution has taken place in close interaction with the microbial environment. There is mounting evidence that commensal microbes acquired during the early postnatal period are required for the development of tolerance both to themselves and to other antigens.[12] For example, Th2-mediated immune responses are not susceptible to oral tolerance induction in germ-free mice.[15] Oral tolerance was induced after the introduction of components of normal microflora in that study.

The gastrointestinal tract of a newborn baby is sterile. Soon after birth, however, it is colonized by numerous types of microorganisms.[16] Colonization is complete after approximately 1 week, but the numbers and species of bacteria fluctuate markedly during the first 3 months of life. Interactions between bacteria and their hosts can be viewed in terms of a continuum of symbiosis, commensalism, and pathogenicity.[13]

The mammalian intestinal epithelium effectively performs its physiological functions in a microbe-rich environment, while the microbes thrive amid efficient host defenses.[17] Thus, a continuous interaction constituting a dynamic ecosystem occurs between the microbial flora and the host. Once established, it is surprisingly stable under normal conditions. Environmental changes such as periods of treatments with antibiotics change the composition of the microflora only temporarily.

It is recognized that interaction with microbes, especially the normal microbial flora of the gastrointestinal tract, is the principal environmental signal for postnatal maturation of T cell function (in particular the Th1 component).[11] Recognition of these signals is mediated by a series of TOLL-like receptors expressed on cells of the innate immune system and other receptors such as CD14, and it is noteworthy that a polymorphism in the CD14 gene has recently been associated with high IgE levels.[18]

Rook and Stanford suggested two major syndromes that could be the results of inadequate microbial stimulation early in life.[14] One is the inadequate priming of T helper cells, leading to an incorrect cytokine balance. The second suggestion was a failure to fine-tune the T cell repertoire in relation to epitopes that are cross-reactive between self and microorganisms. The authors coined the expressions "input deprivation syndrome" and "uneducated T cell regulation syndrome." Their hypothesis could be supported by comparative global studies showing that allergies, type I diabetes, and celiac disease are associated with a "Western life style."[19] Thus, modern society is associated with increasing incidences of diseases considered to be mediated by both Th- and Th2-type immune mechanisms.

Over the past few years, differences have been documented in the composition of the intestinal microflora between healthy infants in countries with low and high prevalences of allergy[20–22] and between allergic and nonallergic infants in both environments.[20–24] These studies indicate that imbalances in the gut flora and differences in indigenous intestinal flora may affect the development and priming of the immune system in early childhood. This in turn could affect the risk for allergy. The fact that differences are present before any clinically manifest disease[10,24] would indicate that the differences between allergic and nonallergic children are not secondary phenomena. Although all the studies conducted to date confirm differences in the composition of the gut flora, no particular protective or potentially harmful bacterial species can yet be identified. This is not surprising because of the enormous number of microbial strains and the complicated ecology of the gut flora.

It is reasonable to suspect that broad-spectrum antibiotics given early in life could affect the establishment of normal gut microbiota. This in turn could theoretically affect the development of normal immune tolerance and other regulatory mechanisms. The putative mechanistic relationship between antibiotic treatment early in life and development of asthma remains speculative, however, as the composition of the normal gut flora is still largely unknown and no experimental studies have proven the concept.

IV. Concluding Remarks

Although it remains to be proven that antibiotics given early in life are risk factors for the development of asthma and other allergic diseases and all Koch's postulates have not been met, it is reasonable to suspect that there is a relationship. Although the epidemiological studies conducted to date are slightly contradictory, studies in which broad-spectrum antibiotics were assessed separately from antibiotics with narrow antimicrobial spectra indicate a modestly increased risk for asthma development after treatment with the former compounds. No animal experiments in which the role of antibiotics was studied directly were reported.

Such studies are complicated, as they would have to be done under gnotobiotic conditions, as any affects of antibiotics on allergy development would likely be mediated indirectly by altering microbial ecology and, furthermore, the composition of the normal gut microbiota is largely unknown. A relationship between antibiotic usage early in life and subsequent development of asthma and other allergies is suggested, however, by epidemiological observations and by the existence of a reasonable mechanism showing how antibiotics may become risk factors for allergy development. Further studies are needed to confirm or refute a relationship, however, and the role of broad-spectrum antibiotics affecting the ecology of the gut microbiota also should be assessed. In the meantime, it is reasonable to consider the possible moderately increased risk for development of asthma and allergy when antibiotics are prescribed to infants.

References

1. Farooqi IS and Hopkin JM. Early childhood infection and atopic disorder. *Thorax* 1998; 53: 927–932.
2. Wickens K, Pearce N, Crane J, and Beasley R. Antibiotic use in early childhood and the development of asthma. *Clin Exp Allergy* 1999; 29: 766–771.
3. Droste JH, Wieringa MH, Weyler JJ, Nelen VJ, Vermeire PA, and Van Bever HP. Does the use of antibiotics in early childhood increase the risk of asthma and allergic disease? *Clin Exp Allergy* 2000; 30: 1547–1553.
4. McKeever TM, Lewis SA, Smith C, Collins J, Heatlie H, Frischer M, and Hubbard R. Early exposure to infections and antibiotics and the incidence of allergic disease: a birth cohort study with the West Midlands General Practice Research Database. *J Allergy Clin Immunol* 2002; 109: 43–50.
5. McKeever TM, Lewis SA, Smith C, and Hubbard R. The importance of prenatal exposures on the development of allergic disease: a birth cohort study using the West Midlands General Practice Database. *Am J Respir Crit Care Med* 2002; 166: 827–832.
6. Ponsonby AL, Couper D, Dwyer T, Carmichael A, and Kemp A. Relationship between early life respiratory illness, family size over time, and the development of asthma and hay fever: a seven-year follow up study. *Thorax* 1999; 54: 664–669.

7. Celedon JC, Litonjua AA, Ryan L, Weiss ST, and Gold DR. Lack of association between antibiotic use in the first year of life and asthma, allergic rhinitis, or eczema at age 5 years. *Am J Respir Crit Care Med* 2002; 166: 72–75.
8. Alm JS, Swartz J, Lilja G, Scheynius A, and Pershagen G. Atopy in children of families with an anthroposophic lifestyle. *Lancet* 1999; 353: 1485–1488.
9. Benn CS, Thorsen P, Jensen JS et al. Maternal vaginal microflora during pregnancy and the risk of asthma hospitalization and use of antiasthma medication in early childhood. *J Allergy Clin Immunol* 2002; 110: 72–77.
10. Björkstén B, Sepp E, Julge K, Voor T, and Mikelsaar M. Allergy development and the intestinal microflora during the first year of life. *J Allergy Clin Immunol* 2001; 108: 516–520.
11. Holt PG, Sly PD, and Björkstén B. Atopic versus infectious diseases in childhood: a question of balance? *Pediatr Allergy Immunol* 1997; 8: 53–58.
12. Brandzaeg P. Development of the mucosal immune system in humans, in *Recent Developments in Infant Nutrition*. Bindels J, Goedhart A, and Visser H, Eds. London: Kluwer Academic Publishers, 1996, pp. 349–376.
13. Hooper L and Gordon J. Commensal host–bacterial relationships in the gut. *Science* 2001; 292: 1115–1118.
14. Rook GA and Stanford JL. Give us this day our daily germs. *Immunol Today* 1998; 19: 113–116.
15. Sudo N, Sawamura S, Tanaka K, Aiba Y, Kubo C, and Koga Y. The requirement of intestinal bacterial flora for the development of an IgE production system fully susceptible to oral tolerance induction. *J Immunol* 1997; 159: 1739–1745.
16. Mevissen-Verhage EA, Marcelis JH, Harmsen-van Amerongen WC, de Vos NM, Berkel J, and Verhoef J. Effect of iron on neonatal gut flora during the first week of life. *Eur J Clin Microbiol* 1985; 4: 14–18.
17. Neish AS. The gut microflora and intestinal epithelial cells: a continuing dialogue. *Microbes Infect* 2002; 4: 309–317.
18. Baldini M, Lohman I, Halonen M, Erickson R, Holt P, and Martinez F. A polymorphism in the 5′ flanking region of the CD14 gene is associated with circulating soluble CD14 levels with total serum IgE. *Am J Resp Cell Mol Biol* 1999; 20: 976–983.
19. Stene LC and Nafstad P. Relation between occurrence of type 1 diabetes and asthma. *Lancet* 2001; 357: 607–608.
20. Adlerberth I, Jalil F, Carlsson B et al. High turnover rate of *Escherichia coli* strains in the intestinal flora of infants in Pakistan. *Epidemiol Infect* 1998; 121: 587–598.
21. Sepp E, Julge K, Vasar M, Naaber P, Bjorksten B, and Mikelsaar M. Intestinal microflora of Estonian and Swedish infants. *Acta Paediatr* 1997; 86: 956–961.
22. Björkstén B, Naaber P, Sepp E, and Mikelsaar M. The intestinal microflora in allergic Estonian and Swedish two-year-old children. *Clin Exp Allergy* 1999; 29: 342–346.
23. Böttcher MF, Nordin EK, Sandin A, Midtvedt T, and Björkstén B. Microflora-associated characteristics in faeces from allergic and nonallergic infants. *Clin Exp Allergy* 2000; 30: 1590–1596.
24. Kalliomäki M, Kirjavainen P, Eerola E, Kero P, Salminen S, and Isolauri E. Distinct patterns of neonatal gut microflora in infants in whom atopy was and was not developing. *J Allergy Clin Immunol* 2001; 107: 129–134.

14

The Atopic March

U. WAHN, R. NICKEL,
C. GRÜBER, S. LAU

Charité-Humboldt University Berlin
Berlin, Germany

S. ILLI

Dr. v. Haunersches Kinderspital
Munich, Germany

I. Introduction and Definition

Atopic diseases such as hay fever, asthma, and eczema are allergic conditions that tend to cluster in families and are associated with the production of specific IgE antibodies to common environmental allergens. The process of sensitization may or may not be associated with the induction of clinical symptoms which alone are characterized by inflammation, corresponding to hyperresponsiveness of skin or mucous membranes.

The term "atopic march" refers to the natural history of atopic manifestations, characterized by a typical sequence of IgE antibody responses and clinical symptoms that appear during a certain age period, persist over years and decades, and often show a tendency for spontaneous remission with age.

II. Assessment of Determinants

In order to identify potential modifiable determinants, epidemiological studies on the development of atopic diseases have received much attention over the past decade.

Cross-sectional studies such as the International Study of Asthma and Allergies in Children (ISAAC) have provided evidence for remarkable differences in the prevalences of certain atopic phenotypes including asthma in children aged 6 and 13 years on continents, in countries, and even within countries.[1,2]

Repeated cross-sectional studies using standard questionnaires and in some studies objective measures of bronchial hyperresponsiveness (BHR) and atopy suggest that the prevalence of some of these phenotypes in defined age groups is increasing and the increase is only in part attributed to changes in public awareness and diagnostic habits.[3,4]

Longitudinal follow-up studies including birth cohorts such as the Children's Respiratory Study in Tucson and the Multicenter Allergy Study in Germany have been designed to clarify the natural history of the disease, describe associations between phenotypes and genetic, environmental, or lifestyle factors, and generate hypotheses for causal relationships.[5–7]

A few **intervention studies** assessing the roles of various environmental factors have been conducted in the United Kingdom, Germany, the Netherlands, Canada, and Australia.[8] A hierarchy of evidence may be extracted from differently designed studies. As far as causal inferences are concerned:

1. Cross-sectional surveys and case control studies can generate hypotheses; in cases of consistent findings across numerous studies, they can suggest causal relationships, particularly if dose response patterns can be observed.
2. Prospective longitudinal cohort studies without intervention are more suggestive in describing a time sequence between potential risk factors and health effects.
3. Controlled longitudinal intervention studies, if applicable and acceptable, provide the most useful information.

One of the important messages from the epidemiological data available to date is that it is obviously meaningful to disentangle various atopic phenotypes and focus on single manifestations in certain age windows because different specific phenotypes (clinical symptoms, sensitization, total serum IgE, and other factors at a certain age) may be induced or modulated by different genetic, environmental or lifestyle factors in various ways (Table 14.1). It is obvious that a prerequisite for any intervention aimed at the prevention of atopic manifestations is the identification of nongenetic determinants such as exposure to environmental,

Table 14.1   Atopic Phenotypes in Childhood

Atopic dermatitis
Seasonal allergic rhinoconjunctivitis
Bronchial hyperresponsiveness
Recurrent wheeze
Elevated concentrations of allergen-specific IgE in serum
Blood eosinophilia
Skin test reactivity to specific allergens
Food allergy
Elevated serum IgE

food-, or lifestyle-related factors that are modifiable on an individual basis or result from public health measures.

III. Natural History of Atopic Manifestations

Although wide individual variations may be observed, atopic diseases tend to be related to the first decades of life, and thereby to the maturation of the immune system. In general, no clinical symptoms are detectable at birth. Although the production of IgE starts in the 11th week of gestation, no specific sensitization to food or inhalant allergens as measured by elevated serum IgE antibodies can be detected in cord blood via standard methods. Early findings describing elevated cord blood IgE concentrations as a predictor for clinical manifestations of atopy could not be confirmed.[9]

Total serum IgE concentrations after birth increase with age and show distribution over a wide range. The 95th percentile achieved by Caucasian children at the age of 1 year is 80 kU/L; it is around 400 kU/L at the age of 6 years (Figure 14.1).

The earliest IgE responses directed to food proteins, particularly to hen's egg and cow's milk, may be observed during the first months of life. Even in completely breast-fed infants, high amounts of specific serum IgE antibodies to hen's egg can be detected. It has been proposed that exposure to hen egg proteins occurs via mother's milk, but this needs further clarification.

Sensitization of humans to environmental allergens from indoor and outdoor sources requires more time and is generally observed between the first and tenth years of life. The annual incidence of early sensitization depends on the amount of exposure. In a longitudinal birth cohort study in Germany (MAS-90), a dose response relationship could be shown between early exposure to cat and mite allergens and the risk of sensitization during the first years of life (Figure 14.2). It has recently been demonstrated that strong infantile IgE antibody

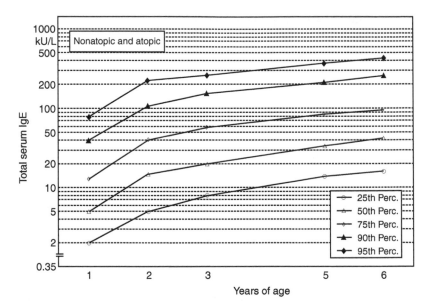

Figure 14.1   Percentiles of total serum IgE in children from 1 to 6 years of age.

responses to food proteins have to be considered as markers for atopic reactivity in general and are predictors of subsequent sensitization to aeroallergens.[10,11]

Regarding clinical symptoms, atopic dermatitis is generally the first manifestation with the highest incidence during the first 3 months of life and the highest period prevalence during the first 3 years (Figure 14.3). Seasonal allergic rhinoconjunctivitis is generally not observed during the first 2 years of life, although a minority of children will develop specific IgE antibodies during this early period. Obviously, two seasons of pollen allergen exposure are required before a classical seasonal allergic rhinoconjunctivitis with typical symptoms in association with specific serum IgE antibodies becomes manifest. Prevalence before the end of the first decade in children is around 15% in Central Europe.

Asthmatic wheezing may be observed during early infancy. The majority of early wheezers turn out to be transiently symptomatic, whereas a minority may continue to wheeze throughout school age and adolescence. Our understanding of the natural history of childhood asthma is limited and several data sets support the existence of various asthma subtypes in childhood. During the first 3 years of life, the manifestation of wheeze is not related to elevated serum IgE levels or specific sensitization. A positive parental history of atopy and asthma seems to be of minor importance during the first 2 years of life. Those who have persistent wheezing show an association with early sensitization to food and

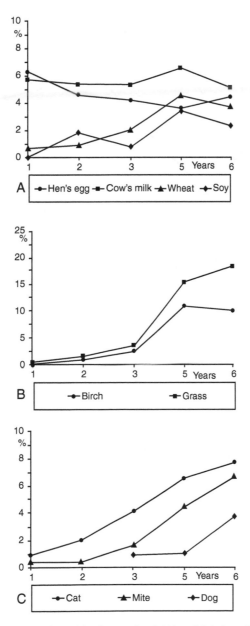

Figure 14.2 Prevalence of sensitization to food (A) and inhalant (B and C) allergens by 6 years of age. Cut-off level 0.7 kU/L (CAP Class 2).

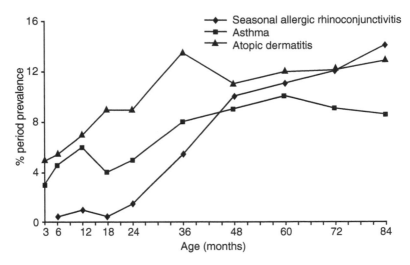

Figure 14.3 Development of atopic dermatitis, asthma, and allergic rhinoconjunctivitis versus age. Data from German Multicenter Atopy Study.

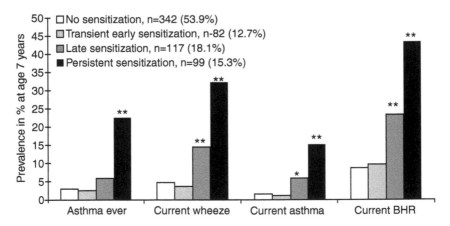

Figure 14.4 Prevalences of asthma and asthmatic symptoms at the age of 7 years, stratified for sensitization patterns. * p <0.05. ** p <0.0001 compared to no sensitization.

subsequent sensitization to aeroallergens (Figure 14.4).[10,11,18] In addition, the association with a positive family history for atopy and asthma in first degree relatives becomes more and more obvious (Figure 14.5).

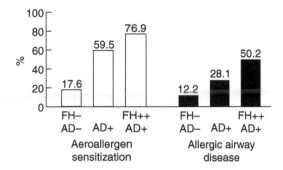

Figure 14.5 Percentage of children with aeroallergen sensitization or manifestation of allergic airway disease at age 5 years according to risk constellation in infancy. AD+/AD– = infants with AD versus infants with AD in first 3 months of life. FH++/FH– = infants with at least two atopic family members or no atopy in their families.

IV. Hereditary Factors

We have known for many years that atopic diseases run in families. The risk of neonates to develop atopic symptoms during the first two decades of life strongly depends on the manifestations of the disease in their parents and siblings. It is already obvious at the phenotype level that there is a closer association between specific symptoms like asthma or atopic dermatitis in the child and the same manifestation in parents or siblings than with other atopic manifestations in the family. These clinical observations suggest the presence of phenotype-specific genes.

During the last two decades, molecular genetic studies have been performed for various allergic diseases including asthma.[13–17] Two approaches have been applied to identify genes related to disease:

1. Positional cloning in which the entire genome is screened using a panel of polymorphic DNA markers. This approach attempts to demonstrate genetic linkages of certain phenotypes and genetic markers of known chromosomal localization.
2. Examination of candidate genes already known to be involved in the pathophysiology contributing to a certain phenotype. The role of candidate genes may be assessed by defining polymorphisms within the respective genes and testing for associations with the disease.

A variety of markers on specific chromosomal regions have been found to be linked to either atopic dermatitis or asthma, whereas other regions seem to be linked to several atopic phenotypes. If genetic studies turn out to be fruitful, they may contribute to the identification of candidates for primary prevention measures and individuals who may respond to certain therapeutic interventions in the future.

V. Nongenetic Factors

During the last two decades, two general hypotheses have been proposed in the literature in connection with the observed increases of atopy and asthma in childhood. New risk factors that were not known several decades ago have become relevant in connection with nutrition, environmental exposure, and lifestyle. Protective factors related to a more traditional lifestyle common in the past have been lost, and this led to greater susceptibility to atopic diseases.

A. Domestic Environment

1. Allergen Exposure

No other environmental factor has been studied as extensively as exposure to environmental allergens as a potential risk for sensitization and manifestation of atopy and asthma. From a number of cross-sectional studies performed in children and in adults, it has become obvious that there is a close association between allergen exposure, particularly in the domestic environment, and sensitization to that specific allergen.[19–20] Longitudinal studies like the MAS study in Germany have clearly demonstrated that during the first years of life there is a dose-response relationship between indoor allergen exposure to dust mite and cat allergens and the risk of sensitization to cat and mites, respectively (Figure 14.6).[25]

As far as the manifestations of atopic dermatitis and asthma are concerned, the situation is much less clear. Early studies performed by Sporik et al. suggested that exposure of sensitized children to dust mite allergens not only determines the risk of asthma, but also the time of onset of the disease.[21] More recent investigations by the same group, however, suggest that other factors besides allergen exposure are important in determining which children develop asthma.[22]

In a comprehensive meta-analysis, Peat[23] evaluated several environmental factors said to be responsible for the incidence and severity of atopic diseases, particularly asthma. Comparing the strengths of the various effects, she concluded that on the basis of the literature, indoor allergen exposure is the environmental component with by far the strongest impact on the manifestation of asthma. In recent years, however, the paradigm that exposure induces asthma with airway inflammation via sensitization has been challenged. In several countries, the prevalence of asthma in children has been increasing independent of allergen exposure.[24]

Data sets obtained from the MAS birth cohort suggest that while domestic allergen exposure is a strong determinant for early sensitization in childhood, it

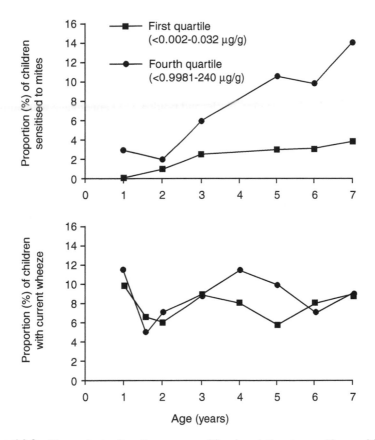

Figure 14.6 House dust mite allergen exposition in relation to specific sensitization and prevalence of weezing at ages 1 through 7 years.[25]

cannot be considered a primary cause of airway hyperresponsiveness or asthmatic symptoms.[25]

A number of intervention studies to examine the effects of indoor allergen elimination on the incidence of asthma are currently being performed in cohorts followed prospectively from birth. The results will have strong impacts on public health policies because they will determine whether considering indoor allergen elimination an important element of primary prevention of various atopic manifestations is meaningful. Even if the result is that other factors play major parts in determining whether an atopic child will develop asthma, so that allergen elimination as a measure of primary prevention is inefficient, a reduction of allergen exposure will still remain a very important element in secondary prevention.

2. Exposure to Endotoxins

The role of endotoxin exposure as a possible element of atopy prevention in early life has recently been discussed. Endotoxins are a family of molecules called lipopolysaccharides (LPS) and are intrinsic parts of the outer membranes of Gram-negative bacteria. LPS and other bacterial wall components that are found abundantly in stables where pigs, cattle, and poultry are kept engage with antigen-presenting cells via CD14 ligation to induce strong interleukin (IL)-12 responses. IL-12, in turn, is regarded as an obligatory signal for the maturation of naïve T cells into TH1 type cells. Endotoxin concentrations were recently found to be highest in stables of farming families and also in dust samples from kitchen floors and mattresses in rural areas in Southern Germany and Switzerland. These findings support the hypothesis that environmental exposure to endotoxins and other bacterial wall components is an important protective determinant related to development of atopic diseases.[26] Indeed, endotoxin levels in samples of dust from children's mattresses were found to be inversely related to the occurrence of hay fever, atopic asthma, and atopic sensitization.[27]

3. Can Early Exposure to Infections Be Protective?

One hypothesis that attracted the most interest is that a decline in certain childhood infections or a lack of exposure to infectious agents during the first years of life associated with smaller families in the middle class environments of industrialized countries may be causal for the recent epidemic in atopic disease and asthma.[28–34] Although this hypothesis is obviously very complex, several pieces of information appear to support it.

Studies from several countries provide indirect evidence for the hypothesis that early exposure to viral infections, although triggering lower airway symptoms during early life, may exert long-lasting protective effects. Children born into families with several, particularly older, siblings, have been found to have reduced risk of allergic sensitization and asthma at school age. Studies in children who attended day care centers during infancy support this concept.

Infections are known to produce long-lasting nonspecific systemic effects on the nature of the immune response to antigens and allergens. For example, recovery from natural measles infection reduces the incidence of atopy and allergic responses to house dust mites to half the rate seen in vaccinated children. Obviously, the fact that certain infections induce a systemic and nonspecific switch to Th1 activities may be responsible for inhibiting the development of atopy during childhood.[35]

Prenatal or perinatal bacterial infections should also be taken into account as potential modulators of the atopic march. Preterm birth in many cases is understood to be a result of bacterial infections during pregnancy. The observation that infants with very low birth weights have lower prevalences of atopic eczema and atopic sensitization could therefore fit this hypothesis.[36]

Although these observations on the relationship of immune responses to infectious agents, atopic sensitization, and disease expression are stimulating and challenging, conclusions regarding the relevance of the atopic march should be drawn with care. In different parts of the world, completely different infectious agents have been addressed in different study settings. It appears to be fashionable to join Rook and Stanford[37] who, in a recent review article in *Immunology Today* pleaded "give us this day our daily germs" — which germ, at what time, under which circumstances, and at what price to be paid?

4. Pollutants and Tobacco Smoke as Adjuvant Factors

Several environmental factors attracted the interest of epidemiologists and experimental researchers. Although they do not serve as allergens, these factors are capable of up-regulating existing IgE responses or leading to disease manifestation or aggravation of symptoms. After guinea pig and mouse experiments suggested an increase of allergic sensitization to ovalbumin after experimental exposure to traffic- or industry-related pollutants,[38] a strong association between allergic rhinitis caused by cedar pollen allergy and exposure to heavy traffic was reported from Japan.[39,40]

Important sociodemographic confounders turned out to be problems in interpreting study results. Other investigators were unable to describe any relationship between traffic exposure and the prevalence of hay fever or asthma.[41] The role of tobacco smoke, a complex mixture of various particles and organic compounds, was studied extensively.[42,43] Recently reviewed studies[44,45] consistently demonstrate that the risk of lower airway diseases such as bronchitis, recurrent wheezing in infants, and pneumonia is increased. Whether passive tobacco smoke exposure is causally related to the development of asthma is still disputed.

Until recently, data about the risk of sensitization has been lacking. The prospective birth cohort MAS in Germany reported that increased risks of sensitization were found only in children whose mothers smoked up to the end of their pregnancies and continued to smoke after birth. In this subgroup of the cohort, a significantly increased sensitization rate of IgE antibodies to food proteins, particularly to hen's eggs and cow's milk, was observed only during infancy. Later sensitization rates were no different from those of children who had never been exposed to tobacco smoke. These observations may be related to the fact that the highest urinary cotinine concentrations in children are detected during the first years of life, when the children spend most of their time close to their mothers.[46]

B. Lifestyle and Development of Atopic Disease

1. *Socioeconomic Status and Anthroposophic Lifestyle*

Taking into account that the risk of atopic sensitization and disease manifestation early in life is particularly high in industrialized Western countries, and that within these countries concomitant variations in the socioeconomic status and the prevalence of atopy are evident, the question arises as to what factor related to Western lifestyle may be responsible for increasing the susceptibility to atopic sensitization?

In a recent Swedish study, the prevalence of atopy in children from anthroposophic families was lower than in children from other types of families. This led the authors to the conclusion that lifestyle factors associated with anthroposophy may lessen the risk of atopy in childhood.[47] Several studies focusing on differences between the former socialist countries and Western European societies reported lower prevalence rates for atopy in the Eastern bloc countries. The differences were particularly striking in areas with few genetic differences such as East and West Germany[48] where it was found that the critical period during which lifestyle mainly influences the development of atopy is probably the first years of life.[29] These observations point in the same direction as studies reporting lower prevalence rates for children born into families that have few siblings.[49]

Recent observations from Germany suggest that within the population of an industrialized country with a Western lifestyle, high socioeconomic status must be considered a risk factor for early sensitization and the manifestations of atopic dermatitis and allergic airway disease.[50,51] Turkish migrants living in Germany exhibited higher prevalences of atopy and asthma after cultural assimilation.[52]

Intestinal microflora may well be the major source of microbial stimulation of the immune system in early childhood.[53-56] The intestinal microflora may enhance Th1-type responses. The results of a comparative study of Estonian and Swedish children demonstrated differences in intestinal microflora. In Estonia, the typical microflora included more lactobacilli and fewer clostridia organisms that are associated with a lower presence of atopic disease.[57]

Intervention studies are needed to demonstrate the relevance of these findings and examine the effects of adding probiotics to infant formulas. In one recently published study from Finland, which unfortunately was not blinded, infants with milk allergy and atopic dermatitis exhibited milder symptoms and fewer markers of intestinal inflammation if their milk formulae were fortified with lactobacilli.[58]

Observations from Japan[59] suggesting that positive tuberculin responses in children predict a lower incidence of asthma, lower serum IgE levels, and cytokine profiles biased toward a Th1 type were supported by animal experiments demonstrating that IgE responses to ovalbumin in mice could be down-regulated by a previous infection with Bacterium Calmette Guerin (BCG).[60,61] Cohort studies from Europe were unable to describe a protective effect of BCG vaccination.[62,63]

Few reports have described an association between the use of antibiotics during the first 2 years of life and increased risks of asthma. It seems too early to draw final conclusions from these publications. Immunizations appear not to influence the risk of early sensitization or development of atopy. Pediatricians therefore should resist questioning successful immunization programs such as those targeting measles.

2. Lifestyle-Related Factors

Obviously, a long list of lifestyle-related factors possibly associated with the apparent allergy and asthma epidemic of the 21st century may have relevance to the atopic march in children. Obesity is a recently proposed factor because studies in the United States associated it with certain types of childhood asthma.[64,65] If obesity and asthma really are associated, the question still remains whether asthma causes obesity or vice versa. Or is it possible both can be explained by a common cause such as lack of physical activity ?

Finally, the hypothesis has been raised that the use of dietary omega-3 versus omega-6 fatty acids in certain populations may be responsible for increased risk of allergic inflammation. Both hypotheses deserve attention, but at this stage preventive advice should not be based on them.

VI. Issues Related to Prevention

It is obvious that in many industrialized countries, the observed increase in prevalence of atopy and asthma has become a serious public health issue. If preventive intervention is to be effective, it should be applied early in life, most probably in early infancy. Unfortunately, our understanding of the natural history of the processes of atopic sensitization, atopic dermatitis, and allergic airway disease is still very limited. The evaluation of risk factors and determinants is a necessary prerequisite for any effective intervention.

A. Primary Prevention

Measures for primary prevention are aimed at a health population that is at risk of the disease. Unfortunately, all predictors investigated to date are insufficient in sensitivity and specificity. Therefore it seems mandatory to recommend possible preventive measures only if they (1) are applicable to the entire population; (2) present no risk; and (3) have low cost.

Although the extent of a preventive effect of breast feeding remains controversial, several other beneficial aspects of breast feeding justify the recommendation for at least 4 months of exclusive breast feeding. If breast milk is not sufficiently available during the first 3 or 4 days, water is recommended. Solid foods should be introduced to the diet after the fourth month. Avoidance of exposure to tobacco smoke should be guaranteed, particularly during pregnancy and infancy. Since children with positive family histories of atopy in first-degree relatives have been shown to be more susceptible for allergic sensitization and the manifestations of atopy and asthma, additional measures for primary prevention have been studied during the last decade for this so called high-risk group.

Most studies aimed at prevention during pregnancy indicate that there is no real evidence for a protective effect of any maternal exclusion diet during that time. The effect of maternal avoidance of potential food allergens (milk, eggs, and fish) during the breast feeding period appears marginal at best. If maternal breast milk is not sufficient, the use of hydrolyzed formulas for atopy prevention has been extensively studied. Some studies indicate that extensively hydrolyzed formulae in combination with avoidance of cow milk proteins and solid foods for at least 4 months in children with positive family histories of atopy produce some preventive effect, but this is related to the avoided food proteins and cannot be considered as a long-lasting method of preventing atopic manifestations of the skin or the airways in general.[66] Extensively and partially hydrolyzed formulae with moderately reduced allergenicity were investigated in a large randomized prospective study (German Infant Nutrition Intervention Study). Compared to standard infant formulae, hydrolysate feeding resulted in a reduction of incidence of atopic dermatitis in infancy.[67]

The introduction of complementary food during the first 4 months of life has been associated with higher risks of atopic dermatitis. It is still not clear how much the risk for atopic sensitization and disease manifestation may be decreased by dietary intervention in early infancy. The majority of studies seem to indicate that the effects are transient and that the development of asthma later in childhood will not be prevented. Since maternal smoking during pregnancy is significantly associated with reduced respiratory function, recurrent wheezing in infancy and early childhood, and the risk of developing IgE responses to food proteins early in life, smoking should be avoided in any case.

B. Secondary Prevention

Measures for secondary prevention are aimed at children who have not yet developed a definite phenotype like allergic airway manifestation, but have developed markers indicating a high risk of subsequent disease manifestation. With regard to atopy, children with positive family histories for asthma who have developed atopic dermatitis or sensitization to food protein in infancy must be considered candidates for secondary prevention. A reduction of indoor allergen exposure by introducing mattress encasings, eliminating wall-to-wall carpets, avoiding damp housing conditions by increasing ventilation, and avoiding furred pets at home has been demonstrated to be a meaningful intervention for secondary prevention.[68]

In young children with atopic dermatitis and positive family histories for atopy, pharmacological intervention with cetirizine led to a significant reduction in the incidence of asthma in a subgroup that developed early sensitization to grass pollen or house dust mites by the second year of life.[69] Before this type of intervention can be recommended generally, confirmatory studies are necessary.

Allergen-specific immunotherapy — demonstrated to be effective for the treatment of seasonal allergic rhinitis — has recently been investigated in young children. The cohort was followed prospectively over a period of 3 years. The early intervention was shown not only to reduce seasonal symptoms of the upper airways, but also reduce the incidence of seasonal asthma.[70]

VII. Conclusion

The increasing prevalence of atopic diseases, particularly atopy-associated asthma, has become a major challenge for allergists and public health authorities in many countries. The understanding of the natural history of the atopic march, including the determinants that are modifiable and may become candidates for preventive intervention, is still very limited. Information provided by cross-sectional studies can only generate hypotheses that must be supported by prospective longitudinal cohort studies. Ultimately, the results of well controlled intervention studies will identify which nutritional, environmental, or lifestyle-related factors should be considered for early intervention that might be useful to reverse the current epidemiological trends.

References

1. International Study of Asthma and Allergies in Childhood (ISAAC) Steering Committee. Worldwide variation in prevalence of symptoms of asthma, allergic rhinoconjunctivitis, and atopic eczema. *Lancet* 1998; 351: 1225–1232.
2. ISAAC Steering Committee. Worldwide variations in the prevalence of asthma symptoms. *Eur Respir J* 1998; 12: 31; 5–335.
3. Burr ML, Butland BK, King S, and Vaughan-Williams E. Changes in asthma prevalence: two surveys 15 years apart. *Arch Dis Child* 1989; 64: 1452–1456.
4. Aberg N, Hesselmar B, Aberg B, and Eriksson B. Increase of asthma, allergic rhinitis and eczema in Swedish schoolchildren between 1979 and 1991. *Clin Exp Allergy* 1995; 25: 815–819.
5. Martinez, FD, Wright AL, Taussig LM, Holberg CJ, Halonen, M, and Morgan WJ. Asthma and wheezing in the first six years of life. *New Engl J Med* 1995, 332; 133–138.
6. Wahn U, Lau S, Bergmann R, Kulig M, Forster J, Bergmann K, Bauer C-P, and Guggenmoos-Holzmann I. Indoor allergen exposure is a risk factor for sensitization during the first three years of life. *J. Allergy Clin Immunol* 1997; 99: 763–769.

7. Bergmann RL, Bergmann KE, Lau-Schadendorf S, and Wahn U. Atopic diseases in infancy: German multicenter atopy study (MAS-90). *Pediatr Allergy Immunol* 1994; 5 (Suppl 1):19–25.

8. Arshad SH, Matthews S, Gant C, and Hide DW. Effect of allergen avoidance on development of allergic disorders in infancy. *Lancet* 1992; 339: 1439–1497.

9. Edenharter G, Bergmann RL, Bergmann KE, Wahn V, Forster J, Zepp F, Wahn U. Cord blood IgE as risk factor and predictor for atopic diseases. *Clin Exp Allergy* 1998; 28: 671–678.

10. Kulig M, Bergmann R, Klettke U, Wahn V, Tacke U, Wahn U and Multicenter Allergy Study Group. Natural course of sensitization to food and inhalant allergens during the first 6 years of life. *J Allergy Clin Immunol* 1999; 103: 1173–1179.

11. Nickel R, Kulig M, Forster J, Bergmann R, Bauer CP, Lau S, Guggenmoos-Holzmann I, and Wahn U. Sensitization to hen's egg at the age of 12 months is predictive for allergic sensitization to common indoor and outdoor allergens at the age of 3 years. *J Allergy Clin Immunol* 1997; 99: 613–617.

12. Illi S, Mutius EV, Bergmann R, Niggemann B, Sommerfeld C, Wahn U, and Multicenter Allergy Study Group. Early childhood infectious diseases and the development of asthma up to school age: a birth cohort study. *Br Med J* 2001; 322: 390–395.

13. Cookson WOCM, Sharp PA, Faux JA, and Hopkin JM. Linkage between immunoglobulin E responses underlying asthma and rhinitis and chromosome 11q. *Lancet* 1989; i: 1292–1295.

14. Shirakawa TS, Li A, Dubowitz M, Dekker JW, Shaw AE, Faux JA, Ra C, Cookson WOCM, and Hopkin JM. Association between atopy and variants of the subunit of the high-affinity immunglobulin E receptor. *Nat Genet* 1994; 7: 125–129.

15. Nickel R, Wahn U, Hizawa N, Maestri N, Duffy DL, Barnes KC, Beyer K, Forster J, Bergmann R, Zepp F, Wahn V, and Marsh DG. Evidence for linkage of chromosome 12q15-q24.1 markers to high total serum IgE concentrations in children of the German Multicenter Atopy Study. *Genomics* 1997; 46: 159–162.

16. Moffatt MF and Cookson WOCM. Gene Identification in asthma and allergy. *Int Arch Allergy Immunol* 1998; 116: 247–252.

17. Martinez FD. Complexities of the genetics of asthma. *Am J Repir Crit Care Med* 1997; 156: 117–122.

18. Sherrill D, Stein R. Kurzius-Spencer M, and Martinez F. On early sensitization to allergens and development of respiratory symptoms. *Clin Exp Allergy* 1999; 29: 905–911.

19. Mahmic A, Tovey ER, Molloy CA, and Young L. House dust mite allergen exposure in infancy. *Clin Exp Allergy* 1998; 28: 1487–1492.

20. Lau S, Falkenhorst G, Weber A et al. High mite-allergen exposure increases the risk of sensitization in atopic children and young adults. *J Allergy Clin Immunol* 1989; 84: 718–725.

21. Sporik R, Holgate ST, Platts-Mills TAE et al. Exposure to house-dust mite allergen (Der p I) and the development of asthma in childhood: a prospective study. *New Engl J Med* 1990; 323: 502–507.

22. Sporik R, Squillace SP, Ingram JM, Rakes G, Honsinger RW, and Platts-Mills ThAE. Mite, cat and cockroach exposure, allergen sensitisation, and asthma in children: a case-control study of three schools. *Thorax* 1999; 54: 675–608.

23. Peat JK and Li J. Reversing the trend: reducing the prevalence of asthma. *J. Allergy Clin Immunol* 1999; 103: 1–10.
24. Ingram JM, Sporik R, Rose G, Honsinger R, Chapman MD, and Platts-Mills TA. Quantitative assessment of exposure to dog (Can f1) and cat (Fel d1) allergens: relation to sensitization and asthma among children living in Los Alamos, New Mexico. *J Allergy Clin Immunol* 1995; 96: 449–456.
25. Lau S, Illi S, Sommerfeld C, Niggemann B, Bergmann R, von Mutius E, Wahn U, and Multicenter Allergy Study Group. Early exposure to house-dust mite and cat allergens and development of childhood asthma: a cohort study. *Lancet* 2000; 356: 1392–1397.
26. Mutius E v, Braun-Fahrländer C, Schierl R, Riedler J, Ehlermann S, Maisch S, Waser M, and Nowak D. Exposure to endotoxin or other bacterial components might protect against the development of atopy. *Clin Exp Allergy* 2000; 30: 1230–1234.
27. Braun-Fährländer, Riedler J, Herz U, Eder W, Waser M, Grize L, Maisch S, Carr D, Gerlach F, Nowak D, and Mutius VE for the Allergy and Endotoxin Study Team. Environmental exposure to endotoxin and its relation to asthma in school-age children. *New Engl J Med* 2002: 347: 869–877.
28. Strachan DP. Allergy and family size: a riddle worth solving. *Clin Exp Allergy* 1997; 27: 235–236.
29. Krämer U, Heinrich J, Wjst M, and Wichmann HE. Age of entry to day nursery and allergy in later childhood. *Lancet* 1999; 353: 450–454.
30. Farooqi IS and Hopkin JM. Early childhood infection and atopic disorder. *Thorax* 1998; 53: 927–932.
31. Shaheen SO, Aaby P, Hall AJ et al. Measles and atopy in Guinea-Bissau. *Lancet* 1996; 347: 1792–1796.
32. Matricardi PM, Rosmini F, Ferrigno L et al. Cross-sectional retrospective study of prevalence of atopy among Italian military students with antibodies against hepatitis A virus. *Br Med J* 1997; 314: 999–1003.
33. Bach, J-F. Effect of infections on susceptibility to autoimmune and allergic diseases. *New Engl J Med* 2002; 347: 911–920.
34. Umetsu D T, McIntire J J, Akbari O, Macaubas C, and DeKruyff R, Asthma: an epidemic of dysregulated immunity. *Nature Immunol* 2002; 3: 715–720.
35. Cookson WOCM and Moffatt MF. Asthma: an epidemic in the absence of infection? *Science* 1997; 275: 41–42.
36. Bührer Chr, Grimmer I, Niggemann B, and Obladen M. Low 1-year prevalence of atopic eczema in very low birthweight infants. *Lancet* 1999; 353: 1674.
37. Rook GAW and Stanford JL: Give us this day our daily germs. *Immunol Today* 1999; 19: 113–117.
38. Riedel F, Krämer M, Scheibenbogen C, and Rieger CHL. Effects of SO_2 exposure on allergic sensitization in the guinea pig. *J Allergy Clin Immunol* 1988; 82: 527–534.
39. Muranaka M, Suzuki S, Koizumi K, Takafuji S, Miyamoto T, Ikemori R, and Tokiwa H. Adjuvant activity of diesel-exhaust particulates for the production of IgE antibody in mice. *J Allergy Clin Immunol* 1986; 77: 616–623.
40. Ishizaki T, Koizumi K, Ikemori R, Ishyama Y, and Kushibiki E. Studies of prevalence of Japanese cedar pollenosis among the residents in a densely cultivated area. *Ann Allergy* 1987; 58: 265.270.

41. Waldron G, Pottle B, and Dod J. Asthma and the motorways: one district's experience. *J Publ Health Med* 1995; 17: 85–89.
42. Tager IB, Ngo L, and Hanrahan JP. Maternal smoking during pregnancy: effects on lung function during the first 18 months of life. *Am J Repir Crit Care Med* 1995; 152: 977–983.
43. Stick SM, Burton PR, Gurrin L, Sly PD, and LeSouef PN. Effects of maternal smoking during pregnancy and a family history of asthma on respiratory function in newborn infants. *Lancet* 1996; 348: 1060–1064.
44. Strachan DP and Cook DG. Health effects of passive smoking. 5. Parental smoking and allergic sensitization in children. *Thorax* 1998; 53: 117–123.
45. Strachan DP and Cook, DG. Health effects of passive smoking. 6. Parental smoking and childhood asthma: longitudinal and case-control studies. *Thorax* 1998; 53: 204–212.
46. Kulig M, Luck W, Lau S, Niggemann B, Bergmann R, Klettke U, Guggenmoos-Holzmann I, Wahn U, and Multicenter Asthma Study Group. Effect of pre-and postnatal tobacco smoke exposure on specific sensitization to food and inhalant allergens during the first 3 years of life. *Allergy* 1999; 54: 220–228.
47. Alm JS, Swartz J, Lilja G, Scheyius A, and Pershagen G. Atopy in children of families with an anthroposophic lifestyle. *Lancet* 1999; 353: 1485–1488.
48. Von Mutius E, Martinez FD, Fritsch C et al. Prevalence of asthma and atopy in two areas of West and East Germany. *Am J Respir Crit Care Med* 1994; 149: 358–364.
49. Mutius E v, Martinez FD, Fritsch C et al. Skin test reactivity and number of siblings. *Br Med J* 1994; 308: 692–695.
50. Heinrich J, Popescu MA, Wjst M, Goldstein IF, and Wichmann HE. Atopy in children and parental social class. *Am J Public Health* 1998; 88: 1319–1324.
51. Bergmann RL, Edenharter G, Bergmann KG, Lau S, and Wahn U. Socioeconomic status is a risk factor for allergy in parents but not in their children. *Clin Exp Allergy* 2000; 30: 1740–1745.
52. Grüber C, Illi S, Plieth A, Sommerfeld C, and Wahn U. Cultural adaptation is associated with atopy and wheezing among children of Turkish origin living in Germany. *Clin Exp Allergy* 2002; 32: 526–531.
53. Björksten B. Allergy priming in early life. *Lancet* 1999; 353: 167–168.
54. Johansson ML, Molin G, Jeppsson B, Nobaek S, Ahrne S, and Bengmark S. Administration of different Lactobacillus strains in fermented oatmeal soup: *in vivo* colonization of human intestinal mucosa and effect on the indigenous flora. *Appl Environ Microbiol* 1993; 59: 15–20.
55. Shida K, Makino K, Morishita A et al. *Lactobacillus casei* inhibits antigen-induced IgE secretion through regulation of cytokine production in murine splenocyte cultures. *Int Arch Allergy Immunol* 1998; 115: 278–287.
56. Murosaki S, Yamamoto Y, Ito K et al. Heat-killed *Lactobacillus plantarum* L-137 suppresses naturally fed antigen-specific IgE production by stimulation of IL-12 production. *J Allergy Clin Immunol* 1998; 102: 57–64.
57. Sepp E, Julge K, Vasar M, Naaber P, Björksten B, and Mikelsaar M. Intestinal microflora of Estonian and Swedish infants. *Acta Paediatr* 1997; 86: 956–961.

58. Majamaa H and Isolauri E. Probiotics: a novel approach in the management of food allergy. *J Allergy Clin Immunol* 1997; 99: 179–185.
59. Shirakawa T, Enomoto T, Shimazu S, and Hopkin JM. The inverse association between tuberculin responses and atopic disorder. *Science* 1997; 275: 77–79.
60. Herz U, Gerhold K, Grüber C, Braun A, Wahn U, Renz H, and Paul K. BCG infection suppresses allergic sensitization and development of increased airway reactivity in an animal model. *J Allergy Clin Immol* 1998; 102: 867–874.
61. Erb JK, Holloway JW, Sobeck A, Heidrun M, and Le Gros G. Infection of mice with BCG suppresses antigen-induced airway eosinophilia. *J Exp Med* 1998; 187: 561–569.
62. Grüber C, Meinschmidt G., Bergmann R, Wahn U, and Stark K. Is early BCG vaccination associated with less atopic disease? An epidemiological study in German preschool children with different ethnic backgrounds. *Pediatr Allergy Immunol* 2002; 13: 177–181.
63. Grüber C and Paul KP. Tuberculin reactivity and allergy. *Allergy* 2002; 57: 277–280.
64. Shaheen SO. Obesity and asthma: a cause for concern? *Clin Exp Allergy* 1998; 29: 291–293.
65. Luder E. Melnik TA. DiMaio M. Association of being overweight with greater asthma symptoms in inner city black and Hispanic children. *J Pediatrics* 1998; 132: 699–703.
66. Zeiger RS, Heller S, Mellon MH, Forsythe AG, O'Connor RD, Hamburger RN, and Schatz M. Effect of combined maternal and infant food-allergen avoidance on development of atopy in early infancy: a randomized study. *J Allergy Clin Immunol* 1989; 84: 72–89.
67. Berg VA, Koletzko S., Grübl, A, Filipiak-Pittroff B, Wichmann H-E, Bauer C P, Reinhardt D, and Berdel D. Effect of hydrolyzed cow's milk formula for allergy prevention in the first year of life: German Infant Nutritional Intervention Study (GINI), a randomized double-blind trial. *J Allergy Clin Immunol* 2003; 111: 467–470.
68. Elnert B, Lau-Schadendorf S, Weber A et al. Reducing domestic exposure to dust mite allergen reduces bronchial hyperreactivity in sensitive children with asthma. *J Allergy Clin Immunol* 1992; 90: 135–138.
69. ETAC Study Group. Allergic factors associated with the development of asthma and the influence of cetirizine in a double-blind, randomised, placebo-controlled trial: first results. *Pediatr Allergy Immunol* 1998; 9: 116–124.
70. Möller Ch, Dreborg St, Ferdousi H, Halken S, Host A, Jacobsen L, Koivikko A, Koller D, Niggemann B, Norberg L, Urbanek R, Valovirta E, and Wahn U. Pollen immunotherapy reduces the development of asthma in children with seasonal rhinoconjunctivitis (PAT Study) *J Allergy Clin Immunol* 2002; 109: 251–265.

15

Stress and Asthma

ROSALIND J. WRIGHT

Brigham and Women's Hospital
and Harvard Medical School
Boston, Massachusetts, U.S.A.

I. Introduction

Scholarly references about the importance of emotional and psychological processes in asthma expression date back to antiquity and include those put forth in
a treatise on asthma by Maimonides, an influential medieval rabbi, philosopher,
and physician in the 12th century.[1] In a medical text that served as the cornerstone
of medical teaching in the late 19th century, Sir William Osler referred to asthma
as "a neurotic affection."[2] Indeed, asthma had long been considered among the
disorders believed to be "purely" psychogenic in origin and was commonly called
asthma nervosa. Early research suggesting that asthma had a psychosomatic
component was strongly dominated by psychoanalytic theory.[3,4] Concurrently,
learning theorists argued that particular emotional experiences reinforced pulmonary physiologic responses, increasing the likelihood of their recurring in the
same context.[5]

Purely psychoanalytic and behavioral formulations eventually gave way to
physiological studies providing more objective support for the idea that emotions
play an important role in asthma. Stress and psychological factors have been
associated with asthma symptomatology[6] and with bronchoconstriction and

reduction in pulmonary flow rates in asthmatic children[7] and adults.[8] When subjected to stressful experiences such as performing mental arithmetic tasks,[9] watching emotionally charged films,[10] and listening to stressful interactions,[11] 15 to 30% of asthmatics respond with increased bronchoconstriction.

Clinical studies demonstrating the efficacies of alternative modalities that reduce stress and alter mood states in treating asthmatics add further support to the hypothesized link of stress and asthma.[12,13] Evidence evolved over the past two decades of important interactions among behavioral, neural, endocrine, and immune processes provides fresh insight into means through which psychosocial stressors may influence the development and expression of inflammatory diseases.[14–17] Collectively, these data led to an integrative paradigm that reconsiders the overlap of biological determinants and psychosocial factors in understanding the rising asthma burden.[18]

To explore potential mechanisms, it is helpful first to consider how environmental and social stressors may influence inflammatory processes in general and second to frame these hypotheses within the current asthma paradigm. This chapter highlights behavioral, neural, endocrine, and immunologic pathways underscoring reciprocal relations that may link psychological factors to both the onset of asthma and exacerbation of established disease. Stress may also affect asthma by influencing the ways children and their families perceive and manage their disease which are not discussed here (for review see Wright et al.[18]). This review of overlapping evidence provides a psychobiological framework that may guide future research priorities.

II. Life Stress Model

A general model of the link between environmental demands as psychological stressors and health has been conceptualized as follows. When confronting environmental demands, an individual cognitively appraises whether an event is threatening or potentially overwhelming to his or her existing coping resources.[14] If environmental demands are found to be taxing or threatening and coping resources are viewed as inadequate, humans perceive themselves as being under stress. This perception is presumed to result in negative emotional states including fear, anger, anxiety, and depression. Changes in behavioral and emotional states that accompany the perception of and the effort to adapt to environmental circumstances are accompanied by complex patterns of neuroendocrine and immunologic changes.[19]

Factors including the type of stressor[19] and the duration and frequency of experienced stress are important determinants of its impact on health.[20] Psychological stress and its biological concomitants can last for a few minutes or for years. Chronicity is to some degree based on the ongoing presence of external stimuli that trigger the stress response, but is also dependent on the long-term success of an individual's coping resources. Events that last a very short time can produce very long-term stress effects and lasting physiological responses thought to be maintained by recurrent "intrusive" thoughts about past events.[20] Variable responses to acute challenges superimposed on chronic stressors may have different implications for disease expression.[21]

III. Asthma Paradigm: Link to Stress

There is an emerging understanding of asthma as a chronic inflammatory process regulated through immune phenomena in which many cells (i.e., mast cells, eosinophils, and T lymphocytes) and associated cytokines play roles. Mechanisms of airway inflammation central to asthma pathophysiology involve a cascade of events that include the release of immunologic mediators triggered by both IgE-dependent and -independent mechanisms. An increasing body of evidence supports the notion that asthma is an epidemic of dysregulated immunity.[22]

The exploration of host and environmental factors that may alter immune expression and potentiate asthma expression is an active area of research. Hormones and neuropeptides released into the circulation when individuals experience stress are thought to be involved in regulating both inflammatory and airway responses.[18,23] Dysregulation of normal homeostatic neural, endocrine, and immunologic mechanisms can occur in the face of chronic stress leading to chronic hyperarousal and/or hyporesponsiveness that may impact asthma expression.

A substantial body of evidence supports the role of complex neural mechanisms and alterations of autonomic nervous system control in the pathophysiology and symptomatology of asthma.[24,25] Autonomic nerves can influence airway caliber and function via effects on airway smooth muscle, bronchial vessels, and mucus glands. Therefore, consideration of recent advances in the field of psychoneuroimmunology — linking psychosocial stress, the central and peripheral nervous system, and alterations in immune and endocrine function — provides plausible biological pathways through which stress may impact asthma expression.

IV. Psychological Stress and Endocrine System

Psychological stressors have been associated with the activation of the sympathetic and adrenomedullary (SAM) system and the hypothalamic–pituitary–adrenocortical (HPA) axis. These systems respond to psychological stress with increased output of adrenaline (epinephrine) and noradrenaline (norepinephrine) from the adrenal medulla.[26] The hormonal responses of the HPA axis have long been thought to represent a nonspecific physiological reaction to excessive stimulation,[27] particularly the emotional arousal associated with appraising situations as stressful.[28]

The hypothalamus produces corticotropin-releasing hormone (CRH) which triggers the anterior pituitary gland to secrete adrenocorticotrophic hormone (ACTH) which, in turn, activates the adrenal cortex to secrete corticosteroids, primarily cortisol in humans (i.e., the so-called generality model). More recent work suggests that negative emotional responses disturb the regulation of the HPA axis system and the SAM; that is, in the face of stress, physiological systems may operate at higher or lower levels than during normal homeostasis. This has been termed allostasis,[28a] a concept that refers to the ability of the body to achieve stability through change.

Immune, metabolic, and neural defensive biological responses important for the short-term response to stress may produce long-term damage if not checked and eventually terminated.[29] The potential detrimental cost of such accommodation to stress has been conceptualized as allostatic load (wear and tear from chronic under- or over-activity of the allostatic system).[29]

For example, relatively pronounced HPA activation is common in depression. Episodes of cortisol secretion are more frequent and of longer duration among depressed than among other psychiatric patients and normal subjects.[30] Shifts in the circadian rhythm of cortisol have also been found among persons in stressful situations.[31] Chronic stress may also induce a state of hyporesponsiveness of the HPA axis whereby cortisol secretion is attenuated, leading to increased secretion of inflammatory cytokines typically counter-regulated by cortisol.

Some populations with post-traumatic stress disorder (PTSD), for example, have lower mean basal plasma cortisol levels throughout the circadian cycle and lower mean 24-hour urinary cortisol excretion.[32] Furthermore, a state of stress-induced HPA hyporesponsiveness has been demonstrated in some research subjects with other inflammatory disorders.[33] A hyporesponsive HPA axis may explain stress-induced exacerbations of asthma in certain subgroups of asthmatics and increased association of asthma with particular psychological states.

Other regulatory pituitary (e.g., corticotropin) and hypothalamic hormones (e.g., [CRH] and arginine vasopressin [AVP]) of the HPA axis exert systemic immunopotentiating and pro-inflammatory effects.[26] Theoharides and colleagues have shown that acute psychological stress (immobilization in rats) results in skin mast cell degranulation, an effect inhibited by anti-CRH serum administered prior to stress.[34] Although hormones of the SAM and HPA systems are most often discussed as the biochemical substances involved in stress responses, alterations in a range of other hormones, neurotransmitters, and neuropeptides found in response to stress may also play a part in the health effects of stress. For example, stressor-associated increases in growth hormone and prolactin secreted by the pituitary gland and in the natural opiate beta-endorphins and enkephalins released in the brain are also thought to play a role in immune regulation.[35]

V. Stress and Autonomic Control of Airways

The argument that psychological stress influences autonomic control of the airways is based primarily on the fact that many of the same autonomic mechanisms thought to play a role in asthma are involved in the activation and regulation of physiological responses to stress. These mechanisms include the release of sympathetic nervous system mediators and the action of adrenergic (sympathetic) and cholinergic (parasympathetic) nerves and the neurotransmitters and neuropeptides they produce.

The parasympathetic nervous system innervates the airways via efferent fibers from the vagus nerve and synapses in ganglia in the airway walls with short postsynaptic fibers directly supplying the airway smooth muscles and submucosal glands.[24] Increased activity of the parasympathetic nervous system was once thought to be the dominant mechanism responsible for the exaggerated reflex bronchoconstriction in asthmatic subjects, although more recent work challenges this idea.[36] In the initial phases, narrowing of the airways in asthma is thought to result primarily from inflammation. Current theory holds that bronchial constriction is due to some combination of vagal input plus inflammation, with the relative importance of these factors dependent upon genetic and environmental influences.

Experimental studies in which asthmatic patients are exposed to stressful situations have focused on stress-induced vagal reactivity as a mediator of emotionally induced bronchoconstriction.[6] Preliminary evidence shows that children with asthma who respond to stressful stimuli with high vagal activation (associated with increased cholinergic activity) have greater impairments of airway reactivity in response to methacholine.[10]

Although human airway smooth muscle is not functionally innervated by adrenergic axons, studies have shown adrenergic innervation of submucosal glands, bronchial blood vessels, and airway ganglia.[37] Adrenergic nerves may influence cholinergic neurotransmission via prejunctional α and β receptors.[24] Depending on the type of agonist (beta or alpha) involved, these changes can variably affect airway smooth muscle, release of inflammatory mediators, cholinergic neurotransmission, mucus secretion, and possibly mucociliary clearance, resulting in either bronchodilation or bronchoconstriction. Adrenoceptors are regulated by noradrenaline released locally from sympathetic nerves and by adrenaline and noradrenaline secreted by the adrenal medulla. The regulatory effects of adrenaline and noradrenaline on adrenoceptors suggest a plausible mechanism by which stress-induced activation of the sympathetic nervous system may influence bronchomotor tone.

It seems paradoxical that activation of the sympathetic nervous system by stress, resulting in release of mediators with a beta agonist effect, should relax airway smooth muscle and that acute psychological stress accompanied by a rapid increase in circulating catecholamines consequently causes bronchodilation. The stress-induced response of the autonomic nervous system is more complex and variable. Once the acute stressor is terminated, levels of adrenaline and noradrenaline quickly return to normal or below normal.[38]

The relative strength of sympathetic versus parasympathetic control in response to certain forms of stress differs with the individual, with some showing predominantly parasympathetic responses. Such individuals may be particularly susceptible to stress-induced bronchoconstriction.[6] It is possible that sympathetic activation itself may contribute to asthma symptoms. For example, increases in circulating levels of adrenaline and noradrenaline are known to alter a number of immune parameters that may contribute to inflammation of the airways. Some evidence suggests long-term elevations or potentiation of the catecholamine response with chronic stress.[20]

Prolonged increases in catecholamine levels under chronic stress may also contribute to asthma severity. Chronic daily use of beta agonists by mild to moderate asthmatics with specific genetic predispositions may increase severity by down-regulating beta receptors.[39] It is possible that chronically increased stress-induced catecholamines do the same among genetically susceptible subgroups. In addition, in those with chronic life stresses, the physiological responses to acute stressors may result in more sustained effects on the immune system, even following sympathetic recovery.[21]

Asthmatic subjects have been characterized by beta-adrenergic hyporesponsiveness and alpha-adrenergic and cholinergic hyperresponsiveness.[40] Defects in the functioning of the autonomic nervous system have also been demonstrated in psychological states including depression, PTSD, and psychomotor agitation.[41–43] In depression and PTSD, studies of central mediators in the brain also demonstrate parasympathetic hyperresponsiveness and beta-adrenergic hyporesponsiveness.[43] While increased α-adrenergic and cholinergic responsiveness distal from the airway has also been demonstrated in asthmatic patients,[44] a similar imbalance in the autonomic nervous system of the central nervous system among asthmatic populations has not been demonstrated. These data raise the question of common biological pathways.

Tachykinins derived from e-NANC nerves influence airway smooth muscle contraction, mucus secretion, vascular leakage, and neutrophil attachment. In experimental studies, tachykinins, especially substance P, have been linked to neurogenic inflammation[45] and regulation of stress hormonal pathways[46] and are implicated in asthma[47,48] and neurogenic skin disorders.[49]

Collectively, these data showing that stress and psychological dysfunction have been associated with modulation of many of the hormones, neurotransmitters, and neuropeptides involved in autonomic control and inflammation of the airways (i.e., common biological mediators) suggest potential common underlying biological mechanisms. Further study of the balance among functional parasympathetic and functional sympathetic activities in relation to stress, emotional stimuli, and immune function in asthmatic populations is needed. Local interactions between the immune system and the autonomic nervous system in the lung are poorly understood, however, and constitute an area of needed research.[50] For example, overlapping evidence demonstrating nerve–mast cell communication in response to stress and the potential import of these interactions in the respiratory system suggest this may be a fruitful area of research relative to stress and asthma.[51]

VI. Stress and Immune Function

A focus on airway inflammation in asthma has drawn attention to the possibility that stress-induced alterations in immune response have implications for development, exacerbation, and triggering of asthma. A substantial literature demonstrating that psychological stress can influence cell trafficking, cell function including mitogen-stimulated blastogenesis and natural killer cell cytotoxicity, and lymphocyte production of cytokines exists.[19] Stress can modulate immune responses through nerve pathways connecting the autonomic nervous and immune systems, by triggering the release of hormones and neuropeptides that interact with immune cells, and through impacts on behaviors such as smoking and drinking alcohol that are adopted as ways of coping with stress.[52]

Subjects exposed to cognitive or social laboratory stressor tasks lasting only a few minutes show suppression of T cell mitogenesis and increased numbers of circulating T suppressor/cytotoxic (CD8) cells and natural killer cells.[53] This phenomenon includes stress-elicited alteration of the production of the cytokines IL-1, IL-2, and interferon (IFN).[54,55] These effects are thought to be mediated by the autonomic nervous system because they occur quite rapidly; have been shown to be associated with increased heart rate, blood pressure, and circulating catecholamines;[56] and are blocked by administration of an adrenoceptor antagonist.[57]

Stress is not expected to have the same effects on immune function in all people. As noted earlier, individual differences in response to stressful events are attributable to interpretation of the event, access to coping resources, and presence of antecedent chronic stress.[58] However, there is also evidence of stable individual differences in immune response that occur independently of psychological response to the stressor. When exposed to multiple acute laboratory stressors over time, some subjects consistently demonstrate stress-elicited alterations in immunity, while others do not.[59] This challenges future investigators designing studies on psychological stress and asthma to consider these factors when choosing susceptible participants. Enrolling subjects experiencing high magnitude or severe chronic stressors (e.g., bereavement, relationship stress, caregiving stress) with

demonstrated psychological impact as well as associations with immune alterations, for example, may be particularly informative.[60] Indeed, studies done prior
to our understanding of the multiple determinants of an individual's susceptibility
to stress in relation to the asthmatic response may be one methodological explanation
for observed small effects in studies linking psychological stress and asthma.

Stress may play a role in the onset of childhood asthma. As highlighted
previously, airway inflammation and hyperresponsiveness are thought to be
orchestrated by activated T lymphocytes and the cytokines they produce. The T
helper cell Th-2 cytokine phenotype promotes IgE production, with subsequent
recruitment of inflammatory cells that may initiate and/or potentiate allergic
inflammation.[61] Prospective seroepidemiologic studies have shown that the newborn period is dominated by Th-2 reactivity in response to allergens,[62] and it is
also evident that the Th-1 memory cells selectively develop shortly after birth (at
3 to 6 months of age) and persist into adulthood in nonatopic subjects.[63] For most
children who become allergic or asthmatic, the polarization of their immune
system into an atopic phenotype probably occurs during early childhood.[64]

These findings have sparked vigorous investigation into the potential influence of early life environmental risk factors for asthma and allergy on the maturation of the immune system, in the hopes of understanding which factors will
potentiate (or protect from) this polarization. For example, Martinez and
colleagues[65] suggest that certain lower respiratory tract infections in early life
(primarily croup) enhance the production of IFN by nonspecifically stimulated
lymphocytes believed to be expressions of the Th-1 phenotype. Although we have
no direct evidence for the influence of stress on Th phenotype differentiation in
the developing immune system, evidence indicates that parental reports of life
stress are associated with subsequent onset of wheezing in children between birth
and 1 year of age.[66]

It has been speculated that stress triggers hormones in the early months of
life, and this may influence Th-2 cell predominance, perhaps through a direct
influence of stress hormones on the production of cytokines thought to modulate
the direction of differentiation. Simultaneous investigation of both host suscep-
tibilty factors and the effect of environmental exposures, including psychosocial
stressors, on the selection process for immunologic memory may provide fresh
insight into the pathogenesis of atopic disorders.

VII. Stress and Infection

A common framework used to link stress and health considers the immunosuppressive effects of stress. Psychological stress may influence the pathophysiology
of asthma by increasing the risk of respiratory infection.[67] The role of respiratory
tract infections in asthma has been widely studied and current evidence indicates

that viral, as opposed to bacterial, infections are the most important infectious agents.[68] Early life lower respiratory viral infections may be associated with an increased risk of developing asthma.[69] Further evidence supports a more complex pathogenetic role for viral infections[65] and suggests that the effects of infection may depend on which pathogen infects the host early in immune development.[70]

One potential consequence of stress-induced changes in immune response is suppression of host resistance to infectious agents, particularly agents that cause upper respiratory disease. The primary evidence for such effects comes from studies of psychological stress as a risk factor for respiratory infections. Increased incidence of upper respiratory infections under stress in these epidemiologic studies may be attributable either to stress-induced increases in exposure to infectious agents or to stress-induced changes in host resistance. Control for exposure is provided by studies in which volunteers are intentionally exposed to a virus — viral-challenge trials. In these prospective studies, psychological stress is assessed before volunteers are exposed to an upper respiratory virus and monitored in quarantine for infection and illness.

Using this paradigm, psychological stress has been associated with the incidence of infection and illness,[71,72] with increasing stress related in a dose response manner to increasing risk of infection.[73] Epidemiological studies also support the relationship of stress, immunity, and respiratory infection. Two prospective studies of preschool-aged children attending day care in California found that children with high autonomic and immune reactivities to stress had higher subsequent rates of respiratory infections during high environmental stress experienced during follow-up.[74,75] Other epidemiological data have linked stress to subsequent respiratory illness in children.[75]

A number of mechanisms may be involved in explaining the exacerbation of asthma, especially wheezing and increased airway responsiveness, by viral respiratory infection. First, viral respiratory infections damage the airway epithelium, causing inflammation. Another mechanism involves the stimulation of the virus-specific IgE antibody. Respiratory syncytial and parainfluenza viruses may potentiate the allergic responses to allergens by increasing the release of inflammatory mediators from mast cells and the subsequent cascade of inflammatory events characteristic of asthma.[76] Finally, viral respiratory infections may also result in the appearance of a late asthmatic response to inhaled antigen;[70,77] that is, viral infections may be "adjuvant" to inflammatory responses and promote the development of airway injuries by enhancing airway inflammation.

VIII. Stress and Glucocorticoid Resistance

An alternative hypothesis linking stress, neuroendocrine and immune function, and inflammatory disease expression considers a glucocorticoid resistance model.[78] As we have come to understand the central role of airway inflammation and immune activation in asthma pathogenesis, asthma treatment guidelines have focused on the use of anti-inflammatory therapy, particularly inhaled glucocorticoids. Asthmatics, however, have shown variable responses to glucocorticoid therapy.[79] Although the majority of patients readily respond to inhaled glucocorticoids, a subset of patients have difficult-to-control asthma even when treated with high doses of oral steroids. The cellular and molecular mechanisms underlying steroid resistance in asthma and other inflammatory diseases have been recently reviewed.[80] Notably, the majority of subjects with glucocorticoid-resistant or glucocorticoid-insensitive asthma have an acquired form of steroid resistance induced by chronic inflammation or immune activation.

Thus, it is important to investigate the factors that may potentiate the development of functional steroid resistance. For example, studies have shown that allergen exposure affects glucocorticoid receptor binding affinity in T lymphocytes from atopic asthmatics.[81] It has been proposed that chronic psychological stress, resulting in prolonged activation of the HPA and SAM axes, may result in a counter-regulatory response in stimulated lymphocytes and consequent down-regulation of the expression and/or functioning of glucocorticoid receptors, leading to functional glucocorticoid resistance.[78] Examination of mechanisms for steroid resistance in asthmatics related to chronic stress may provide further insight into the mechanisms underlying the link between stress and asthma. Moreover, research in this area may point to new directions for future strategies in the management of chronic asthma.[13]

IX. Psychological Stress and Oxidative Stress

Another potential mechanism linking stress to asthma is through oxidative stress pathways. A common feature of inflammation in living organisms is that it is frequently mediated by reactive oxygen species (ROS), acquired exogenously or as by-products of normal metabolism. The bronchial airway is particularly susceptible to ROS as it is directly exposed not only to molecular oxygen, but also to exogenous oxidative toxins such as particulate matter and ozone. While certain endogenous processes are designed to protect the respiratory epithelium from oxidative stress, individuals may nonetheless differ in their abilities to deal with oxidant burdens due to genetic or environmental factors that induce or augment oxidative stress. It has been proposed that differences in host detoxification provide the basis for either resolution or progression of inflammation in atopic individuals after exposure to environmental triggers.[82]

Spiteri and colleagues postulate that the inability to detoxify ROS species among atopic subjects leads to the release of chemotactic factors, the activation and recruitment of immune effector cells, prolonged inflammation, and the stimulation of bronchoconstricting mechanisms.[82] Theoretically, atopic subjects who are unable to detoxify ROS or overwhelmed by a chronic elevated burden of ROS develop the onset or aggravation of respiratory symptoms. Suggested factors that predispose susceptible subjects to asthma include chronic exposure to oxidative toxins (tobacco smoke, air pollution). An extension of the oxidative stress hypothesis is that psychological stress may be an additional environmental factor that may augment oxidative toxicity and increase airway inflammation.

There is evidence that psychological stress has pro-oxidant properties that augment oxidative toxicity. Emotionally stressed rats have increased levels of 8-deoxy-hydroxy-guanosine (8-OhdG), a commonly used biomarker of oxidative stress.[83] Similarly, staying awake all night increased the levels of thiobarbituric acid reactive substances (an indicator of lipid peroxidation) in humans.[84] Psychological stress has been noted to decrease DNA repair[85] and will inhibit radiation-induced apoptosis in human blood cells. These findings suggest that psychological stress may increase the likelihood of oxidative stress-induced pathology. Irie and colleagues[86] used classical conditioning to illustrate the roles of chronic stress and oxidative damage. Rats treated with ferric nitrilotriacetate, an oxidant, and conditioned to associated treatment with taste aversion therapy had increased 8-OhdG levels with further taste therapy than unconditioned animals.

Evidence also supports the notion that psychological stress modifies the host response to inflammatory oxidative toxins.[87] Psychological stress has been demonstrated to increase the activities of hepatic enzymes that activate polycyclic aromatic hydrocarbons in rats.[88,89] Similarly, chronic stress has been shown to increase the levels of lipoperoxides in rat livers and plasma, and decrease levels of reduced glutathione in erythrocytes and liver.[90] Moreover, evidence indicates that stress can induce enzymes that activate exogenous toxins to influence health outcomes.

In a birth cohort followed in mainland China, women with self-reported moderate to high levels of occupational stress had offspring with modest reductions in birthweights.[91] Similar independent effects of occupational benzene exposure were also reported. Upon further analysis, subjects who underwent *both stress and benzene exposure* had average reductions of 184 g in the birthweights of their children. Subjects exposed only to benzene had only 15-g reductions and subjects with only maternal stress exposure had 19-g reductions.

Benzene, a cyclic aromatic hydrocarbon, is an oxidative toxin that is activated and ultimately detoxified by the hepatic P450 enzyme system in conjunction with phase II enzymes. These results suggest that the interaction may be due to induction of benzene activation by maternal stress. In the same cohort of mother–infant pairs, genetic susceptibilities to benzene and decreased gestation were also described.[92] Mothers with the CYP1A1 HincII polymorphism AA and occupational exposure to benzene had statistically significant decreased gestational periods. CYP1A1 is a phase I enzyme that activates polycyclic aromatic hydrocarbons.

The association between the AA genotype and benzene exposure was postulated to be due to increased activation of benzene in the AA genotype subjects. The interaction of maternal stress with benzene exposure in the study by Chen and colleagues[91] may be similar to the interaction between the AA genotype and benzene in predicting gestational age reported by Wang and others.[92] While the A variant has no increased activity relative to the lower-case *a* variant, the A variant does have increased inducibility, and stress has been demonstrated to induce P450 enzyme systems.

A study conducted in mice parallels these findings. Among mice exposed to chronic intermittent restraint stress, total P450 content was decreased; however, the presence of both stress and the toxic benzene derivative 1,4-bis [2-(3,5-dicholoropyridyloxy)]benzene (TCPOBOP) *increased* total P450 content.[93] Furthermore, a seven-fold decrease in glutathione content was noted in the lungs of the TCPOBOP-treated mice after stress, whereas glutathione levels in the unstressed TCPOBOP-treated mice were unaffected. This animal study together with the study by Chen and coauthors suggests that stress is a pro-oxidant exposure that modifies the host response to inflammatory oxidative toxins and that stress may interact both with environmental oxidative toxins and/or with genetic polymorphisms within candidate genes that activate or detoxify oxidative toxins.

Environmental exposures that may interact with stress through these pathways include air pollution and tobacco smoke. While epidemiologic evidence suggests that asthma symptoms can be worsened by air pollution, air pollution has not been clearly associated with increased risk of sensitization and induction of disease.[94] Several investigators suggested that the ability of air pollution to generate ROS may explain its role in asthma and other respiratory diseases.[95–97]

While the mechanisms by which air pollution produces respiratory toxicity are likely to be multifactorial, the evidence that oxidative toxicity plays a role is quite strong. Ultrafine particles (<0.1 micron in diameter) have been demonstrated to increase oxidatively mediated inflammation in the lungs of rats.[98,99] *In vitro* studies demonstrate that PM10 is responsible for the production and release of inflammatory cytokines by the respiratory tract epithelium as well as the activation of the transcription factor Nf kappa B and that these properties are mediated by the production of ROS.[99] Air pollution contains other oxidative toxins, such as reactive quinones and polycyclic aromatic hydrocarbons.[97] Ozone, a gaseous component of air pollution, is also a highly reactive oxygen species and has been associated with 37% increased emergency department visits for asthma in urban children.[100]

Tobacco smoke also contains a number of compounds with oxidative potential, at least 50 of which are pro-carcinogens.[101] These include polycyclic aromatic hydrocarbons (PAHs).[101–103] Several components of tobacco smoke undergo activation by enzymes of the P450 superfamily. The metabolism of a PAH leads to the formation of an oxidative intermediate that is detoxified by glutathione conjugation in phase II metabolism. These reactive compounds sometimes initiate carcinogenesis, but more frequently induce inflammatory responses that can exacerbate respiratory problems such as infections, asthma, and chronic obstructive pulmonary disease. Elevated levels of biomarkers linked to oxidative stress have been found among smokers relative to nonsmokers.[104,105] Young children who are exposed to environmental tobacco smoke have increased levels of 8-OhdG, a biomarker of oxidative toxicity in infants.[106]

The glutathione transferase (GST) enzyme family consists of four main classes (alpha, mu, pi, and theta), each of which has one or more isoforms. Their primary role is as phase II enzymes catalyzing the addition of a glutathione moiety to a wide variety of exogenous and endogenous compounds. The GST enzymes are expressed in all tissues. Of particular interest in respiratory epidemiology are GST- M1 and GST-T1, each containing a null allele that is highly prevalent, and GST-P1 containing a functional variant with decreased activity (Val105Ile). The polymorphism in the GST-P1 Ile[105] has been associated with increased risk of asthma.[107,108]

These data support yet another pathway linking stress to asthma. The effects of environmental toxins (air pollution, tobacco smoke) on asthma may be mediated by the common pathway of oxidative stress, a process that may be potentiated by chronic psychological stress. Further research is needed to examine these relationships.

X. Genetics

Most advances in our knowledge of the genetic and molecular events underlying the neurobiology of the stress response have come from animal models.[109] These animal data along with the discussions elsewhere in this chapter suggest that studies to determine the role of genetics in modifying the risk of the social and physical environment experienced through psychological stress may further inform pathways through which stress may impact asthma expression. Genetic factors of potential import include those that influence immune development and airway inflammation in early life, corticosteroid regulatory genes, adrenergic system regulatory genes, biotransformation genes, and cytokine pathway genes.

XI. Epidemiological Evidence

Growing evidence in prospective population-based studies supports the role of differential life stress experiences and asthma expression. A prospective study of 150 genetically predisposed children from Colorado (14 of whom developed asthma) found that parental difficulties measured at age 3 weeks predicted an increased risk of asthma onset by age 3 years after controlling for frequent illness and 6-month IgE levels.[110]

In a prospective birth cohort study, our laboratory demonstrated that greater levels of maternal caregiver-perceived stress were associated with subsequent risk of recurrent wheeze episodes (two or more) in early childhood.[66] Higher levels of caregiver-perceived stress remained independent predictors of early childhood wheeze in these analyses even when controlling for standard variables that may have been related to stress (i.e., birth weight, parental asthma, race/ethnicity, and socioeconomic status), indicating that caregiver stress was not simply a marker of these other factors. Moreover, higher levels of caregiver stress predicted an increased risk of wheeze in the index children even after adjusting for potential mediators (i.e., maternal smoking, lower respiratory illness (LRI), allergen levels, and breast feeding) suggesting that the relation between stress and early childhood repeated wheeze may not be primarily mediated through these caregiver behaviors or susceptibility to lower respiratory infections.

A plausible alternative hypothesis may be that there is a more direct effect on airway inflammation through influences on the immune system that may promote airway obstruction and wheeze. Sandberg and colleagues[111] found an increased risk of asthma exacerbation among children aged 6 to 13 years associated with acute severe life events. This effect was enhanced in the context of chronic ongoing stress.

XII. Socioeconomic Status (SES) and Asthma Disparities

Extending our knowledge of the influence of stress on asthma morbidity may also help explain socioeconomic and racial or ethnic disparities in disease burden. Asthma prevalence and the associated morbidity are increasing worldwide.[112] These trends disproportionately affect nonwhite children living in urban areas and children living in poverty in the United States.[113] Higher rates of asthma prevalence, hospitalization, and mortality have also been described among poor individuals and members of minority groups worldwide[114] A graded association between SES and asthma prevalence, morbidity, and mortality has been demonstrated in the United States.[115–117]

Many proposed explanations for the association between SES and health focus on factors associated with poverty (i.e., poor nutrition, suboptimal housing). However, these explanations would predict a threshold effect for SES; above a certain level of SES, inadequate housing and malnutrition should not be problems and individuals above this threshold should benefit from similar good health.[115] The data actually suggest that health outcomes worsen in a graded or linear fashion with decreasing SES; not only those in poverty are at risk. Such a gradient might be explained by access to higher quality health care with each increase in

SES although the SES gradient persists in countries with universal health insurance. Another suggested explanation is that lower SES individuals engage in more risky health behaviors (e.g., smoking, poor diet). However, the linear relationship between SES and health remains after controlling for such health behaviors.[115]

A similar graded association between SES and asthma morbidity and mortality has been demonstrated. In the United States, children living at greater economic disadvantage and those whose parents have lower education or occupational class have higher prevalence rates of asthma with gradient effects seen in many studies.[113]

It has been proposed that direct biological effects of differential life stress may help explain health inequalities.[118,119] Research shows that emotions are responses to power and status differentials embedded within social situations.[120] An individual's biological reactivity then may also vary by the social context in which he or she lives. A series of relevant experiments demonstrate relationships between social status and biological and behavioral processes. Social stress models analogous to human circumstances developed in animal research may be particularly informative. The most widely used social stressors include low social status or dominance hierarchies, defeat in aggressive encounters, social isolation, crowding for males, and social instability for females (alternating crowding with isolation phases). Interesting parallels in animal and human research have already begun to emerge. For example, in the Whitehall cohort, the same lipoprotein and apolipoprotein gradients demonstrated across employment grade in male civil servants parallel observations in male baboons relative to social dominance: low status associated with low HDL cholesterol and apolipoprotein AI.[121,122]

Chen and Matthews[123] recently reported on the development and validation of a series of videos designed to assess adolescent cognitive appraisals and understanding of social events (CAUSE). This methodology was designed based on the premise that individuals from low SES backgrounds who may have more stressful and unpredictable environments may develop tendencies toward making threat interpretations when presented with ambiguous situations compared with their higher SES counterparts. These authors and others hypothesize that this tendency to overinterpret life events as threatening (even when ambiguous) may translate into greater physiologic reactivity in these situations and may have long-term adverse consequences.[124]

Using this paradigm, Chen and colleagues are beginning to explore differential immune responses among adolescent asthmatics relative to SES and emotional responses to their environments. In a study of adolescent asthmatics, these authors demonstrated differential cytokine expression in mitogen-stimulated T cells in the low SES group (i.e., higher IL-5 and IFN-gamma) and lower morning cortisol levels compared with their higher SES counterparts.[125] These authors also found that low SES adolescents experienced greater stress and that stress partially explained the relationship between SES and IL-5/IFN-gamma. Further research in this area may buttress the hypothesis that differential life stress may, in part, explain asthma disparities.

Community-level variables are receiving increased attention for their potential role in determining inequalities across several health outcomes including asthma. Lower SES and minority group status may predispose individuals to pervasive chronic stressors. For example, the broader political and economic forces that result in marginalization of minority populations in disadvantaged inner city neighborhoods may lead to increased stress experienced by these populations and thus greater disease morbidity.[113]

High magnitude stressors such as violence and crime prevalent in high risk urban populations are receiving increased attention in health research. Violent crime undermines social cohesion[126–128] and is associated with the erosion of social capital and community resilience. Crime is most prevalent in societies that permit large disparities in the material standards of living of their citizens.[126] Thus, in addition to direct impacts on community residents, crime and violence (or the lack of them) can be used as indicators of collective well-being, social relations, and social cohesion within a community or society. Furthermore, the conditions known to be associated with violence exposure are related to experienced stress.[129] Chronic violence exposure has been conceptualized as a pervasive environmental stressor imposed on already vulnerable populations.[130] Studies are beginning to explore the health effects of living in a violent environment with a chronic pervasive atmosphere of fear and perceived threats of violence.[131–135]

Violence exposure has been associated with asthma.[136] In a population-based study in Boston, lifetime exposure to violence was ascertained retrospectively through parental report interview questionnaires administered to 416 caregivers and their children who were followed longitudinally for respiratory health outcomes, including asthma. Preliminary analyses suggest a link of high lifetime exposure to community violence and increased risks of asthma and wheeze syndromes and prescription bronchodilator use among these inner city children.[137]

Community violence exposure has been linked to asthma morbidity among children aged 9 to 12 years in the Inner-City Asthma Study. Greater violence exposure was independently associated with asthma morbidity after simultaneous adjustment for income, employment status, caretaker education, housing problems, and other adverse life events, suggesting that violence was not merely a marker for these other factors. Psychological stress and caretaker behaviors (keeping children indoors, smoking, and skipping medications) partially explained the association between higher violence and increased asthma morbidity, although the greatest attenuation occurred among those reporting lower level violence, suggesting that other mechanisms are operating between high level violence exposure and childhood asthma morbidity.[138]

Future studies need to examine the links among neighborhood disadvantage (ND), minority group status, low levels of social capital, violence exposure, and other social influences (and the heightened stress they may elicit) as risk factors for childhood asthma analogous to physical environmental exposures to allergens, tobacco smoke, and air pollution. Such studies are likely to further our understanding of the increased asthma burdens on populations of children living in poverty in urban areas or other disadvantaged communities.

XIII. Summary

Environmental stressors may impact asthma morbidity through neuroimmunologic mechanisms that are adversely impacted and/or buffered by social circumstances and psychological functioning. While earlier psychosomatic models have supported a role for psychological stress in contributing to variable asthma morbidity among those with existing disease, a growing appreciation of the interactions of behavioral, neural, endocrine, and immune processes suggest a role for these psychosocial factors in the genesis of asthma as well. While a causal link between stress and asthma has not been established, this review provides a framework in which we can begin to see links between these systems that might provide new insights to guide future explorations. To simplify the discussion we have arbitrarily chosen to review the relationships of stress, psychological dysfunction, endocrine function, neural function, immune function, and behavior separately in order to explore the influence of environmental stress on asthma morbidity.

We understand that this is a rudimentary approach, as contemporary attempts to apply the biopsychosocial model to disease emphasize that a unidirectional model is too simplistic; causality is at least bidirectional or reciprocal and more probably cyclic in complexity.[139] The complexity of these interactions underscores the need for a multidisciplinary and truly integrative approach as research in this area moves ahead. It also emphasizes the need for careful attention to explicit theoretical frameworks in designing future research and as a potential target for asthma prevention.[60]

Acknowledgment

During preparation of this manuscript, Dr. Wright was supported by the National Heart, Lung, and Blood Institute Grant K08 HL04187.

References

1. Rosner F. Moses Maimonides' treatise on asthma. *Thorax* 1981; 36: 245–251.
2. Osler W. *The Principles and Practice of Medicine*. Edinburgh: YJ Pentland, 1892.

3. Freud S. *Inhibitions, Symptoms, and Anxiety*, 20th ed. London: Hogarth Press; 1948.

4. Alexander F, French TM, and Pollock GH. *Psychosomatic Specificity, Vol 1: Experimental Study and Results*. Chicago: University of Chicago Press, 1968.

5. Fenichel O. Nature and classifications of the so-called psychosomatic phenomena. *Psychoanal Q* 1945; 14: 287.

6. Lehrer PM, Isenberg S, and Hochron SM. Asthma and emotion: a review. *J Asthma* 1993; 30: 5–21.

7. Isenberg SA, Lehrer PM, and Hochron SM. The effects of suggestion and emotional arousal on pulmonary function in asthma: a review and a hypothesis regarding vagal mediation. *Psychosomatic Med* 1992; 54: 192–216.

8. Affleck G, Apter A, Tennen H, Reisine S, Barrows E, Willard A, Unger J, and Zuwallack R. Mood states associated with transitory changes in asthma symptoms and peak expiratory flow. *Psychosomatic Med* 2000; 62: 61–68.

9. Miklich DR, Rewey HH, Weiss JH, and Kolton S. A preliminary investigation of psychophysiological responses to stress among different subgroups of asthmatic children. *J Psychosomatic Res* 1973; 17: 1–8.

10. Miller B and Wood B. Psychophysiologic reactivity in asthmatic children: a cholinergically mediated confluence of pathways. *J Am Acad Child Adolescent Psychiatr* 1994; 33: 1236–1245.

11. Tal A and Miklich DR. Emotionally induced decrease in pulmonary flow rates in asthmatic children. *Psychosomatic Med* 1976; 38: 190–200.

12. Kellner R. Psychotherapy in psychosomatic disorders: a survey of controlled studies. *Arch Gen Psychiatr* 1975; 32: 1021–1028.

13. Wright RJ. Alternative modalities for asthma that reduce stress and modify mood states: evidence for underlying psychobiological mechanisms. *Ann Allergy Asthma Immun* 2004; 93(Supl. 1): S18–23.

14. Ader R, Cohen N, and Felten D. Psychoneuroimmunology: interactions between the nervous system and the immune system. *Lancet* 1995; 345: 99–103.

15. McEwen BS. Protective and damaging effects of stress mediators. *New Engl J Med* 1998; 338: 171–179.

16. Holgate ST. Asthma: a dynamic disease of inflammation and repair, in *Rising Trends in Asthma*, Chadwick DJ and Cardew G, Eds. West Chichester: John Wiley & Sons. 1997, pp. 5–34.

17. Busse WW and Rosenwasser LJ. Mechanisms of asthma. *J Allergy Clin Immunol* 2003; 111: S799–S804.

18. Wright R, Rodriguez M, and Cohen S. Review of psychosocial stress and asthma: an integrated biopsychosocial approach. *Thorax* 1998; 53: 1066–1074.

19. Herbert T and Cohen S. Stress and immunity in humans: a meta-analytic review. *Psychosomatic Med* 1993; 55: 364–379.

20. Baum A, Cohen L, and Hall M. Control and intrusive memories as possible determinants of chronic stress. *Psychosomatic Med* 1993; 55: 274–286.

21. Pike JL, Smith TL, Hauger RL, Nicassio PM, Patterson TL, McClintick J et al. Chronic life stress alters sympathetic, neuroendocrine, and immune responsivity to an acute psychological stressor in humans. *Psychosomatic Med* 1997; 59: 447–457.

22. Umetsu DT, McIntire JJ, Akbari O, Macaubas C, and DeKruyff RH. Asthma: an epidemic of dysregulated immunity. *Nature Immunol* 2002; 3: 715–720.

23. Moran MG. Psychological factors affecting pulmonary and rheumatologic diseases: a review. *Psychosomatics* 1991; 32: 14–23.
24. Barnes PJ. Is asthma a nervous disease? *Chest* 1995; 107: 119S–125S.
25. Barnes PJ. Airway inflammation and autonomic control. *Eur J Respir Dis* 1986; 69: 80–87.
26. Chrousos GP. The hypothalamic–pituitary–adrenal axis and immune-mediated inflammation. *New Engl J Med* 1995; 332: 1351–1362.
27. Selye H. *The Stress of Life*. New York: McGraw-Hill, 1956.
28. Mason JW. A re-evaluation of the concept of "non-specificity" in distress theory. *J Psychiatr Res* 1971; 8: 323–333.
28a. Sterling P. Principles of allostasis: optimal design, predictive regulation, pathophysiology, and rational therapeutics. In: Schulkin, J *Allostasis, Homeostasis, and the Cost of Physiologic Adaptation*. Cambridge, U.K.: Cambridge University Press; 2004; 17–65.
29. McEwen BS. Stress, adaptation, and disease: allostasis and allostatic load. *Ann NY Acad Sci* 1998; 840: 33–44.
30. Pariante CM. Depression, stress and the adrenal axis. *J Neuroendocrinol* 2003; 15: 811–812.
31. Ockenfels MC, Porter L, Smyth J, Kirschbaum C, Hellhammer DH, and Stone AA. Effect of chronic stress associated with unemployment on salivary cortisol: overall cortisol levels, diurnal rhythm, and acute stress reactivity. *Psychosomatic Med* 1995; 57: 460–467.
32. Yehuda R, Teicher MH, Trestman RL, Levengood RA, and Siever LJ. Cortisol regulation in posttraumatic stress disorder and major depression: a chronobiological analysis. *Biol Psychiatr* 1996; 40: 79–88.
33. Buske-Kirschbaum A, Jobst S, Wustmans A, Kirschbaum C, Rauh W, and Hellhammer D. Attenuated free cortisol response to psychosocial stress in children with atopic dermatitis. *Psychosomatic Med* 1997; 59: 419–426.
34. Theoharides TC, Singh LK, Boucher W, Pang X, Letourneau R, Webster E et al. Corticotropin-releasing hormone induces skin mast cell degranulation and increased vascular permeability: a possible explanation for its proinflammatory effects. *Endocrinology* 1998; 139: 403–413.
35. Rabin BS, Cohen S, Ganguli R, Lysle DT, and Cunnick JE. Bidirectional interaction between the central nervous system and the immune system. *Crit Rev Immunol* 1989; 9: 279–312.
36. Barnes PJ, Baraniuk JN, and Belvisi MG. Neuropeptides in the respiratory tract. *Am Rev Respir Dis* 1991; 144: 1187–1198, 1391–1399.
37. Barnes PJ. Neural control of human airways in health and disease. *Am Rev Respir Dis* 1986; 134: 1289–1314.
38. Dimsdale JE and Moss J. Short-term catecholamine response to psychological stress. *Psychosomatic Med* 1980; 42: 493–497.
39. Drazen JM, Irsrael E, Boushey HA, Chinchilli VM, Fahy JV, Fish JE et al. Comparison of regularly scheduled with as-needed use of albuterol in mild asthma. *New Engl J Med* 1996; 335: 841–847.
40. Lemanske RF and Kaliner MA. Autonomic nervous system abnormalities and asthma. *Am Rev Respir Dis* 1990; 141: S157–S161.

41. Mann JJ, Brown RP, Halper JP, Sweeney JA, Kocsis JH, Stokes PE et al. Reduced sensitivity of lymphocyte beta-adrenergic receptors in patients with endogenous depression and psychomotor agitation. *New Engl J Med* 1985; 313: 715–720.

42. Fritze J. The adrenergic-cholinergic imbalance hypothesis of depression: a review and a perspective. *Rev Neurosci* 1993; 4: 63–93.

43. Charney DS, Deutch AY, Krystal JH, Southwick SM, and Davis M. Psychobiologic mechanisms of posttraumatic stress disorder. *Arch Gen Psychiatr* 1993; 50: 295–305.

44. Davis PB. Pupillary responses and airway reactivity in asthma. *J Allergy Clin Immunol* 1986; 77: 667–672.

45. Weinstock JV. *Substance P and the Immune System.* New York: Taylor & Francis, 2003.

46. Jessop DS, Renshaw D, Larsen PJ, Chowdrey HS, and Harbuz MS. Substance P is involved in terminating the hypothalamo-pituitary-adrenal axis response to acute stress through centrally located neurokinin-1 receptors. *Stress* 2000; 3: 209–220.

47. Ichinose M, Miura M, Yamauchi H, Kageyama N, Tomaki M, Oyake T et al. A neurokinin 1-receptor antagonist improves exercise-induced airway narrowing in asthmatic patients. *Am J Respir Crit Care Med* 1996; 153: 936–941.

48. Tomaki M, Ichinose M, Miura M, Hirayama Y, Yamauchi H, Nakajima N et al. Elevated substance P content in induced sputum from patients with asthma and patients with chronic bronchitis. *Am J Respir Crit Care Med* 1995; 151: 613–617.

49. Singh LK, Pang X, Alexacos N, Letourneau R, and Theoharides TC. Acute immobilization stress triggers skin mast cell degranulation via corticotropin releasing hormone, neurotensin, and substance P: a link to neurogenic skin disorders. *Brain Behavior Immun* 1999; 13: 225–239.

50. Undem BJ and Weinreich D. Neuroimmune interactions in the lung, in *Autonomic Neuroimmunology*, Bienenstock J, Goetzle EJ, and Blennerhassett MG, Eds. New York: Taylor & Francis, 2003, pp. 279–294.

51. van der Kleij HPM, Blennerhassett MG, and Bienenstock J. Nerve–mast cell interactions: partnership in health and disease, in *Autonomic Neuroimmunology*, Bienenstock J, Goetzl JE, and Blennerhassett MG, Eds. New York: Taylor & Francis; 2003, pp. 139–170.

52. Cohen S and Herbert T. Health psychology: psychological factors and physical disease from the perspective of human psychoneuroimmunology. *Annu Rev Psychol* 1996; 47: 113–142.

53. Kiecolt-Glaser JK, Cacioppo JT, Malarkey WB, and Glaser R. Acute psychological stressors and short-term immune changes: what, why, for whom, and to what extent? *Psychosomatic Med* 1992; 54: 680–685.

54. Dobbin JP, Harth M, McCain GA, Martin RA, and Cousin K. Cytokine production and lymphocyte transformation during stress. *Brain Behavior Immun* 1991; 5: 339–348.

55. Glaser R, Kennedy S, Lafuse WP, Bonneau RH, Speicher C, Hillhouse J et al. Psychological stress-induced modulation of interleukin-2 receptor gene expression and interleukin-2 production in peripheral blood leukocytes. *Arch Gen Psychiatr* 1990; 47: 707–712.

56. Herbert TB, Cohen S, Marsland AL, Bachen EA, Rabin BS, Muldoon MF et al. Cardiovascular reactivity and the course of immune response to an acute psychological stressor. *Psychosomatic Med* 1994; 56: 337–344.

57. Bachen EA, Manuck SB, Cohen S, Muldoon MF, Raible R, Herbert TB et al. Adrenergic blockade ameliorates cellular immune responses to mental stress in humans. *Psychosomatic Med* 1995; 57: 366–372.

58. McEwen BS. From molecules to mind: stress, individual differences, and the social environment. *Ann NY Acad Sci* 2001; 935: 42–49.

59. Marsland AL, Manuck SB, Fazzari TV, Stewart CJ, and Rabin BS. Stability of individual differences in cellular immune responses to acute psychological stress. *Psychosomatic Med* 1995; 57: 295–298.

60. Miller GE and Cohen S. Psychological interventions and the immune system: a meta-analytic review and critique. *Health Psychol* 2001; 20: 47–63.

61. Romagnani S. Induction of Th1 and Th2 responses: a key role for the 'natural' immune response? *Immunol Today* 1992; 13: 379–381.

62. Prescott SL, Macaubas C, Holt BJ, Smallacombe TB, Loh R, Sly PD et al. Transplacental priming of the human immune system to environmental allergens: universal skewing of initial T cell responses toward the Th2 cytokine profile. *J Immunol* 1998; 160: 4730–4737.

63. Holt PG. Immunoprophylaxis of atopy: light at the end of the tunnel. *Immunol Today* 1994; 15: 484–489.

64. Yabuhara A, Macaubas C, and Prescott SL. Th-2 polarised immunological memory to inhalant allergens in atopics is established during infancy and early childhood. *Clin Exp Allergy* 1997; 27: 1261–1269.

65. Martinez FD. Role of viral infection in the inception of asthma and allergies during childhood: could they be protective? *Thorax* 1994; 49: 1189–1191.

66. Wright RJ, Cohen S, Carey V, Weiss ST, and Gold DR. Parental stress as a predictor of wheezing in infancy: a prospective birth-cohort study. *Am J Respir Crit Care Med* 2002; 165: 358–365.

67. Cohen S and Rodriguez M. Stress, viral respiratory infections and asthma, in *Asthma and Respiratory Infection*, Skoner DP, Ed. New York: Marcel Dekker; 2003.

68. Gern JE. Viral and bacterial infections in the development and progression of asthma. *J Allergy Clin Immunol* 2000; 105: S497–S502.

69. Sherman CB, Tosteson TD, Tager IB, Speizer FE, and Weiss ST. Early childhood predictors of asthma. *Am J Epidemiol* 1990; 132: 83–95.

70. Folkerts G, Busse WW, Nijkamp FP, Sorkness R, and Gern JE. Virus-induced airway hyperresponsiveness and asthma. *Am J Respir Crit Care Med* 1998; 157: 1708–1720.

71. Stone AA, Bovbjerg DH, Neale JM, Napoli A, Valdimarsdottir H, Cox D et al. Development of common cold symptoms following experimental rhinovirus infection is related to prior stressful life events. *Behavioral Med* 1992; 18: 115–120.

72. Cohen S, Frank E, Doyle WJ, Skoner DP, Rabin BS, and Gwaltney JM, Jr. Types of stressors that increase susceptibility to the common cold in healthy adults. *Health Psychol* 1998; 17: 214–223.

73. Cohen S, Tyrrell DAJ, and Smith AP. Psychological stress and susceptibility to the common cold. *New Engl J Med* 1991; 325: 606–612.

74. Boyce TW, Chesney M, Alkon A, Tschann JM, Adams S, Chesterman B et al. Psychobiologic reactivity to stress and childhood respiratory illnesses: results of two prospective studies. *Psychosomatic Med* 1995; 57: 411–422.

75. Graham NMH, Woodward AJ, Ryan P, and Douglas RM. Acute respiratory illness in Adelaide children. II: Relationship of maternal stress, social supports and family functioning. *Int J Epidemiol* 1990; 19: 937–944.

76. Busse WW. Respiratory infections: their role in airway responsiveness and the pathogenesis of asthma. *J Allergy Clin Immunol* 1990; 85: 671–683.

77. Weiss ST, Tager IB, Munoz A, and Speizer FE. The relationship of respiratory infections in early childhood to the occurrence of increased levels of bronchial responsiveness and atopy. *Am Rev Respir Dis* 1985; 131: 573–578.

78. Miller GE, Ritchey AK, and Cohen S. Chronic psychological stress and regulation of pro-inflammatory cytokines: a glucocorticoid-resistance model. *Health Psychol* 2002; 21: 531–541.

79. Lee TH, Brattsand R, and Leung DYM. Corticosteroid action and resistance in asthma. *Am J Respir Cell Mol Biol* 1996; 154: S1–S79.

80. Leung DYM. Update on glucocorticoid action and resistance. *J Allergy Clin Immunol* 2003; 111: 3–22.

81. Nimmagadda S, Spahn J, Surs W, Szefler S, and Leung D. Allergen exposure decreases glucocorticoid receptor binding affinity and steroid responsiveness in atopic asthmatics. *Am J Respir Crit Care Med* 1997; 155: 97–93.

82. Spiteri MA, Bianco A, Strange RC, and Freyer AA. Polymorphisms at the glutathione S-transferase, GSTP1 locus: a novel mechanism for susceptibility and development of atopic airway inflammation. *Allergy* 2000; 55: 15–20.

83. Adachi S, Kawamura K, and Takemoto K. Oxidative damage of nuclear DNA in liver of rats exposed to psychological stress. *Cancer Res* 1993; 53: 4153–4155.

84. Kosugi H, Enomoto H, Ishizuka Y, and Kikugawa K. Variations in the level of urinary thiobarbituric acid reactant in healthy humans under different physiological conditions. *Biol Pharm Bull* 1994; 17: 1645–1650.

85. Tomei LD, Kiecolt-Glaser JK, Kennedy S, and Glaser R. Psychological stress and phorbol ester inhibition of radiation-induced apoptosis in human peripheral blood leukocytes. *Psychiatr Res* 1990; 33: 59–71.

86. Irie M, Asami S, Nagata S, Miyata M, and Kasai H. Classical conditioning of oxidative DNA damage in rats. *Neurosci Lett* 2000; 288: 13–16.

87. Moller P, Wallin H, and Knudsen LE. Oxidative stress associated with exercise, psychological stress and life-style factors. *Chem Biol Interactions* 1996; 102: 17–36.

88. Capel ID. The effect of isolation stress on some hepatic drug and carcinogen metabolising enzymes in rats. *J Env Pathol Toxicol* 1980; 4: 337–344.

89. Capel ID, Jenner M, Pinnock MH, Dorrell HM, and Williams DC. The effect of overcrowding stress on carcinogen-metabolizing enzymes of the rat. *Env Res* 1980; 23: 162–169.

90. Capel ID, Dorrell HM, and Smallwood AE. The influence of cold restraint stress on some components of the antioxidant defence system in the tissues of rats of various ages. *J Toxicol Env Health* 1983; 11: 425–436.

91. Chen D, Cho SI, Chen C, Wang X, Damokosh AI, Ryan L et al. Exposure to benzene, occupational stress, and reduced birth weight. *Occ Env Med* 2000; 57: 661–667.

92. Wang X, Chen D, Niu T, Wang Z, Wang L, Ryan L et al. Genetic susceptibility to benzene and shortened gestation: evidence of gene-environment interaction. *Am J Epidemiol* 2000; 152: 693–700.
93. Konstandi M, Marselos M, Radon-Camus AM, Johnson E, and Lang MA. The role of stress in the regulation of drug metabolizing enzymes in mice. *Eur J Drug Metabol Pharmacokin* 1998; 23: 483–490.
94. Peden DB. Air pollution in asthma: effect of pollutants on airway inflammation. *Ann Allergy Asthma Immunol* 2001; 87: 12–17.
95. Prahalad AK, Inmon J, Dailey LA, Madden MC, Ghio AJ, and Gallagher JE. Air pollution particles mediated oxidative DNA base damage in a cell free system and in human airway epithelial cells in relation to particulate metal content and bioreactivity. *Chem Res Toxicol* 2001; 14: 879–887.
96. Ghio AJ, Carter JD, Richards JH, Crissman KM, Bobb HH, and Yang F. Diminished injury in hypotransferrinemic mice after exposure to a metal-rich particle. *Am J Physiol Lung Cell Mol Physiol* 2000; 278: L1051–1061.
97. Donaldson K, Gilmour MI, and MacNee W. Asthma and PM10. *Respir Res* 2000; 1: 12–15.
98. Oberdorster G. Pulmonary effects of inhaled ultrafine particles. *Int Arch Occ Env Health* 2001; 74: 1–8.
99. Baeza-Squiban A, Bonvallot V, Boland S, and Marano F. Airborne particles evoke an inflammatory response in human airway epithelium: activation of transcription factors. *Cell Biol Toxicol* 1999; 15: 375–380.
100. White MC, Etzel RA, Wilcox WD, and Lloyd C. Exacerbations of childhood asthma and ozone pollution in Atlanta. *Env Res* 1994; 65: 56–68.
101. Ford JG, Li Y, O'Sullivan MM, Demopoulos R, Gartc S, Taioli E et al. Glutathione S-transferase M1 polymorphism and lung cancer risk in African-Americans. *Carcinogenesis* 2000; 21: 1971–1975.
102. Kelsey KT, Spitz MR, Zuo ZF, and Wiencke JK. Polymorphisms in the glutathione S-transferase class mu and theta genes interact and increase susceptibility to lung cancer in minority populations (Texas, United States). *Cancer Causes Control* 1997; 8: 554–559.
103. Rahman I and MacNee W. Oxidative stress and regulation of glutathione in lung inflammation. *Eur Respir J* 2000; 16: 534–554.
104. Lodovici M. Levels of 8-hydroxydeoxyguanosine as a marker of DNA damage in human leukocytes. *Free Radical Biol Med* 2000; 28: 13–17.
105. Zhou JF, Yan XF, Guo FZ, Sun NY, Qian ZJ, and Ding DY. Effects of cigarette smoking and smoking cessation on plasma constituents and enzyme activities related to oxidative stress. *Biomed Env Sci* 2000; 13: 44–55.
106. Hong YC, Kim H, Im MW, Lee KH, Woo BH, and Christiani DC. Maternal genetic effects on neonatal susceptibility to oxidative damage from environmental tobacco smoke. *J Natl Cancer Inst* 2001; 93: 645–647.
107. Spiteri MA, Bianco A, Strange RC, and Fryer AA. Polymorphisms at the glutathione S-transferase, GSTP1 locus: a novel mechanism for susceptibility and development of atopic airway inflammation. *Allergy* 2000; 55: S15–S20.
108. Fryer AA, Spiteri MA, Bianco A, Hepple M, Jones PW, Strange RC et al. The −403 G → A promoter polymorphism in the RANTES gene is associated with atopy and asthma. *Genes Immun* 2000; 1: 509–514.

109. Steckler T. The molecular neurobiology of stress: evidence from genetic and epigenetic models. *Behav Pharmacol* 2001; 12: 381–427.

110. Mrazek DA, Klinnert M, Mrazek PJ, Brower A, McCormick D, Rubin B et al. Prediction of early-onset asthma in genetically at-risk children. *Pediatr Pulmonol* 1999; 27: 85–94.

111. Sandberg S, Paton JY, McCann DC, McGuiness D, Hillary CR, and Oja H. The role of acute and chronic stress in asthma attacks in children. *Lancet* 2000; 356: 982–987.

112. Wright R and Weiss S. Epidemiology of allergic disease, in *Allergy*, 2nd ed., Holgate S, Church M, and Lichtenstein L, Eds. London: Harcourt; 2000.

113. Wright RJ and Fisher EB. Putting asthma into context: influences on risk, behavior, and intervention, in *Neighborhoods and Health*. Kawachi I and Berkman LF, Eds. New York: Oxford University Press, 2003, pp. 233–262.

114. McElmurry B, Buseh A, and Dublin M. Health education program to control asthma in multiethnic, low-income urban communities: Chicago Health Corps Asthma Program. *Chest* 1999; 116: 198S–199S.

115. Chen E, Matthew K, and Boyce W. Socioeconomic differences in children's health: how and why do these relationships change with age? *Psychol Bull* 2002; 128: 295–329.

116. Bor W, Najman J, Anderson M, Morrison J, and Williams G. Socioeconomic disadvantage and child morbidity: an Australian longitudinal study. *Soc Sci Med* 1993; 9: 27–30.

117. Weiss K, Gergen PJ, and Wagener DK. Breathing better or wheezing worse? The changing epidemiology of asthma morbidity and mortality. *Annu Rev Publ Health* 1993; 14: 491–513.

118. Brunner E. Socioeconomic determinants of health: stress and biology of inequality. *Br Med J* 1997; 314: 1472–1476.

119. Kemeny ME. Psychobiology of stress. *Curr Dir Psychol Sci* 2003; 12: 124–129.

120. Kemper TD. Sociological models in the explanation of emotions, in *Handbook of Emotions*, Lewis M and Haviland JM, Eds. New York: Guilford Press, 1993, pp. 41–52.

121. Brunner EJ, Marmot MG, and White IR. Gender and employment grade differences in blood cholesterol, apolipoproteins and haemostatic factors in the Whitehall II study. *Atherosclerosis* 1993; 102: 195–207.

122. Sapolsky RM and Mott GE. Social subordinance in wild baboons is associated with suppressed high density lipoprotein cholesterol concentrations: the possible role of chronic social stress. *Endocrinology* 1987; 121: 1605–1610.

123. Chen E and Matthews KA. Development of the Cognitive Appraisal and Understanding of Social Events (CAUSE) videos. *Health Psychol* 2003; 22: 106–110.

124. Chen E and Matthews KA. Cognitive appraisal biases: an approach to understanding the relation between socioeconomic status and cardiovascular reactivity in children. *Ann Behav Med* 2001; 23: 101–111.

125. Chen E, Fisher EB, Bacharier LB, and Strunk RC. Socioeconomic status, stress, and immune markers in adolescents with asthma. *Psychosomatic Med* 2003; 65(6): 984–992.

126. Kawachi I. Social capital and community effects on population and individual health. *Ann NY Acad Sci* 1999; 896: 120–130.

127. Kennedy B, Kawachi I, Prothrow-Smith D, Lochner K, and Gupta V. Social capital, income inequality, and firearm violent crime. *Soc Sci Med* 1998; 47: 7–17.
128. Sampson R, Raudenbush S, and Earls F. Neighborhoods and violent crime: a multilevel study of collective efficacy. *Science* 1997; 277: 918–924.
129. Breslau N, Davis G, Andreski P, and Petersen E. Traumatic events and posttraumatic stress disorder in an urban population of young adults. *Arch Gen Psychiatr* 1991; 48: 216–222.
130. Isaacs M. *Violence: The Impact of Community Violence on African American Children and Families.* Arlington, VA: National Center for Educational Maternal and Child Health, 1992.
131. Boney-McCoy S and Finkelhor D. Psychosocial sequelae of violent victimization in a national youth sample. *J Consult Clin Psychol* 1995; 63: 726–736.
132. Herman A. Political violence, health, and health services in South Africa. *Am J Public Health* 1988; 8: 767–768.
133. Martinez P and Richters J. The NIMH Community Violence Project II: children's distress symptoms associated with violence exposure. *Psychiatry* 1993; 56: 22–35.
134. Yach D. The impact of political violence on health and health services in Capetown, South Africa, 1986: methodological problems and preliminary results. *Am J Public Health* 1988; 78: 772–776.
135. Zapata B, Rebolledo A, Atalah E, Newman B, and King M. The influence of social and political violence on the risk of pregnancy complications. *Am J Public Health* 1992; 82: 685–690.
136. Wright R and Steinbach S. Violence: an unrecognized environmental exposure that may contribute to greater asthma morbidity in high risk inner city populations. *Env Health Perspectives* 2001; 109: 1085–1089.
137. Wright RJ, Hanrahan JP, and Tager I. Effect of the exposure to violence on the occurrence and severity of childhood asthma in an inner city population. *Am J Respir Crit Care Med* 1997; 155: A972.
138. Wright RJ, Mitchell H, Visness CM, Cohen S, Stout J, Evan R et al. Community violence and asthma morbidity in the Inner City Asthma Study. *Am J Publ Health* 2004; 94(4): 625–632.
139. Engel GL. Clinical application of the biopsychosocial model. *Am J Psychiatr* 1980; 137: 535–544.

16

Infant Feeding Practices and Prevention of Asthma

ANNE L. WRIGHT

Arizona Respiratory Center
University of Arizona
Tucson, Arizona, U.S.A.

I. Introduction

Infant feeding practices have the potential to influence risk for the development of asthma in childhood through several pathways. First, human milk is a complex substance that provides both potentially protective compounds such as secretory IgA and growth factors, as well as inflammatory and anti-inflammatory cytokines, all of which may influence susceptibility to infection. Whatever food is given to a newborn provides early and prolonged exposure to potential antigens including allergens. Finally, substances taken by an infant by mouth interact with the largest immunologic organ in the human body, the intestinal mucosa. It has been speculated[1,2] that substances in human milk may exert immunomodulatory effects either through interactions with the gut-associated lymphoid tissue or at distal locations, after crossing the mucosal barrier and migrating to susceptible organs.

Despite this potential, the relationship between infant feeding practices and asthma remains controversial. This chapter will review existing knowledge of the relationship, identify methodological issues that may contribute to the continuing controversy, and discuss possible mechanisms that might underlie the observed relationships. Finally, it will consider the potential role of breast feeding in the prevention of asthma.

II. Background

A. Existing Evidence of Relationship of Infant Feeding and Asthma

Tables 16.1 and 16.2 summarize the studies[3–18] that assessed the relationship of infant feeding practices and the development of asthma. Only studies that adjusted for confounders are considered because mothers who breast feed differ from those who formula feed in many respects, some of which likely influence risk for the development of asthma. In addition, only studies with a minimum of 100 subjects that were unselected with regard to parental history of asthma and assessed incidence and/or prevalence (not severity) of asthma were included. It is evident that a wide range of findings exists. Some studies showed protective effects of breast feeding for various periods, some found no relation, and some cited potential deleterious effects.

Numerous methodological factors may influence the results of studies, including sample sizes, definitions of asthma, and compositions of populations, particularly with reference to proportions of subjects with allergic parents. Wide variability also exists among results of studies of the prevalence of asthma — rates are as low as 2.0%[17] and as high as 14.3%.[18] In addition, many studies do not consider whether breast feeding is the exclusive feeding method. Even small amounts of formula given early in life can induce sensitization, and misclassification of subjects in this regard could alter findings.

B. Age as a Determinant of the Relationship of Breast Feeding and Asthma

The one consistent factor that appears to influence the relationship of infant feeding practices to asthma is age at which asthma is ascertained. This is critically important because it has become apparent during the past decade that not all the different wheezing phenotypes observed throughout childhood are synonymous with allergic asthma.[19,20] Wheeze is common in early life, and is generally a transient condition associated with viral infection. Early wheeze may be the first indication of later allergic asthma for only a minority of children. Classic IgE-mediated asthma becomes the predominant form of wheezing only after the first decade of life. Between these two periods (i.e., in the early school years), wheezing syndromes overlap substantially, with wheeze occurring both in nonatopic, nonasthmatic children and in those who will go on to develop classic allergic asthma.

Table 16.1 Studies Showing Protective Effects of Breast Feeding against Asthma

Reference	N	Age at Outcome	Study Type	Asthma Definition	Population	Adjusted Effect of Breast Feeding[a]
Chulada et al. 2003 [2a]	7766	6 yr	Retrospective	MD diagnosis	U.S.	Ever BF protective
Dell and To 2001 [3]	2184	1–2 yr	Retrospective	MD diagnosis; wheeze past year	Canada	BF >9 months protective
Haby et al. 2001 [4]	974	3–5 yr	Retrospective	MD diagnosis with current symptoms and asthma meds	Australia	Ever BF protective
Karunasekera et al. 2001 [5]	600	1–10 yr	Case control	Asthma hospitalization and ≥2 prior episodes	Sri Lanka	BF ≥6 months protective
McConnochie and Roughman 1986 [6]	234	6–10 yr	Historical cohort	Wheeze in the past 2 years	Rochester, NY	BF >6 months protective
Oddy et al. 1999 [7]	2187	6 yr	Prospective cohort	MD diagnosis and ≥3 wheezing episodes after 1 yr	Western Australia	Exclusive BF >4 months protective
Tariq et al. 1998 [8]	1218	4 yr	Prospective cohort	≥3 episodes of wheeze lasting ≥3 days	Isle of Wight, U.K.	Exclusive BF >3 months protective
Wilson et al. 1998 [9]	545	7 yr	Prospective cohort	MD diagnosis or current use of asthma meds	Dundee, Scotland	BF >15 weeks protective
Wright et al. 1995 [10]	988	6 yr	Prospective cohort	≥4 episodes of wheeze in past year	U.S.	Any BF protective (nonatopic children)

Note: See text for inclusion criteria.

[a] After adjustment for confounders, as defined by the authors

Table 16.2 Studies Showing No Significant Effects or Deleterious Effects of Breast Feeding on Asthma

Reference	N	Age at Outcome	Study Type	Asthma Definition	Population	Adjusted Effect of Breast Feeding[a]
Infante-Rivard et al. 2001 [11]	1,114	9–11 yr	Case control	MD diagnosis	Montreal, Canada	No relation
Lewis et al. 1996 [12]	20,528	16 yr	Birth cohort	Self-reported asthma or wheezy bronchitis	U.K.	No relation
Romieu et al 2000 [13]	5,182	7–14 yr	Retrospective	MD diagnosis	Brazil	No significant relation
Schwartz et al. 1990 [14]	5,672	6 mo–11 yr	Retrospective (national sample)	MD diagnosis	U.S.	No relation
Sears et al. 2002 [15]	1,037	9–21 yr	Prospective cohort	Current asthma, BHR	Dunedin, New Zealand	BF >4 mo adverse
Takemura et al. 2001 [16]	23,828	6–15 yr	Case control	MD diagnosis, ≥2 attacks of SOB	Japan	Exclusive BF ≥3 mo adverse
Taylor et al. 1983 [17]	12,473	5 yr	Retrospective (national sample)	MD diagnosis	U.K.	No relation
Wright et al. 2001 [18]	926	13 yr	Prospective birth cohort	MD diagnosis and wheeze in past year	U.S.	No relation overall; adverse effects in atopic children of asthmatic mothers

Note: See text for inclusion criteria. BHR = bronchial hyperresponsiveness. SOB = Shortness of breath.
a After adjustment for confounders, as defined by the authors.

Virtually all the studies following children to age 6 or 7 years show protective effects of breast feeding against asthma. However, it is extremely difficult to differentiate early onset allergic asthma from transient wheezing early in life, even after careful consideration of numerous risk factors.[21] This means that the label of asthma in the first years of life refers primarily to the nonallergic infection-related form that predominates early in life. Indeed, few of the studies that find protective effects show a relation with skin test responses or other objective indicators of atopy that would indicate that the outcome considered is IgE-mediated asthma. Thus, these results are consistent with the well-documented protective effect of breast feeding against infectious wheezing[22-25] rather than any protection from allergic asthma.

Results of studies of children between 6 and 8 years of age are more mixed, with most showing no relation between infant feeding practices and asthma. Studies that continue to show protective effects in these years[6] tend to be substantially smaller than those that show no relation.[17] However, the conflicting results may also reflect differences between populations in, for example, the overall susceptibility to allergic asthma including genetic predisposition for asthma and general risk factors for infectious respiratory illness.

Finally, all studies that assessed asthma in children above 8 years of age showed either no relation or an adverse effect of breast feeding on asthma. One commonly cited exception to this observation is a study by Saarinen and Kajosaari[26] of 150 children followed to age 17 years. However, the outcome of this study was designated "respiratory allergy," and included atopic eczema, doctor-diagnosed "allergic asthma" with observable bronchodilator response, and rhinoconjunctivitis, either seasonal or in association with animal contact. Only 10 of the 67 children identified as having respiratory allergies in this population had asthma, so the finding cannot be said to pertain specifically to asthma.

Two studies provide internal support for an age-dependent relation of breast feeding and asthma. Infante-Rivard et al.[11] differentiated children with diagnoses of asthma into two groups: those with persistent symptoms 6 to 7 years after the original diagnosis and those whose symptoms had remitted. Breast feeding duration of less than 4 months showed no relation to case–control status for persistent symptoms. However, a trend toward a protective effect against doctor-diagnosed asthma was noted among children whose symptoms had remitted, suggesting that breast feeding protects only against early wheezing illnesses. Our own studies suggest a similar effect. We had previously shown that breast feeding was associated with a lower prevalence of recurrent wheeze at age 6.[10] However, when physician-diagnosed asthma with current symptoms from ages 8 to 13 years was considered,[18] there was no relation between duration of exclusive breast feeding and asthma for the group as a whole. In addition, we found that the relation differed depending on maternal asthma status: while breast feeding was unrelated to asthma among children of nonasthmatic mothers, it was associated with a significantly elevated risk of asthma among children who were atopic at age 6 and whose mothers had asthma.

III. Possible Explanations for Conflicting Observations

A. Explaining Protective Effects in Early Life

Because infections provide the stimuli for most wheezing in the first years of life, it is likely that the anti-infective components of human milk play a major role in the protection against early asthma. These components, most of which are not found in infant formulas, provide specific as well as nonspecific defenses against infectious agents.

1. Specific Defense Mechanisms

Human milk has been shown to have specific antibody and cellular immune reactivity against many etiologic agents associated with respiratory tract infections. Maternal immunity is transferred to an infant via secretory IgA antibodies in milk, assuring that the infant is protected against the specific pathogens likely to be encountered. Secretory IgA (sIgA) is produced in the intestinal tract except during the first 4 to 6 weeks of life, during which time sIgA is provided in a highly concentrated form through colostrum and milk. Tsutsumi et al.[27] have shown that colostrum and early milk contain sIgA to respiratory syncytial virus (RSV), the most common etiologic agent associated with lower respiratory illnesses in infancy. Andersson et al.[28] found that the sIgA in human milk blocks the attachment to retropharyngeal cells of *Streptococcus pneumoniae* and of *Hemophilus influenzae*, two other common causes of early respiratory illness.

2. Nonspecific Defenses

Other components of human milk, such as lysozyme, lactoferrin, oligosaccharides, and mucins, play roles in protecting an infant from infection at a time when the infant defense system is poorly developed.[29,30] These elements typically render microbes ineffective or alter their ability to replicate.

Milk also contains numerous biologically active peptides, including several types of growth factors, some of which have been shown in animal models to accelerate growth of the lungs and the intestines.[31] These growth factors may account for our finding[32] that breast-fed infants have more mature lungs prior to respiratory infections, based on measures of airway conductance derived from the shapes of breathing curves obtained in the first 2 months of life. This finding has direct relevance to wheeze in infancy because we have also shown that infants with reduced lung function early in life had increased risk of lower respiratory illness (LRI) before their first birthdays[33] It raises the possibility that lower rates of respiratory illness in the first few years of life among breast-fed infants may be due in part to the greater maturity of their lungs.

3. Possible Immunoregulatory Effects

Finally, it has been postulated that the infant immune system may be modulated by exposure to immunologically active components in human milk, including cytokines produced by immunocompetent cells.[34] It has been shown, for example, that breast-fed infants produce higher levels of interferon-α in response to RSV infection.[35] Little research has been done on the effects of cytokines in milk, but we have recently shown that the dose of transforming growth factor (TGF)-β received through breast feeding is significantly inversely associated with wheeze in infancy,[36] even after adjusting for duration of breast feeding. Evidence from animal models[37] indicates that at least some of components of milk may be absorbed into systemic circulation and reach distal organs. It is this aspect of human milk that may provide long-lasting effects against respiratory and other types of illness. Clearly, the mechanisms by which breast milk may provide protection against respiratory illness are multiple, diverse, and complex.

B. Lack of Association or Deleterious Effects of Breast Feeding on Later Asthma

Several mechanisms may account for the lack of association or deleterious effect of breast feeding on asthma shown in studies of older children. If the hygiene hypothesis discussed below is true, some of the beneficial effects of breast feeding in early life may paradoxically increase the risk for asthma by reducing the stimulus for development of Th1 responses. Components of human milk may also differ based on the mother's allergic status and that may affect the infant's susceptibility to asthma beyond any genetic influence.

1. Breast Feeding May Reduce Stimulus for Development of Th1 Response

It has been hypothesized[38] that one cause of the worldwide increase in asthma may be global changes in exposures to infectious organisms through access to clean water, plumbing, and the use of antibiotics to treat illness and in foods. In particular, it has been hypothesized[39] that exposure early in life to bacteria and their products fosters dendritic cell maturation and production of interleukin (IL)-12, which stimulates a Th1 response. Epidemiologic studies support the hygiene hypothesis by showing lower prevalence of asthma and atopy in association with high exposure to Gram-negative bacteria, for example, among children raised on farms.[40–42] Similarly, we have shown that early life exposure to other children, often considered a surrogate marker for increased microbial burden, is associated with frequent wheezing in early life and a significantly lower prevalence of asthma beginning after age 6.[43] It is well established that breast feeding is protective against a range of infectious illnesses including lower respiratory tract infections, otitis media, and gastrointestinal illnesses.[44] However, this protection may reduce the stimulus for maturation of dendritic cells in the context of reduced exposure to microbes, thereby attenuating or delaying development of a Th1 response.

Alternatively, breast feeding may alter risk for asthma through another pathway: bacterial colonization of the intestinal tract. A major impetus for immune system development comes from microorganisms in the intestinal tract where 70% of all immune cells are located.[45] It has been postulated that gut colonization may influence susceptibility to asthma.[39,46] This speculation is consistent with the finding that the gut flora of infants in the industrialized world (where asthma prevalence is high) are less diverse and lower in Gram-negative organisms than gut flora of infants in the developing world, where asthma prevalence is low.[47,48] Others[46] have shown differences in early gut microflora, depending on whether a child develops atopic sensitization by 12 months of age. Finally, Matricardi et al.[49] revealed that serologic evidence of past infection with orofecal and foodborne organisms was associated with lower prevalence of asthma; no similar protective effect was shown for infections with airborne organisms.

These findings are relevant to the relation of breast feeding and asthma because infants who are breast fed exclusively have lower levels of Gram-negative enterobacteria in their gastrointestinal tracts[50,51] and less diversity of colonizing species. These differences are partially responsible for the well-documented reduction in gastroenteritis among breast-fed infants[52] that is particularly critical to infant health in settings of poor sanitation. Nevertheless, by altering gut flora, breast feeding may reduce the stimulus for immune system development in neonates. Either the protection from infection or the differences in gut flora associated with breast feeding may have particular consequences for asthma risk among infants genetically predisposed to asthma.

2. Variability in Components of Human Milk in Relation to Maternal Asthma Status

The milk of allergic mothers may differ from milk of nonallergic mothers in ways that affect subsequent allergic susceptibility. This speculation is supported by *in vitro* experiments[53] showing that cord blood lymphocytes stimulated with supernatants from the milk of atopic mothers were significantly more likely to produce IgE than lymphocytes stimulated with supernatants from nonatopic mothers.

Several components of human milk are potential candidates for a differential effect, depending on asthma maternal status. Asthma has been characterized as a Th2 disease,[39] associated with a preponderance of the IL-4, -5, and -13 cytokines. If the cytokines present in milk[2,54] differed by maternal atopic status, they might influence the polarization of the infant's immune response. Bottcher et al.[55] have shown that concentrations of IL-4 in colostrum are higher in allergic rather than nonallergic mothers; similar trends were found for IL-5 and IL-13. These authors also demonstrated elevated IL-8 in both colostrum and mature milk of allergic mothers,[56] To our knowledge, however, the relation of the amount of these cytokines in milk to respiratory or allergic symptoms in the infant has not yet been investigated.

Human milk also contains large amounts of soluble CD14,[57] a bacterial pattern recognition receptor shown to be inversely associated with total IgE at age 11.[58] If sCD14 levels vary by atopic status in milk as they do in serum, this variability may influence subsequent immune system development in a child. Variability in sCD14 levels would be consistent with our previous finding[59] that the association between breast feeding and total serum IgE in a child depends on maternal IgE level. We reported that IgE was elevated in children of mothers with high IgE only if they were breast fed, whereas IgE was lower in children of mothers with lower IgE only if they were breast fed. We assessed the amount of sCD14 in milk from healthy nonselected women (n = 219) enrolled in the Infant Immune Study at 11 days postpartum. Preliminary analyses indicated that sCD14 levels among mothers with active physician-diagnosed asthma tended to be in the lower half of the distribution for age-adjusted CD14 levels, but the difference was not statistically significant (p <0.09, unpublished data).

Finally, it has been shown[60] that levels of long-chain polyunsaturated fatty acid levels in milk differ depending on the atopic status of the mother. While this is intriguing, the relation of fat consumption to asthma has not been established. The presence of allergens or allergen-specific antigens may also differ by maternal atopic status, but this has not, to our knowledge, been studied.

IV. Implications for Prevention

Based on the paradoxical relations between infant feeding practices and childhood asthma, it is difficult to formulate a clear proposal for using breast feeding as a prophylaxis measure for asthma. However, several points should be made.

The first point is that the composition of all mammalian milk is species specific. For example, among sub-Antarctic fur seals whose body fat is critical to survival, lipids comprise 43% of milk volume,[61] compared with less than 4% for human milk. Like other milks, human milk has been specifically adapted through evolutionary pressures operating over millennia to suit the unique needs of our species. Human milk is rich both in factors that protect from infection in infancy and in long-chain polyunsaturated fatty acids that appear critical to the development of the growing brain.[62] It contains agents that affect the growth, development, and the functions of the gastrointestinal tract.[63] Breast feeding also provides optimal nutrition, benefits maternal health, and fosters bonding between mother and infant. Obviously, these effects of breast feeding were more critical to infant survival than any potential effect of human milk on risk for the development of later asthma. Given these multiple benefits, any deleterious effect of breast feeding on child health would have to be much more persuasive than what has been shown for asthma to date, before one would question the American Academy of Pediatrics' recommendation[64] that infants be exclusively breast fed for 4 to 6 months.

Based on this commitment to the benefits of breast feeding, it would be ideal if potential deleterious effects could be mitigated. Accumulating evidence for the hygiene hypothesis and the recognition that intestinal microflora may influence early immune system development led to an interest in exploring the role of probiotics, bacterial cultures that are ingested to foster the growth of healthy gut flora, as possible prophylaxis against allergic disease. Because breast feeding provides direct transference of whatever is in the mother's system to the infant, several promising studies have investigated the effects of administration of probiotics through lactating mothers. Rautava et al.[65] showed in a small double-blind study that administering probiotics to pregnant or lactating women increased the concentrations of TGF-β in milk. Further, maternal intake of probiotics was associated with a significant reduction in atopic eczema in their infants (15 versus 47% of mothers receiving the placebo). In a study of infants at risk of allergic disease, Kalliomaki et al.[66] also showed that the risk for developing atopic eczema was half for infants whose mothers received probiotics compared with the placebo group (relative risk = 0.51; confidence interval 0.32–0.84). If additional research shows that probiotics alter the risk of developing asthma, lactation may provide a safe, effective route of administration of these substances to infants at a critical time in the development of their immune systems.

V. Conclusions

To summarize, it appears that breast feeding is associated with a reduction in the nonallergic form of asthma that predominates in early in life, consistent with the protective effect of breast feeding against infection. However, as children age and asthma becomes predominantly IgE-mediated, there is either no relation to or adverse relation of breast feeding with asthma.

The apparent paradoxical findings regarding asthma and wheeze suggest that two mechanisms may be at work. Numerous factors in milk provide both specific and nonspecific protection against respiratory infection in early life and likely account for the relation with asthma prior to age 6 years. Paradoxically, this protection or the beneficial effect of breast feeding on gut flora may reduce some of the stimulus for the maturation of the Th1 response in early life, thereby increasing risk for later allergic asthma. Future prevention efforts may include administration of probiotics to lactating mothers, which may provide a safe way to maintain the benefits of breast feeding while adding protection against asthma.

References

1. Pabst H. Immunomodulation by breast feeding. *Pediatr Infect Dis J* 1997; 16: 991–995.
2. Goldman A, Chheda S, Garofalo R, and Schmalstieg FC. Cytokines in human milk: properties and potential effects upon the mammary gland and the neonate. *J Mammary Gland Biol Neoplasia* 1996; 1: 251–258.
2a. Chulada PC, Arbes SJ Jr, Dunson D, Zeldin DC. Breast-feeding and the prevalence of asthma and wheeze in children: analyses from the Third National Health and Nutrition Examination Survey, 1988–1994. *J Allergy Clin Immunol* 2003 Feb; 111(2): 328–336.
3. Dell S and To R. Breast feeding and asthma in young children. *Arch Pediatr Adolescent Med* 2001; 155: 1261–1266.
4. Haby M, Peat JK, Marks GB, Woolcock AJ, and Leeder SR. Asthma in preschool children: prevalence and risk factors. *Thorax* 2001; 56: 589–595.
5. Karunasekera K, Jayasinghe CT, and Alwis LW. Risk factors of childhood asthma: a Sri Lankan study. *J Trop Pediatr* 2001. 47: 142–145.
6. McConnochie K and Roghmann KJ. Breast feeding and maternal smoking as predictors of wheezing in children age 6 to 10 years. *Pediatr Pulmonol* 1986; 2: 260–268.
7. Oddy W, Holt PG, Sly PD, Read AW, Landau LI, Stanley FJ, Kendall GE, and Burton PR. Association between breast feeding and asthma in 6-year-old children: findings of a prospective birth cohort study. *Br Med J* 1999; 319: 815–819.
8. Tariq S, Matthews SM, Hakim EA, Stevens M, Arshad SH, and Hide DW. Prevalence of and risk factors for atopy in early childhood: a whole population birth cohort study. *J Allergy Clin Immunol* 1998; 101: 587–593.
9. Wilson A, Forsyth JS, Greene SA, Irvine L, Hau C, and Howie PW. Relation of infant diet to childhood health: seven-year follow-up of cohort of children in Dundee infant feeding study. *Br Med J* 1998; 316: 21–26.
10. Wright A, Holberg CJ, Taussig LM, and Martinez FD. Relationship of infant feeding to recurrent wheezing at age 6 years. *Arch Pediatric Adolescent Med* 1995; 149: 758–763.
11. Infante-Rivard C, Amre D, Gautrin D, and Malo JL. Family size, day-care attendance, and breast feeding in relation to the incidence of childhood asthma. *Am J Epidemiol* 2001; 153: 653–658.
12. Lewis S, Butland B, Strachan D, Bynner J, Richards D, Butler N, and Britton J. Study of the aetiology of wheezing illness at age 16 in two national British birth cohorts. *Thorax* 1996; 51: 670–676.
13. Romieu I, Werneck G, Velasco SR, White M, and Hernandez M. Breast feeding and asthma among Brazilian children. *J Asthma* 2000; 37: 575–583.

14. Schwartz J, Gold D, Dockery DW, Weiss ST, and Speizer FE. Predictors of asthma and persistent wheeze in a national sample of children in the United States: association with social class, perinatant events, and race. *Am Rev Respir Dis* 1990; 142: 555–562.

15. Sears M, Greene JM, Willan AR, Taylor DR, Flannery EM, Cowan JO, Herbison GP, and Poulton R. Long-term relation between breast feeding and development of atopy and asthma in children and young adults: a longitudinal study. *Lancet* 2002; 360: 901–907.

16. Takemura Y, Sakurai Y, Honjo S, Kusakari A, Hara T, Gibo M, Tokimatsu A, and Kugai N. Relation between breast feeding and the prevalence of asthma: Tokorozawa Childhood Asthma and Pollinosis Study. *Am J Epidemiol* 2001; 154: 115–119.

17. Taylor B, Wadsworth J, Golding J, and Butler N. Breast feeding, eczema, asthma, and hayfever. *J Epidemiol. Commun Health* 1983; 37: 95–99.

18. Wright A, Holberg CJ, Taussig LM, and Martinez FD. Factors influencing the relation of infant feeding to asthma and recurrent wheeze in childhood. *Thorax* 2001; 56: 192–197.

19. Martinez F, Wright AL, Taussig LM, Holberg CJ, Halonen M, and Morgan WJ. Asthma and wheezing in the first six years of life. *New Engl J Med* 1995; 332: 133–138.

20. Stein R, Holberg CJ, Morgan WJ, Wright AL, Lombardi E, Taussig L, and Martinez FD. Peak flow variability, methacholine responsiveness and atopy as markers for detecting different wheezing phenotypes in childhood. *Thorax* 1997; 52: 946–952.

21. Castro-Rodriguez J, Holberg C, Wright AL, and Martinez, FD. An index to define signs of asthma in young children with recurrent wheezing. *Am J Respir Crit Care Med* 2000; 162: 1403–1406.

22. Cushing A, Samet JM, Lambert WE, Skipper BJ, Hunt WC, Young SA, and McLaren, LC. Breast feeding reduces risk of respiratory illness in infants. *Am J Epidemiol* 1998; 147: 863–870.

23. Holberg C, Wright AL, Martinez FD, Ray CG, Taussig LM, and Lebowitz MD. Risk factors for respiratory syncytial virus-associated lower respiratory illnesses in the first year of life. *Am J Epidemiol* 1991; 133: 1135–1151.

24. Howie TM, Forsyth JS, Ogston SA, Clark A, Florey CD. Protective effect of breast feeding against infection. *Br Med J* 1990; 300: 11–16.

25. Wright A, Holberg CJ, Martinez FD, Morgan WJ, and Taussig L. Breast feeding and lower respiratory tract illness in the first year of life. *Br Med J* 1989; 299: 946–949.

26. Saarinen U and Kajosaari M. Breast feeding as prophylaxis against atopic disease: prospective follow-up study until 17 years old. *Lancet* 1995; 346: 1065–1069.

27. Tsutsumi H, Honjo T, Nagai K, Chiba Y, Chiba S, and Tsugawa S. Immunoglobulin A antibody response to respiratory syncytial virus structural proteins in colostrum and milk. *J Clin Microbiol* 1989; 27: 1949–1951.

28. Andersson B, Porras O, Hanson LA, Svanborg-Eden C, and Leffler H. Non-antibody-containing fractions of breast milk inhibit epithelial attachment of *Streptococcus pneumoniae* and *Haemophilus influenzae*. *Lancet* 1985; 1: 643.

29. Goldman A. The immune system of human milk: antimicrobial, antiinflammatory and immunomodulating properties. *Pediatr Infect Dis J* 1993; 12: 664–671.

30. Hamosh M, Peterson JA, Henderson TR, Scallan CD, Kiwan R, and Ceriani RL, Armand M, and Mehta NR. Protective function of human milk: the milk fat globule. *Sem Perinatol* 1999; 23: 242–249.

31. Chinoy MR, Zgleszewski SE, Cilley RE, Blewett CJ, Krummel TM, Reisher, SR and Feinstein SI. Influence of epidermal growth factor and transforming growth factor beta-1 on patterns of fetal mouse lung branching morphogenesis in organ culture. *Pediatr Pulmonol* 1998; 25: 244–256.
32. Martinez F, Morgan WJ, Wright AL, and Taussig LM. Diminished lung function as a predisposing factor for wheezing respiratory illness in infants. *New Engl J Med* 1998; 319: 1112–1117.
33. Martinez F, Morgan WJ, Wright AL, and Taussig, LM. Breast feeding, lung function and lower respiratory tract illnesses during the first year of life. *Am Rev Respir Dis* 1988; 137: 405.
34. Brandtzaeg J. Development of the mucosal immune system in humans, in *Recent Developments in Infant Nutrition*, Bindels JG, Goedhart AC, and Visser HKA, Eds. London: Kluwer Academic, 1996, pp. 349–376.
35. Chiba Y, Minagawa T, Mito K, Nakane A, Suga K, Honjo T, and Nakao T. Effect of breast feeding on responses of systemic interferon and virus-specific lymphocyte transformation in infants with respiratory syncytial virus infection. *J Med Virol* 1987; 21: 7–14.
36. Oddy W, Halonen M, Martinez FD, Lohman IC, Stern DA, Kurzius-Spencer M, Guerra S, and Wright, AL. TGF-beta in human milk is associated with wheeze in infancy. *J Allergy Clin Immunol*. 2003; 112: 723–728.
37. Tuboly S and Bernath S. Intestinal absorption of colostral lymphoid cells in newborn animals: integrating population outcomes, biological mechanisms and research methods, in *The Study of Human Milk and Lactation*, Davis MK et al., Eds., New York: Kluwer Academic/Plenum, 2002.
38. Strachan D. Hay fever, hygiene, and household size. *Br Med J* 1989; 299: 1259–1260.
39. Holt P, Sly PD, and Bjorksten B. Atopic versus infectious diseases in childhood: a question of balance? *Pediatr Allergy Immunol* 1997; 8: 53–58.
40. Braun-Fahrlander C, Gassner M, Grize L, Neu U, Sennhauser FH, Varonier HS, Vuille JC, and Wuthrich B. Prevalence of hay fever and allergic sensitization in farmers' children and their peers living in the same rural community: Swiss study on childhood allergy and respiratory symptoms with respect to air pollution. *Clin Exp Allergy* 1999; 29: 28–34.
41. Riedler J, Braun-Fahrlander B, Eder W, Schreuer M, Waser M, Maisch S, Carr D, Schierl R, Nowak D, and von Mutis, E. Exposure to farming in early life and development of asthma and allergy: a cross-sectional survey. *Lancet* 2001; 358: 1129–1133.
42. Von Ehrenstein O, Von Mutius E, Illi S, Baumann L, Bohm O, and von Kries R. Reduced risk of hay fever and asthma among children of farmers. *Clin Exp. Allergy* 2000; 30: 187–193.
43. Ball T, Castro-Rodriguez JA, Griffith KA, Holberg CJ, Martinez FD, and Wright, AL. Siblings, day-care attendance, and the risk of asthma and wheezing during childhood. *New Engl J Med* 2000; 343: 538–543.
44. Oddy W. Breast feeding protects against illness and infection in infants and children: review of the evidence. *Breast Feeding Rev* 2001; 9: 11–18.

45. Gaskins H. Immunological aspects of host/microbiota interactions at the intestinal epithelium, in *Gastrointestinal Microbiology*, Vol 2, Mackie RI, White BA, and Isaacson RE, Eds. New York: International Thompson Publishing, 1997, pp. 537–587.

46. Kalliomaki M, Kirjavainen P, Eerola E, Kero P, Salminen S, and Isolauri, E. Distinct patterns of neonatal gut microflora in infants in whom atopy was and was not developing. *J Allergy Clin Immunol* 2001; 107: 129–134.

47. Sepp E, Julge K, Vasar M, Naaber P, Bjorksten B, and Mikelsaar M. Intestinal microflora of Estonian and Swedish infants. *Acta Paediatr* 1997; 86: 956–961.

48. Bjorksten B, Naaber P, Sepp E, and Mikelsaar M. Intestinal microflora in allergic Estonian and Swedish 2-year-old children. *Clin Exp Allergy* 1999; 29: 342–346.

49. Matricardi P, Rosmini F, Riondino S, Fortini M, Ferrigno L, Rapicetta M, and Bonini S. Exposure to foodborne and orofecal microbes versus airborne viruses in relation to atopy and allergic asthma: epidemiological study. *Br Med J* 2000; 320: 412–417.

50. Day A and Sherman PM. Normal intestinal flora: pathobiology and clinical relevance. *Int Sem Paediatr Gastroenterol Nutr* 1998; 7: 2–7.

51. Yoshioka H, Iseki K, and Fujita K. Development and differences of intestinal flora in the neonatal period in breast-fed and bottle-fed infants. *Pediatrics* 1983; 72: 317–321.

52. Molbak K, Gottschau A, Aaby P, Hojlyng N, Ingholt L, and da Silva, A. Prolonged breast feeding, diarrheal disease, and survival of children in Guinea-Bissau. *Br Med J* 1994; 308: 1403–1406.

53. Allardyce R and Wilson A. Breast milk cell supernatants from atopic donors stimulate cord blood IgE secretion *in vitro*. *Clin Allergy* 1984; 14: 259–267.

54. Eglinton B, Roberton DM, and Cumins AG. Phenotype of T cells, their soluble receptor levels, and cytokine profile of human breast milk. *Immunol Cell Biol* 1994; 72: 306–313.

55. Bottcher M, Jenmalm MC, Bjorksten B, and Garofalo R Chemoattractant factors in breast milk from allergic and nonallergic mothers. *Pediatr Res* 2000; 47: 592–597.

56. Bottcher M, Jenmalm MC, Garofalo RP, and Bjorksten, B. Cytokines in breast milk from allergic and nonallergic mothers. *Pediatr Res* 2000; 41: 157–162.

57. Labeta M, Vidal K, Nores JE, Arias M, Vita N, Morgan BP, Guillemot JC, Loyaux D, Ferrara P, Schmid D, Affolter M, Borysiewicz LK, Donnet-Hughes A, and Schiffrin EJ. Innate recognition of bacteria in human milk is mediated by a milk-derived highly expressed pattern recognition receptor, soluble CD14. *J Exp Med* 2000; 191: 1807–1812.

58. Baldini M, Lohman IC, Halonen M, Erickson RP, Holt PG, and Martinez FD. A polymorphism in the 5' flanking region of the CD14 gene is associated with circulating soluble CD14 levels and with total serum immunoglobulin E. *Am J Respir Cell Mol Biol* 1999; 20: 976–983.

59. Wright A, Sherrill D, Holberg CJ, Halonen M, and Martinez FD. Mechanisms of allergy: breast feeding, maternal IgE, and total serum IgE in childhood. *J Allergy Clin Immunol* 1999; 104: 589–594.

60. Duchen K, Yu G, and Bjorksten B. Atopic sensitization during the first year of life in relation to long chain polyunsaturated fatty acid levels in human milk. *Pediatr Res* 1998; 44: 478–484.

61. Georges J, Groscolas R, Guinet C, and Robin J. Milking strategy in subantarctic fur seals *Arctocepyhalus tropicalis* breeding on Amsterdam Island: evidence from changes in milk composition. *Physiol Biochem Zool* 2001; 74: 548–559.
62. Koletzko B, Rodriguez-Palmero M, Demmelmair H, Fidler N, Jensen R, and Sauerwald T. Physiological aspect of human milk lipids. *Early Hum Dev* 2001; 65: S3–S18.
63. Goldman AS. Modulation of the gastrointestinal tract of infants by human milk: interfaces and interactions: an evolutionary perspective. *J Nutr* 2000; 130: S426–S431.
64. American Academy of Pediatrics Work Group on Breast Feeding. Breast feeding and the use of human milk. *Pediatrics* 1997; 100: 1035–1039.
65. Rautava S, Kalliomaki M, and Isolauri E. Probiotics during pregnancy and breast feeding might confer immunomodulatory protection against atopic disease in the infant. *J Allergy Clin Immunol* 2002; 109: 119–121.
66. Kalliomaki M, Salminen S, Arvilommi H, Kero P, Koskinen P, and Isolauri E. Probiotics in primary prevention of atopic disease: a randomised placebo-controlled trial *Lancet* 2001; 357: 1076–1079.

IV

Treatment

17

Asthma in the Inner City

KRISTIN M. BURKART, MEGAN T. SANDEL, and GEORGE T. O'CONNOR

Boston University School of Medicine
Boston, Massachusetts, U.S.A.

I. Excess Burden of Asthma in the Inner City

Asthma, one of the most common chronic diseases in all socioeconomic groups in the United States, imposes a particularly heavy burden on residents of inner cities. The dimensions of this excess burden include asthma prevalence, morbidity, and mortality.[1–8] Inner city residence, low socioeconomic status (SES), and racial and ethnic minority group status are closely intertwined in the United States. This intermingling makes it difficult, if not impossible, to fully disentangle the independent relationship of each of these characteristics to asthma.

National and regional population-based surveys indicate a higher prevalence of asthma in inner city communities than in the nation as a whole. Data collected in the Second National Health and Nutritional Examination Survey (NHANES II) reported that inner city residents are 1.58 times more likely to have asthma compared with non-inner city residents.[9] Population-based surveys of children in inner city areas of New York City[10] and Chicago[11] demonstrate a prevalence of ever having asthma between 14.3 and 17.4% and a prevalence of symptomatic asthma within the past 12 months between 8.6 and 14.3%. Among first graders in inner city Baltimore, the cumulative prevalences of parent-reported asthma were 8.6% for girls and 13.6% for boys.[12] These rates are two to three times the national average. In Boston, community surveys indicate strikingly high prevalence of self-reported asthma, ranging from 26 to 40% among adults in some urban public housing developments.[13,14] One survey revealed that 41% of households in inner city Buffalo report histories of asthma in at least one family member.[15]

Many studies have indicated that racial and ethnic minority groups and persons of lower SES have a higher asthma prevalence than their white, non-Hispanic, and more affluent counterparts. Data from the Hispanic Health and Nutritional Examination Survey (HHANES) reveal that children of Puerto Rican ancestry have a prevalence of questionnaire-reported asthma of 20.1%, nearly four times that of white children.[16] Data from NHANES II indicate asthma prevalences in black children and adults of nearly three times the rates in white children and adults.[6,9] Interestingly, Mexican American school children have been reported to have lower asthma prevalence rates than non-Mexican American white school children (1.9 versus 6.5%) in a rural community in Arizona.[17] How much race *per se* influences the risk of developing asthma remains unclear based on these population studies.

Relatively few investigators have attempted to tease apart the independent effects of inner city residence, race or ethnicity, and SES on asthma prevalence. Schwartz and coworkers analyzed asthma data from a sample of children 6 months to 11 years of age collected for NHANES II.[9] In this national sample, unadjusted asthma prevalence was significantly higher among blacks compared with whites (7.2 versus 3.0%). In multiple logistic regression analysis, poverty, inner city residence, and black race were all independently associated with asthma after controlling for age and sex, and the adjusted odds ratio for blacks was 1.68.[9] In a similar analysis using data from NHANES II, Turkeltaub and Gergen[6] studied subjects 12 through 74 years of age and found that blacks had significantly higher prevalence of asthma compared with whites even after adjusting for age, smoking, sex, low SES, and inner city residence.

These analyses suggest that the increased risk of asthma among blacks may be due partially to inner city residence and lower SES, but that these factors alone do not account for all of the racial effects noted. Data from the 1988 Child Health Supplement (CHS) to the National Health Interview Survey (NHIS), however, did not confirm this conclusion.

In an analysis of subjects from birth through 17 years of age, Aligne and coworkers[18] examined race, poverty, and urban residence as independent variables with parental report of current asthma serving as the outcome variable. Unadjusted data supported the findings that black children have higher prevalences of asthma than white children. After adjustment for either urban residence or poverty, however, black race was no longer significantly associated with asthma. The association of asthma and urban residence remained significant despite controlling for race and poverty.[18] This analysis suggests that urban residence, and not race *per se*, is associated with increased risk of childhood asthma.

Inner city and minority communities suffer excess burdens of asthma hospitalizations and mortality that are out of proportion to the increases in asthma prevalence seen in these communities. Inner city blacks in Chicago[4] and inner city blacks and Hispanics in New York City[3] experience hospitalization and asthma death rates 3 to 5.5 times the rate for the entire country; the prevalence of asthma in these communities is 2 to 3 times the national prevalence.

Carr et al.[3] investigated asthma hospitalization rates for residents up to 34 years of age in New York City from 1982 to 1986. Blacks, Hispanics, and non-Hispanics accounted for 81.8% of all asthma hospitalizations; their average annual hospitalization rates were five times the hospitalization rates of white patients. Between 1982 and 1986, the asthma hospitalization rate increased by 17.4% in New York City. Subgroup analysis demonstrated a 21.1% increase in asthma hospitalizations for blacks and non-Hispanics during that period compared with an 8.0% increase for Hispanics and a 5.1% increase for white non-Hispanics.[3]

Asthma hospitalization rates varied significantly within the New York City boroughs. East Harlem, where 93% of the population is black or Hispanic and of lower SES, had a significantly higher hospitalization rate for asthma (115.0 per 10,000) than Greenwich Village–Soho in Manhattan (7.2 per 10,000), an area that has a predominantly white population of higher SES.[3] Gottlieb and coworkers[19] report the asthma hospitalization rate for the city of Boston to be twice the age- and gender-adjusted Massachusetts rate. The rates of some inner city communities were nearly five times the state average. The six areas within Boston with the highest asthma hospitalization rates had higher proportions of low-SES and minority residents than other areas of the city.[19]

Despite improved preventive asthma medications, asthma death rates have increased over the past few decades, especially in urban communities with lower SES and largely minority populations.[3,4,7,20,21] In New York City between 1982 and 1987, black non-Hispanics accounted for 50% of asthma-related deaths; 27% were attributed to Hispanics.[3] Data from the National Center for Health Statistics (NCHS) revealed that the annual national asthma mortality rate among persons 5 to 34 years of age rose by 6.2% from 1982 to 1985, and an alarming 80.2% of asthma deaths occurred in urban communities.

The national asthma mortality rate of 3.5 per million per year was exceeded by the rates in many inner city populations including New York City (10.1 per million per year); Cook County, Illinois (6.6 per million per year); Maricopa County, Arizona (6.1 per million per year); and Fresno County, California (7.1 per million per year). These analyses suggest that a substantial proportion of asthma mortality nationwide is accounted for by the disproportionate mortality rates in large cities.

While the national asthma mortality rate increased from 2.8 per million per year in the early 1970s (averaged over 4 years, 1970 through 1973) to 3.5 per million per year in the early 1980s (averaged over 4 years, 1982 through 1985), more impressive increases in asthma mortality rates were noted in many inner city populations including New York (5.9 to 10.1 per million per year) and Cook County, Illinois (3.6 to 6.6 per million per year).[7] Carr et al.[3] reported that 45% of asthma-related deaths in New York City from 1982 through 1987 occurred in 6 of 41 neighborhoods although the 6 neighborhoods accounted only for 21% of city's population. Race and ethnicity remained independent risk factors for asthma hospitalization and mortality when controlled for poverty.[3]

The relative importance of urban residence, low SES, and minority (particularly black and Hispanic) status as independent risk factors for increased asthma morbidity and morality remains controversial. These three risk factors remain tightly woven in the U.S. and may exert synergistic effects on asthma morbidity and mortality.

II. Causes of Excess Burdens of Asthma in Inner Cities

The causes of excess burdens of asthma in inner city communities are not fully understood, and it is likely that multiple factors play contributing roles (Table 17.1). Possible causes of these excess burdens, many of which remain speculative, are discussed below.

A. Genetic Factors

As noted in earlier chapters, asthma is considered a familial condition. Twin studies provided early evidence of the importance of genetic factors in asthma susceptibility,[22–24] but the mode of inheritance is complex and not yet fully understood.[25,26] Segregation analysis suggests that a single-gene model is unlikely to explain asthma's mode of inheritance;[27] asthma appears to be a complex genetic trait. Genome-wide linkage studies of asthma phenotypes in families and diverse ethnic populations have identified multiple chromosomal loci associated with susceptibility to asthma.[28–35] Multiple candidate genes, suggested by current models of asthma pathogenesis and/or linkage findings, have been investigated. The "cytokine gene cluster" on chromosome 5q31-33, in particular, the polymorphisms of interleukin (IL)-13, IL-4Rα, the β_2 adrenergic receptor gene on chromosome 5q,[36–50] and chromosome 11q13 with polymorphisms in the β chain of the high affinity receptor for IgE,[51–54] have received particular attention.

Gene–environment interactions, race-specific susceptibility, and identification of genes and gene products of potential therapeutic importance are the most intriguing prospects for genetic investigations in inner cities. The multicenter Collaborative Study on the Genetics of Asthma (CSGA) collected data from

Table 17.1 Potential Causes of Excess Burdens of Asthma in Inner Cities

Perinatal factors
Young maternal age
Prematurity
Low birth weight
Environmental exposures
Indoor allergens (cockroach, dust mite, rodent, mold)
Environmental tobacco smoke
Outdoor air pollution (e.g., diesel exhaust particles)
Obesity and decreased physical activity
Stress and psychosocial factors
Stress related to poverty, exposure to violence
Depression
Drug abuse

families from three U.S. ethnic groups: whites (European Americans), African Americans, and Hispanics. Linkages to chromosomal regions varied among the different ethnic groups.[36,55] Ethnic-specific analysis revealed linkages at 6p21 in the European American population, at 11q21 in the African American population, and at 1p32 in the Hispanic population.[36]

Huang et al. performed fine mapping of the 11q21 region in 91 African American families and demonstrated significant linkage with a peak non-parametric linkage (NPL) score of 4.38.[56] Following fine mapping, they performed family-based association tests (FBATs) and transmission disequilibrium tests (TDTs) that demonstrated significant association between asthma and several individual markers in the region. These analyses suggest that chromosome 11q may contain susceptibility genes for asthma in that population of African American families.[36,55,56]

Data from the CSGA have suggested racial differences in the familial aggregation of asthma. For example, a significantly greater number of African American asthmatics had other family members afflicted with asthma compared with European Americans and Hispanics (39 versus 25 versus 26%; p = 0.001). This may be in part due to environmental influences, but it suggests that specific alleles may be more frequent or have different degrees of penetration in various ethnic groups.[55] Lester et al. also reported variability in allergen responsiveness among the ethnic groups studied in the CSGA.[55] Sensitization to cockroach allergens varied significantly among ethnic groups (African American, 53%; European American, 17%; Hispanic, 46%) after adjusting for site differences (p = 0.001).

Linkage to the β_2 adrenergic receptor (ADRB2) and possible therapeutic implications of this region led to further investigations of this candidate gene.

The ADBR2 is encoded on chromosome 5q31-32 and two common polymorphisms (Arg16 to Gly and Gln27 to Glu) have been described.[57–61] Multiple studies revealed significant differences in allelic, genotypic, and haplotype frequencies of ADRB2 polymorphisms among different ethnic groups.[57,58,62]

Caucasian Americans have greater Gly16 allelic frequencies compared with African Americans,[62,63] and the Glu27 allele is seen more frequently in Caucasian Americans than in African Americans.[58,62] Racial differences in allele and genotype frequencies of the ADRB2 polymorphisms may explain differences in airway responsiveness to inhaled β-adrenergic agonists. *In vitro* studies using mutagenesis and recombinant expression in cells[64,65] and experiments with transgenic mice[66] demonstrated differences in signaling and regulation after chronic exposure to β agonists.

Martinez et al.[61] reported that homozygotes for Arg16 were 5.3 times more likely and heterozygotes for Arg16 were 2.3 times more likely to respond to single-use bronchodilators compared with homozygotes for Gly16 (95% confidence intervals [CI] 1.6–17.7 and 1.3–4.2, respectively). Bronchodilator response was not related to the Gln27–Glu polymorphism. Israel et al.[60] performed a 16-week trial comparing asthmatics who regularly used albuterol and those who used it as needed. They demonstrated that homozygous Arg16 genotypes were more likely to show small but significant decreases in their morning peak flow measurements during regular use of albuterol, and suggest that tachyphylaxis to inhaled β agonists may be more likely in patients who are homozygous for Arg16.

Four major haplotype groups have been investigated and their frequencies varied significantly among Caucasian, African American, Asian, and Hispanic Latino ethnic groups.[59] *In vivo* investigation of these major haplotypes was performed to assess variability in bronchodilator responses to β agonists. The study demonstrated significant differences in response to bronchodilators among various haplotypes that were not observed for various single-nucleotide polymorphisms (SNPs).[59] These studies suggest that differences among racial and ethnic groups in the frequency of specific polymorphisms and/or haplotypes may influence both susceptibility to asthma and its clinical expression.

The U.S. Food and Drug Administration (FDA) recently released an alert announcing the results of a prospective study of the impact of salmeterol, a long-acting β agonist, on asthma mortality.[67] Subgroup analysis revealed a statistically significant increase in respiratory-related deaths and life-threatening respiratory events in African American patients in the salmeterol group compared with the placebo group. No differences were noted among the two groups of Caucasian patients.[67] Although the mechanisms underlying the observed effect remain unknown, such findings raise the intriguing possibility that racial differences in asthma mortality rate may be mediated in part by genetically determined responses to a pharmacologic agent.

B. Perinatal Factors

Multiple studies have linked prenatal and perinatal factors to asthma. The factors most frequently included are young maternal age, prematurity, and low or very low birth weights that are frequently seen in urban and African American populations.[9,68–73] Data from NHANES II revealed that low birth weight (defined as less than 3800 grams), prematurity, and young maternal age all have statistically significant associations with asthma (odds ratio [OR] values were 1.31, 1.28, and 1.41, respectively).[9]

Cross-sectional analysis of data from the 1988 National Maternal–Infant Health Survey and 1991 longitudinal follow-up survey revealed the prevalence of very low birth weight (below 1500 g) to be disproportionately increased in African American children compared with white children (1.8 versus 0.6%).[73]

Two additional studies were designed specifically to investigate the association of low birth weight and asthma in urban African American populations. A case control study of African American children in the inner city found that asthmatic children are more likely than non-asthmatic children to have lower birth weights, younger gestational age, and mothers who smoked during pregnancy.[69] In Michigan, the Southfield Childhood Allergy Study cohort data were analyzed to determine whether an increase in asthma prevalence among African Americans could be explained by low birth weight independent of race. Low birth weight remained a statistically significant independent risk factor associated with asthma after adjusting for race.[70]

The influence of breast feeding on the development of atopy and/or asthma remains controversial[9,74–78] and must be investigated further. The rate of breast feeding has declined in recent years, and inner city mothers who are black, young, and poorly educated and deliver low birth weight infants have particularly low rates.[79] The relationship of decreased breastfeeding and asthma burdens in inner cities has not yet been studied.

C. Environmental Exposures in Homes and Communities

1. Hygiene Hypothesis

The hygiene hypothesis states that early life infections and exposures to bacterial products such as endotoxins may activate the Th1 immune response pathway, inhibiting the development of Th2 responses involved in allergy.[80–83] Although this hypothesis is suggested by asthma prevalence patterns outside the United States (poor rural populations have lower asthma prevalence rates compared with wealthier urban populations), the excess burden of asthma seen in low-income urban communities in the United States does not appear consistent with this hypothesis at first glance.

Inner city children do not necessarily live in more hygienic conditions or suffer fewer infections than children from other socioeconomic groups. They do not generally experience the exposures to farm animals that protect against asthma and atopy in European populations,[80,84,85] but neither do most suburban children in the United States.

The relevance of the hygiene hypothesis to the excess asthma seen in inner cities remains uncertain and is the subject of ongoing investigations.

2. Indoor Allergens

IgE-mediated hypersensitivity to environmental allergens is present in most children and young adults with asthma, and exposure to allergens appears to be involved in the initial development of asthma and the exacerbation of existing asthma.[86] These pathophysiologic mechanisms are not unique to asthma in inner cities, but the specific indoor allergens and intensities of exposures encountered in the inner cities differ from those encountered in other environments.[87–90]

Cockroach allergen is an important allergen associated with asthma, especially in low-income urban communities. The German cockroach (*Blatella germanica*) is the most common species infesting homes in United States cities.[91–93] The two major German cockroach allergens have been designated Bla g 1 and Bla g 2, and a high proportion of cockroach-allergic patients produce specific IgE against both.[94,95] Cockroach allergen is more frequently encountered in urban homes than in rural homes, and the concentrations encountered in urban homes cover a wide range. In the northeastern United States, high levels of Bla g 1 and Bla g 2 in house dust are associated with low SES, African American race, and urban residence.[96]

A high percentage of low-income inner city residences have detectable cockroach allergens in vacuumed house dust.[87,88,96] For example, 71% of urban homes sampled in Atlanta, Georgia, showed detectable levels of Bla g 1 in vacuumed dust.[97] Data from the National Cooperative Inner City Asthma Study (NCICAS) indicate that the homes of 85% of urban asthmatic children in the northeastern United States cities had detectable Bla g 1 in bedroom dust; 50% of the homes had levels exceeding 8 U/g of cockroach allergen present in sampled dust.[98]

In the Inner City Asthma Study (ICAS) conducted in seven sites across the United States, 58% of the families of urban asthmatic children reported seeing cockroaches in their homes.[99] In other studies, the highest cockroach allergen levels were found in kitchens, followed by bedding, bedroom floors, and upholstered furniture.[100,101] Homes without obvious cockroach infestation may still harbor cockroach allergens. For example, in Wilmington, Delaware, 20% of homes without visible evidence of cockroach infestation had detectable levels of *Bla g* 2 in at least one room.[87]

Many asthmatic and allergic patients who reside in inner cities demonstrate immediate cutaneous hypersensitivity to cockroach extract.[98,102–105] Among 81 asthmatic children in Baltimore, the levels of cockroach allergens (Bla g 1 and Bla g 2) in their bedrooms were significantly associated with skin test reactivity to cockroach extract, even after adjustment for covariants including age, race, and SES.[96] Eighty percent of asthmatic children with bedroom levels of Bla g 1 or Bla g 2 greater than 1 U/g of dust exhibited positive skin tests to cockroach extract. In this study, urban children were more likely to test positive to cockroach extract than suburban children. African American ethnicity and low SES were independently associated with skin test reactivity to cockroach extract.[96]

In Washington, DC, positive allergy skin tests to *B. germanica* extract were seen in 28% of unselected allergy patients compared with only 7.5% of healthy control subjects.[106] In New York City, 44% of 589 patients seen at hospital-based allergy clinics had positive skin test reactions to German cockroach extract.[97]

Other studies suggest an increased prevalence of sensitization to cockroach proteins among Puerto Ricans,[97] African Americans,[96,97,107] and Mexican Americans[107] compared with non-Hispanic whites. Studies of general community samples revealed striking variations in the prevalence of skin test reactivities to cockroach extracts among racial and ethnic groups. A New York City study revealed that 59% of Puerto Rican patients and 47% of African American patients seen in allergy clinics were sensitized to cockroach extract compared with 17% of white non-Hispanic allergic patients.[97] Data from NHANES III (1988 through 1984) indicated that among children 6 to 16 years of age who underwent skin testing, African American children had 2.5 times the odds and Mexican American had 1.9 times the odds of having cockroach sensitivity compared with white children.[107]

Cockroach allergens and allergen sensitivity are commonly found in inner city environments and are powerful triggers for asthma. Bronchial provocation studies show that most asthmatics with positive skin tests to cockroach extract develop acute asthmatic responses upon inhalation of cockroach extract aerosols as well as late asthmatic reactions hours later. In contrast, cockroach skin test-negative asthmatics do not react to inhaled cockroach extract aerosols.[91,108]

Cockroach allergy is associated with severe and chronic asthma in children.[109,110] The NCICAS examined skin test sensitivity, bedroom dust allergen levels, and asthma morbidity among 476 asthmatic children.[111] Those with positive skin test reactions to cockroach extract and bedroom levels of Bla g 1 exceeding 8 U/g of dust underwent significantly more hospitalizations for asthma, unscheduled medical visits, and parent-reported wheezing. A combination of exposure and sensitization to cockroach allergens markedly increases the risk of morbidity from asthma. This combination seems more prevalent in inner cities and may explain some of the disparity in asthma severity in inner city populations.

A birth cohort study in Boston showed that exposure to cockroach allergen and sensitization are associated with increased incidence of wheeze in the first year of life[112] and incident asthma among siblings of the index children.[113] These studies suggest that exposure to cockroach allergens in inner city homes places children at a greater risk for developing asthma.

Dust mite allergen exposure is a major environmental risk factor for asthma in many settings including inner cities. Dust mites from the Dermatophagoides genus deposit feces in many household sites, including bedding, drapes, upholstered furniture, and carpets. Two allergens derived from the *Dermatophagoides pteronyssinus* mite, Der p I and Der p II,[114] are potent allergens. Direct inhalation causes immediate decreases in FEV_1 levels and late phase responses in sensitized asthmatics.[115]

Residential dust mite infestation varies from region to region. Regions with high levels of humidity and moderate climates throughout the year have higher Der p I allergen levels.[116–118] Additionally, seasonal temperature and humidity differences result in dust mite allergen levels that vary with season and peak in the late summer months.[118] Dust mite exposure may be particularly high in inner city areas where crowding, high indoor humidity due to water leaks and poor ventilation, and older carpeting, bedding, and upholstered furniture provide excellent conditions for mite proliferation.[119]

Studies have revealed varying rates of dust mite sensitization among urban asthmatics.[98,99,111] For example, in NCICAS, 31% of asthmatic children had allergen sensitivity to *D. pteronyssinus*.[98] The ICAS revealed that 57.1% of atopic asthmatic children were allergic to *D. pteronyssinus*.[99]

In the northeastern cities included in NCICAS, dust mite allergen exposures were not as important as cockroach allergen exposures as risk factors for asthma morbidity.[111] Mite allergens appear to be more important risk factors in other geographic locales such as the southeastern United States. Exposure to house dust mite allergen may be a risk factor for the development of childhood asthma. Case control studies and a birth cohort study demonstrated that exposure to dust mite allergens early in life is associated with an increased risk of asthma in later childhood.[120–122]

Mouse and rat allergens are widely distributed in inner city homes and may exert important effects on inner city children with allergy and asthma, but few data are available to address this issue. The NCICAS found detectable mouse allergens in at least one room in 95% of homes studied; 33% of inner city homes contained detectable rat allergens.[90,123]

Forty-nine percent of the homes reported mice infestation in the year preceding the study[90] and 47% reported problems with rats. Homes that reported mouse infestation were three times as likely to contain detectable rat allergens.[123] The highest allergen levels were found in the kitchens, followed by bedrooms and living/television rooms.[90]

The association of IgE-mediated hypersensitivity with mouse and rat allergens is well documented in occupational settings.[124] In NCICAS, mouse sensitivity was noted in 18% of inner city asthmatic children and was seen in 28% of atopic inner city asthmatic children in ICAS.[90,98,99] No statistically significant association was noted among mouse allergen exposure, sensitization, and asthma morbidity in inner city asthmatic children studied in NCICAS.[89]

Rat allergen sensitivity was seen in 19% of children in both the ICAS and NCICAS studies.[98,99] Perry[123] demonstrated that rat allergen sensitization and exposure were statistically significantly associated with asthma morbidity in inner city children. These studies demonstrate that rat and mouse allergens are commonly found in urban housing and suggest that increased asthma morbidity may be associated with rodent sensitization.

3. Environmental Tobacco Smoke (ETS)

The prevalence of cigarette smoking remains high in inner city areas despite an overall decrease in the tobacco use in United States in the past decade.[8] Passive exposure to ETS is more common in low-income urban communities than in other demographic groups. For example, 48% of urban asthmatic children enrolled in ICAS and 59% enrolled in NCICAS lived in houses with at least one cigarette smoker.[98,99] In NCICAS, a household member smoked during 10% of the home visits, and 48% of urine samples collected from asthmatic children had cotinine/creatine ratios consistent with significant tobacco smoke exposure within 24 hours.[98]

Exposure to ETS appears to constitute a risk factor for the development of asthma in early childhood[125–129] and an aggravating factor that increases morbidity among asthmatics.[9,69,127,130–134] A survey of 15- to 69-year-old residents of a medium-sized city revealed a significant association between physician-diagnosed asthma in non-smokers and a history of childhood ETS exposure.[132] Additionally, ETS was the most commonly reported asthma trigger in this sample. Prospective cohort studies demonstrated a dose–response relationship between ETS exposure and the risk of asthma and wheezing in early childhood.[125,126] Maternal smoking during pregnancy appeared to be an even stronger risk factor for wheezing and early childhood asthma than postnatal ETS exposure.[69,130,131]

An extensive scientific review published in 1992 by the U.S. Environmental Protection Agency concluded that there is strong evidence that ETS exposure due to parental smoking is associated with a small but significant decrease in lung function, an increase in the frequency and severity of asthma exacerbations, and increased risk of developing asthma.[127] A more recent metanalysis[135] confirmed the conclusion that parental smoking is associated with more severe disease among children with established asthma. It also indicated that parental smoking is a risk factor for the development of non-allergic wheezy bronchitis in early childhood, although it may not be a risk factor for allergic asthma that persists into later childhood.[135] Childhood ETS exposure does not appear to be a risk factor for allergic sensitization.[136] This suggests that ETS may exert its major role directly on the airways rather than on the immune system.

4. Outdoor Air Pollution

In time series analyses of population samples, day-to-day increases in outdoor air pollution were associated with increases in asthma-related energy department (ED) visits[137-139] and asthma-related hospitalizations.[140,141] Time series studies of panels of asthmatics demonstrated that short-term air pollution exposure is associated with pulmonary function decrements, increased respiratory symptoms, and increased need for asthma medications.[142] Although these effects are not limited to residents of inner cities, many urban areas have high concentration pollution-emitting industrial facilities, and all urban areas have high densities of motor vehicle traffic. Mobile source emissions, i.e., pollution from motor vehicle exhaust systems, are major sources of air pollution in inner cities.[143] Prevalence studies demonstrate increases in respiratory symptoms in individuals who live near heavily traveled roads.[144-147]

In a case–control study, Venn et al.[148] reported increased risks of wheezing in children aged 11 to 16 years who lived within 90 m of major roadways. Another case control study revealed an association between increased traffic (measured by high traffic flow) and hospitalization for wheezing and asthma in children under 5 years of age.[149]

While considerable evidence indicates that individuals with asthma experience increased morbidity upon exposure to outdoor air pollution,[150] it is less clear whether exposure to outdoor air pollution is a risk factor for the initial development of asthma.[151] In a birth cohort study, a slightly positive association between estimated exposure to traffic-related pollution and physician-diagnosed asthma was not statistically significant.[152] In a prospective cohort study, the baseline prevalence of asthma in first graders was not associated with air pollution, but after 6 years of follow-up, asthma was associated with exposure to NO_2 and particulate matter with an aerodynamic diameter smaller than 10 μm (PM_{10}). The risk of asthma in that cohort of children increased with increasing concentrations of NO_2 and PM_{10}. The odds ratios (for most polluted community, with the least polluted community as a referent) for NO_2 and PM_{10} were 3.62 and 2.84, respectively, after adjusting for sex, history of allergic disease, and maternal smoking habits.[153] Neither study achieved statistical significance but they suggest a possible role for outdoor air pollution in the development of asthma.

Particular interest has recently focused on the potential role of exposure to diesel exhaust particles (DEPs) as risk factors for asthma or for the aggravation of asthma symptoms. In a cross-sectional study, van Vliet et al.[155] investigated the effect of motor vehicle exhaust from freeways on the respiratory health of children. Truck traffic intensity and the concentration of black smoke, a marker of DEP, were associated with chronic cough, wheeze, and asthma attacks in children. This study suggested that DEPs and not NO_2 may be the factors responsible for traffic-related respiratory effects.[155] DEPs are 0.2 to 0.3 μm in size[156] and penetrate to the lower airways.[152,154,156]

The particles are relatively biologically stable and mutagenic, and they remain for long periods in the lower respiratory tract.[154] Many inner city neighborhoods are dependent on bus transportation, both for work and school, and those neighborhoods disproportionately house buses that primarily use diesel fuel. For example, in New York City, six of seven bus terminals in Manhattan are housed above 125th Street and over 2000 buses are housed in Harlem.[152] In Detroit, one area in close proximity to heavy industrial sites is associated with increased levels of both $PM_{2.5}$ and PM_{10} compared with another Detroit community further from that site.[143]

Laboratory research has shown alarming effects of DEPs on the immune system.[157–161] Human and animal studies have shown that DEPs increase IgE production — the hallmark of allergic disease.[157–161] In a mouse model, direct inhalation of DEPs resulted in increased airway inflammation and hyperresponsiveness after exposure to the ovalbumin allergen.[158] In *in vitro* studies, human bronchial epithelial cells (BECs) from atopic asthmatic patients demonstrated exaggerated releases of inflammatory mediators when exposed to DEPs compared with BECs from non-asthmatics.[159]

Diaz-Sanchez et al.[161] performed *in vivo* nasal provocation challenges with aerosolized DEPs sprayed into the nostrils of healthy volunteers to analyze local immune response in nasal lavages. They reported significant increases in IgE production and concomitant increases in expression of mRNA that codes for the IgE epsilon heavy chain in nasal lavage fluid. In a second study,[160] they demonstrated that individuals sensitized to ragweed exhibited excess allergic responses to ragweed allergens when the exposure was accompanied by DEPs. These studies suggest that exposure to DEPs may increase allergic responses when sensitized individuals are exposed to allergens. The heavy burden of diesel exhaust exposure present in inner cities may explain in part the increased prevalence and severity of asthma in urban populations, but additional research is needed.

D. Obesity, Physical Activity, and Diet

The prevalence of obesity in children and adults is increasing within the United States[162,163] and analysis of NHANES III data reveals non-Hispanic black and Mexican American adolescents to be disproportionately affected.[162] Multiple studies have reported an association between obesity and chronic respiratory diseases including asthma and airway hyperresponsiveness.[9,164–169]

In the NHANES III population-based sample, the prevalence of asthma increased significantly with increasing quartiles of body mass index (BMI) ranging from 8.7% (lowest quartile) to 14.9% (highest quartile). A significant odds ratio of 1.77 remained between the asthma and highest quartile BMIs even after controlling for confounders (age, sex, ethnicity, household size and ETS, birth weight, breastfeeding).[166]

Two urban-based studies investigated the association of asthma and BMI in urban minority children.[165,166] Both studies demonstrated significant positive associations between the degree of obesity and asthma prevalence. In a predominantly Hispanic population (78%), Gennuso et al.[165] reported that 31% of asthmatic children were very obese (>95th BMI percentile) compared with 11% of controls (p = 0.004) and that the degree of obesity did not appear to influence the severity of asthma. Data from Luder et al.[167] confirmed the association of asthma and obesity and also found obesity to be significantly associated with moderate to severe asthma.

Although these cross-sectional studies show an association between obesity and asthma, it is not clear whether respiratory compromise from asthma results in decreased activity and thus leads to increased obesity or whether obesity has a causative role in the development of asthma. A prospective cohort study of female registered nurses in the United States (Nurses' Health Study II) was designed to determine whether obesity increased the risk of developing asthma. The study demonstrated that BMI at the beginning of the study had a strong, independent, and positive association with the development of asthma during the follow-up period of 4 years, suggesting that obesity is a causative factor of asthma and not due limited to physical activity from dyspnea.[170] If obesity is indeed an independent risk factor for the development of asthma, then low income minority populations that have high prevalences of obesity[171] would be particularly affected.

E. Stress and Psychosocial Factors

Psychological stressors in the inner city exist at both individual and community levels and include poverty, unemployment, depression, and violence. Exposure to these forms of stress affects both adults and children, and increasing evidence suggests that such stress may predispose individuals to the development of asthma and aggravate existing asthma.

Urban adults with asthma have higher-than-expected rates of depression that exert major impacts on their daily functional status.[172] Among inner city children with asthma, parental psychosocial problems are associated with increased asthma morbidity.[173,174] Sly[20] reported that asthma deaths in inner city populations are often related to family dysfunction resulting in medical non-adherence and limited understanding of asthma severity with consequent delay in seeking treatment.

In addition to the impact of psychosocial dysfunction on the treatment of asthma, growing evidence indicates that psychological stress may have neuroendocrine and immunologic effects that aggravate established asthma and increase the risk that a child will develop asthma. In many inner city communities in the United States, disturbingly high numbers of children have been exposed to various forms of violence.[175,176] Wright and Steinbach[177] describe four cases of inner city children with established asthma in which temporal exposure to violence precipitated asthma exacerbation. The exposures to violence included physical abuse of the asthmatic child, witnessing domestic violence, and hearing gunshots.[177]

Exposure to emotional stress such as violence is under investigation as a potential factor that influences the initial development of asthma. A birth cohort study revealed that family stress in early childhood was associated with increased allergen-induced lymphocyte proliferation.[178] Klinnert and coworkers[179] observed that children whose parents had parenting difficulties were more likely to develop asthma. It has been proposed that stress may produce immune system effects that promote activation of Th2 pathways, thereby leading to allergic sensitization and asthma.[180,181] This risk factor could be especially potent for inner city children who face combinations of stress, exposure to environmental tobacco smoke, and high degrees of exposure to indoor allergens such as cockroach allergen.

Drug abuse is a problem that is widespread throughout society in the United States, and it takes an especially heavy toll on many inner city communities. Between 1.5 and 5.7 individuals are estimated to use cocaine regularly, and approximately 40% of the users freebase or smoke crack cocaine.[182-186] Cocaine use, and crack cocaine use in particular, has been shown to have a temporal association with life-threatening asthma exacerbation and increases in durations of hospital stays.[185,187,188]

In one small study of inner city asthmatics, 116 of 167 patients presenting to emergency rooms with asthma exacerbation agreed to provide urine samples for drug screening. Thirteen (11%) tested positive for cocaine, and five required hospitalization. Three patients in the study required intubation with mechanical ventilation and two of them tested positive for cocaine. This study suggests that asthma exacerbation associated with cocaine use may be particularly severe, but the value of this report is limited by the high refusal rate.[185]

Heroin use is also on the rise. Younger users report insufflation (snorting) and inhalation as the preferred methods of delivery.[189] Case series and retrospective case–control studies have demonstrated a temporal relationship between insufflation or inhalation of heroin and life-threatening asthma exacerbation.[190,191] In addition to directly provoking potentially life-threatening asthma exacerbation, drug abuse often poses substantial barriers to optimal health care.

Table 17.2   Potential Barriers to Health Care in Inner Cities

Risk factors associated with decreased access to health care
Lack of health insurance
Lack of transportation to health care facilities
Need for child care for other children
Barriers at health care facilities (long waiting times, inconvenient hours, limited
   telephone access)
Economic barriers
Direct financial costs (medications, physician office visits)
Indirect financial costs (transportation, child care for other children, lost days of work)
Educational barriers
Minimal education, low levels of literacy
Poor insight into disease severity
Poor understanding of asthma medications
Ineffective problem-solving skills

F.   Barriers to Health Care

The excess morbidity and mortality experienced by asthmatics who live in inner
cities are undoubtedly due in part to barriers to effective health care including
care obtained from health providers, care provided by family members, and self
care. These barriers to health care may be divided into three broad interrelated
categories: (1) barriers related to health care facilities including access to care,
continuity of care, and quality of care; (2) economic barriers including the
inability to afford medical care, medications, and adequate home environments;
(3) educational barriers; and (4) cultural barriers. (Table 17.2)

1.   Access

Many asthmatics living in inner cities do not receive routine health care and rely
instead on emergency department visits at times of crisis.[12,192–196] Sixty-two percent of patients seeking care in an urban public hospital reported that they had
no routine health care. Almost 50% of patients with new medical problems waited
2 days before obtaining medical care. That study[192] reported that independent risk
factors related to lack of routine care were lack of health insurance (odds ratio
[OR] 2.2), lack of transportation (OR 1.44), exposure to violence (OR 1.21), and
living in a supervised setting or shelter (OR 1.5).

   Asthma is a disease that requires reliable and in some cases frequent access
to ongoing health care. The NCICAS investigators observed that the most frequently perceived barrier to health care was difficulty accessing the system.[193]
Specifically, the most frequent barriers to health care reported by parents were
needs for child care for their other children (24%), long waits for appointment

dates (19.6%), and lack of transportation (18.6%). Additional access issues related to health care facilities included excessive waits in offices, too much time spent on hold when attempting to call for appointments, and inconvenient clinic hours.[193]

For those with asthma, particularly severe asthma, emergency health care service and follow-up care subsequent to acute care are as important as routine health care. In inner city populations, African American children with asthma are more likely to use emergency departments than white children with asthma.[12,194,196,197] For example, African American children on Medicaid in Seattle, Washington were more likely to use the emergency department (ED) and had fewer office visits for preventive asthma care than white children on Medicaid.[196] Use of the ED to obtain routine care for inner city children with severe asthma was more frequent compared with use for mild asthma.[195,196,198] In several inner city studies, commonly cited reasons for use of the ED were difficulty obtaining care at a doctor's office, inconvenient clinic hours, and inability to reach staff by telephone.[12,193,196]

In contrast, a few studies reported that visits to primary care clinicians within 6 months were associated with greater use of the ED.[197,198] Ford and coworkers[198] reported that adult asthmatics in the Harlem section of New York City frequently used EDs in addition to, rather than in lieu of, routine health care. In addition to difficulties obtaining routine care, many inner city studies throughout the United States demonstrated that follow-up care for inner city child and adult asthmatics was equally difficult to obtain after admission to a hospital or care in an ED.[193–195,199] In NCICAS, as many as 50% of patients were unable to obtain follow-up care; only 23% were able to speak to health care providers via telephone.[193]

In many urban populations, the majority of routine health care is obtained from a hospital-based practice with residents in training as the providers. Relatively few poor inner city communities have many private physicians or HMO practices. Services that are often absent or limited in hospital-based practices include telephone advice from trained asthma nurses, evening hours, and the ability to refill medications by telephone. In NCICAS, close to a third of the participants reported that these services were not available to them.[193]

Along with these limitations to health care access, the quality of available medical care for asthma may be suboptimal in many low-income urban communities.[194,199,200] Many inner city asthma patients are not taught the correct techniques for using metered-dose inhalers. Additionally, under-utilization of spacers, inhaled anti-inflammatory medications, peak flow meters, and written action plans is relatively common.[193–195,199,200] The National Asthma Education and Prevention Program (NAEPP II) guidelines recommend inhaled corticosteroids in conjunction with beta agonists as first line treatments and theophylline as a third line treatment.[201]

Many studies demonstrated that inappropriately prescribed inhaler regimens and non-adherence are common in inner city asthma populations.[194,197,199,200,202,203] Hartert and coworkers[199] reported that many moderate to severe adult asthmatics seen in inner city Baltimore during 1992 and 1993 had suboptimal treatment. For example, only 45% of patients were prescribed inhaled corticosteroids and 68% were prescribed oral theophylline. Additionally, of the 27% of patients on oral corticosteroids, one third had never been prescribed inhaled corticosteroids.[199] In 1992, only 3.5% of urban African American children with asthma in Washington, D.C., and inner city Baltimore reported use of inhaled corticosteroids.[197] The health care providers' underestimates of the severity of their patients' asthma may, in part, explain the underuse of anti-inflammatory inhalers.[204]

In addition to anti-inflammatory treatment, the NAEPP II recommends using a written plan for daily management of asthma and management of an acute exacerbation.[201] In 1993, 0 to 28% of patients in New Orleans and inner city Baltimore received written action plans from their physicians,[194,199] and a disturbing 60% of asthmatics who spoke with their physicians during acute exacerbations had no changes made in their inhaler regimens and did not receive systemic corticosteroids.[199]

2. Economic Barriers

Asthma places significant financial burdens on inner city families, and lack of health insurance is an independent risk factor for not obtaining routine care.[192] Direct financial costs include medications, physician office visits, copayments, and hospitalizations. Most families must pay some portion of these costs.[193,205,206] Fifty-two percent of patients in NCICAS paid some portions of the direct costs of asthma health care.[193] In addition to the direct costs, indirect costs are incurred for transportation, child care for well children, and lost days of work for patients or parents of children with asthma.[192,196,197]

The combination of these financial demands exerts significant impacts on inner city families and their ability to obtain preventive medicine and health care. The HHANES reports that the cost significantly prevented adult Mexican Americans from obtaining health care.[205] Vance and Taylor[206] reported that between 1965 and 1968 in Los Angeles and Orange County, California, families spent between 2.1 and 30% of their annual incomes on direct medical costs for their children's asthma. These estimates did not include indirect costs for transportation, lost work, and child care.

3. Educational Barriers

NAEPP guidelines state that education is a key component of asthma management.[201] Limited literacy, lack of knowledge about medications, and poor understanding of asthma severity are all educational barriers that may place inner city asthmatics at higher risk. Minimal education and low levels of literacy are common in inner city populations.[194,207,208] For example, among urban asthmatics in Atlanta, Georgia, 27% were found to read at high-school level, 33% at seventh and eighth grade levels, 27% at fourth through sixth grade levels, and 13% below third grade level.[207]

This high prevalence of limited literacy strongly correlated with poor knowledge of asthma and improper MDI technique.[207] Many asthmatics and their caregivers do not understand the serious sequelae of asthma, including the possibility of a fatal outcome,[194,202,209] and many do not understand the roles of the medications prescribed. For example, parents of asthmatic children were interviewed about commonly used asthma medications, including inhaled beta agonists, cromolyn, and inhaled and oral corticosteroids. On average, fewer than 50% of the parents understood the mechanisms of action, side effects, or when to use the medications.[210]

In a telephone survey, parental caretakers were given a scenario that involved an acute asthma exacerbation. No parent mentioned referring to written plans, only one of 220 parents would have measured peak flow (PF), only 36% would have administered β agonists, and only 4% would have contacted their clinicians.[203]

NCICAS investigators evaluated cognitive and behavioral factors believed to affect the management of asthma, including knowledge of the disease and problem-solving skills. They observed that children of caregivers with ineffective problem-solving skills experienced significantly more days of wheezing and poorer functional status.[208] These studies suggest that lack of knowledge of the disease and its medications and limited problem-solving skills contribute to increased morbidity among inner city asthmatic children.

4. Cultural and Language Barriers

Cultural and language barriers to effective asthma care are common in urban populations. Analysis of data from the 1982–1984 HHANES focused on the importance of two predictors of preventive health care: access to services (health insurance coverage, type of facility, travel time, and regular clinic or health care provider) and acculturation (language, ethnic identification). The analysis demonstrated that utilization of preventive health services was more strongly associated with access to health care than with acculturation.[211]

Health insurance was positively associated with obtaining preventive health care in regression analysis. Among Hispanic immigrant populations, Mexican Americans are less likely than Cuban Americans and Puerto Rican Americans to have health insurance. Cuban Americans are more likely to have private insurance and Puerto Rican Americans are more likely to have Medicaid coverage compared with Mexican Americans.[211] HHANES data indicated that 33% of Mexican Americans reported one or more barriers to health care, and 73% of them did not receive care due to the barriers.[205] The most frequent barriers they reported were economic issues and decreased access to health care.[205,211] These barriers represent a common theme also seen in other inner city populations.[193,205,211]

In Hispanic communities in the southwestern United States, Kirkman-Liff and Mondragon[212] reported that the language (English versus Spanish) of health care visits was related to health status, health care access, satisfaction with care, and barriers to care despite the availability of Spanish-speaking providers. This telephone survey revealed that the combination of Hispanic ethnicity and inability to speak English was associated with decreased education, poverty, and decreased access to care.[212] These findings suggest that language preference is a marker of functional societal integration that may predict utilization of health services.[205,211]

III. Asthma Prevention Strategies for Inner Cities

A. Primary Prevention Strategies

The primary prevention of asthma in inner city children is a subject of considerable research interest. The epidemiologic findings discussed earlier suggested the potential utility of approaches including the avoidance of allergens, ETS, and DEPs and/or the administration of non-harmful forms of endotoxins in early infancy. At present, however, no clinical trials of primary prevention interventions have been undertaken among inner city populations.

B. Secondary Prevention Strategies

In contrast, a number of secondary prevention strategies to reduce morbidity and complications among urban children and adults with existing asthma have been assessed in clinical trials. They have taken the form of clinical, educational, environmental, and hybrid interventions, and well-designed trials have established the efficacy of a number of measures.

Trials of clinical strategies for preventing morbidity among inner city asthmatics have a variety of forms. Two randomized clinical trials (RCTs) in inner city asthmatics assessed interventions that reduced barriers to follow-up asthma care by assisting patients in making appointments, placing reminder phone calls, obtaining transportation vouchers, and using other means. These interventions increased the likelihood that both urban children[213] and adults[214] with asthma would follow up with primary care providers.

Another placebo-controlled RCT tested an intervention that attempted to overcome barriers to care by prescribing long-term inhaled corticosteroid treatment to inner city asthmatics aged 18 to 50 years at the time of acute asthma care in an ED.[215] The study noted no apparent clinical benefit of the intervention after 24 days of follow-up, suggesting that the initiation of inhaled corticosteroid alone without follow-up care to encourage its use may produce relatively little impact on outcome.

Other clinical interventions included intensive outpatient asthma care programs. For example, hospitalized adult asthmatics were enrolled in an RCT with a crossover arm at Bellevue Hospital, New York City. They were randomly assigned to an intensive outpatient clinic or to continued care with their previous outpatient clinics. The intensive outpatient clinical care resulted in a three-fold decrease in readmission rate (p <0.004) for the primary intervention, with similar results seen in the crossover arm (p <0.004). The intervention also resulted in a two-fold decrease in hospital days used (p <0.02).[216]

Another RCT of hospitalized adult asthmatics in inner city Philadelphia demonstrated that a program including both asthma education and enrollment in an outpatient asthma program resulted in fewer ED visits and hospitalizations during the 6 months after randomization.[217] In inner city New York, an RCT among asthmatic children aged 2 to 17 years revealed that care in a specialty clinic that provided intensive medical and environmental control, education, close monitoring, and 24-hour availability was associated with fewer ED visits and hospitalizations during the first year of treatment compared with children receiving routine care.[218]

Asthma education programs represent another secondary prevention strategy tested in many populations, including low-income inner city communities. Interventional studies used a variety of educational tools to improve both the parents' and asthmatics' knowledge of the disease, its medications, and common management issues ranging from daily medication use to action plans for exacerbations. Educational programs for self-management by children and adolescents have been found to improve pulmonary function, enhance self-efficiency, and reduce school absenteeism, restricted activity, and emergency visits.[219] School-based asthma education programs in inner cities have led to improved asthma knowledge, enhanced self-efficiency, and reduced symptoms.[220,221]

One RCT enrolled asthmatic children from low-income urban communities in New York City.[222] The intervention group received health education programs for children and parents and attended monthly sessions incorporating management of asthma exacerbation, inhaler technique, allergen avoidance in the home, and communications with physicians. Overall, the outcome for the intervention group did not differ from that for the control group, but an analysis restricted to children with one or more hospitalizations in the preceding year revealed that children in the intervention arm experienced significant decreases in hospitalizations compared with controls.[222]

An RCT in inner city Chicago, however, demonstrated no significant impact of an educational intervention for asthmatic children on subsequent ED visits.[223] Overall, educational interventions for inner city asthmatic children appear to provide a number of benefits although the evidence of important effects of education alone on emergency visit and hospitalization rates remains limited.

In addition to traditional educational pathways, interest in computer-based learning tools that can be used in clinic waiting areas and homes is growing. Most programs have demonstrated some degree of improved asthma knowledge although data available on improved clinical outcomes associated with improved knowledge are limited.[224–226] The computer programs range from games[225] to an interactive question-and-answer system that permits ongoing monitoring.[227]

The latter system, called the Health Buddy, is an interactive device designed for inner city children with asthma. It incorporates self-management and education programs that provide immediate responses for routine questions and allow the information to be reviewed the following day by a health care provider. In an RCT, inner city children with asthma were assigned to the Health Buddy or a control arm. Children who used the Health Buddy demonstrated significantly improved clinical outcomes, decreases in activity limitations, improved pulmonary function, and fewer urgent calls to hospitals compared with the control group. In another RCT, inner city children with asthma who used a computer-assisted instructional game to track asthma symptoms did not experience reductions in asthma symptoms compared with the control group.[228]

Secondary prevention approaches based on environmental remediation, usually focused on allergen avoidance, have also been investigated in low-income urban communities. The efficacy of allergen avoidance in the treatment of asthma is a controversial subject. Many clinical trials of allergen avoidance have focused on dust mite allergens. Although some revealed evidence of short-term efficacy,[229–233] others have not done so.[234,235]

Relatively few trials of allergen avoidance have been conducted in inner city settings where older and often poorly maintained housing stock and limited financial resources pose barriers to environmental remediation. One inner city intervention study demonstrated significant decreases in dust mite allergen concentrations with the use of impermeable bed coverings, professional laundering of bedding, or instructions to wash bedding in hot water. These decreases in allergen concentrations persisted throughout the 8-week sampling period.[236]

In a recent RCT,[237] asthmatic children in inner city Atlanta, Georgia, were randomized to three groups: (1) an avoidance arm involving allergen-impermeable covers for mattresses and bedding, instructions to launder bedding weekly in hot water, use of active roach traps, and instructions on cleaning methods to control dust mites and cockroaches; (2) a placebo arm involving allergen-permeable covers for mattresses and bedding, ineffective roach traps, and instructions to continue current cold water laundering practices; and (3) a control arm involving no home visits or interventions. No differences were noted between the active intervention and placebo groups in allergen levels or asthma morbidity during the follow-up interval. The children enrolled in both the active intervention and placebo arms showed significant decreases in numbers of acute visits compared with children in the control arm (p <0.001), demonstrating out the potential importance of attention effects in studies of asthma interventions.[237] The Inner City Asthma Study[99] undertook an RCT of a multidimensional home-based environmental intervention and the results will be available soon.

Cockroach infestation and allergen sensitization are common problems for inner city asthmatics. Environmental remediation trials that did not involve clinical outcomes demonstrated that home cockroach allergen concentrations can be reduced by aggressive interventions.[238,239] In the NCICAS trial of a multifaceted intervention, a significant decrease in Bla g 1 levels was noted at the 6-month visits; however, by the 12-month visits, the allergen levels returned to or exceeded baseline levels.[240]

In the environmental intervention trial conducted by Carter and coworkers mentioned earlier,[237] a low intensity cockroach remediation intervention did not produce significant reductions in cockroach allergen levels or significant effects on asthma morbidity. No RCTs published to date demonstrate that home interventions to reduce cockroach allergen levels can improve clinical outcomes among inner city asthmatics.

Other environmental interventions have focused on avoidance of exposure to ETS but few concentrated on reducing ETS exposure among asthmatic children. Most of these trials involved behavioral counseling sessions that continued over 3- to 6-month periods and follow-up intervals as long as 30 months. These studies based on reports of parents along with concurrent monitoring of air nicotine or urine cotinine levels in asthmatic children revealed significant decreases of ETS exposure of the children in their homes.[241–245]

Similar studies specifically designed for Hispanic children with asthma[246] and ethnically diverse low-income households with healthy children[243] produced similar results. Few studies were designed to evaluate the impact of decreased ETS exposure on the frequency of asthma exacerbation. In one RCT, predominantly minority children of low SES who had asthma were enrolled in an ETS reduction trial.[244] The primary outcome measures were urinary cotinine levels and number of acute asthma visits. The intervention arm involved three nurse-led sessions covering behavior-changing tactics, basic asthma education, and feedback based on the children's urinary cotinine levels. Children in the intervention arm had significantly lower risks of acute asthma visits in the follow-up year than children in the control group.[244] These studies demonstrate that counseling may lead to decreased ETS levels in homes of asthmatic children and potentially improved clinical outcomes.

Some investigators tested secondary prevention strategies for inner city asthmatics in multifaceted trials that included clinical, educational, and environmental components. In one RCT,[247] inner city children with asthma were randomized to receive care at a specialty clinic or continue with current outpatient management. The specialty clinic adjusted medication regimens in accordance with national guidelines, taught peak flow meter use, created asthma emergency plans, and performed allergy skin tests on all participants. Atopic subjects received education in environmental avoidance measures. Allergen-impermeable covers for mattresses and pillows were provided for dust mite-allergic children who could not afford them. Participants in the intervention arm had fewer emergency visits and hospitalizations compared with the control group.[247]

Another RCT[248] examined the effects of an asthma outreach and case management program in children with asthma. This study demonstrated significant decreases in emergency visits and hospitalizations for children randomized to the outreach program.

NCICAS investigators conducted an RCT of a multifaceted intervention designed specifically for inner city children with asthma.[249] This multicenter study recruited 5- to 11-year-old children with moderate to severe asthma living in an inner city. The interventions were implemented by counselors (master's level social workers) trained to assist families with asthma care. At the beginning of the intervention, the asthma counselors helped obtain written action plans from the medical providers and assisted the families in implementing the plans. Asthma management education for the caretakers of the children included two group sessions and one individual meeting covering common asthma triggers, environmental controls, asthma physiology, and strategies for problem solving. The asthma counselors also focused on providing the caretakers with the means to help improve communication with the children's physicians. If necessary, the asthma counselors facilitated referrals for additional services such as smoking cessation programs and psychological counseling.

Environmental interventions involved allergen-impermeable pillow and mattress covers and professional application of baited gel insecticides for children with cockroach sensitization. The asthma counselors met with caretakers every 2 months and spoke with the caretakers by telephone in alternate months. The number of contacts and material discussed varied based on the individual needs of the family.[250]

Children in the intervention arm had significant decreases in symptom days and fewer hospitalizations over the first 12 months compared with the control group, an effect that was even more striking among the children with the most severe asthma. These improvements were maintained during the second year of the study, i.e., for a year after the end of the 12-month asthma counselor intervention.[249]

Sullivan et al.[250] evaluated the data from NCICAS and reported that the intervention arm was cost-effective for inner city children, with an average additional cost of $9.20 per symptom-free day gained. The NCICAS intervention and the other studies reviewed above suggest that multifaceted interventions tailored to an individual asthmatic's needs are successful in decreasing emergent health care utilization and increasing symptom-free days for asthmatic children in inner cities.

IV. Summary

Residents of low-income urban communities in the United States experience disproportionate burdens of asthma prevalence, morbidity, and mortality. The causes of these disproportionate burdens are not fully understood. Multiple social, environmental, and possibly genetic factors may all contribute to the burdens. Inner city asthmatics constitute a high-risk subgroup that warrants particular attention in terms of intervention efforts. A number of secondary intervention strategies have been tested among inner city children and adults with asthma and some have proven efficacious in well-designed clinical trials. At present, the primary prevention of inner city asthma remains a goal for future investigations.

References

1. Mannino DM, Homa DM, Pertowski CA, Ashizawa A, Nixon LL, Johnson CA, Ball LB, Jack E, and Kang DS. Surveillance for asthma: United States, 1960–1995. *Morbidity & Mortality Weekly Report* 1998; 47: 1–27.
2. Evans R, Mullaly DI, Wilson RW, Gergen PJ, Rosenberg HM, Grauman JS, Chevarley FM, and Feinleib M. National trends in the morbidity and mortality of asthma in the U.S.: prevalence, hospitalization and death from asthma over two decades: 1965–1984. *Chest* 1987; 91: 65S–74S.
3. Carr W, Zeitel L, and Weiss K. Variations in asthma hospitalizations and deaths in New York City. *American Journal of Public Health* 1992; 82: 59–65.
4. Marder D, Targonski P, Orris P, Persky V, and Addington W. Effect of racial and socioeconomic factors on asthma mortality in Chicago. *Chest* 1992; 101: 426S–429S.
5. Gerstman BB, Bosco LA, Tomita DK, Gross TP, and Shaw MM. Prevalence and treatment of asthma in the Michigan Medicaid patient population younger than 45 years, 1980–1986. *Journal of Allergy & Clinical Immunology* 1989; 83: 1032–1039.
6. Turkeltaub PC and Gergen PJ. Prevalence of upper and lower respiratory conditions in the U.S. population by social and environmental factors: data from the second National Health and Nutrition Examination Survey, 1976 to 1980 (NHANES II). *Annals of Allergy* 1991; 67: 147–154.
7. Weiss KB and Wagener DK. Changing patterns of asthma mortality: identifying target populations at high risk. *Journal of the American Medical Association* 1990; 264: 1683–1687.
8. Weitzman M, Gortmaker S, and Sobol A. Racial, social, and environmental risks for childhood asthma. *American Journal of Diseases of Children* 1990; 144: 1189–1194.
9. Schwartz J, Gold D, Dockery DW, Weiss ST, and Speizer FE. Predictors of asthma and persistent wheeze in a national sample of children in the United States: association with social class, perinatal events, and race. *American Review of Respiratory Disease* 1990; 142: 555–562.

10. Crain EF, Weiss KB, Bijur PE, Hersh M, Westbrook L, and Stein RE. An estimate of the prevalence of asthma and wheezing among inner city children. *Pediatrics* 1994; 94: 356–362.

11. Joseph CL, Foxman B, Leickly FE, Peterson E, and Ownby D. Prevalence of possible undiagnosed asthma and associated morbidity among urban schoolchildren. *Journal of Pediatrics* 1996; 129: 735–742.

12. Mak H, Johnston P, Abbey H, and Talamo RC. Prevalence of asthma and health service utilization of asthmatic children in an inner city. *Journal of Allergy & Clinical Immunology* 1982; 70: 367–372.

13. Hynes HP, Brugge D, Watts J, and Lally J. Public health and the physical environment in Boston public housing: a community-based survey and action agenda. *Planning Practice and Research* 2000; 15: 31–39.

14. Brugge D et al. Housing conditions and respiratory health in a Boston public housing community. *New Solutions* 2001; 11: 149–164.

15. Lwebuga-Mukasa JS, Wojcik R, Dunn-Georgiou E, and Johnson C. Home environmental factors associated with asthma prevalence in two Buffalo inner city neighborhoods. *Journal of Health Care for the Poor and Underserved* 2002; 13: 214–228.

16. Carter-Pokras OD and Gergen PJ. Reported asthma among Puerto Rican, Mexican American, and Cuban children, 1982 through 1984. *American Journal of Public Health* 1993; 83: 580–582.

17. Dodge R. A comparison of the respiratory health of Mexican-American and non-Mexican-American white children. *Chest* 1983; 84: 587–592.

18. Aligne CA, Auinger P, Byrd RS, and Weitzman M. Risk factors for pediatric asthma: contributions of poverty, race, and urban residence. *American Journal of Respiratory & Critical Care Medicine* 2000; 162: 873–877.

19. Gottlieb DJ, Beiser AS, and O'Connor GT. Poverty, race, and medication use are correlates of asthma hospitalization rates: a small area analysis in Boston. *Chest* 1995; 108: 28–35.

20. Sly RM. Mortality from asthma in children 1979–1984. *Annals of Allergy* 1988; 60: 433–443.

21. Marwick C. Inner city asthma control campaign under way. *Journal of the American Medical Association* 1995; 274: 1004.

22. Clarke JR, Jenkins MA, Hopper JL, Carlin JB, Mayne C, Clayton DG, Dalton MF, Holst DP, and Robertson CF. Evidence for genetic associations between asthma, atopy, and bronchial hyperresponsiveness: a study of 8- to 18-year old twins. *American Journal of Respiratory & Critical Care Medicine* 2000; 162: 2188–2193.

23. Duffy DL, Martin NG, Battistutta D, Hopper JL, and Mathews JD. Genetics of asthma and hay fever in Australian twins. *American Review of Respiratory Disease* 1990; 142: 1351–1358.

24. Hopper JL, Hannah MC, Macaskill GT, and Mathews JD. Twin concordance for a binary trait: III. A bivariate analysis of hay fever and asthma. *Genetic Epidemiology* 1990; 7: 277–289.

25. Ober C and Moffatt MF. Contributing factors to the pathobiology and genetics of asthma. *Clinics in Chest Medicine* 2000; 21: 245–261.

26. Sibbald B, Horn ME, Brain EA, and Gregg I. Genetic factors in childhood asthma. *Thorax* 1980; 35: 671–674.
27. Lawrence S, Beasley R, Doull I, Begishvili B, Lampe F, Holgate ST et al. Genetic analysis of atopy and asthma as quantitative traits and ordered polychotomies. *Annals of Human Genetics* 1994; 58: 359–368.
28. Xu J, Meyers DA, Ober C, Blumenthal MN, Mellen B, Barnes KC et al. Genome-wide screen and identification of gene–gene interactions for asthma-susceptibility loci in three U.S. populations: collaborative study on the genetics of asthma. *American Journal of Human Genetics* 2001; 68: 1437–1446.
29. Daniels SE, Bhattacharrya S, James A, Leaves NI, Young A, Hill MR et al. A genome-wide search for quantitative trait loci underlying asthma. *Nature* 1996; 383: 247–250.
30. Hizawa N, Freidhoff LR, Chiu YF, Ehrlich E, Luehr CA, Anderson JL et al. Genetic regulation of *Dermatophagoides pteronyssinus*-specific IgE responsiveness: a genome-wide multipoint linkage analysis in families recruited through two asthmatic sibs. *Journal of Allergy & Clinical Immunology* 1998; 102: 436–442.
31. Ober C, Tsalenko A, Parry R, and Cox NJ. A second generation genome-wide screen for asthma susceptibility alleles in a founder population. *American Journal of Human Genetics* 2000; 67: 1154–1162.
32. Wjst M, Fischer G, Immervoll T, Jung M, Saar K, Rueschendorf F et al. A genome-wide search for linkage to asthma. *Genomics* 1999; 58: 1–8.
33. Dizier MH, Besse-Schmittler C, Guilloud-Bataille M, Annesi-Maesano I, Boussaha M, Bousquet J et al. Genome screen for asthma and related phenotypes in the French EGEA study. *American Journal of Respiratory & Critical Care Medicine* 2000; 162: 1812–1818.
34. Koppelman GH, Stine OC, Xu J, Howard TD, Zheng SL, Kauffman HF et al. Genome-wide search for atopy susceptibility genes in Dutch families with asthma. *Journal of Allergy & Clinical Immunology* 2002; 109: 498–506.
35. Haagerup A, Bjerke T, Schiotz PO, Binderup HG, Dahl R, and Kruse TA. Asthma and atopy : a total genome scan for susceptibility genes. *Allergy* 2002; 57: 680–686.
36. Xu J, Meyers DA, Ober C, Blumenthal MN, Mellen B, Barnes KC et al. Genomewide screen and identification of gene-gene interactions for asthma-susceptibility loci in three U.S. populations: collaborative study on the genetics of asthma. *American Journal of Human Genetics* 2001; 68: 1437–1446.
37. Postma DS, Bleecker ER, Amelung PJ, Holroyd KJ, Xu J, Panhuysen CM et al. Genetic susceptibility to asthma: bronchial hyperresponsiveness coinherited with a major gene for atopy. *New England Journal of Medicine* 1995; 333: 894–900.
38. Marsh DG, Neely JD, Breazeale DR, Ghosh B, Freidhoff LR, Ehrlich-Kautzky E et al. Linkage analysis of IL4 and other chromosome 5q31.1 markers and total serum immunoglobulin E concentrations. *Science* 1994; 264: 1152–1156.
39. Palmer LJ, Daniels SE, Rye PJ, Gibson NA, Tay GK, Cookson WO et al. Linkage of chromosome 5q and 11q gene markers to asthma-associated quantitative traits in Australian children. *American Journal of Respiratory & Critical Care Medicine* 1998; 158: 1825–1830.

40. Noguchi E, Shibasaki M, Arinami T, Takeda K, Maki T, Miyamoto T et al. Evidence for linkage between asthma/atopy in childhood and chromosome 5q31-q33 in a Japanese population. *American Journal of Respiratory & Critical Care Medicine* 1997; 156: 1390–1393.

41. Meyers DA, Postma DS, Panhuysen CI, Xu J, Amelung PJ, Levitt RC et al. Evidence for a locus regulating total serum IgE levels mapping to chromosome 5. *Genomics* 1994; 23: 464–470.

42. Walley AJ, Wiltshire S, Ellis CM, and Cookson WO. Linkage and allelic association of chromosome 5 cytokine cluster genetic markers with atopy and asthma associated traits. *Genomics* 2001; 72: 15–20.

43. Burchard EG, Silverman EK, Rosenwasser LJ, Borish L, Yandava C, Pillari A et al. Association between a sequence variant in the IL-4 gene promoter and FEV(1) in asthma. *American Journal of Respiratory & Critical Care Medicine* 1999; 160: 919–922.

44. Zhu S, Chan-Yeung M, Becker AB, Dimich-Ward H, Ferguson AC, Manfreda J et al. Polymorphisms of the IL-4, TNF-alpha, and Fc epsilon RI beta genes and the risk of allergic disorders in at-risk infants. *American Journal of Respiratory & Critical Care Medicine* 2000; 161: 1655–1659.

45. Heinzmann A, Mao XQ, Akaiwa M, Kreomer RT, Gao PS, Ohshima K et al. Genetic variants of IL-13 signalling and human asthma and atopy. *Human Molecular Genetics* 2000; 9: 549–559.

46. Graves PE, Kabesch M, Halonen M, Holberg CJ, Baldini M, Fritzsch C et al. A cluster of seven tightly linked polymorphisms in the IL-13 gene is associated with total serum IgE levels in three populations of white children. *Journal of Allergy & Clinical Immunology* 2000; 105: 506–513.

47. Liu X, Nickel R, Beyer K, Wahn U, Ehrlich E, Freidhoff LR et al. An IL13 coding region variant is associated with a high total serum IgE level and atopic dermatitis in the German multicenter atopy study (MAS-90). *Journal of Allergy & Clinical Immunology* 2000; 106: 167–170.

48. Howard TD, Whittaker PA, Zaiman AL, Koppelman GH, Xu J, Hanley MT et al. Identification and association of polymorphisms in the interleukin-13 gene with asthma and atopy in a Dutch population. *American Journal of Respiratory Cell & Molecular Biology* 2001; 25: 377–384.

49. Holberg CJ, Halonen M, Solomon S, Graves PE, Baldini M, Erickson RP et al. Factor analysis of asthma and atopy traits shows two major components, one of which is linked to markers on chromosome 5q. *Journal of Allergy & Clinical Immunology* 2001; 108: 772–780.

50. Howard TD, Koppelman GH, Xu J, Zheng SL, Postma DS, Meyers DA et al. Gene–gene interaction in asthma: IL4RA and IL13 in a Dutch population with asthma. *American Journal of Human Genetics* 2002; 70: 230–236.

51. Shirakawa T, Li A, Dubowitz M, Dekker JW, Shaw AE, Faux JA et al. Association between atopy and variants of the beta subunit of the high-affinity immunoglobulin E receptor. *Nature and Genetics* 1994; 7: 125–129.

52. Sandford AJ, Shirakawa T, Moffatt MF, Daniels SE, Ra C, Faux JA et al. Localisation of atopy and beta subunit of high-affinity IgE receptor (Fc epsilon RI) on chromosome 11q [comment]. *Lancet* 1993; 341: 332–334.

53. van Herwerden L, Harrap SB, Wong ZY, Abramson MJ, Kutin JJ, Forbes AB et al. Linkage of high-affinity IgE receptor gene with bronchial hyperreactivity, even in absence of atopy. *Lancet* 1995; 346: 1262–1265.

54. Trabetti E, Cusin V, Malerba G, Martinati LC, Casartelli A, Boner AL et al. Association of the Fc epsilon RI beta gene with bronchial hyperresponsiveness in an Italian population. *Journal of Medical Genetics* 1998; 35: 680–681.

55. Lester LA, Rich SS, Blumenthal MN, Togias A, Murphy S, Malveaux F et al. Ethnic differences in asthma and associated phenotypes: collaborative study on the genetics of asthma. *Journal of Allergy & Clinical Immunology* 2001; 108: 357–362.

56. Huang SK, Mathias RA, Ehrlich E, Plunkett B, Liu X, Cutting GR et al. Evidence for asthma susceptibility genes on chromosome 11 in an African-American population. *Human Genetics* 2003; 113: 71–75.

57. Xie HG, Stein CM, Kim RB, Xiao ZS, He N, Zhou HH et al. Frequency of functionally important beta-2 adrenoceptor polymorphisms varies markedly among African-American, Caucasian and Chinese individuals. *Pharmacogenetics* 1999; 9: 511–516.

58. Snieder H, Dong Y, Barbeau P, Harshfield GA, Dalageogou C, Zhu H et al. Beta2-adrenergic receptor gene and resting hemodynamics in European and African American youth. *American Journal of Hypertension* 2002; 15: 973–979.

59. Drysdale CM, McGraw DW, Stack CB, Stephens JC, Judson RS, Nandabalan K et al. Complex promoter and coding region beta 2-adrenergic receptor haplotypes alter receptor expression and predict *in vivo* responsiveness. *Proceedings of the National Academy of Sciences of the United States of America* 2000; 97: 10483–10488.

60. Israel E, Drazen JM, Liggett SB, Boushey HA, Cherniack RM, Chinchilli VM et al. Effect of polymorphism of the beta (2) adrenergic receptor on response to regular use of albuterol in asthma. *International Archives of Allergy & Immunology* 2001; 124: 183–186.

61. Martinez FD, Graves PE, Baldini M, Solomon S, and Erickson R. Association between genetic polymorphisms of the beta 2-adrenoceptor and response to albuterol in children with and without a history of wheezing. *Journal of Clinical Investigation* 1997; 100: 3184–3188.

62. Weir TD, Mallek N, Sandford AJ, Bai TR, Awadh N, Fitzgerald JM et al. Beta 2-adrenergic receptor haplotypes in mild, moderate and fatal/near fatal asthma. *American Journal of Respiratory & Critical Care Medicine* 1998; 158: 787–791.

63. Snieder H, Dong Y, Barbeau P, Harshfield GA, Dalageogou C, Zhu H et al. Beta 2-adrenergic receptor gene and resting hemodynamics in European and African American youth. *American Journal of Hypertension* 2002; 15: 973–979.

64. Green SA, Turki J, Innis M, and Liggett SB. Amino-terminal polymorphisms of the human beta 2-adrenergic receptor impart distinct agonist-promoted regulatory properties. *Biochemistry* 1994; 33: 9414–9419.

65. Green SA, Cole G, Jacinto M, Innis M, and Liggett SB. A polymorphism of the human beta 2-adrenergic receptor within the fourth transmembrane domain alters ligand binding and functional properties of the receptor. *Journal of Biological Chemistry* 1993; 268: 23116–23121.

66. Turki J, Lorenz JN, Green SA, Donnelly ET, Jacinto M, and Liggett SB. Myocardial signaling defects and impaired cardiac function of a human beta 2-adrenergic receptor polymorphism expressed in transgenic mice. *Proceedings of the National Academy of Sciences of the United States of America* 1996; 93: 10483–10488.

67. FDA Talk Paper: labeling changes for drug products that contain salmeterol. U.S. Food and Drug Administration, August 14, 2003 (electronic citation).

68. Palta M, Sadek-Badawi M, Sheehy M, Albanese A, Weinstein M, McGuinness G et al. Respiratory symptoms at age 8 years in a cohort of very low birth weight children. *American Journal of Epidemiology* 2001; 154: 521–529.

69. Oliveti JF, Kercsmar CM, and Redline S. Pre- and perinatal risk factors for asthma in inner city African-American children. *American Journal of Epidemiology* 1996; 143: 570–577.

70. Joseph CL, Ownby DR, Peterson EL, and Johnson CC. Does low birth weight help to explain the increased prevalence of asthma among African-Americans? *Annals of Allergy, Asthma & Immunology* 2002; 88: 507–512.

71. Ekwo EE and Moawad A. Maternal age and preterm births in a black population. *Paediatric and Perinatal Epidemiology* 2000; 14: 145–151.

72. Amini SB, Dierker LJ, Catalano PM, Ashmead GG, and Mann LI. Trends in an obstetric patient population: an 18-year study. *American Journal of Obstetrics & Gynecology* 1994; 171: 1014–1021.

73. Brooks AM, Byrd RS, Weitzman M, Auinger P, and McBride JT. Impact of low birth weight on early childhood asthma in the United States. *Archives of Pediatrics & Adolescent Medicine* 2001; 155: 401–406.

74. Fergusson DM, Horwood LJ, and Shannon FT. Asthma and infant diet. *Archives of Disease in Childhood* 1983; 58: 48–51.

75. Oddy WH, Peat JK, and de Klerk NH. Maternal asthma, infant feeding, and the risk of asthma in childhood. *Journal of Allergy & Clinical Immunology* 2002; 110: 65–67.

76. Oddy WH, de Klerk NH, Sly PD, and Holt PG. The effects of respiratory infections, atopy, and breastfeeding on childhood asthma. *European Respiratory Journal* 2002; 19: 899–905.

77. Sears MR, Greene JM, Willan AR, Taylor DR, Flannery EM, Cowan JO et al. Long-term relation between breast feeding and development of atopy and asthma in children and young adults: a longitudinal study. *Lancet* 2002; 360: 901–907.

78. Leventhal JM, Shapiro ED, Aten CB, Berg AT, and Egerter SA. Does breastfeeding protect against infections in infants less than three months of age? *Pediatrics* 1986; 78: 896–903.

79. Ryan AS, Rush D, Krieger FW, and Lewandowski GE. Recent declines in breast feeding in the United States, 1984 through 1989. *Pediatrics* 1991; 88: 719–727.

80. Braun-Fahrlander C, Gassner M, Grize L, Neu U, Sennhauser FH, Varonier HS et al. Prevalence of hay fever and allergic sensitization in farmers' children and their peers living in the same rural community. *Clinical & Experimental Allergy* 1999; 29: 28–34.

81. Braun-Fahrlander C, Riedler J, Herz U, Eder W, Waser M, Grize L et al. Environmental exposure to endotoxin and its relation to asthma in school-age children. *New England Journal of Medicine* 2002; 347: 869–877.
82. Holt PG, Sly PD, and Bjorksten B. Atopic versus infectious diseases in childhood: a question of balance? *Pediatric Allergy & Immunology* 1997; 8: 53–58.
83. Martinez FD. Maturation of immune responses at the beginning of asthma. *Journal of Allergy & Clinical Immunology* 1999; 103: 355–361.
84. Von Ehrenstein OS, von Mutius E, Illi S, Baumann L, Bohm O, and von Kries R. Reduced risk of hay fever and asthma among children of farmers. *Clinical & Experimental Allergy* 2000; 30: 187–193.
85. Riedler J, Eder W, Oberfeld G, and Schreuer M. Austrian children living on a farm have less hay fever, asthma and allergic sensitization. *Clinical & Experimental Allergy* 2000; 30: 194–200.
86. Burrows B, Martinez FD, Halonen M, Barbee RA, and Cline MG. Association of asthma with serum IgE levels and skin-test reactivity to allergens. *New England Journal of Medicine* 1989; 320: 271–277.
87. Call RS, Smith TF, Morris E, Chapman MD, and Platts-Mills TE. Risk factors for asthma in inner city children. *Journal of Pediatrics* 1992; 121: 862–866.
88. Gelber LE, Seltzer LH, Bouzoukis JK, Pollart SM, Chapman MD, and Platts-Mills TE. Sensitization and exposure to indoor allergens as risk factors for asthma among patients presenting to hospital. *American Review of Respiratory Disease* 1993; 147: 573–578.
89. Phipatanakul W, Eggleston PA, Wright EC, and Wood RA. National Cooperative Inner City Asthma Study: mouse allergen II: the relationship of mouse allergen exposure to mouse sensitization and asthma morbidity in inner city children with asthma. *Journal of Allergy & Clinical Immunology* 2000; 106: 1075–1080.
90. Phipatanakul W, Eggleston PA, Wright EC, and Wood RA. National Cooperative Inner City Asthma Study: mouse allergen I: the prevalence of mouse allergen in inner city homes. *Journal of Allergy & Clinical Immunology* 2000; 106: 1070–1074.
91. Twarog FJ, Picone FJ, Strunk RS, So J, and Colten HR. Immediate hypersensitivity to cockroach: isolation and purification of the major antigens. *Journal of Allergy & Clinical Immunology* 1976; 59: 154–160.
92. Stankus RP and O'Neil CE. Antigenic/allergenic characterization of American and German cockroach extracts. *Journal of Allergy & Clinical Immunology* 1988; 81: 563–570.
93. Stankus RP, Horner WE, and Lehrer SB. Identification and characterization of important cockroach allergens. *Journal of Allergy & Clinical Immunology* 1990; 86: 781–786.
94. Schou C, Lind P, Fernandez-Caldas E, Lockey RF, and Lowenstein H. Identification and purification of a cross-reacting, acidic allergen from American (*Periplaneta americana*) and German (*Blattella germanica*) cockroach. *Journal of Allergy & Clinical Immunolology* 1990; 86: 935–946.

95. Pollart SM, Mullins DE, Vailes LD, Hayden ML, Platts-Mills TA, Sutherland WM et al. Identification, quantitation, and purification of cockroach allergens using monoclonal antibodies. *Journal of Allergy & Clinical Immunology* 1991; 87: 511–521.

96. Sarpong SB, Hamilton RG, Eggleston PA, and Adkinson NF, Jr. Socioeconomic status and race as risk factors for cockroach allergen exposure and sensitization in children with asthma. *Journal of Allergy & Clinical Immunology* 1996; 97: 1393–1401.

97. Bernton HS and Brown H. Cockroach allergy II. *Southern Medical Journal* 1967; 60: 852–855.

98. Kattan M, Mitchell H, Eggleston P, Gergen P, Crain E, Redline S et al. Characteristics of inner city children with asthma: National Cooperative Inner City Asthma Study. *Pediatric Pulmonology* 1997; 24: 253–262.

99. Crain EF, Walter M, O'Connor GT, Mitchell H, Gruchalla RS, Kattan M et al. Home and allergic characteristics of children with asthma in seven U.S. urban communities and design of an environmental intervention: the Inner City Asthma Study. *Environmental Health Perspectives* 2002; 110: 939–945.

100. Schou C, Fernandez-Caldas E, Lockey RF, and Lowenstein H. Environmental assay for cockroach allergens. *Journal of Allergy & Clinical Immunology* 1991; 87: 828–834.

101. de Blay F, Sanchez J, Hedelin G, Perez-Infante A, Verot A, Chapman M et al. Dust and airborne exposure to allergens derived from cockroach (*Blattella germanica*) in low-cost public housing in Strasbourg (France). *Journal of Allergy & Clinical Immunology* 1997; 99: 107–112.

102. Kang B and Sulit N. A comparative study of skin hypersensitivity to cockroach and house dust antigens. *Annals of Allergy* 1978; 41: 333–336.

103. Hulett AC and Dockhorn RJ. House dust mite (*D. farinae*) and cockroach allergy in a midwestern population. *Annals of Allergy* 1979; 42: 160–165.

104. Kang BC, Johnson J, and Veres-Thorner C. Atopic profile of inner city asthma with a comparative analysis on the cockroach-sensitive and ragweed-sensitive subgroups. *Journal of Allergy & Clinical Immunology* 1993; 92: 802–811.

105. Christiansen SC, Martin SB, Schleicher NC, Koziol JA, Hamilton RG, and Zuraw BL. Exposure and sensitization to environmental allergen of predominantly Hispanic children with asthma in San Diego's inner city. *Journal of Allergy & Clinical Immunology* 1996; 98: 288–294.

106. Bernton HS and Brown H. Preliminary studies of the cockroach. *Allergy* 1964; 35: 506–513.

107. Stevenson LA, Gergen PJ, Hoover DR, Rosenstreich D, Mannino DM, and Matte TD. Sociodemographic correlates of indoor allergen sensitivity among United States children. *Journal of Allergy & Clinical Immunology* 2001; 108: 747–752.

108. Broder I, Higgins MW, Mathews KP, and Keller JB. Epidemiology of asthma and allergic rhinitis in a total community, Tecumseh, Michigan. *Journal of Allergy & Clinical Immunology* 1974; 53: 127–138.

109. Kang BC. Ubiquitous dwelling infestation of cockroaches makes allergies more prevalent than previously recognized, particularly in the urban atopic population. *American Journal of Asthma & Allergy for Pediatricians* 1990; 3: 228–233.

110. Kang B, Jones J, Johnson J, and Kang IJ. Analysis of indoor environment and atopic allergy in urban populations with bronchial asthma. *Annals of Allergy* 1989; 62: 30–34.
111. Rosenstreich DL, Eggleston P, Kattan M, Baker D, Slavin RG, Gergen P et al. The role of cockroach allergy and exposure to cockroach allergen in causing morbidity among inner city children with asthma. *New England Journal of Medicine* 1997; 336: 1356–1363.
112. Gold DR, Burge HA, Carey V, Milton DK, Platts-Mills TA, and Weiss S. Predictors of repeated wheeze in the first year of life: relative role of cockroach, birth weight, acute lower respiratory illness and maternal smoking. *American Journal of Respiratory & Critical Care Medicine* 1999; 160: 227–236.
113. Litonjua AA, Carey VJ, Burge HA, Weiss ST, and Gold DR. Exposure to cockroach allergen in the home is associated with incident doctor-diagnosed asthma and recurrent wheezing. *Journal of Allergy & Clinical Immunology* 2001; 107: 41–47.
114. Chapman MD and Platts-Mills TA. Purification and characterization of the major allergen from *Dermatophagoides pteronyssinus* antigen P1. *Journal of Immunology* 1980; 125: 587–592.
115. Cockcroft DW, Ruffin RE, Frith PA, Cartier A, Juniper EF, Dolovich J et al. Determinants of allergen-induced asthma: dose of allergen, circulating IgE antibody concentration, and bronchial responsiveness to inhaled histamine. *American Review of Respiratory Disease* 1979; 120: 1053–1058.
116. Platts-Mills TA and Chapman MD. Dust mites: immunology, allergic disease, and environmental control. *Journal of Allergy & Clinical Immunology* 1987; 80: 755–775.
117. Platts-Mills TA, Hayden ML, Chapman MD, and Wilkins SR. Seasonal variation in dust mite and grass-pollen allergens in dust from the houses of patients with asthma. *Journal of Allergy & Clinical Immunology* 1987; 79: 781–791.
118. Lintner TJ and Brame KA. The effects of season, climate, and air-conditioning on the prevalence of Dermatophagoides mite allergens in household dust. *Journal of Allergy & Clinical Immunology* 1993; 91: 862–867.
119. Platts-Mills TA. How environment affects patients with allergic disease: indoor allergens and asthma. *Annals of Allergy* 1994; 72: 381–384.
120. Sporik R, Holgate ST, Platts-Mills TAE, and Cogswell JJ. Exposure to house-dust mite allergen (der p I) and the development of asthma in childhood. *New England Journal of Medicine* 1990; 323: 502–507.
121. Korsgaard J. Mite asthma and residency: a case-control study on the impact of exposure to house-dust mites in dwellings. *American Review of Respiratory Disease* 1983; 128: 231–235.
122. Finn PW, Boudreau JO, He H, Wang Y, Chapman MD, Vincent C et al. Children at risk for asthma: home allergen levels, lymphocyte proliferation, and wheeze. *Journal of Allergy & Clinical Immunology* 2000; 105: 933–942.
123. Perry T. The prevalence of rat allergen in inner city homes and its relationship to sensitization and asthma morbidity. *Journal of Allergy & Clinical Immunology* 2003; 112: 346–352.

124. Bush RK, Wood RA, and Eggleston PA. Laboratory animal allergy. *Journal of Allergy & Clinical Immunology* 1998; 102: 99–112.

125. Martinez FD, Cline M, and Burrows B. Increased incidence of asthma in children of smoking mothers. *Pediatrics* 1992; 89: 21–26.

126. Neuspiel DR, Rush D, Butler NR, Golding J, Bijur PE, and Kurzon M. Parental smoking and post-infancy wheezing in children: a prospective cohort study. *American Journal of Public Health* 1989; 79: 168–171.

127. U.S. Environmental Protection Agency. Respiratory Health Effects of Passive Smoking: Lung Cancer and Other Disorders, EPA/600/6-90/006F, 1993.

128. Weiss ST, Tager IB, Speizer FE, and Rosner B. Persistent wheeze: its relation to respiratory illness, cigarette smoking, and level of pulmonary function in a population sample of children. *American Review of Respiratory Disease* 1980; 122: 697–707.

129. Dekker C, Dales R, Bartlett S, Brunekreef B, and Zwanenburg H. Childhood asthma and the indoor environment. *Chest* 1991; 100: 922–926.

130. National Research Council. *Environmental Tobacco Smoke*. Washington, D.C.: National Academies Press, 1986.

131. Ehrlich RI, Du TD, Jordaan E, Zwarenstein M, Potter P, Volmink JA et al. Risk factors for childhood asthma and wheezing: importance of maternal and household smoking. *American Journal of Respiratory & Critical Care Medicine* 1996; 154: 681–688.

132. Larsson ML, Frisk M, Hallstrom J, Kiviloog J, and Lundback B. Environmental tobacco smoke exposure during childhood is associated with increased prevalence of asthma in adults. *Chest* 2001; 120: 711–717.

133. Colley JR, Douglas JW, and Reid DD. Respiratory disease in young adults: influence of early childhood lower respiratory tract illness, social class, air pollution, and smoking. *British Medical Journal* 1973; 3: 195–198.

134. Eisner MD, Yelin EH, Trupin L, and Blanc PD. Asthma and smoking status in a population-based study of California adults. *Public Health Reports* 2001; 116: 148–157.

135. Strachan DP and Cook DG. Health effects of passive smoking. 6. Parental smoking and childhood asthma: longitudinal and case-control studies. *Thorax* 1998; 53: 204–212.

136. Strachan DP and Cook DG. Health effects of passive smoking. 5. Parental smoking and allergic sensitisation in children. *Thorax* 1998; 53: 117–123.

137. Schwartz J, Slater D, Larson TV, Pierson WE, and Koenig JQ. Particulate air pollution and hospital emergency room visits for asthma in Seattle. *American Review of Respiratory Disease* 1993; 147: 826–831.

138. Norris G, Larson T, Koenig J, Claiborn C, Sheppard L, and Finn D. Asthma aggravation, combustion, and stagnant air. *Thorax* 2000; 55: 466–470.

139. Atkinson RW, Anderson HR, Sunyer J, Ayres J, Baccini M, Vonk JM et al. Acute effects of particulate air pollution on respiratory admissions: results from APHEA 2 project. *American Journal of Respiratory & Critical Care Medicine* 2001; 164: 1860–1866.

140. Tseng RY, Li CK, and Spinks JA. Particulate air pollution and hospitalization for asthma. *Annals of Allergy* 1992; 68: 425–432.

141. Petroeschevsky A, Simpson RW, Thalib L, and Rutherford S. Associations between outdoor air pollution and hospital admissions in Brisbane, Australia. *Archives of Environmental Health* 2001; 56: 37–52.

142. Pope CA, Dockery DW, Spengler JD, and Raizenne ME. Respiratory health and PM10 polution. *American Review of Respiratory Disease* 1991; 144: 668–674.

143. Keeler GJ, Dvonch T, Yip FY, Parker EA, Isreal BA, Marsik FJ et al. Assessment of personal and community-level exposures to particulate matter among children with asthma in Detroit, Michigan, as part of Community Action Against Asthma (CAAA). *Environmental Health Perspectives* 2002; 110: 173–181.

144. Wjst M, Reitmeir P, Dold S, Wulff A, Nicolai T, Loeffelholz-Colberg EF et al. Road traffic and adverse effects on respiratory health in children. *British Medical Journal* 1993; 307: 596–600.

145. Nitta H, Sato T, Nakai S, Maeda K, Aoki S, and Ono M. Respiratory health associated with exposure to automobile exhaust. I. Results of cross-sectional studies in 1979, 1982, and 1983. *Archives of Environmental Health* 1993; 48: 53–58.

146. Weiland SK, Mundt KA, Ruckmann A, and Keil U. Self-reported wheezing and allergic rhinitis in children and traffic density on street of residence. *Annals of Epidemiology* 1994; 4: 243–247.

147. Hirsch T, Weiland SK, von Mutius E, Safeca AF, Grafe H, Csaplovics E et al. Inner city air pollution and respiratory health and atopy in children. *European Respiratory Journal* 1999; 14: 669–677.

148. Venn AJ, Lewis SA, Cooper M, Hubbard R, and Britton J. Living near a main road and the risk of wheezing illness in children. *American Journal of Respiratory & Critical Care Medicine* 2001; 164: 2177–2180.

149. Edwards J, Walters S, and Griffiths RK. Hospital admissions for asthma in pre-school children: relationship to major roads in Birmingham, United Kingdom. *Archives of Environmental Health* 1994; 49: 223–227.

150. von Mutius E. The environmental predictors of allergic disease. *Journal of Allergy & Clinical Immunology* 2000; 105: 9–19.

151. Wardlaw AJ. The role of air pollution in asthma. *Clinical & Experimental Allergy* 1993; 23: 81–96.

152. Brauer M, Hoek G, Van Vliet P, Meliefste K, Fischer PH, Wijga A et al. Air pollution from traffic and the development of respiratory infections and asthmatic and allergic symptoms in children. *American Journal of Respiratory & Critical Care Medicine* 2002; 166: 1092–1098.

153. Shima M, Nitta Y, Ando M, and Adachi M. Effects of air pollution on the prevalence and incidence of asthma in children. *Archives of Environmental Health* 2002; 57: 529–535.

154. Zaebst DD, Clapp DE, Blade LM, Marlow DA, Steenland K, Hornung RW et al. Quantitative determination of trucking industry workers' exposures to diesel exhaust particles. *American Industrial Hygiene Association Journal* 1991; 52: 529–541.

155. Van Vliet P, Knape M, de Hartog J, Janssen N, Harssema H, and Brunekreef B. Motor vehicle exhaust and chronic respiratory symptoms in children living near freeways. *Environmental Research* 1997; 74: 122–132.

156. McClellan RO, Mauderly JL, Jones RK, and Cuddihy RG. Health effects of diesel exhaust: a contemporary air pollution issue. *Postgraduate Medicine* 204; 78: 199–201.

157. Nel AE, Diaz-Sanchez D, Ng D, Hiura T, and Saxon A. Enhancement of allergic inflammation by the interaction between diesel exhaust particles and the immune system. *Journal of Allergy & Clinical Immunology* 1998; 102: 539–554.

158. Miyabara Y, Ichinose T, Takano H, Lim HB, and Sagai M. Effects of diesel exhaust on allergic airway inflammation in mice. *Journal of Allergy & Clinical Immunology* 1998; 102: 805–812.

159. Bayram H, Devalia JL, Khair OA, Abdelaziz MM, Sapsford RJ, Sagai M et al. Comparison of ciliary activity and inflammatory mediator release from bronchial epithelial cells of nonatopic nonasthmatic subjects and atopic asthmatic patients and the effect of diesel exhaust *particles in vitro. Journal of Allergy & Clinical Immunology* 1998; 102: 771–782.

160. Diaz-Sanchez D, Tsien A, Fleming J, and Saxon A. Combined diesel exhaust particulate and ragweed allergen challenge markedly enhances human in vivo nasal ragweed-specific IgE and skews cytokine production to a T helper cell 2-type pattern. *Journal of Immunology* 1997; 158: 2406–2413.

161. Diaz-Sanchez D, Dotson AR, Takenaka H, and Saxon A. Diesel exhaust particles induce local IgE production *in vivo* and alter the pattern of IgE messenger RNA isoforms. *Journal of Clinical Investigation* 1994; 94: 1417–1425.

162. Ogden CL, Flegal KM, Carroll MD, and Johnson CL. Prevalence and trends in overweight among U.S. children and adolescents, 1999–2000. *Journal of the American Medical Association* 2002; 288: 1728–1732.

163. Flegal KM, Carroll MD, Ogden CL, and Johnson CL. Prevalence and trends in obesity among U.S. adults, 1999–2000. *Journal of the American Medical Association* 2002; 288: 1723–1727.

164. Shaheen SO, Sterne JA, Montgomery SM, and Azima H. Birth weight, body mass index and asthma in young adults. *Thorax* 1999; 54: 396–402.

165. Gennuso J, Epstein LH, Paluch RA, and Cerny F. The relationship between asthma and obesity in urban minority children and adolescents. *Archives of Pediatrics & Adolescent Medic*ine 1998; 152: 1197–1200.

166. von Mutius E, Schwartz J, Neas LM, Dockery D, and Weiss ST. Relation of body mass index to asthma and atopy in children: the National Health and Nutrition Examination Study III. *Thorax* 2001; 56: 835–838.

167. Luder E, Melnik TA, and DiMaio M. Association of being overweight with greater asthma symptoms in inner city black and Hispanic children. *Journal of Pediatrics* 1998; 132: 699–703.

168. Arif AD. Prevalence and risk factors of asthma and wheezing among U.S. adults: an analysis of NHANES III data. *European Respiratory Journal* 2003; 21: 827–833.

169. Chen Y, Dales R, Krewski D, and Breithaupt K. Increased effects of smoking and obesity on asthma among female Canadians: the National Population Health Survey, 1994–1995. *American Journal of Epidemiology* 1999; 150: 255–262.

170. Camargo CA, Jr., Weiss ST, Zhang S, Willett WC, and Speizer FE. Prospective study of body mass index, weight change, and risk of adult-onset asthma in women. *Archives of Internal Medicine* 1999; 159: 2582–2588.

171. Clark JM, Bone LR, Stallings R, Gelber AC, Barker A, Zeger S et al. Obesity and approaches to weight in an urban African-American community. *Ethnicity & Disease* 2001; 11: 676–686.

172. Goethe JW, Maljanian R, Wolf S, Hernandez P, and Cabrera Y. The impact of depressive symptoms on the functional status of inner city patients with asthma. *Annals of Allergy, Asthma & Immunology* 2001; 87: 205–210.

173. Weil CM, Wade SL, Bauman LJ, Lynn H, Mitchell H, and Lavigne J. The relationship between psychosocial factors and asthma morbidity in inner city children with asthma. *Pediatrics* 1999; 104: 1274–1280.

174. Bartlett SJ, Kolodner K, Butz AM, Eggleston P, Malveaux FJ, and Rand CS. Maternal depressive symptoms and emergency department use among inner city children with asthma. *Archives of Pediatrics & Adolescent Medicine* 2001; 155: 347–353.

175. Taylor L, Zuckerman B, Harik V, and Groves BM. Witnessing violence by young children and their mothers. *Journal of Developmental & Behavioral Pediatrics* 1994; 15: 120–123.

176. Sheehan K, DiCara JA, LeBailly S, and Christoffel KK. Children's exposure to violence in an urban setting. *Archives of Pediatrics & Adolescent Medicine* 1997; 151: 502–504.

177. Wright RJ and Steinbach SF. Violence: an unrecognized environmental exposure that may contribute to greater asthma morbidity in high risk inner city populations. *Environmental Health Perspectives* 2001; 109: 1085–1089.

178. Wright RJ. Allergen-induced lymphocyte proliferation in early childhood: role of stress. *American Journal of Respiratory & Critical Care Medicine* 2001; 163: A22.

179. Klinnert MD, Nelson HS, Price MR, Adinoff AD, Leung DY, and Mrazek DA. Onset and persistence of childhood asthma: predictors from infancy. *Pediatrics* 2001; 108: E69.

180. Marshall GD, Jr. and Agarwal SK. Stress, immune regulation, and immunity: applications for asthma. *Allergy & Asthma Proceedings* 2000; 21: 241–246.

181. Wright RJ, Rodriguez M, and Cohen S. Review of psychosocial stress and asthma: an integrated biopsychosocial approach. *Thorax* 1998; 53: 1066–1074.

182. Leikin JB, Morris RW, Warren M, and Erickson T. Trends in a decade of drug abuse presentation to an inner city ED. *American Journal of Emergency Medicine* 2001; 19: 37–39.

183. Drug Abuse Warning Network. *Semiannual Report: Trend Data through January–July 1988*. Rockville, MD: U.S. Department of Health & Human Services, Publication ADM89-1607, 2003.

184. National Institute on Drug Abuse. *Research Report: Cocaine Abuse and Addiction*, 1999. Bethesda, MD: National Institutes of Health, Publication 99-4342, 2003.

185. Rome LA, Lippmann ML, Dalsey WC, Taggart P, and Pomerantz S. Prevalence of cocaine use and its impact on asthma exacerbation in an urban population. *Chest* 2000; 117: 1324–1329.

186. McNagny SE and Parker RM. High prevalence of recent cocaine use and the unreliability of patient self-report in an inner city walk-in clinic. *Journal of the American Medical Association* 1992; 267: 1106–1108.
187. Rubin R and Neugarten J. Cocaine-associated asthma. *American Journal of Medicine* 1990; 88: 438–439.
188. Rebhun J. Association of asthma and freebase smoking. *Annals of Allergy* 1988; 60: 339–342.
189. Community Epidemiologic Work Group. *Epidemiologic Trends in Drug Abuse, 1999*, Vol. 1. Rockville, MD: National Institute on Drug Abuse, Publication 00-4529, 2003.
190. Cygan J, Trunsky M, and Corbridge T. Inhaled heroin-induced status asthmaticus: five cases and a review of the literature. *Chest* 2000; 117: 272–275.
191. Krantz AJ, Hershow RC, Prachand N, Hayden DM, Franklin C, and Hryhorczuk DO. Heroin insufflation as a trigger for patients with life-threatening asthma. *Chest* 2003; 123: 510–517.
192. Rask KJ, Williams MV, Parker RM, and McNagny SE. Obstacles predicting lack of a regular provider and delays in seeking care for patients at an urban public hospital. *Journal of the American Medical Association* 1994; 271: 1931–1933.
193. Crain EF, Kercsmar C, Weiss KB, Mitchell H, and Lynn H. Reported difficulties in access to quality care for children with asthma in the inner city. *Archives of Pediatrics & Adolescent Medicine* 1998; 152: 333–339.
194. Farber HJ, Johnson C, and Beckerman RC. Young inner city children visiting the emergency room (ER) for asthma: risk factors and chronic care behaviors. *Journal of Asthma* 1998; 35: 547–552.
195. Murray MD, Stang P, and Tierney WM. Health care use by inner city patients with asthma. *Journal of Clinical Epidemiology* 1997; 50: 167–174.
196. Lozano P, Connell FA, and Koepsell TD. Use of health services by African-American children with asthma on Medicaid. *Journal of the American Medical Association* 1995; 274: 469–473.
197. Rand CS, Butz AM, Kolodner K, Huss K, Eggleston P, and Malveaux F. Emergency department visits by urban African American children with asthma. *Journal of Allergy & Clinical Immunology* 2000; 105: 83–90.
198. Ford JG, Meyer IH, Sternfels P, Findley SE, McLean DE, Fagan JK et al. Patterns and predictors of asthma-related emergency department use in Harlem. *Chest* 2001; 120: 1129–1135.
199. Hartert TV, Windom HH, Peebles RS, Jr., Freidhoff LR, and Togias A. Inadequate outpatient medical therapy for patients with asthma admitted to two urban hospitals. *American Journal of Medicine* 1996; 100: 386–394.
200. Bosco LA, Gerstman BB, and Tomita DK. Variations in the use of medication for the treatment of childhood asthma in the Michigan Medicaid population, 1980 to 1986. *Chest* 1993; 104: 1727–1732.
201. National Asthma Education and Prevention Program. *Expert Panel Report 2. Guidelines for the Diagnosis and Management of Asthma*. Rockville, MD: U.S. Department of Health & Human Services, Publication 97-4051.

202. Birkhead G, Attaway NJ, Strunk RC, Townsend MC, and Teutsch S. Investigation of a cluster of deaths of adolescents from asthma: evidence implicating inadequate treatment and poor patient adherence with medications. *Journal of Allergy & Clinical Immunology* 1989; 84: 484–491.

203. Warman KL, Silver EJ, McCourt MP, and Stein RE. How does home management of asthma exacerbations by parents of inner city children differ from National Heart, Lung and Blood Institute guideline recommendations? *Pediatrics* 1999; 103: 422–427.

204. Halterman JS, Yoos HL, Kaczorowski JM, McConnochie K, Holzhauer RJ, Conn KM et al. Providers underestimate symptom severity among urban children with asthma. *Archives of Pediatrics & Adolescent Medicine* 2002; 156: 141–146.

205. Estrada AL, Trevino FM, and Ray LA. Health care utilization barriers among Mexican Americans: evidence from HHANES 1982–1984. *American Journal of Public Health* 1990; 80: 27–31.

206. Vance VJ and Taylor WF. The financial cost of chronic childhood asthma. *Annals of Allergy* 1971; 29: 455–460.

207. Williams MV, Baker DW, Honig EG, Lee TM, and Nowlan A. Inadequate literacy is a barrier to asthma knowledge and self-care. *Chest* 1998; 114: 1008–1015.

208. Wade SL, Holden G, Lynn H, Mitchell H, and Ewart C. Cognitive-behavioral predictors of asthma morbidity in inner city children. *Journal of Developmental & Behavioral Pediatrics* 2000; 21: 340–346.

209. Conway T, Hu TC, Bennett S, and Niedos M. A pilot study describing local residents' perceptions of asthma and knowledge of asthma care in selected Chicago communities. *Chest* 1999; 116: 229S–234S.

210. Donnelly JE, Donnelly WJ, and Thong YH. Inadequate parental understanding of asthma medications. *Annals of Allergy* 1989; 62: 337–341.

211. Solis JM, Marks G, Garcia M, and Shelton D. Acculturation, access to care, and use of preventive services by Hispanics: findings from HHANES 1982–1984. *American Journal of Public Health* 1990; 80: 11–19.

212. Kirkman-Liff B and Mondragon D. Language of interview: relevance for research of southwest Hispanics. *American Journal of Public Health* 1991; 81: 1399–1404.

213. Zorc JJ, Scarfone RJ, Li Y, Hong T, Harmelin M, Grunstein L et al. Scheduled follow-up after a pediatric emergency department visit for asthma: a randomized trial. *Pediatrics* 2003; 111: 495–502.

214. Baren JM, Shofer FS, Ivey B, Reinhard S, DeGeus J, Stahmer SA et al. A randomized, controlled trial of a simple emergency department intervention to improve the rate of primary care follow-up for patients with acute asthma exacerbations. *Annals of Emergency Medicine* 2001; 38: 115–122.

215. Brenner BE, Chavda KK, and Camargo CA, Jr. Randomized trial of inhaled flunisolide versus placebo among asthmatic patients discharged from the emergency department. *Annals of Emergency Medicine* 2000; 36: 417–426.

216. Mayo PH, Richman J, and Harris HW. Results of a program to reduce admissions for adult asthma. *Annals of Internal Medicine* 1990; 112: 864–871.

217. George MR, O'Dowd LC, Martin I, Lindell KO, Whitney F, Jones M et al. A comprehensive educational program improves clinical outcome measures in inner city patients with asthma. *Archives of Internal Medicine* 1999; 159: 1710–1716.

218. Harish Z, Bregante AC, Morgan C, Fann CS, Callaghan CM, Witt MA et al. A comprehensive inner city asthma program reduces hospital and emergency room utilization. *Annals of Allergy, Asthma, & Immunology* 2001; 86: 185–189.
219. Guevara JP, Wolf FM, Grum CM, and Clark NM. Effects of educational interventions for self management of asthma in children and adolescents: systematic review and meta-analysis. *British Medical Journal* 2003; 326: 1308–1309.
220. Christiansen SC, Martin SB, Schleicher NC, Koziol JA, Mathews KP, and Zuraw BL. Evaluation of a school-based asthma education program for inner city children. *Journal of Allergy & Clinical Immunology* 1997; 100: 613–617.
221. Evans D, Clark NM, Feldman CH, Rips J, Kaplan D, Levison MJ et al. A school health education program for children with asthma aged 8–11 years. *Health Education Quarterly* 1987; 14: 267–279.
222. Clark N and Feldman D. Impact of health education on frequency and cost of health care use by low income children with asthma. *Journal of Allergy & Clinical Immunology* 1986; 78: 108–115.
223. Shields MC, Griffin KW, and McNabb WL. The effect of a patient education program on emergency room use for inner city children with asthma. *American Journal of Public Health* 1990; 80: 36–38.
224. Bartholomew LK, Shegog R, Parcel GS, Gold RS, Fernandez M, Czyzewski DI et al. Watch, Discover, Think, and Act: a model for patient education program development. *Patient Education & Counseling* 2000; 39: 253–268.
225. Bartholomew LK, Gold RS, Parcel GS, Czyzewski DI, Sockrider MM, Fernandez M et al. Watch, Discover, Think, and Act: evaluation of computer-assisted instruction to improve asthma self-management in inner city children. *Patient Education & Counseling* 2000; 39: 269–280.
226. Shegog R, Bartholomew LK, Parcel GS, Sockrider MM, Masse L, and Abramson SL. Impact of a computer-assisted education program on factors related to asthma self-management behavior. *Journal of the American Medical Informatics Association* 2001; 8: 49–61.
227. Guendelman S, Meade K, Benson M, Chen YQ, and Samuels S. Improving asthma outcomes and self-management behaviors of inner city children: a randomized trial of the Health Buddy interactive device and an asthma diary. *Archives of Pediatrics & Adolescent Medicine* 2002; 156: 114–120.
228. Huss K, Winkelstein M, Nanda J, Naumann PL, Sloand ED, and Huss RW. Computer game for inner city children does not improve asthma outcomes. *Journal of Pediatric Health Care* 2003; 17: 72–78.
229. Ehnert B, Lau-Schadendorf S, Weber A, Beuttner P, Schou C, and Wahn U. Reducing domestic exposure to dust mite allergen reduces bronchial hyperreactivity in sensitive children with asthma. *Journal of Allergy & Clinical Immunology* 1992; 90: 135–138.
230. Rijssenbeek-Nouwens LH, Oosting AJ, Bruin-Weller MS, Bregman I, de Monchy JG, and Postma DS. Clinical evaluation of the effect of anti-allergic mattress covers in patients with moderate to severe asthma and house dust mite allergy: a randomised double blind placebo controlled study. *Thorax* 2002; 57: 784–790.

231. Frederick JM, Warner JO, Jessop WJ, Enander I, and Warner JA. Effect of a bed covering system in children with asthma and house dust mite hypersensitivity. *European Respiratory Journal* 1997; 10: 361–366.

232. Shapiro GG, Wighton TG, Chinn T, Zuckrman J, Eliassen AH, Picciano JF et al. House dust mite avoidance for children with asthma in homes of low-income families. *Journal of Allergy & Clinical Immunology* 1999; 103: 1069–1074.

233. Cloosterman SG, Schermer TR, Bijl-Hofland ID, van der Heide S, Brunekreef B, Van Den Elshout FJ et al. Effects of house dust mite avoidance measures on Der p 1 concentrations and clinical condition of mild adult house dust mite-allergic asthmatic patients using no inhaled steroids. *Clinical & Experimental Allergy* 1999; 29: 1336–1346.

234. Gotzsche PC, Hammarquist C, and Burr M. House dust mite control measures in the management of asthma: meta-analysis. *British Medical Journal* 1998; 317: 1105–1110.

235. Woodcock A, Forster L, Matthews E, Martin J, Letley L, Vickers M et al. Control of exposure to mite allergen and allergen-impermeable bed covers for adults with asthma. *New England Journal of Medicine* 2003; 349: 225–236.

236. Vojta PJ, Randels SP, Stout J, Muilenberg M, Burge HA, Lynn H et al. Effects of physical interventions on house dust mite allergen levels in carpet, bed, and upholstery dust in low-income, urban homes. *Environmental Health Perspectives* 2001; 109: 815–819.

237. Carter MC, Perzanowski MS, Raymond A, and Platts-Mills TA. Home intervention in the treatment of asthma among inner city children. *Journal of Allergy & Clinical Immunology* 2001; 108: 732–737.

238. Arbes SJ, Jr., Sever M, Archer J, Long E, Gore J, Schal C et al. Abatement of cockroach allergen (Bla g 1) in low-income, urban housing: a randomized controlled trial. *Journal of Allergy & Clinical Immunology* 2003; 112: 339–345.

239. Eggleston PA, Wood RA, Rand C, Nixon WJ, Chen PH, and Lukk P. Removal of cockroach allergen from inner city homes. *Journal of Allergy & Clinical Immunology* 1999; 104: 842–846.

240. Gergen PJ, Mortimer KM, Eggleston PA, Rosenstreich D, Mitchell H, Ownby D et al. Results of the National Cooperative Inner City Asthma Study (NCICAS) environmental intervention to reduce cockroach allergen exposure in inner city homes. *Journal of Allergy and Clinical Immunology* 1999; 103: 501–506.

241. Hovell MF, Meltzer SB, Zakarian JM, Wahlgren DR, Emerson JA, Hofstetter CR et al. Reduction of environmental tobacco smoke exposure among asthmatic children: a controlled trial. *Chest* 1994; 106: 440–446.

242. Wahlgren DR, Hovell MF, Meltzer SB, Hofstetter CR, and Zakarian JM. Reduction of environmental tobacco smoke exposure in asthmatic children. A two-year follow-up. *Chest* 1997; 111: 81–88.

243. Emmons KM, Hammond SK, Fava JL, Velicer WF, Evans JL, and Monroe AD. A randomized trial to reduce passive smoke exposure in low-income households with young children. *Pediatrics* 2001; 108: 18–24.

244. Wilson SR, Yamada EG, Sudhakar R, Roberto L, Mannino D, Mejia C et al. A controlled trial of an environmental tobacco smoke reduction intervention in low-income children with asthma. *Chest* 2001; 120: 1709–1722.

245. Hovell MF, Zakarian JM, Matt GE, Hofstetter CR, Bernert JT, and Pirkle J. Effect of counselling mothers on their children's exposure to environmental tobacco smoke: randomised controlled trial. *British Medical Journal* 2000; 321: 337–342.

246. Hovell MF, Meltzer SB, Wahlgren DR, Matt GE, Hofstetter CR, Jones JA et al. Asthma management and environmental tobacco smoke exposure reduction in Latino children: a controlled trial. *Pediatrics* 2002; 110: 946–956.

247. Harish Z, Bregante AC, Morgan C, Fann CS, Callaghan CM, Witt MA et al. A comprehensive inner city asthma program reduces hospital and emergency room utilization. *Annals of Allergy, Asthma, & Immunology* 2001; 86: 185–189.

248. Greineder DK, Loane KC, and Parks P. Reduction in resource utilization by an asthma outreach program. *Archives of Pediatric & Adolescent Medicine* 1995; 149: 415–420.

249. Evans R, III, Gergen PJ, Mitchell H, Kattan M, Kercsmar C, Crain E et al. A randomized clinical trial to reduce asthma morbidity among inner city children: results of the National Cooperative Inner City Asthma Study. *Journal of Pediatrics* 1999; 135: 332–338.

250. Sullivan SD, Weiss KB, Lynn H, Mitchell H, Kattan M, Gergen PJ et al. The cost effectiveness of an inner city asthma intervention for children. *Journal of Allergy & Clinical Immunology* 2002; 110: 576–581.

18

Therapeutic Approaches to Childhood Asthma

STANLEY J. SZEFLER

National Jewish Medical and Research Center
and University of Colorado Health Sciences Center
Denver, Colorado, U.S.A.

I. Introduction

The trend of increasing asthma mortality and morbidity has fortunately reached a plateau over the past several years[1] and we now have an opportunity to see a decline in morbidity and mortality. Perhaps a more proactive approach that facilitates the identification of patients at risk for developing persistent asthma and effective interventions will be successful. It will also be important to identify methods to alter the natural history of asthma and long-term outcomes related to asthma.

Inhaled glucocorticoids are now identified as the cornerstones for managing persistent asthma even in children under 5 years of age.[2–4] New medications and delivery systems have been introduced including a nebulized inhaled glucocorticoid and a leukotriene antagonist for asthma therapy in children as young as 1 year of age.[5,6] These initiatives have now made it possible to intervene at a very early age and thus improve the overall management of childhood asthma.[7,8]

Current methods applied in the management of asthma in children include early diagnosis and intervention via environmental control in allergen-sensitized patients or administration of long-term control therapy.[9,10] This direction in management may result in improved methods for diagnosing asthma and identifying

Table 18.1 Risks Related to Under-Treatment of Asthma

Mortality
Respiratory arrest
Hospitalization
Acute exacerbation
  Emergency department visits
  Course of systemic glucocorticoid therapy
Nocturnal symptoms
Breakthrough symptoms — spontaneous or activity induced
Variability in pulmonary function due to airway sensitivity
School absence
Reduced quality of life, for example, reduced activity level and poor self-image
Progression as indicated by loss of pulmonary function, increasing symptoms, and
  increasing medication requirements
Persistent inflammation
Airway remodeling and irrecoverable loss of pulmonary function
Adverse effects related to overuse of rescue therapy, for example, bronchodilators and
  systemic glucocorticoids

methods to effectively intervene in the natural history of asthma. Although inhaled glucocorticoid therapy improves asthma control, it is not clear whether this treatment can prevent all long-term outcomes (Table 18.1), especially those related to asthma progression and airway remodeling.[11,12]

This review will summarize the currently applied approaches to asthma management in children and the population of patients who may benefit from early intervention with anti-inflammatory therapy. New information related to variable responses to asthma treatment will be discussed since pursuing mechanisms for variability in response could lead to even better methods to tailor therapy for individual patients based on their unique asthma presentations.

II. Managing Asthma in Children

Current guidelines for asthma management place emphasis on the identification of asthma triggers, environmental control, pulmonary function monitoring, education, and therapeutic intervention.[2–4] Asthma is now categorized as intermittent, mild persistent, moderate persistent, and severe persistent based on the frequency of daytime and nighttime symptoms and level and variability of pulmonary function. The Global Initiative for Asthma and the National Heart, Lung, and Blood Institute (NHLBI) Guidelines for the Diagnosis and Management of Asthma have recently been updated.[2,3] The recently updated guidelines of the National Asthma Education and Prevention Program (NAEPP) address the needs of childhood asthma through a careful evidence-based review of critical issues such as the time of intervention, the safety and limitations of inhaled glucocorticoids, and the preferred medication for additive therapy to inhaled glucocorticoids.[3,4]

Information related to asthma management for children below 5 years of age is still sparse due to the small number of studies covering this important age group. Therefore, many assumptions for designing treatment regimens for young children are still based primarily on adult studies. Hopefully, investigators and the pharmaceutical industry will fill the information gaps and also develop new medications for younger children.

Inhaled glucocorticoids are the preferred first-line treatments for both children and adults.[2,3] The preferred additive therapy for inadequate control with low-to-medium dose inhaled glucocorticoid is a long-acting β-adrenergic agonist.[3] Leukotriene antagonists along with cromolyn, nedocromil, and theophylline are considered alternative first-line therapies to inhaled glucocorticoids and alternative additive therapies to long-acting β2-adrenergic agonists once inhaled glucocorticoids have been initiated.[3]

Several recent studies solidify the role of inhaled glucocorticoids as first-line therapy in the management of persistent asthma and also identify some limitations in the efficacy of inhaled glucocorticoids such as a failure to eradicate acute exacerbations and prevent losses in pulmonary function.[8,12] Treatment strategies must address the limitations of inhaled glucocorticoids in preventing asthma progression and reversing pulmonary function in long-standing poorly controlled asthma.

A long-term outcome study from the NHLBI's Childhood Asthma Management Program (CAMP) Research Group established the efficacy of inhaled glucocorticoids as first-line long-term control therapies in children 5 to 12 years of age with mild to moderate persistent asthma.[12] The CAMP clinical trial was initiated in 1991 to determine whether continuous long-term treatment with either an inhaled glucocorticoid (budesonide) or an inhaled nonsteroid (nedocromil) control medication could improve lung growth safely over a 4- to 6-year treatment period as compared with placebo (treatment based only on the management of symptoms with albuterol and oral prednisone as needed).

For clinical outcomes examined in the CAMP study, the most significant treatment effect was observed with the inhaled glucocorticoid treatment arm as compared with placebo. The number of acute exacerbations as indicated by hospitalizations, urgent care visits, and prednisone courses was reduced by approximately 45% in the inhaled budesonide group as compared with the placebo group. The inhaled budesonide group also had better asthma control as indicated by significantly lower symptom scores, higher numbers of episode-free days per month, and fewer albuterol inhalations per week as compared with the placebo group. For the inhaled nedocromil group, reductions only in urgent care visits and prednisone courses compared to the placebo group were observed. No differences were noted in the other clinical outcome measures when the inhaled nedocromil group was compared to the placebo group.

The time to the first significant asthma exacerbation that required systemic glucocorticoid (prednisone) therapy and the time for adding supplementary inhaled glucocorticoid therapy were longer for the inhaled budesonide group as compared to the placebo group, with no difference noted for this indicator when the nedocromil group was compared to the placebo group (Figure 18.1D). The proportion of patients necessitating intervention with oral prednisone or supplementary inhaled glucocorticoid therapy was much lower in the inhaled budesonide group as compared to placebo, while results for the inhaled nedocromil group again were comparable to the placebo group for this measure of control.

The primary measure of lung growth selected for this study was post-bronchodilator $FEV_1\%$ predicted because it reflects maximal lung capacity. The CAMP trial showed that the inhaled glucocorticoid treatment increased post-bronchodilator $FEV_1\%$ predicted from a mean 103.2% predicted to 106.8% predicted within the first 2 months. However, post-bronchodilator $FEV_1\%$ predicted gradually diminished to 103.8% predicted by the end of the treatment period (Figure 18.1A) and surprisingly was comparable to the results that occurred in the placebo and nedocromil groups. Post-bronchodilator $FEV_1\%$ predicted in the nedocromil group was similar to that measured in the placebo group throughout the study period, indicating that this treatment had no significant effect on lung growth.

The finding that neither budesonide nor nedocromil provided significant benefit over placebo for the post-bronchodilator predicted $FEV_1\%$ was an unexpected result compared to data reported from an earlier study by Agertoft and Pedersen.[13] This study reported that early intervention with inhaled glucocorticoids in childhood asthma may prevent irrecoverable loss in pulmonary function. However, this study did not specifically examine post-bronchodilator FEV_1 as an outcome measure, and it was not conducted in a randomized, placebo-controlled design. Since a decline in $FEV_1\%$ predicted did not occur in the placebo group, the CAMP study results raise questions whether airway remodeling actually occurs in this population of mild to moderate persistent asthma and/or whether inhaled glucocorticoids have any effects on preventing this alteration in airway pathology.

The decline in post-bronchodilator $FEV_1\%$ predicted noted in the budesonide treatment arm along with the evolving requirement for supplementary therapy in the CAMP study population suggest that asthma may be progressing despite continuous therapy. Ongoing analysis in the CAMP study population will determine whether this observed evidence of progression could be due to poor adherence with the study medication during the treatment period and whether progression continues after the study medication is discontinued.

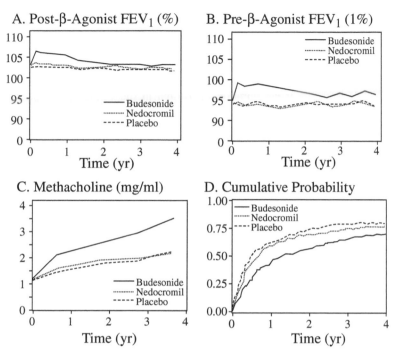

Figure 18.1 Results of Childhood Asthma Management Program (CAMP) study. A: Changes in post-bronchodilator FEV_1 during the duration of the study. Initial improvement occurred in post-bronchodilator FEV_1 in patients receiving budesonide, but by the end of the study, no differences existed among the three treatment groups. B: Changes with pre-bronchodilator therapy. Budesonide produced a modest but statistically significant improvement in pre-bronchodilator FEV_1 throughout the treatment period compared to placebo. C: Changes in methacholine responsiveness over time. All subjects showed improvements in bronchial hyperresponsiveness (BHR) as indicated by the increase in methacholine PC_{20} values over the 4 to 6 years of the trial. Patients randomized to budesonide had significantly greater reductions in BHR compared to placebo-treated patients. D: Kaplan–Meier curve describing the cumulative probability of a first course of prednisone during 4 years of follow-up in the budesonide, nedocromil, and placebo-treated children. (From Agertoft, L and Pedersen, S *New Engl J* Med 2000; 343: 1054–1063. With permission.).

Since a decline in post-bronchodilator FEV_1% predicted was not observed in the placebo group of the CAMP study, questions have been raised on whether airway remodeling is occurring in this patient population. It is possible that FEV_1 % predicted may not be sufficiently sensitive to detect the process of airway remodeling. It is also possible that the study did not include patients who were the most susceptible to airway remodeling since patients with severe asthma were excluded. Therefore, patients who were potentially most susceptible to a progressive loss in $FEV_1\%$ predicted may have been excluded from this study. It is also possible that the most significant effect on FEV_1 decline occurred prior to initiation of the study as indicated in two previous long-term studies on the natural history of asthma.[14,15] Indeed, the mean duration of asthma in the CAMP participants was 5 years and it is conceivable that the most significant effects on airway structures occurred shortly after the onset of the disease. Thus, significant irrecoverable loss in pulmonary function was already established. If these early events are proved to be correct, earlier diagnosis and prompt, effective intervention would be necessary to prevent airway remodeling and the long-term consequences of airway inflammation such as impairment in lung growth or airway hyperresponsiveness.

Other measures of post-bronchodilator pulmonary function were not significantly different upon completion of the treatment phase of CAMP. In contrast, in the treatment group, several measurements of pulmonary function obtained *prior to* bronchodilator administration were different from placebo results. The difference in pre-bronchodilator $FEV_1\%$ predicted following inhaled budesonide treatment as compared to baseline exceeded the level in the placebo group (2.9 versus 0.9, p = 0.02; Figure 18.1B). This observation may be an indicator that the functional airway caliber in the budesonide group was greater than that detected in the placebo group. Although the difference was indeed statistically significant, the magnitude of effect was small.

For inhaled nedocromil, the only difference in any measure of pulmonary function when compared to the placebo group was pre-bronchodilator FEV_1 (liters). Of significant interest was the observation that all of the pulmonary function values were similar for all of the treatment groups 4 months after the active study medication was discontinued. This important observation suggests that any beneficial effect observed on pulmonary function outcome measures due to active treatment is lost in only a short time following treatment cessation. Moreover, these results indicate that inhaled glucocorticoids do not have long-term effects on altering the natural history of asthma if administered too late in the course of the disease. Taken together, these CAMP results reinforce the need to perform very early intervention studies to determine whether long-term efficacy can be realized.

The most remarkable effect of inhaled glucocorticoid treatment on a measure of pulmonary function in CAMP was the significant reduction in airway hyperresponsiveness that persisted throughout the treatment period (Figure 18.1C). Inhaled nedocromil exerted no effect on airway hyperresponsiveness when compared to placebo. Although inhaled budesonide reduced airway hyperresponsiveness during treatment, all three groups had similar methacholine PC_{20} levels after study medication was discontinued. These results further reinforce the concept that long-term outcomes of asthma may not be altered by even the current best treatment options. However, continued prospective evaluation of CAMP participants is ongoing to evaluate the effects of intense long-term treatment courses with anti-inflammatory therapy on maximal lung function and airway hyperresponsiveness as these children approach adulthood.

The CAMP results support the effects of inhaled glucocorticoids on reducing asthma morbidity.[11] However, they differ significantly from observations obtained from studies of shorter duration, for example a year or less, particularly in measures of pulmonary function and body growth. The CAMP study showed that the only detectable adverse effect of long-term treatment with inhaled budesonide was a transient (persistent but not progressive) reduction in growth velocity limited to 1 cm in the first year of treatment. Based on an estimation of final growth evaluated by bone age and height at the end of the treatment period, the height projected in all three treatment groups would be similar once the participants reached final adult height. Agertoft and Pedersen confirmed this estimate with a report of follow-up in young adults who received inhaled glucocorticoid therapy during childhood.[16] However, long-term follow-up in a prospective study population such as CAMP will still be necessary to relieve the lingering concerns regarding persistent effects of inhaled glucocorticoid therapy on final height.

Importantly, the medications studied in the CAMP trial did not completely eliminate the morbidity, for example, hospitalizations and urgent care visits, associated with asthma and the need for improvement in overall asthma management continues. While the CAMP study attenuated concerns about the long-term effects of inhaled glucocorticoid therapy on linear growth, it still raised questions regarding the effects of inhaled glucocorticoids on the natural history of asthma. A greater effect in reducing exacerbations could be achieved conceivably through the use of combination therapy with available medications such as long-acting β_2-adrenergic agonists as observed in adults,[17] through the introduction of new medications such as immunomodulators[18] or through earlier interventions with available medications such as inhaled glucocorticoids or even leukotriene antagonists.[6,8,19] Some of these various therapeutic alternatives are currently under evaluation in prospective clinical trials.

III. Managing Asthma in Young Children

As noted earlier, issues related to the appropriate time to intervene with anti-inflammatory therapy and the efficacy of such treatment are currently under study. Several medications are now labeled and thus approved for use in young children, specifically nebulized budesonide for children 1 year of age or older and montelukast for children 2 years of age or older.[5,6] A new formulation of montelukast is now approved for use by children over 1 year of age. Several key pivotal studies substantiate the efficacy of nebulized budesonide in children under 5 years of age.[5] The approval for montelukast in young children was based primarily on safety data along with pharmacokinetic data demonstrating that the formulations indicated for use in children provided blood levels comparable to those derived from formulations used in adults. Specific parameters for evaluating the efficacy of montelukast remain to be defined for young children. At present, no long-acting β-adrenergic agonist is specifically labeled for use in children below 4 years of age.

Since current treatment plans are based on the assumptions that chronic inflammation is a core feature of asthma and that persistent asthma can occur early in life, current interest focuses on identifying reliable methods for earlier diagnosis and earlier intervention. It remains to be seen whether these strategies for early recognition and early treatment will indeed alter the natural history of asthma and prevent irrecoverable loss of pulmonary function and persistent symptoms. As indicated in the recent update to the NAEPP asthma guidelines, this question calls for the design of prospective, randomized controlled intervention studies with environmental control, pharmacotherapy, immune modulation measures, or a combination of these alternatives.[3]

Currently, asthma management in young children is based primarily on experience derived from studies conducted in older children and adults.[2,3,10,19] These limitations are primarily due to challenges related to the diagnosis of early onset asthma and the assessment of asthma control in young children. Although challenging, measurements of pulmonary function in young children are possible, albeit restricted predominantly to research settings in which these types of assessments are routinely performed.

Pharmacotherapy in young children can be complicated further by the difficulties of properly administering inhaled medication and the dependence of this administration on the skill of the caregiver.[19] As noted, information regarding the appropriate doses of medications for children under 5 years of age is available for some, but not all, medications. These issues have been addressed in the recent update to the NAEPP guidelines for the diagnosis and management of asthma.[3]

The updated asthma guidelines suggest that first-line therapy can start with low-dose inhaled glucocorticoid administered via nebulizer or alternatively a spacer or holding chamber and face mask.[3] A nebulized budesonide preparation is now approved for use in children as young as 1 year of age and includes dosage guidelines for this age group.[5] Other alternatives include a montelukast formulation that can be administered to children as young as 1 year of age. Comparative studies are needed to determine whether an inhaled glucocorticoid administered by a pressurized metered dose inhaler along with a spacer and face mask is as effective as control attained through nebulized administration. No inhaled glucocorticoid in a dry powder or metered dose inhaler formulation available in the United States is approved currently for use in children under 4 years of age. Understandably, it is rare that a dry powder formulation will be administered to a young child because the device requires the generation of a sufficient inspiratory flow rate to generate particle distribution to the lungs. In addition, it is likely that the current pressurized metered dose formulations with the chlorofluorocarbon propellants will be removed from the market once the alternative devices are fully accepted. It will therefore be important to evaluate the new hydrofluoroalkane-based metered dose inhalers along with the spacer–face mask devices for appropriate use (including dose definition and safety) in young children.

Following the publication of the updated asthma guidelines,[3] a published report compared nebulized budesonide to cromolyn inhaled via nebulizer.[8] This study by Leflein et al. clearly demonstrated superiority in asthma control by the nebulized budesonide formulation group with all measures of symptom control and time for supplementary medication as compared to the cromolyn group. However, the number of hospitalizations and emergency department visits were similar for both treatment groups.[8]

For the treatment of moderate persistent asthma in young children, the asthma guidelines recommend either a medium dose of inhaled glucocorticoid or the addition of a long-acting β-adrenergic agonist to low or medium dose inhaled glucocorticoid.[4] These recommendations are clearly based on conclusions derived from adult studies in lieu of adequate controlled studies performed in children. However, no long-acting β-adrenergic agonist formulation has been approved for use in children below 4 years of age. The result is the use of long-acting β_2-adrenergic agonists, specifically metered dose inhaler formulations along with spacers, for such children. Admittedly, no dosing guidelines that would assure safety exist. Therefore, it is important to test the available chlorofluoro-carbon-based formulation in young children or develop and test a hydrofluoro-alkane preparation or nebulized form of a long-acting β-adrenergic agonist. An alternative would be to utilize the approved form of a leukotriene antagonist for supplementary therapy with an inhaled glucocorticoid. A combination of a high dose inhaled glucocorticoid and a long-acting β_2-adrenergic agonist is recommended for more severe asthma. If needed, a systemic glucocorticoid can be added. The dose should be adjusted to the lowest dose required to minimize symptoms.

The updated asthma guidelines also address criteria to consider for early intervention in young children, namely those at risk for persistent asthma.[3] Recent work by the Tucson Children's Respiratory Study following analysis of respiratory patterns in children for the first 15 years of life reported that children who wheezed during lower respiratory tract illnesses in the first 3 years of life and still wheezed at age 6 ("persistent wheezers") had lower levels of pulmonary function than children who had no wheezing illnesses before the age of 6 years.[21] The researchers reported that the lowest levels of lung function in early childhood were observed among children who wheezed before age 3 and were not current wheezers at age 6. These patients are considered transient wheezers; persistent wheezers have comparably normal pulmonary functions in the first 3 years of life and lower pulmonary function thereafter.[14,21] This raises the question whether the observed decline in pulmonary function of persistent wheezers can be prevented with early utilization of either environmental control or anti-inflammatory therapy.

This natural history study was also useful in determining risk factors for the development of persistent asthma. An Asthma Predictive Index (API) introduced by Castro-Rodriguez et al.[22] revealed that frequent wheezing during the first 3 years of life associated with either one major risk factor (parental history of asthma or eczema in the child) or two of three minor risk factors (eosinophilia (>4%), wheezing without cold, and allergic rhinitis) significantly increased the risk of developing asthma by age 6.

It has also been suggested that a loss of pulmonary function over time is associated with airway remodeling.[23] This loss of pulmonary function is comparable to the pattern observed in chronic obstructive pulmonary disease in adults and cystic fibrosis in children except that asthma retains a reversible component. It thus appears that patients differ considerably in both clinical presentation and susceptibility to impairment in lung growth. It remains to be seen whether early intervention with anti-inflammatory therapy, such as an inhaled glucocorticoid, can alter the natural history of asthma, especially the component of progressive loss of pulmonary function. Nevertheless, it is already clear that intervention with inhaled glucocorticoids improves asthma control based on well-controlled studies in young and older children including adolescents.[8,12]

The NHLBI Childhood Asthma Research and Education Network is now conducting an early intervention study with inhaled glucocorticoid therapy in young children at risk for childhood asthma that applies the API[22] as an entry criterion. The results of this study should be available in approximately 2 years and promise to answer a number of questions relating to the effect of early intervention with anti-inflammatory therapy on altering clinical and pulmonary function features associated with the development of asthma.

IV. When to Initiate Long-Term Controller Therapy in Children

The revised NAEPP asthma guidelines now recommend intervention at several points.[3] First, bronchodilators should be administered for symptoms and systemic glucocorticoids for significant exacerbations regardless of patient age. Second, intervention with long-term control therapy has been recommended for children with symptoms that occur more than twice per week, nocturnal symptoms that occur more than two times per month, and pulmonary function below 80% predicted or within day PEF variability that exceeds 20% (Figure 18.2 and Figure 18.3).

	Symptoms**	Nighttime Symptoms	Lung Function
STEP 4 **Severe** **Persistent**	■ Continual symptoms ■ Limited physical activity ■ Frequent exacerbations	Frequent	■ FEV_1/PEF ≤60% predicted ■ PEF variability >30%

STEP 3
Moderate
Persistent
	■ Daily symptoms
	■ Daily use of inhaled short-acting ß2
	  agonist
	■ Exacerbations affect activity
	■ Exacerbations ≥2 times a week;
	  may last days
		> 1 time a week	■ FEV_1/PEF ≤60% - <80%
			  predicted
			■ PEF variability >30%

STEP 2 **Mild** **Persistent**	■ Symptoms >2 times a week, but <1 time a day ■ Exacerbations may affect activity	≥ 2 times a month	■ FEV_1/PEF ≥80% predicted ■ PEF variability >20-30%

Mild
Intermittent
	■ Symptoms ≥2 times a week
	■ Asymptomatic and normal PEF
	  between exacerbations
	■ Exacerbations brief (from a few
	  hours to a few days), intensity may
	  vary
		≤ 2 times a month	■ FEV_1/PEF ≥80% predicted
			■ PEF variability <20%

Figure 18.2 Classification of asthma severity. (NIH Guidelines for the Diagnosis and Management of Asthma, 1997.)

In addition, the guidelines suggest that intervention with long-term controller therapy should be considered in young children who have significant acute exacerbations that recur within 6 weeks. The updated guidelines also suggest a consideration for intervention with long-term therapy in young children at risk for persistent asthma based on frequent episodes of wheezing and major or minor risk factors that comprise the API as described previously.[22]

V. Evolution of Asthma Therapy and Potential for Future Developments

The treatment of asthma less than 50 years ago originally focused on alleviating episodes of bronchospasm by using short-acting bronchodilators that included epinephrine, isoproterenol, and eventually metaproterenol. Structural modifications of epinephrine led the way to the currently recognized and preferred β_2-adrenergic agonists, albuterol, terbutaline, and pirbuterol. Within the past 20 years, theophylline, a long-acting bronchodilator, was the preferred maintenance therapy for asthma. Alteration of the oral release characteristics resulted in the development of products that facilitated twice- and even once-daily administration and also offered benefits in reducing the number of nighttime asthma episodes. Subsequently, it was recognized that inhaled cromolyn offered advantages in attenuating early and late pulmonary responses to allergen challenges in sensitized patients, and the concept of preventative therapy was introduced. Cromolyn also blocked the development of airways hyperresponsiveness that followed allergen challenges in sensitized patients.

Classify Severity: Clinical Features Before Treatment or Adequate Control			Medications Required to Maintain Long-Term Control
	Symptoms/Day or FEV₁ **Symptoms/Night Variability**	**PEF** **PEF**	**Daily Medications**
Step 4 **Severe Persistent**	Continual Frequent	≤ 60% ≥ 30%	**Preferred treatment:** - High-dose inhaled corticosteroids AND -Long-acting inhaled beta₂-agonists AND, if needed, -Corticosteroid tablets or syrup long term (2 mg/kg/day, generally do not exceed 60 mg per day). (Make repeat attempts to reduce systemic corticosteroids and maintain control with high-dose inhaled corticosteroids.)
Step 3 **Moderate Persistent**	Daily > 1 night/week	> 60% - < 80% > 30%	**Preferred treatment:** - Low-to-medium dose inhaled corticosteroids and long-acting inhaled beta₂-agonists. **Alternate treatment (listed alphabetically):** - Increased inhaled corticosteroids within medium-dose range OR - Low-to-medium dose inhaled corticosteroids and either leukotriene modifier or theophylline ········· If needed (particularly in patients with recurring severe exacerbations): **Preferred treatment:** - Increased inhaled corticosteroids within medium-dose range, and add long-acting inhaled beta₂-agonists. **Alternate treatment (listed alphabetically):** - Increased inhaled corticosteroids in medium-dose range, and add either leukotriene modifier or theophylline.
Step 2 **Mild Persistent**	> 2/week but < 1x/day > 2 nights/month	≥ 80% 20-30%	**Preferred treatment:** - Low dose inhaled corticosteroids. **Alternate treatment (listed alphabetically):** - Cromolyn, leukotriene modifier, nedocromil, OR Sustained release theophylline to serum concentration of 5-15 mcg/mL.
Step 1 **Mild Intermittent**	≤ 2 days/weeks ≤ 2 nights/month	≥ 80% < 20%	No daily medication needed. Severe exacerbations may occur, separated by long periods of normal lung function and no symptoms. A course of systemic corticosteroids is recommended.

All Patients:	• Short-acting bronchodilator: 2-4 puffs short-acting inhaled beta₂-agonists as needed for symptoms. • Intensity of treatment will depend on severity of exacerbation; up to 3 treatments at 20-minute intervals or a single nebulizer treatment as needed. Course of systemic corticosteroids may be needed. • Use of short-acting inhaled beta₂-agonists on a daily basis, or increasing use, indicates the need to initiate or increase long-term control therapy.

Step Down

Review treatment every 1 to 6 months; a gradual stepwise reduction in treatment may be possible.

Note

The stepwise approach is meant to assist, not replace, the clinical decision making required to meet individual patient needs.

Classify severity: assign patient to most severe step in which any feature occurs (PEF is % of personal best; FEV₁ is % predicted).

Gain control as quickly as possible (consider a short course of systemic corticosteroids); then step down to the least medication necessary to maintain control.

Provide education on self-management and controlling environmental factors that make asthma worse (e.g., allergens and irritants).

Refer to an asthma specialist if there are difficulties controlling asthma or if step 4 care is required. Referral may be considered if step 3 care is required.

· Minimal or no chronic symptoms day or night · Minimal or no exacerbations · No limitations on activities; no school/work missed	· PEF > 80% of personal best · Minimal use of inhaled short-acting beta₂-agonist (< 1x per day) · Minimal or no adverse effects from medications

Figure 18.3 Guidelines: Stepwise approach for managing asthma in adults and children older than 5 years of age: Treatment. (NIH Guidelines for the Diagnosis and Treatment of Asthma — Update on Selected Topics 2002).

Although the benefits of inhaled glucocorticoid therapy dosing were recognized in the late 1970s, they were not considered preferred therapy until the clear documentation of efficacy in the long-term management of asthma for both adults and children.[10] Several new classes of medications were introduced in the past 5 years including long-acting β_2-adrenergic agonists and leukotriene modifiers. The long acting β_2-adrenergic agonists, specifically salmeterol and formoterol, have 12-hour durations of bronchodilator action and are now approved for use in children 4 years of age and older. Montelukast, an oral leukotriene antagonist, has emerged as the most popular first-line long-term control therapy in children with asthma due to the availability of product information regarding dosage and the demonstration of safety in children as young as 1 year of age.

To limit the adverse effects of short-acting β-agonists, levalbuterol, a stereoisomer of albuterol, was developed and introduced.[24] Renewed interest centers on combinations of medications in one formulation, such as an inhaled steroid and a long-acting β-adrenergic agonist, based on evidence of additive effects, convenience for the patient, and the potential to further reduce the risks of significant exacerbation.[17] Each medication included in this combination exerts unique benefits including bronchodilator, bronchoprotective, and anti-inflammatory effects (Table 18.2). Combination therapy is now approved for use in children aged 4 and older. Physicians now have opportunities to individualize their patients' treatment plans by selecting potent medications that can address concerns of cost, taste, and ease of administration.

A. Variable Responses to Treatment and Relevance of Asthma Phenotype

The NHLBI's Asthma Clinical Research Network (ACRN) recently reported on the significant variability in responses associated with inhaled glucocorticoid therapy in adults with compromised pulmonary function and persistent asthma.[25] The effects of increasing doses of inhaled glucocorticoids on improvement in pulmonary function and reduction in airway hyperresponsiveness were evaluated in 30 adult participants with persistent asthma and FEV_1 percents predicted between 55 and 85%.

Several key observations were reported related to measures of response. Near maximal FEV_1 and methacholine PC_{20} changes were obtained with low to medium doses of both inhaled glucocorticoids evaluated (fluticasone propionate and beclomethasone dipropionate) administered with metered dose inhalers and spacer devices. The highest dose of each inhaled glucocorticoid did not result in a further increase in efficacy for either outcome measure, but did produce increased systemic effects as determined by overnight plasma cortisol levels. Of interest was the significant variability in responses among the participants and

Table 18.2 Comparative Effects of Asthma Medications

	Bronchodilator	Protection		Resolution
		Allergen	Histamine/EIB	
β-adrenergic				
albuterol, terbutaline	+++	I	+++	—
pirbuterol				
salmeterol	+++	I, L	+++	—
(long duration)				
Anticholinergic	+	—	ND	ND
Theophylline	++	I, L	+	+
Cromolyn	—	I, L, AR	—	++
Nedocromil	—	I, I, AR	—	++
Inhaled glucocorticoid	—	L, AR	—	+++
Leukotriene modifiers				
Zileuton	++	I, L	ND	ND
Zafirlukast	±	I, L	ND	ND
Montelukast	++	I, L	++	ND

+++, marked effect; ++, moderate effect; +, some effect; —, no effect; ND, no data available.

Blocks immediate (I) or late (L) pulmonary response to allergen challenge or consequent airway hyperresponsiveness (AR). EIB = exercise-induced bronchospasm.

Resolution is defined as a reduction in airways hyperresponsiveness, number of inflammatory cells or thickness of subepithelial layer below basement membrane following continuous therapy.

Source: Szefler SJ. Asthma — the new advances. *Adv Pediatr* 2000; 47: 273–308.

this observation occurred with both inhaled glucocorticoids evaluated. The investigators cautioned that it is possible that higher doses of inhaled glucocorticoids may be necessary to manage more severe patients or prevent significant asthma exacerbations.

About one third of the subjects had good pulmonary responses as determined by greater than 15% improvements in FEV_1. Another third produced marginal responses — increases of FEV_1 between 5 and 15%. The final third failed to respond and showed less than 5% increases in FEV_1. A similar pattern was observed with reductions in methacholine PC_{20}.

FEV_1 improvement did not correlate to the PC_{20} improvement. Patients were able to improve one measure of response without showing an effect from the other measure of response. Thus, the type of response and the magnitude of effect varied from patient to patient. It was observed that certain biomarkers (exhaled nitric oxide and sputum eosinophils) along with asthma characteristics including duration of asthma and bronchodilator responses could be associated with these two response parameters.[25] The ACRN will conduct additional studies to determine the mechanisms of poor response to inhaled glucocorticoid therapy.

In addition, the NHLBI's Childhood Asthma Research and Education (CARE) Network is currently conducting a study to determine whether poor responses to inhaled glucocorticoid therapy can occur in children and whether the biomarkers that predict responses in adults are similar in children. A unique feature of this study will be to determine whether the response to an inhaled glucocorticoid is proportional to the response to a leukotriene antagonist. An assessment of asthma phenotypic characteristics similar to that conducted by the ACRN in adults as well as a genotypic analysis will be conducted in children participating in the CARE Network study to further identify predictors of response to these two medications.

B. Steroid-Resistant Asthma

A review by Payne and Balfour-Lynn provided an approach to the management of severe persistent asthma in children.[26] Interestingly, they proposed that tools to measure airway inflammation such as exhaled nitric oxide, induced sputum, bronchoalveolar lavage, and biopsy could be used to assist with decisions regarding alternative anti-inflammatory and bronchodilator therapy. Other components of airway inflammation, such as interleukin (IL)-4 and interferon-, can be measured in exhaled condensates.[27] The field of biomarker measurement has progressed rapidly, particularly with the ability to measure carbon monoxide, pH, and even leukotrienes in exhaled condensates.[28–31]

Biomarkers can also be measured in induced sputum. For example, levels of matrix metalloproteinase (MMP)-9 and the tissue inhibitor of matrix metalloproteinase (TIMP)-1 can be measured in induced sputum.[32] The balance of MMP-9 and TIMP has been associated with the airway remodeling process. Thus, opportunities to incorporate biomarkers in the assessment of disease control, potential prediction of medication response, and indications of treatment effect on inflammation control and long-term sequelae of uncontrolled inflammation are growing. These measures could also be applied to investigate the mechanisms associated with treatment failure.

However, little evidence indicates that these markers or indicators of airway inflammation can be reliably applied to clinical management in children. In an innovative study conducted by Sont et al.[33] it was observed that a treatment plan based on measures of methacholine PC_{20} along with the guidelines approach could lead to better asthma control as compared to the guidelines approach alone. They also observed a greater reduction in subepithelial fibrosis in the airway hyperresponsiveness-based group, suggesting a potential reversal in airway remodeling.

The ACRN studies[25] provide a note of caution in applying this approach since patients may not be able to reduce airway hyperresponsiveness or improve pulmonary function with inhaled glucocorticoid doses beyond the medium dose range. This raises the question whether patients who failed to respond had persistent inflammation as previously recognized or perhaps structural airway changes that were unresponsive to any form of available anti-inflammatory therapy. It is possible that new medications or approaches need to be developed to treat these refractory patients.

A similar study conducted by Green et al.[34] utilized sputum eosinophil counts as guides to adjustments in asthma therapy as compared to a conventional guidelines approach. Of interest, the investigators reported a six-fold reduction in asthma exacerbations with a treatment strategy directed at normalization of the induced sputum eosinophils. Curiously, it did not result in a greater need for additional anti-inflammatory therapy. Therefore, this approach stimulates interest in treatment strategies directed at reducing markers of inflammation.

Chan et al.[35] reported that patients classified as having severe steroid-resistant asthma showed at least two different patterns of pulmonary function in the presence of optimal therapy. One group of patients with low pulmonary function had fixed patterns of pulmonary function despite high dose systemic glucocorticoid therapy. Another group had a pattern of variable pulmonary function. Of interest is the observation that African Americans had greater prevalences of steroid-resistant asthma, as defined by failure to improve FEV_1, as compared to Caucasians. It will therefore be important to obtain further information on the mechanisms for these two patterns of apparent steroid resistance along with the reason for the higher prevalence of steroid resistance in the African American population.

C. Immunomodulator Therapy

The discoveries based on studies of bronchoscopy, bronchoalveolar lavage, biopsy, molecular biology, and noninvasive measures of airway inflammation stimulated new considerations for the use of approved medications and bases for developing new entities. For example, the observation that certain mediators such as IL-4, IL-5, IL-13 and interferon- are present in airway inflammation generated the development and clinical trial evaluation of drugs that block or enhance these mediators.[36] Another concept being evaluated is a DNA vaccine therapy with antisense oligonucleotides to block inflammatory responses.[37] Currently, the immunomodulator nearest to approval is anti-IgE. Several reports have indicated that anti-IgE has the potential to reduce the frequency of acute exacerbations and improve asthma control.[38–41] Phosphodiesterase-4 inhibitors are also undergoing early clinical trials.

D. Pharmacogenetics

The area of pharmacogenetics may provide additional information about the relationship of genetics and medication responses.[42-44] Advances in this area could be useful in defining asthma phenotypes and genotypes for associations with good or poor responses to medications and assist clinicians in selecting treatment approaches tailored for individual patients. The responses to medications could be related to specific genetic polymorphisms that alter drug responses at the receptor or cellular level, influence drug metabolism pathways,44 or modify asthma-associated disease features, such as increased IgE production, that could influence the levels of responses to available asthma medications.[45-54] This information could provide unique opportunities for understanding variability in drug responses as well as new methods for selecting medications to optimize responses.

VI. Conclusions

The long-term CAMP clinical trial has provided evidence-based support for the benefits of continuous long-term use of inhaled glucocorticoids on asthma control in childhood asthma. Based on the limitations of effects identified in CAMP and other studies, clinical trials are now in progress to determine whether earlier interventions with inhaled glucocorticoids can influence the progression of asthma. Data are also being generated that help define the patient at risk for persistent asthma and thus identify the best candidates for early intervention. With the correct medication and patient profile, it is conceivable that remission could be induced. Unfortunately, patients with established severe asthma already have low pulmonary function that is difficult to reverse. Perhaps early intervention with effective therapy will also reduce the prevalence and morbidity of severe asthma.

Even the best therapy will not be successful without appropriate attention to all levels of asthma care, including access to health care. Although it is encouraging to see that the rise in asthma mortality and morbidity has reached a plateau[1] significant racial and ethnic disparities affect asthma health care utilization and mortality.[55]

We should now strive for reductions in asthma morbidity and mortality in these groups of patients. For example, a high proportion of asthma morbidity among inner city children appears to be related to nonadherence. Therefore, targeting management approaches to improve adherence should reduce morbidity.[56] Programs that would integrate available resources in the United States to improve overall asthma outcomes for children have been suggested and should be considered in the overall strategy to reduce the burden of illness related to asthma.[57]

Acknowledgment

I would to thank Gretchen Czapla for assistance in the manuscript preparation. This work was supported in part by Public Health Services Research Grants 1NO1-HR-16048, HL36577, and HL 51834, General Clinical Research Center Grant 5 MO1 RR00051 from the Division of Research Resources, and NICHHD Pediatric Pharmacology Research Unit Network Grant 1-U01-HD37237.

References

1. Mannino DM, Homa DM, Akinbami LJ, Moorman JE, Gwynn C, and Redd SC. Surveillance for asthma, United States, 1980–1999. *MMWR* 2002; 51:1–513.
2. National Institutes of Health, National Heart, Lung, and Blood Institute. Global Initiative for Asthma: Global Strategy for Asthma Management and Prevention: Workshop Report. 2002.
3. National Asthma Education and Prevention Program Report. Guidelines for the Diagnosis and Management of Asthma: Update on Selected Topics, 2002. *J Allergy Clin Immunol* 2002; 110: S141–S219.
4. Busse WW, Lenfant C, and Lemanske RF. Asthma guidelines: changing paradigm to improve asthma care. *J Allergy Clin Immunol* 2002; 110: 703–705.
5. Szefler SJ and Eigen H. Budesonide inhalation suspension: a nebulized corticosteroid for persistent asthma. *J Allergy Clin Immunol* 2002; 109: 730–742.
6. Knorr B, Franchi LM, Bisgaard H et al. Montelukast, a leukotriene receptor antagonist, for the treatment of persistent asthma in children aged 2 to 5 years. *Pediatrics* 2001; 108: 1–10.
7. Szefler SJ. Meeting the needs of the modernization act: challenges in developing pediatric therapies. *J Allergy Clin Immunol* 2000; 106: 115–117.
8. Leflein JG, Szefler SJ, Murphy KR, Fitzpatrick S, Cruz-Rivera M, Miller CJ, and Smith JA. Nebulized budesonide inhalation suspension compared with cromolyn sodium nebulizer solution for asthma in young children: results of a randomized outcome trial. *Pediatrics* 2002; 109: 866–872.
9. Naspitz C, Szefler SJ, Tinkelman D, and Warner JO, Eds. *Textbook of Pediatric Asthma*. London: Martin-Dunitz, 2001.
10. Spahn JD and Szefler SJ. Childhood asthma: new insights into management. *J Allergy Clin Immunol* 2002; 109: 3–13.
11. Suissa S and Ernst P. Inhaled corticosteroids: impact on asthma morbidity and mortality. *J Allergy Clin Immunol* 2001; 107: 937–944.
12. Childhood Asthma Management Program Research Group. Long-term effects of budesonide or nedocromil in children with asthma. *New Engl J Med* 2000; 343: 1054–1063.
13. Agertoft L and Pedersen S. Effects of long-term treatment with an inhaled corticosteroid on growth and pulmonary function in asthmatic children. *Respir Med* 1994; 88: 373–381.

14. Martinez FD, Wright AL, Taussig LM, Holberg CJ, Halonen M, and Morgan WJ. Asthma and wheezing in the first six years of life. *New Engl J Med* 1995; 332: 133–138.
15. Phelan PD, Robertson CF, and Olinsky A. The Melbourne Asthma Study: 1964–1999. *J Allergy Clin Immunol* 2002; 109: 189–194.
16. Agertoft L and Pedersen S. Effect of long-term treatment with inhaled budesonide on adult height in children with asthma. *New Engl J Med* 2000; 343: 1064–1069.
17. Matz J, Emmett A, Rickard K, and Kalberg C. Addition of salmeterol to low-dose fluticasone versus higher-dose fluticasone: an analysis of asthma exacerbations. *J Allergy Clin Immunol* 2001; 107: 783–789.
18. Soler M, Matz, J, Townley R, Buhl R, O'Brien J, Fox H, Thirlwell J, Gupta N, and Della Cioppa G. The anti-IgE antibody omalizumab reduces exacerbations and steroid requirement in allergic asthmatics. *Eur Respir J* 2001; 18: 254–261.
19. Spahn JD, Covar RA, Gleason MC, Tinkelman DG, and Szefler SJ. Pharmacologic management of asthma in infants and small children, in Naspitz CK, Szefler SJ, Tinkelman D, and Warner JO, Eds. *Textbook of Pediatric Asthma*. London: Martin Dunitz, 2001, pp. 121–147.
20. Liu AH. Endotoxin exposure in allergy and asthma: reconciling a paradox. *J Allergy Clin Immunol* 2002; 109: 379–392.
21. Martinez FD. Development of wheezing disorders and asthma in preschool children. *Pediatrics* 2002; 109: 362–367.
22. Castro-Rodriguez JA, Holberg CJ, Wright AL, and Martinez FD. A clinical index to define risk of asthma in young children with recurrent wheezing. *Am J Respir Crit Care Med* 2000; 162: 1403–1406.
23. Rasmussen F, Taylor DR, Flannery EM, Cowan JO, Greene JM, Herbison GP, and Sears M. Risk factors for airway remodeling in asthma manifested by a low post-bronchodilator FEV_1 vital capacity ratio. *Am J Respir Crit Care Med* 2002; 165: 1480–1488.
24. Milgrom H, Skoner DP, Bensch G, Kim KT, Claus R, and Baumgartner RA. Low-dose levalbuterol in children with asthma: safety and efficacy in comparison with placebo and racemic albuterol. *J Allergy Clin Immmunol* 2001; 108: 938–945.
25. Szefler SJ, Richard J. Martin RJ et al. Significant variability in response to inhaled corticosteroids for persistent asthma. *J. Allergy Clin Immunol* 2002; 109: 410–418.
26. Payne DNR and Balfour-Lynn IM. Children with difficult asthma: a practical approach. *J Asthma* 2001; 38: 189–203.
27. Shahid SK, Kharitinov SA, Wilson NM, Bush A, and Barnes PJ. Increased inter-leukin-4 and decreased interferon- in exhaled breath condensate of children with asthma. *Am J Respir Crit Care Med* 2002; 165: 1290–1293.
28. Zanconato S, Scollo M, Zaramella C, Landi L, Zacchello F, and Baraldi E. Exhaled carbon monoxide levels after a course of oral prednisone in children with asthma exacerbation. *J Allergy Clin Immunol* 2002; 109: 440–445.
29. Terashima T, Amakawa K, Matsumaru A, and Yamaguchi K. Correlation between cysteinyl leukotriene release from leukocytes and clinical response to a leukotriene inhibitor. *Chest* 2002; 122: 1566–1570.

30. Csoma Z, Kharitonov SA, Baliant B, Bush A, Wilson NM, and Barnes PJ. Increased leukotrienes in exhaled breath condensate in childhood asthma. *Am J Respir Crit Care Med* 2002; 166: 1345–1349.

31. Antczak A, Montuschi P, Kharitonov S, Gorski P, and Barnes PJ. Increased exhaled cysteinyl-leukotrienes and 8-isoprostane in aspirin-induced asthma. *Am J Respir Crit Care Med* 2002; 166: 301–306.

32. Cataldo DD, Bettiol J, Noel A, Bartsch P, Foidart J-M, and Louis R. Matrix metalloproteinase-9, but not tissue inhibitor of matrix metalloproteinase-1, increases in the sputum from allergic asthmatic patients after allergen challenge. *Chest* 2002; 122: 1553–1559.

33. Sont JK, Willems LNA, Bel EH, van Krieken JHJM, Vendenbroucke JP, Sterk PJ, and AMPUL Study Group. Clinical control and histopathologic outcome of asthma when using airway hyperresponsiveness as an additional guide to long-term treatment. *Am J Respir Crit Care Med* 1999; 159: 1043–1051.

34. Green RH, Brightling CE, McKenna S, Hargadon B, Parker D, Bradding P, Wardlaw AJ, and Pavord I. Asthma exacerbations and sputum eosinophil counts: a randomized controlled trial. *Lancet* 2002; 360: 1715–1721.

35. Chan MT, Leung DYM, Szefler SJ, and Spahn JD. Difficult-to-control asthma: clinical characteristics of steroid-insensitive asthma. *J Allergy Clin Immunol* 1998; 101: 594–601.

36. Barnes P. New targets for future asthma therapy, in Yeadon M and Diamont Z, Eds., *New and Exploratory Therapeutic Agents for Asthma: Lung Biology in Health and Disease*. New York: Marcel Dekker, 2000. pp. 361–389.

37. Kline JN. DNA therapy for asthma. *Curr Opin Allergy Immunol* 2002; 2: 69–73.

38. Milgrom H, Fick RB, Su JQ et al. Treatment of allergic asthma with monoclonal anti-IgE antibody. *New Engl J Med* 1999; 341: 1966–1973.

39. Holgate S, Bousquet J, Wenzel S, Fox H, Liu J, and Castellsague J. Efficacy of omalizumab, an anti-immunoglobulin E antibody, in patients at high risk of serious asthma-related morbidity and mortality. *Current Med Res Opinions* 2001; 17: 233–240.

40. Soler M, Matz J, Townley R, Buhl R, O'Brien J, Fox H, Thirlwell J, Gupta N, and Della Cioppa G. The anti-IgE antibody omalizumab reduces exacerbations and steroid requirement in allergic asthmatics. *Eur Respir J* 2001; 18: 254–261.

41. Lemanske RF, Nayak A, McAlary M, Everhard F, Fowler-Taylor A, and Gupta N. Omalizumab improves asthma-related quality of life in children with allergic asthma. *Pediatrics* 2002; 110: 55. ⟨http://www.pediatrics.org/cgi/content/full/110/5/e55⟩.

42. Ober C and Moffatt ME. Contributing factors to the pathobiology: genetics of asthma. *Clin Chest Med* 2000; 21: 245–261.

43. Fenech A and Hall IP. Pharmacogenetics of asthma. *Br J Clin Pharmacol* 2002; 53: 2–15.

44. Palmer LJ, Silverman ES, Weiss ST, and Drazen JM. Pharmacogenetics of asthma. *Am J Respir Crit Care Med* 2002; 165: 861–866.

45. Marsh DG, Neely JD, Breazeale DR, Ghosh B, Freidhoff LR, Ehrlich-Kautzky E, Schou C, Krishnaswamy G, and Beaty TH. Linkage analysis of IL4 and other chromosome 5q31.1 markers and total serum immunoglobulin E concentrations. *Science* 1994; 264: 1152–1156.

46. Borish L, Mascali JJ, Klinnert M, Leppert M, and Rosenwasser LJ. SSC polymorphisms in interleukin genes. *Hum Mol Genet* 1995; 4: 974.

47. Rosenwasser LJ, Klemm DJ, Dresback JK, Inamura H, Mascali JJ, Klinnert M, and Borish L. Promoter polymorphisms in the chromosome 5 gene cluster in asthma and atopy. *Clin Exp Allergy* 1995; 25: 74–78, 95–96.

48. Burchard EG, Silverman EK, Rosenwasser LJ, Borish L, Yandava C, Pillari A, Weiss ST, Hasday J, Lilly CM, Ford JG, and Drazen JM. Association between a sequence variant in the IL-4 gene promoter and FEV(1) in asthma. *Am J Respir Crit Care Med* 1999; 160: 919–922.

49. Hershey GK, Friedrich MF, Esswein LA, Thomas ML, and Chatila TA. The association of atopy with a gain-of-function mutation in the alpha subunit of the interleukin-4 receptor. *New Engl J Med* 1997; 337: 1720–1725.

50. Rosa-Rosa L, Zimmermann N, Bernstein JA, Rothenberg ME, Khurana and Hershey GK. The R576 IL-4 receptor alpha allele correlates with asthma severity. *J Allergy Clin Immunol* 1999; 104: 1008–1014.

51. Martinez FD. Maturation of immune responses at the beginning of asthma. *J Allergy Clin Immunol* 1999; 103: 355–361.

52. Spahn JD, Szefler SJ, Surs W, Doherty DE, Nimmagadda SR, and Leung DYM. A novel action of IL-13: induction of diminished monocyte glucocorticoid receptor-binding affinity. *J Immunol* 1996; 157: 2654–2659.

53. Kam JC, Szefler SJ, Surs W, Sher ER, and Leung DYM. Combination IL-2 and IL-4 reduces glucocorticoid receptor binding affinity and T cell response to glucocorticoids. *J Immunol* 1993; 151: 3460–3466.

54. Sher ER, Leung DYM, Surs W, Kam JC, Zieg, G, Kamada AK, and Szefler SJ. Steroid-resistant asthma: cellular mechanisms contributing to inadequate response to glucocorticoid therapy. *J Clin Invest* 1994; 93: 33–39.

55. Akinbami LJ and Schoendorf KC. Trends in childhood asthma: prevalence, health care utilization, and mortality. *Pediatrics* 2002; 110: 315–322.

56. Bauman LJ, Wright E, Leickly FE, Crain E, Kruszon-Moran D, Wade SL, and Visness CM. Relationship of adherence to pediatric asthma morbidity among inner-city children. *Pediatrics* 2002; 110. ⟨http://www.pediatrics.org/cgi/content/full/110/1/e6⟩.

57. Lara M, Rosenbaum S, Rachelefsky G et al. Improving childhood asthma outcomes in the United States: blueprint for policy action. *Pediatrics* 2002; 109: 919–930.

19

Allergen Avoidance

JACQUELINE PONGRACIC

Northwestern University Feinberg School of Medicine
and Children's Memorial Hospital
Chicago, Illinois, U.S.A.

I. Introduction

Because the combination of sensitization and exposure to inhaled environmental allergens is related to both the development of asthma and elicitation of symptoms, it follows that avoidance of allergens would exert beneficial effects in the prevention and control of the disease. Allergens may, however, be difficult to avoid, and despite the advances in knowledge surrounding allergens, our understanding of the threshold levels of exposure required for sensitization and induction of symptoms is limited. These problems complicate the investigation of allergen reduction and its clinical efficacy. Most studies have focused upon allergen reduction as a primary endpoint. Fewer studies have been designed to specifically address clinical efficacies of allergen avoidance interventions. This chapter will review what is known about allergen avoidance with attention to specific indoor allergens and strategies for reducing exposure.

II. Principles of Allergen Avoidance

Allergen avoidance measures should incorporate several key principles. Selection of appropriate target allergens, effective interventions, practicable strategies, and

Table 19.1 Allergen Levels Associated with
Sensitization and Asthma Symptoms

Allergen	Sensitization Level	Asthma Symptom Level
Der p 1	2 µg/g dust	10 µg/g
Bla g 1	2 U/g dust	8 U/g dust
Fel d 1	1 µg/g	8 µg/g
Can f 1	2 µg/g	10 µg/g

cost effectiveness should guide recommendations to patients and families. Lifestyle changes, especially in home construction, have been associated with increased time spent indoors. Americans have been reported to spend as much as 90% of their time indoors.[1] With this observation in mind, it is logical to focus upon developing strategies to reduce exposure to indoor allergens. Although their relative distributions vary geographically, the most common indoor allergens are dust mites, animals, molds, and cockroaches. Dust mites are the best studied of these allergens. Cats are the most dominant indoor allergens in many Westernized countries. In inner city homes, cockroaches are especially prevalent, but rodents (mice and rats) may also be present.

In order to establish the effectiveness of an intervention, adequate sampling methods to measure allergens must be available. Most studies analyzed allergen concentrations in settled dust, but this type of analysis has been criticized for being a poor estimate of inhalational exposure. Nonetheless, it is a measure of an indoor allergen burden that is relatively easy to obtain. Fewer trials have been performed with airborne allergen sampling because the procedure is more difficult. Table 19.1 presents allergen levels of clinical importance in settled dust. Table 19.2 describes current understanding of their airborne characteristics. Determination of efficacy of allergen avoidance should also assess clinical responses to interventions. This is complicated by many factors such as other contributors to asthma morbidity (infections, pollutants, adherence), exposures to other relevant allergens that are difficult to avoid, and sufficient duration of the study observation period. Strategies that are costly, complicated, or difficult to implement are less likely to be embraced; interventions should target simple, cost-effective measures.

A. Dust Mites

Dust mites (Dermatophagoides spp.) are microscopic members of the spider (Acaridae) family. Their primary food source is human skin scales. Because they thrive at room temperature (70°F) and in relatively humid (70 to 80%) conditions, they commonly inhabit homes.[2,3] Originating from fecal particles, major dust mite allergens (Der p 1 and Der f 1) are rather large (10 µm) and are not generally present in undisturbed ambient air. Mite allergens are found in settled dust and

Table 19.2 Aerobiology of Indoor Allergens

Type	Major Allergen	Airborne Particle Size (microns)
Dust Mites		
Dermatophagoides	Der f 1	<2.5 to 10
	Der p 1	(15% <5)
Cockroaches		
Blatella germanica	Bla g 1	75% ≥10
Animals		
Felis domesticus	Fel d 1	<2.5 to 10 (15% <5)
Canis familiaris	Can f 1	20% <5
Mus musculus	Mus m 1	3.3 to 18
Rattus norvegicus	Rat n 1	<1 to >20 (most <7)

can be detected in the air only in association with a disturbance.[4] In Europe and the U.S., levels of dust mites appear to vary both regionally and from home to home.[5,6] Within homes, dust mite concentrations are usually highest in bedrooms, especially in mattresses, but carpets are the largest reservoirs.[7] Other reservoirs include pillows, fabric window treatments, stuffed toys, upholstered furniture, and even clothing.[4] Home characteristics associated with high levels of dust mites include ground floor residence,[8–10] low rates of ventilation.[9,11–13] dampness,[8] concrete floors,[10] dog in the home,[14] and high numbers of occupants.[12,14] Carpeting has a similar effect, especially if it is old[10,12] or made of wool.[15]

An inverse relationship exists between high altitudes and dust mite levels.[16–18] Clinical trials to reduce exposure to dust mites have been based upon this observation. Mite-allergic individuals were moved to high altitudes in the Alps[19–22] and prolonged (8 months) dust mite avoidance was associated with improvements in pulmonary function and bronchial hyperresponsiveness with associated reductions in medication use.[19] Basophil histamine release and serum IgE to mites decreased[23] and serum markers of eosinophil activation improved.[24]

Bronchial hyperresponsiveness was shown to improve within 1 month at high elevation[20] and within 3 months in other studies.[22] Decreased epithelial shedding[25] and T helper lymphocyte activation[21] were also demonstrated. Biomarkers that improved in the high altitude studies included sputum eosinophilia[26] and exhaled nitric oxide.[27] Improvement in symptoms and IgE responses did not persist after the study subjects returned home. A recent study, however, demonstrated some sustained benefit over 6 weeks in conjunction with continuation of inhaled corticosteroids.[28] Decreased bronchial hyperreactivity was also demonstrated after mite-allergic individuals who had asthma were moved to mite-free in-patient units in hospitals.[29]

Because changing residences is neither practicable nor cost effective, a variety of alternative dust mite interventions have been developed and evaluated.

A meta-analysis of 27 controlled trials failed to show a significant effect on asthma.[30] The result is not surprising because most published trials of mite interventions have not achieved significant reductions in allergen levels. Of the citations in the meta-analysis that decreased allergen exposures for at least 6 months, five of six studies demonstrated clear improvements in the intervention groups.[31]

Most trials to date have focused on bedrooms and carpets. A study performed in the 1980s, in which aggressive dust mite control measures were implemented in the bedrooms of children with asthma, showed significant improvements in wheezing and medication use, fewer low peak expiratory flow rate (PEFR) days, and a four-fold increase in PC_{20}.[32] Allergen measurements were not performed.

A trial of education found good compliance with installation of dust mite encasements. Although allergen measurements were not made, improved symptom scores, symptom-free days, and quality of life were demonstrated.[33] When dust mite allergen-impermeable covers were implemented in conjunction with instructions on home cleaning and hot water washing of bed linens, significant reductions in mite allergen levels were achieved.[34,35] The reductions did not occur in another trial in which no such instructions were given.[36]

Low baseline mite allergen levels (<2 µg/g dust) were common in this study population so that significant reductions in allergen would be unlikely to occur, which may also explain the lack of clinical improvement in the treatment group. In contrast, use of encasements reduced mattress mite allergens and was associated with reductions in inhaled corticosteroid dose, improved PEFR, and modest increases in PC_{20}.[37] A year-long encasement intervention involving adults with asthma resulted in improvements in FEV_1, PEFR, PC_{20}, and symptoms.[38] Encasings are currently available for pillows, mattresses, and box springs. Those that are air- and water-permeable are recommended because they are more comfortable than impermeable fabrics.[39]

Hot water washing of sheets and blankets at temperatures 55°C kills mites and removes allergens.[40] In the U.S., such temperatures may be achieved with commercial but not residential washers. Using cooler water to launder bedding and clothing helps remove over 90% of mite allergens, but it is less efficient in killing mites.[40] Adding essential oils and benzyl benzoate for final concentrations of 0.2% and 0.03%, respectively, has been shown to kill mites at less extreme water temperatures.[41]

Other methods of laundering, such as dry cleaning, kill mites but are expensive.[42] Drying for 10 minutes at settings over 55°C is effective for killing mites.[43] For more delicate toys and fabrics, placement in a domestic freezer for 24 hours is also an effective way to kill mites.[44] The use of electric blankets is associated with decreased mite exposure, but is expensive and impractical.[45] Avoiding the use of sheepskins and down comforters, pillows, and stuffed toys is both practical and effective.[46]

Many carpet interventions have been evaluated. Because carpets are the largest reservoirs for mites, removal may be the best option for heavy infestation.[39] Carpet removal is effective for decreasing mite allergen concentrations in settled dust, but is not always an acceptable or feasible option. Vacuuming has been shown to reduce allergen levels if performed daily, but this is laborious[47] and other studies have not found it to be beneficial.[48]

One study demonstrated reductions in allergen levels as long as 4 weeks after a single intensive vacuuming using a device with a high efficiency particulate air (HEPA) filter.[34] Vacuum cleaner use is associated with increased airborne allergens, but devices with double-ply bags and HEPA filters do not leak allergens.[49] Steam cleaning kills mites and reduces allergens, but only transiently, perhaps due to residual moisture or failure to reach deeply into carpeting.[50] Dry steam cleaning followed by vacuuming reduces mite levels up to 2 months.[34] Sun exposure also reduces allergens[51] but is impractical for large rugs.

Treating carpets with chemical agents that kill (acaricides such as benzyl benzoate) or denature (tannic acid) dust mite allergens or perform both functions (benzyl–tannate complex) has produced variable results. Trials have involved different intervention strategies, many of which implemented comprehensive approaches including chemical applications, dust mite encasements, cleaning, hot water washing of bed linens, and carpet removal. Given the approaches, it is not surprising that results have varied.

Acaricide use has been shown to reduce allergen levels in carpet dust in some studies[52–55] and not in others.[56–59] Reductions in airborne mite allergens were demonstrated in one study.[60] Studies of tannic acid demonstrated moderate but transient declines in mite allergens in settled dust.[55,61–63] Although a prompt reduction of allergens occurred, it appeared that repeated applications may be necessary to sustain the effects. In a 1-year pediatric trial of tannic acid applied every 2 months combined with encasements, dust mite levels decreased and bronchial hyperresponsiveness improved.[64] Interestingly, the effects of tannic acid may be inhibited by the concurrent presence of Fel d 1; one study found that the presence of a cat in a home was associated with a lack of effect of tannic acid on mite allergens.[61]

Benzyl–tannate complex treatment is associated with reductions in mite allergens[65–67] and modest effects on cat allergens.[65] However, other controlled studies have not demonstrated clear benefits.[68,69] Liquid nitrogen applied to carpeting kills mites but requires professional application.[70] A trial of an anti-mite shampoo showed no impact on allergens.[71] Of the studies that evaluated both allergen effects and asthma clinical outcomes, benzyl benzoate was associated with clinical improvement (including pulmonary function) when reductions in carpet and furniture allergen levels were achieved.[54]

A study of benzyl benzoate found reductions in Der p 1, Der f 1, symptoms, rescue bronchodilator use, and bronchial hyperresponsiveness.[59] No clinical response occurred when allergen levels did not fall.[56,57] A trial of tannic acid applied to carpet combined with dust mite encasement was shown to reduce mite antigen in mattresses by more than 90% and also reduced bronchial hyperresponsiveness.[56] Quarterly application of tannic acid to living and family room carpets along with removal of bedroom carpeting and encasement of pillows, mattresses, and box springs resulted in a three-fold decrease in allergen levels and improved PEFR in children with asthma. No changes in FEV_1 or methacholine responsiveness were seen.[63] The benzyl–tannate complex did not affect allergen levels or clinical measures.[68] Liquid nitrogen application was associated with decreased numbers of live mites and improved symptoms, PEFR, and PC_{20} in adults with asthma.[72]

Reducing indoor relative humidity below 50% was shown to reduce mites in some studies[73,74] but not others.[75–78] The use of HEPA air cleaners and ionizers was not found to be effective[65,79,80] although one study[81] demonstrated a 70% decline in airborne particulates and a modest effect on symptoms. The combination of air cleaner and dust mite encasements produced a slight clinical improvement.[82]

These generally negative results are to be expected because mite allergens are heavy and only transiently airborne following a disturbance. Improving home ventilation appeared to reduce allergens and showed a trend toward decreasing bronchial responsiveness; this effect was somewhat enhanced by daily vacuuming.[83] Some authors proposed changes in house design and construction as means to reduce indoor mite allergen loads.[13,84] Although impractical as short-term solutions, such changes warrant further consideration. Table 19.3 provides an overview of the effects of dust mite interventions.

B. Animals

It is estimated that 100 million domestic animals live in or in close proximity to American households.[85,86] In the United Kingdom, one household of four has a pet.[87] As many as 2 million cat-allergic Americans live with cats.[86] The high prevalence of pet ownership combined with the incidence of animal allergy makes allergen avoidance a challenging component of allergy treatment. Cats and dogs account for the majority of pets, and cats are the most studied. It is important to note that other furred mammals such as hamsters, gerbils, guinea pigs, mice, rats, and rabbits are also kept as pets, and they also produce allergens. No doubt more creatures will join this list as people search for new and unusual pets. Some mammals, specifically mice and rats, are unwanted pests that manage to infest homes, particularly multi-unit dwellings in inner cities of the United States.[88]

The major allergen of cats is Fel d 1. It is produced in varying amounts by all breeds of cats. Its production is under hormonal control. Males produce higher levels than females, and castration causes a three- to five-fold reduction in allergen

Table 19.3 Dust Mite Reduction Strategies

Strategy	Kills Mites or Reduces Allergen?	Practical? Y/N	Expensive? Y/N
Bedroom			
Dust mite encasement	R	Y	+/–
Washing bed linens (55°C)	K, R	N	N
Regular washing (home washer)	R	Y	N
Regular washing + benzyl benzoate (0.03%)	K, R	Y	N
Regular washing + essential oils (0.2%)	K, R	Y	N
Tumble drying (55°C, 10 min)	K, R	Y	N
Dry cleaning	K, R	N	N
Freezing (24 h)	K	+/–	N
Electric blankets	K	N	+/–
Removal of stuffed toys, soft furnishings	R	Y	N
Carpet			
Removal	R	N	Y
Daily vacuuming	R	N	N
Steam cleaning	K, R	N	Y
Sun exposure	K	N	N
Benzyl benzoate (applied q 3 mos)	K	N	+/–
Tannic acid (applied q 3 mos)	R	N	+/–
Benzyl–tannate complex	K, R	N	+/–
General Measures			
Dehumidification	K (mattress only)	Y	Y
Ventilation	K (mattress only)	Y	Y
Air cleaners	Neither	Y	Y
Change in home design/construction	R	N	Y

K = kills mites. R = allergen reduction. Y = yes. N = no. +/– =

that can be restored with testosterone replacement.[89,90] Produced primarily by sebaceous glands, the allergen is also secreted from salivary and anal glands and is found in fur, skin, and saliva.

Allergen particle size varies from <2.5 to 10 μm.[91] Cat allergen has been found in homes without cats.[87,92,93] It has also been detected in public places such as nurseries, schools, theaters, airplanes, hotels, and even hospitals.[94–101] In these settings, the highest levels of allergen have been found on upholstered seats in theaters, airplanes, and hospitals.[94,96,97]

It has been hypothesized that Fel d 1 is passively transported on shoes and clothing.[102] This is supported by the finding that cat allergen is present at higher levels in the clothing of cat owners than nonowners.[103] This may in part be related to the "stickiness" of the allergen.[104] The allergen is widely distributed in homes. It has been measured on walls,[104] but the highest levels are found in upholstered furniture; the next highest levels are found in living room carpets.[105] Upholstered furniture appears to be the primary reservoir in homes with and without cats and in public places.

Can f 1 and albumin are the major allergens of dogs. Can f 1 is found in fur and saliva. Its production varies among breeds. Can f 1 has been measured in settled dust and air samples.[106] Its airborne particle size is similar to the size of Fel d 1. Can f 1 has also been detected in public areas, in furniture, settled dust, and ambient air.[95,97–99,101]

Rodent allergens have been less well studied. Mus m 1, the major mouse allergen, is found in urine and has 80% homology with the major rat allergen, Rat n 1. The size of airborne mouse allergen ranges from 3.3 to 10 µm.[107] Rat n 1 has a broader size range but most particles are smaller than 7 µm.[108,109] Mus m 2 is found in hair and skin. Ninety-five percent of inner city homes exhibited measurable levels of Mus m 1, with the highest levels present in kitchens.[88] Higher levels of mouse allergen were associated with the presence of cockroaches in the home.[88]

Animal riddance or eradication is generally recommended as the preferred avoidance method for individuals with animal allergies. Surprisingly, no evidence in the literature covers the clinical benefits of animal removal or allergen reduction measures in the home. Most affected individuals are emotionally attached or otherwise dependent upon their pets and often will not remove the pets from their homes.

Studies have evaluated a variety of allergen reduction strategies. Removing cats from living rooms has been reported to reduce airborne levels by over 60% only 2 days after removal, mainly due to reductions of large particles.[105] The same study found that using a HEPA air cleaner for 4 and 8 hours was associated with a five-fold reduction in airborne Fel d 1. It is important to note that the clinical effects of cat removal may not be seen for months, perhaps longer, because allergens persist for 4 to 6 months in settled dust[110] and may persist longer than 5 years in mattresses.[111]

Antigen levels in dust will fall more quickly if measures such as carpet and furniture removal followed by vigorous cleaning are also undertaken.[110] Because cat allergen is found in schools and many other public places, aggressive interventions may be necessary to reduce exposure.[112] If such exposures outside the home are not addressed, home allergen interventions may be futile.[113]

Several studies evaluated strategies for reducing allergen levels when cats remain in homes. Studies of air cleaners demonstrated mixed clinical results. A pediatric study of air cleaners showed a reduction in bronchial hyperresponsiveness in children with cat allergies and asthma.[114] Another study showed that the combination of HEPA air cleaners and dust mite encasements did not affect symptoms even though airborne Fel d 1 levels were reduced.[115] Several trials of cat washing produced conflicting results. One study found decreased airborne Fel d 1 with washing[116] and others noted no benefits from washing or from using Allerpet/C.[117,118] Reductions in airborne cat allergens lasted only a week.[119] When washing was combined with air filtration, vacuuming, and furniture removal, signification reductions in airborne Fel d 1 were reported.[116]

Evaluations of interventions for dog allergy have been limited. Removal of the dog is generally recommended. One study that looked at the effects of dog washing found that allergen reductions were transient and recommended twice-weekly washing.[120] HEPA air cleaners were shown to reduce Can f 1 levels by 90%.[121] Vacuum cleaners equipped with HEPA filters and double-thickness bags prevented generation of airborne dog allergens usually seen with disturbances related to cleaning.[122] Because both dog and cat allergens are present in public areas, complete avoidance may be unachievable.

Home-based rodent-specific interventions in the treatment of asthma and allergic diseases are lacking and sorely needed. In laboratory animal asthma, airborne allergen avoidance may be reduced by avoiding certain tasks such as feeding and cleaning of cages.[123] Reducing the concentration of rodent stock housed in a facility, improving ventilation, and using HEPA air cleaners may also be helpful.[124]

C. Molds

Mold allergens are poorly understood. Molds (fungi) are multicellular microorganisms that take on different forms during their life cycles. Most genera include more than one species and their characteristics often differ. Mold allergens are thought to be enzymes liberated during spore germination. Multiple allergens have been described for each of the best understood allergenic molds. Quantitative measurements of molds and their allergens are difficult. Mold spore and colony counts of $1000/m^3$ or higher have been proposed to indicate indoor fungal contamination.[125] Investigators have also used fungal elements such as ergosterol and $(1 \rightarrow 3)$-β-D-glucan as markers for the presence of mold. Mold exposure may occur both outdoors and indoors, and indoor levels are correlated positively with outdoor weather.[126] The most common indoor molds include Aspergillus, Penicillium, and Cladosporium.[127,128]

Although the literature in the area of mold abatement is sparse, several studies focused upon residential characteristics associated with indoor mold. Interventions that remediate these factors are likely to reduce indoor mold growth and allergen levels, but controlled studies of clinical benefit are sorely needed. Fungal substrates include wood, paper, gypsum board and other high cellulose materials, and water.[129] Water is a key requirement. Buildings with high humidity or water damage are especially problematic. Factors associated with lower levels of airborne fungi indoors include ceiling fans, lack of visible mold, frequent vacuuming, closed windows, and use of a solid fuel fire within a year.[127] Pets also are associated with increased indoor fungi levels.[130,131] In settled dust, several studies have shown that presence of wall-to-wall carpet plays a major role[84,132,133] and that ventilation is also important.[134] Air cleaners also reduce airborne fungi.[84,130,135]

Based on these findings, specific measures for mold abatement have been empirically recommended. Efforts directed at reducing sources of moisture should include reduction of indoor relative humidity below 50%, sealing leaks, using a sump pump,[136] and minimizing houseplants.[137] Although ventilation is important, the data are in conflict because keeping windows and doors closed reduces infiltration from the outdoors.[127] Other recommendations include using air conditioning because it has been shown to reduce infiltration;[138] ventilating bathrooms, kitchens, and laundry rooms (outdoor vents for dryers); and heating all rooms including household storage areas. Clean-up of contaminated HVAC systems including ducts and filters is recommended.[139] Electronic air cleaners and negative ionizers modestly reduce spore counts.[135] Vacuuming may be helpful for reducing indoor mold, but removal of wall to wall carpeting may be more effective. Pet avoidance should be considered. Removal of aquariums and living Christmas trees may be helpful. Removing paneling and wallpaper or using a 5% bleach solution to them are other suggestions.[125] The same authors suggest wearing well-fitted masks that will filter particulates down to 1 μm in size during exposures such as cleaning, vacuuming, handling compost, and raking leaves.

D. Cockroaches

Cockroaches have become well-recognized asthma allergens. *Blatella germanica* is the most prevalent domestic species in the United States. *Periplaneta americana* is most common species in the tropics. Cockroaches inhabit environments that provide water sources and favor damp indoor conditions. German cockroaches favor crevices and may infest appliances, heaters, and plumbing fixtures in kitchens, laundry rooms, and bathrooms.[140] They will eat nearly anything including glue, soap, and grease and can survive for days without food and water. Although generally associated with urban areas, cockroaches also inhabit substandard housing in rural and suburban areas.[141] Cockroach allergens are found in feces, salivas, and bodies. Allergen particles tend to be large (>10 μm). Home analysis reveals that the allergens are primarily found in the kitchen, with lower levels measured in beds, on bedroom floors, and in furniture.[142-144] Cockroach allergen has also been detected in day care centers, schools, and dormitories, especially in food preparation and eating areas.[145-147]

A number of pesticides are available in spray, powder, aerosol, emulsion, granule, gel, and bait station forms. Abatement trials have shown mixed results.

Extermination is effective for reducing cockroach populations but effectiveness is shorter than 3 months[148] and cockroach allergens persist after extermination.[145,149]

Thorough vacuuming effectively removes allergens after extermination.[150,151] In integrated pest management (IPM), the targeted application of gels and baits using agents such as abamectin and hydramethylnon has been found to reduce cockroach populations and allergen levels. A study of professional extermination using abamectin combined with professional cleaning revealed decreased cockroaches and allergen levels, although the level of Bla g 1 remained >20 μ/g dust — higher than estimated thresholds associated with symptoms.[150]

A trial of hydramethalnon resulted in successful extermination but persistence of allergen.[151] The National Cooperative Inner City Asthma Study (NCICAS) implemented a strategy that included professional extermination with abamectin, education about house cleaning, and allergen reduction measures for children who were skin test positive to cockroach allergen. Extermination was performed in kitchens and other rooms with evidence of infestation. A two-fold decrease in Bla g 1 was seen in kitchen dust 2 months after extermination; at 12 months, levels increased to baseline or higher.

Of note, only 50% of families performed cleaning tasks as instructed.[152] In NCICAS, the intervention group improved, but this was not felt to be associated with the allergy intervention. An ongoing study in New York City is evaluating an integrated approach involving intensive cleaning and repair; use of pesticides in kitchens, bedrooms, bathrooms, and hallways; and one-on-one education.[153] It will be interesting to learn the results of this trial, especially in light of the many obstacles the investigators and intervention families have reported.

Because of the lack of evidence-based data, the following recommendations may be considered for cockroach abatement. A recent review promoted this comprehensive approach.[140] Beginning with inspection, identify the type of pest along with its eating, travel, and living habits. Observation of living roaches, the brown stains (digestive secretions) left on surfaces, and body parts indicates their presence, living or dead. Because of their nutritional needs, focus should be on areas with water sources, especially leaks, and kitchens (open food containers, grease, and trash receptacles). Cockroaches may even infest pet food.

After hiding places and other sources are identified, insecticides and thorough cleaning should be instituted. IPM is preferred because it reduces the likelihood of human and pet exposure to the toxins. Bait traps are also helpful, but may not work for heavy infestations. Gels and baits are more effective if roaches have no access to other food sources, so cleaning before placement of gels and baits is advised. Following IPM, practices that include eating only in designated areas, sealed food storage, and good housekeeping may help sustain the effects of intervention.

III. Environmental Control and Primary Prevention

Relationships between allergen exposure and development of childhood asthma, such as those seen for dust mites in the United Kingdom[154] led investigators to consider clinical trials of early environmental interventions for the primary prevention of asthma and allergic disorders. The Isle of Wight study, a prospective, prenatally randomized, controlled trial, implemented a postnatal intervention composed of dust mite intervention and food allergen avoidance in the first 9 months of life.[155] A 75% reduction in mite allergen was achieved in homes of high-risk infants in the intervention group. Prevalences of dust mite sensitization and atopic manifestations were lower in the intervention group at ages 1, 2, and 4 years. Despite a trend, no significant difference in asthma prevalence was seen at ages 2 and 4 years.[156,157]

The National Asthma Campaign Manchester Asthma and Allergy Study is another prospective, prenatally randomized, controlled cohort study of pre- and postnatal environmental dust mite intervention.[158] Dust mite allergen levels in the intervention group were more than 30 times lower than those found in the Isle of Wight study. This study was also significantly larger, with over 500 participants completing follow-up at 1 year. A decreased relative risk was found for respiratory symptoms in the intervention group, especially for severe wheeze with shortness of breath; wheeze with exertion, play, or crying; and in use of prescription medications for treatment of "wheezy attacks." The overall prevalence of wheeze was the same for both groups, but the trend was toward reduced respiratory symptoms separate from viral infections in the active treatment group.[159]

The Prevention and Incidence of Asthma and Mite Allergy birth cohort study has been in progress since 1996.[160] One arm of this study is a double-blind placebo-controlled trial in high-risk children to evaluate the use of mite encasements for pillows and mattresses given to participating families 1 to 2 months before births of their children. The interventions had a modest effect on allergen levels in settled dust.[161] No effects on atopic manifestations were observed when the children reached 2 years of age.[162]

Other trials of allergen avoidance for primary prevention are in progress and their results are eagerly awaited. Long-term follow-up of the participants is critical in order to ascertain whether primary prevention is effective.

IV. Summary

Allergen avoidance in the management of asthma is a complicated but attractive strategy. Although the evidence for the effectiveness of dust mite avoidance is conflicting, substantial evidence indicates that reducing allergen loads over prolonged periods may be associated with clinical improvement. Although pet riddance is recommended frequently, it is impractical and intolerable to many individuals; additional techniques for reducing exposures to pet allergens are necessary for successful collaborative management of asthma triggered by animal allergies. Despite advances in our knowledge of allergens, fungal antigens remain poorly understood. This problem adversely affects the design and assessment of environmental intervention strategies. Cockroach abatement remains a formidable challenge, particularly in crowded, urban housing. Solutions to these problems are urgently needed to determine whether environmental manipulation for primary and secondary prevention of asthma is feasible and effective.

References

1. Moschandreas DJ. Exposure to pollutants and daily time budgets of people. *Bull NY Acad Med* 1981; 57: 845–849.
2. Solomon WR and Platts-Mills TAE. Aerobiology and inhalant allergens, in *Allergy Principles and Practice*, 5th ed. Middleton E, Reed CE, Ellis EF, Adkinson NF, Yunginger JW, Busse WW, Eds. St. Louis, MO: Mosby, 1998, pp. 367–403.
3. Korsgaard J. House dust mites and absolute indoor humidity. *Allergy* 1983; 38: 85–92.
4. Tovey ER, Chapman MD, Wells CW, and Platts-Mills TA. The distribution of dust mite allergen in the houses of patients with asthma. *Am Rev Respir Dis* 1981; 124: 630–635.
5. Lowenstein H, Gravesen S, Larsen L, and Schwartz B. Indoor allergens. *J Allergy Clin Immunol* 1986; 78: 1035–1039.
6. Chew GL, Higgins KM, Gold DR, Muilenberg ML, and Burge HA. Monthly measurements of indoor allergens and the influence of housing type in a northeastern U.S. city. *Allergy* 1999; 54: 1058–1066.
7. Tovey ER. Allergen exposure and control. *Exp Appl Acarol* 1992; 16: 181–202.
8. Kuehr J, Frishcher T, and Karmaus W. Natural variation in mite antigen density in house dust and relationship to residential factors. *Clin Exp Allergy* 1994; 24: 229–237.
9. Sundall J, Wickman M, Pershagen G, and Nordvall S. Ventilation in homes infested with house dust mites. *Allergy* 1995; 50: 106–112.
10. Luczynska C, Sterne J, Bond J, Azima H, and Burney P. Indoor factors associated with concentrations of house dust mite allergen, Der p 1, in a random sample of houses in Norwich, U.K. *Clin Exp Allergy* 1998; 28: 1201–1209.
11. Harving H, Korsgarrd J, and Dahl R. House dust mites and associated environmental conditions in Danish homes. *Allergy* 1993; 48: 106–109.
12. Van Strien RT, Verhoeff AP, Brunekreef B, and Van Wijnen JH. Mite antigen in house dust: relationship with different housing characteristics in the Netherlands. *Clin Exp Allergy* 1994; 24: 843–853.
13. Harving H, Korsgaard J, and Dahl R. Clinical efficacy of reduction in house dust mite exposure in specially designed, mechanically ventilated "healthy' homes. *Allergy* 1994; 49: 866–870.

14. Van de Hoeven WAD, Boer R, and Bruin J. The colonisation of new houses by house dust mites (Acari: Pyroglyphidae). *Exp Appl Acarol* 1992; 16: 75–84.
15. Price JA, Pollock I, Little SA, Longbottom JL, and Warner JO. Measurement of airborne mite antigen in homes of asthmatic children. *Lancet* 1990; 336: 895–897.
16. Voorhorst R, Spieksma FTM, and Varekamp N. *House Dust Mite Atopy and the House Dust Mite* (Dermatophagoides pterronyssinus). Leiden: Stafleu's Scientific Publishing, 1969.
17. Vervloet D, Penaud A, Razzouk H, Senft M, Arnaud A, Boutin C, and Charpin J. Altitude and house dust mites. *J Allergy Clin Immunol* 1982; 69: 290–296.
18. Charpin D, Birnbaum J, Haddi E, Genard G, Lanteaume A, Toumi M, Faraj F, Van der Brempt X, and Vervloet D. Altitude and allergy to house-dust mites: paradigm of the influence of environmental exposure on allergic sensitization. *Am Rev Respir Dis* 1991; 143: 983–986.
19. Boner AL, Niero E, Antolini I, Valletta EA, and Gaburro D. Pulmonary function and bronchial hyperreactivity in asthmatic children with house dust mite allergy during prolonged stay in the Italian Alps (Misurina, 1756 m). *Ann Allergy* 1985; 54: 42–45.
20. van Velzen E, van den Bos JW, Benckhuijsen JA, van Essel T, de Bruijn R, and Aalbers R. Effect of allergen avoidance at high altitude on direct and indirect bronchial hyperresponsiveness and markers of inflammation in children with allergic asthma. *Thorax* 1996; 51: 582–584.
21. Simon HU, Grotzer M, Nikolaizik WH, Blaser K, and Schoni MH. High altitude climate therapy reduces peripheral blood T lymphocyte activation, eosinophilia, and bronchial obstruction in children with house-dust mite allergic asthma. *Pediatr Pulmonol* 1994; 17: 304–311.
22. Peroni DG, Boner Al, Vallone G, Antolini I, and Warner JO. Effective allergen avoidance at high altitude reduces allergen-induced bronchial hyperresponsiveness. *Am J Respir Crit Care Med* 1994; 149: 1442–1446.
23. Piacentini GL, Martinati L, Fornari A, Comis A, Carcereri L, Boccagni P, and Boner AL. Antigen avoidance in a mountain environment: influence on basophil releasability in children with allergic asthma. *J Allergy Clin Immunol* 1993; 92: 644–650.
24. Boner AL, Peroni DG, Piacentini GL, and Venge P. Influence of allergen avoidance at high altitude on serum markers of eosinophil activation in children with allergic asthma. *Clin Exp Allergy* 1993; 23: 1021–1026.
25. Piacentini GL, Vicentini L, Mazzi P, Chilosi M, Martinati L, and Boner AL. Mite antigen avoidance can reduce bronchial epithelial shedding in allergic asthmatic children. *Clin Exp Allergy* 1998; 28: 561–567.
26. Piacentini GL, Martinati L, Mingoni S, and Boner AL. Influence of allergen avoidance on the eosinophil plase of airway inflammation in children with allergic asthma. *J Allergy Clin Immunol* 1996; 97: 1079–1084.
27. Piacentini GL, Bodini A, Costella S, Vicentini L, Peroni D, Zanolla L, and Boner AL. Allergen avoidance is associated with a fall in exhaled nitric oxide in asthmatic children. *J Allergy Clin Immunol* 1999; 104: 1323–1324.

28. Grootendorst DC, Dahlen SE, Van Den Bos JW, Duiverman EJ, Veselic-Charvat M, Vrijlandt EF, O'Sullivan S, Kumlin M, Sterk PJ, and Roldaan AC. Benefits of high altitude allergen avoidance in atopic adolescents with moderate to severe asthma, over and above treatment with high dose inhaled steroids. *Clin Exp Allergy* 2001; 31: 400–408.

29. Platts-Mills TA, Tovey ER, Mitchell EB, Moszoro H, Nock P, and Wilkins SR. Reduction of bronchial hyperreactivity during prolonged allergen avoidance. *Lancet* 1982; 2: 675–678.

30. Gotzcshe PC, Hammarquist C, and Bur M. House dust mite control measures in the management of asthma: meta-analysis. *Br Med J* 1998; 317: 1105–1110.

31. Platts-Mills TA, Chapman MD, and Wheatley LM. Control of house dust mite in managing asthma: conclusions of meta-analysis are wrong. *Br Med J* 1999; 318: 870–871.

32. Murray AB and Ferguson AC. Dust-free bedrooms in the treatment of asthmatic children with house dust or house dust mite allergy: a controlled trial. *Pediatrics* 1983; 71: 418–422.

33. Cote J, Cartier A, Robichaud P, Boutin H, Malo JL, Rouleau M, and Boulet LP. Influence of asthma education on asthma severity, quality of life and environmental control. *Can Respir J* 2000; 7: 395–400.

34. Vojta PJ, Randels SP, Stout J, Muilenberg M, Burge HA, Lynn H, Mitchell H, O'Connor GT, and Zeldin DC. Effects of physical interventions on house dust mite allergen levels in carpet, bed, and upholstery dust in low-income, urban homes. *Env Health Perspec* 2001; 109: 815–819.

35. Terreehorst I, Hak E, Oosting AJ, Tempels-Pavlica Z, de Monchy JGR, Bruijnzeel-Koomen CAFM, Aalberse RC, and Gerth van Wijk R. Evaluation of impermeable covers for bedding in patients with allergic rhinitis. *New Engl J Med* 2003; 349: 237–246.

36. Woodcock A, Forster L, Matthews E, Martin J, Letley L, Vickers M, Britton J, Strachan D, Howarth P, Altmann D, Frost C, and Custovic A. Control of exposure to mite allergen and allergen impermeable bed covers for adults with asthma. *New Engl J Med* 2003; 349: 225–236.

37. Halken S, Niklassen U, Hansen LG, Nielsen F, Host A, Osterballe O, Verggerby MC, and Poulsen LK. Encasing mattresses in children with asthma and house dust mite allergy. *J Allergy Clin Immunol* 1997; 99: S320.

38. Walshaw MJ and Evans CC. Allergen avoidance in house dust mite sensitive adult asthma. *Q J Med* 1986; 58: 199–215.

39. Platts-Mills TA, Vervloet D, Thomas WR, Aalberse RC, and Chapman MD. Indoor allergens and asthma: report of the Third International Workshop. *J Allergy Clin Immunol* 1997; 100: S2–S24.

40. McDonald LG and Tovey E. The role of water temperature and laundry procedures in reducing house dust mite populations and allergen content of bedding. *J Allergy Clin Immunol* 1992; 90: 599–608.

41. McDonald LG and Tovey E. The effectiveness of benzyl benzoate and some essential plant oils as laundry additives for killing house dust mites. *J Allergy Clin Immunol* 1993; 92: 771–772.

42. Vandenhove T, Soler M, Birnbaum J, Charpin D, and Vervloet D. Effect of dry cleaning on mite allergen levels in blankets. *Allergy* 1993; 48: 264–266.

43. Miller JD and Miller A. Ten minutes in a clothes dryer kills all mites in blankets. *J Allergy Clin Immunol* 1986; 90: 962a, 423.

44. Dodin A and Rak H. Influence of low temperature (–30°C) on the different stages of the human allergy mite *Dermatophagoides pteronyssinus* (Acari: Epidermoptidae). *J Med Entomol* 1993; 30: 810–811.

45. Mosbech H, Korsgaard J, and Lind P. Control of house dust mites by electrical heating blankets. *J Allergy Clin Immunol* 1988; 81: 706–710.

46. Nagakura T, Yasueda H, Obata T, Kanmuri M, Masaki T, Ihara N, and Maekawa K. Major Dermatophagoides mite allergen, Der 1, in soft toys. *Clin Exp Allergy* 1996; 26: 585–589.

47. de Boer R. The control of house dust mite allergens in rugs. *J Allergy Clin Immunol* 1990; 86: 808–814.

48. Wassenaar DP. Effectiveness of vacuum cleaning and wet cleaning in reducing house-dust mites, fungi and mite allergen in a cotton carpet: a case study. *Exp Appl Acarol* 1988; 4: 53–62.

49. Vaughan JW, Woodfolk JA, and Platts-Mills TA. Assessment of vacuum cleaners and vacuum cleaner bags recommended for allergic subjects. *J Allergy Clin Immunol* 1999; 104: 1079–1083.

50. Colloff MJ, Taylor C, and Merrett TG. The use of domestic steam cleaning for the control of house dust mites. *Clin Exp Allergy* 1995; 25: 1061–1066.

51. Tovey ER and Woolcock AJ. Direct exposure of carpets to sunlight can kill all mites. *J Allergy Clin Immunol* 1994; 93: 1072–1074.

52. Lau-Schadendorf S, Rusche AF, Weber AK, Buettner-Goetz P, and Wahn U. Short-term effect of solidified benzyl benzoate on mite-allergen concentrations in house dust. *J Allergy Clin Immunol* 1991; 87: 41–47.

53. Hayden ML, Rose G, Diduch KB, Domson P, Chapman MD, Heymann PW, and Platts-Mills TA. Benzyl benzoate moist powder: investigation of acaricidal activity in cultures and reduction of dust mite allergens in carpets. *J Allergy Clin Immunol* 1992; 89: 536–545.

54. Dietemann A, Bessot JC, Hoyet C, Ott M, Verot A, and Pauli G. A double-blind, placebo controlled trial of solidified benzyl benzoate applied in dwellings of asthmatic patients sensitive to mites: clinical efficacy and effect on mite allergens. *J Allergy Clin Immunol* 1993; 91: 738–746.

55. Woodfolk JA, Hayden ML, Couture N, and Platts-Mills TA. Chemical treatment of carpets to reduce allergen: comparison of the effects of tannic acid and other treatments on proteins derived from dust mites and cats. *J Allergy Clin Immunol* 1995; 96: 325–333.

56. Ehnert B, Lau-Schadendorf S, Weber A, Buettner P, Schou C, and Wahn U. Reducing domestic exposure to dust mite allergen reduces bronchial hyperreactivity in sensitive children with asthma. *J Allergy Clin Immunol* 1992; 90: 135–138.

57. Huss RW, Huss K, Squire EN Jr, Carpenter GB, Smith LJ, Salata K, and Hershey J. Mite allergen control with acaricide fails. *J Allergy Clin Immunol* 1994; 94: 27–32.

58. Weeks J, Oliver J, Birmingham K, Crewes A, and Carswell F. A combined approach to reduce mite allergen in the bedroom. *Clin Exp Allergy* 1995; 25: 1179–1183.
59. Carswell F, Birmingham K, Oliver J, Crewes A, and Weeks J. The respiratory effects of reduction of mite allergen in the bedrooms of asthmatic children: a double-blind controlled trial. *Clin Exp Allergy* 1996; 26: 386–396.
60. Carswell F, Oliver J, and Weeks J. Do mite avoidance measures affect mite and cat airborne allergens? *Clin Exp Allergy* 1999; 29: 193–200.
61. Woodfolk JA, Hayden ML, Miller JD, Rose G, Chapman MD, and Platts-Mills TA. Chemical treatment of carpets to reduce allergen: a detailed study of the effects of tannic acid on indoor allergens. *J Allergy Clin Immunol* 1994; 94: 19–26.
62. Christiansen SC, Martin SB, Schleicher NC, Koziol JA, Hamilton RG, and Zuraw BL. Exposure and sensitization to environmental allergen of predominantly Hispanic children with asthma in San Diego's inner city. *J Allergy Clin Immunol* 1996; 98: 288–294.
63. Hayden ML, Perzanowski M, Matheson L, Scott P, Call RS, and Platts-Mills TA. Dust mite allergen avoidance in the treatment of hospitalized children with asthma. *Ann Allergy Asthma Immunol* 1997; 79: 437–442.
64. Shapiro GG, Wighton TG, Chin T, Zuckerman J, Eliassen H, Picciano JF, and Platts-Mills TAE. House dust mite avoidance for children with asthma in homes of low income families. *J Allergy Clin Immunol* 1999; 103: 1069–1074.
65. Warner JA, Marchant JL, and Warner JO. Allergen avoidance in the homes of atopic asthmatic children: the effect of Allersearch DMS. *Clin Exp Allergy* 1993; 23: 279–286.
66. Tovey ER, Marks GB, Matthews M, Green WF, and Woolcock A. Changes in mite allergen Der p I in house dust following spraying with a tannic acid/acaricide solution. *Clin Exp Allergy* 1992; 22: 67–74.
67. Green WF, Nicholas NR, Salome CM, and Woolcock AJ. Reduction of house dust mites and mite allergens: effects of spraying carpets and blankets with Allersearch DMS, an acaricide combined with an allergen reducing agent. *Clin Exp Allergy* 1989; 19: 203–207.
68. Marks GB, Tovey ER, Green W, Shearer M, Salome CM, and Woolcock AJ. House dust mite allergen avoidance: a randomized controlled trial of surface chemical treatment and encasement of bedding. *Clin Exp Allergy* 1994; 24: 1078–1083.
69. Tan BB, Weald D, Strickland I, and Friedmann PS. Double-blind controlled trial of effect of house dust-mite allergen avoidance on atopic dermatitis. *Lancet* 1996; 347: 15–18.
70. Colloff MJ. Use of liquid nitrogen in the control of house dust mite populations. *Clin Allergy* 1986; 16: 41–47.
71. Sporik R, Hill DJ, Thompson PJ, Stewart GA, Carlin JB, Nolan TM, Kemp AS, and Hosking CS. The Melbourne House Dust Mite Study: long-term efficacy of house dust mite reduction strategies. *J Allergy Clin Immunol* 1998; 101: 451–456.
72. Dorward AJ, Colloff MJ, MacKay NS, McSharry C, and Thomson NC. Effect of house dust mite avoidance measures on adult asthma. *Thorax* 1988; 43: 98–105.

73. Cabrera P, Julia-Serda G, Rodriguez de Castro F, Caminero J, Barber D, and Carrillo T. Reduction of house-dust mite allergens after dehumidifier use. *J Allergy Clin Immunol* 1995; 95: 635–636.

74. Arlian LG, Neal JS, and Vyszenski-Moher DZ. Reducing relative humidity to control the house dust mite *Dermatophagoides farinae*. *J Allergy Clin Immunol* 1999; 104: 852–856.

75. Custovic A, Taggart SCO, Kennaugh JK, and Woodcock A. Portable dehumidifiers in the control of house-dust mites and mite allergens. *Clin Exp Allergy* 1995; 25; 312–316.

76. Fletcher AM, Pickering CAC, Custovic A, Simpson J, Kennaugh J, and Woodcock A. Reduction in humidity as a method of controlling mites and mite allergens: the use of mechanical ventilation in British domestic dwellings. *Clin Exp Allergy* 1996; 26: 1051–1056.

77. Niven R, Fletcher AM, Pickering AC, Custovic A, Sivour JB, Preece AR, Oldham LA, and Francis HC. Attempting to control mite allergens with mechanical ventilation and dehumidification in British homes. *J Allergy Clin Immunol* 1999; 103: 756–762.

78. Hyndman SJ, Vickers LM, Htut T, Maunder JW, Peock A, and Higenbottam TW. A randomized trial of dehumidification in the control of house dust mite. *Clin Exp Allergy* 2000; 30: 1172–1180.

79. Antonicelli L, Bilo MB, Puca S, Shov C, and Bonifazi F. Efficacy of an air-cleaning device equipped with a high efficiency particulate air filter in house dust mite respiratory allergy. *Allergy* 1991; 46: 594–600.

80. Warburton CJ, Niven RM, Pickering CA, Fletcher AM, Hepworth J, and Frances HC. Domiciliary air filtration units, symptoms and lung function in atopic asthmatics. *Respir Med* 1994; 88: 771–776.

81. Reisman R, Mauriello P, Davis G, Georgitis JW, and DeMasi JM. A double-blind study of the effectiveness of a high-efficiency particulate air (HEPA) filter in the treatment of patients with perennial allergic rhinitis and asthma. *J Allergy Clin Immunol* 1990; 85: 1050–1059.

82. Van der Heide S, Kauffman HF, Dubois AEF, and de Monchy JGR. Allergen reduction measures in houses of allergic asthmatic patients: effects of air-cleaners and allergen-impermeable mattress covers. *Eur Resp J* 1997; 10: 1217–1223.

83. Warner JA, Frederick JM, Bryant TN, Weich C, Raw GJ, Hunter C, Stephen FR, McIntyre DA, and Warner JO. Mechanical ventilation and high-efficiency vacuum cleaning: a combined strategy of mite and mite allergen reduction in the control of mite-sensitive asthma. *J Allergy Clin Immunol* 2000; 105: 75–82.

84. Wickman M, Emenius G, Egmar AC, Axelsson G, and Pershagen G. Reduced mite-allergen levels in dwellings with mechanical exhaust and supply ventilation. *Clin Exp Allergy* 1994; 24: 109–114.

85. Knysak D. Animal allergens. *Immunol Allergy Clin N Amer* 1989; 9(2): 357–364.

86. Ledford DK. Indoor allergens. *J Allergy Clin Immunol* 1994; 94: 327–334.

87. Custovic A, Simpson A, Pahdi H, Green RM, Chapman MD, and Woodcock A. Distribution, aerodynamic characteristics, and removal of the major cat allergen Fel d 1 in British homes. *Thorax* 1998; 53: 33–38.

88. Phipatanakul W, Eggleston PA, Wright EC, and Wood RA. Mouse allergen. I. Prevalence of mouse allergen in inner-city homes. *J Allergy Clin Immunol* 2000; 106: 1070–1074.

89. Zielonka TM, Charpin D, Berbis P, Luciani P, Casanova D, and Vervloet D. Effects of castration and testosterone on Fel d I production by sebaceous glands of male cats. I. Immunological assessment. *Clin Exp Allergy* 1994; 24: 1169–1173.

90. Charpin C, Zielonka TM, Charpin D, Ansaldi JL, Allasia C, and Vervloet D. Effects of castration and testosterone on Fel d I production by sebaceous glands of male cats. II. Morphometric assessment. *Clin Exp Allergy* 1994; 24: 1174–1178.

91. Luczynska CM, Li Y, Chapman MD, and Platts-Mills TA. Airborne concentrations and particle size distribution of allergen derived from domestic cats (*Felis domesticus*): measurements using cascade impactor, liquid impinger, and a two-site monoclonal antibody assay for Fel d I. *Am Rev Respir Dis* 1990; 141: 361–367.

92. Bollinger ME, Eggleston PA, Flanagan E, and Wood RA. Cat antigen in homes with and without cats may induce allergic symptoms. *J Allergy Clin Immunol* 1996; 97: 907–914.

93. Bollinger ME, Wood RA, Chen P, and Eggleston PA. Measurement of cat allergen levels in the home by use of an amplified ELISA. *J Allergy Clin Immunol* 1998; 101: 124–125.

94. Custovic A, Taggart SCO, and Woodcock A. House dust mite and cat allergen in different indoor environments. *Clin Exp Allergy* 1994; 24: 1164–1168.

95. Dornelas de Andrade A, Charpin D, Birnbaum J, Lanteaume A, Chapman M, and Vervloet D. Indoor allergen levels in day nurseries. *J Allergy Clin Immunol* 1995; 95: 1158–1163.

96. Martin IR, Wicken K, Patchett K, Kent R, Fitzharris P, Siebers R, Lewis C, Holbrook N, and Smith S. Cat allergen levels in public places in New Zealand. *NZ Med J* 1998; 111: 356–358.

97. Custovic A, Fletcher A, Pickering CAC, Francis HC, Green R, Smith A, Chapman M, and Woodcock A. Domestic allergens in public places. III. House dust mite, cat, dog and cockroach allergens in British hospitals. *Clin Exp Allergy* 1993; 28: 53–59.

98. Perzanowski MS, Ronmark E, Nold B, Lundback B, and Platts-Mills TA. Relevance of allergens from cats and dogs to asthma in the northernmost province of Sweden: schools as a major site of exposure. *J Allergy Clin Immunol* 1999; 103: 1018–1024.

99. Wickman M, Egmar AC, Emenius G, Almqvist C, Berglind N, Larsson P, Van and Hage-Hamsten M. Fel d 1 and Can f 1 in settled dust and airborne Fel d 1 in allergen avoidance day-care centres for atopic children in relation to number of pet owners, ventilation and general cleaning. *Clin Exp Allergy* 1999; 29: 626–632.

100. Karlsson AS, Renstrom A, Hedren M, and Larsson K. Comparison of four allergen-sampling methods in conventional and allergy prevention classrooms. *Clin Exp Allergy* 2002; 32: 1776–1781.

101. Custovic A, Green R, Taggart SC, Smith A, Pickering CA, Chapman MD, and Woodcock A. Domestic allergens in public places. II. Dog (Can f1) and cockroach (Bla g 2) allergens in dust and mite, cat, dog and cockroach allergens in the air in public buildings. *Clin Exp Allergy* 1996; 26: 1246–1252.

102. Enberg RN, Shamie SM, McCullough J, and Ownby DR. Ubiquitous presence of cat allergen in cat-free buildings: probable dispersal from human clothing. *Ann Allergy* 1993; 70: 471–474.

103. D'Amato G, Liccardi G, Russo M, Barber D, D'Amato M, and Carreira J. Clothing is a carrier of cat allergens. *J Allergy Clin Immunol* 1997; 99: 577–578.

104. Wood RA, Mudd KE, and Eggleston PA. The distribution of cat and dust mite allergens on wall surfaces. *J Allergy Clin Immunol* 1992; 89: 126–130.

105. Custovic A, Simpson A, Pahdi H, Green RM, Chapman MD, and Woodcock A. Distribution, aerodynamic characteristics, and removal of the major cat allergen Fel d I in British homes. *Thorax* 1998; 53: 33–38.

106. Custovic A, Green R, Fletcher A, Smith A, Pickering CA, Chapman MD, and Woodcock A. Aerodynamic properties of the major dog allergen Can f 1: distribution in homes, concentration, and particle size of allergen in the air. *Am J Respir Crit Care Med* 1997; 155: 94–98.

107. Ohman JL, Jr, Hagberg K, MacDonald MR, Jones RR, Jr, Paigen BJ, and Kacergis JB. Distribution of airborne mouse allergen in a major mouse breeding facility. *J Allergy Clin Immunol* 1994; 94: 810–817.

108. Platts-Mills TA, Heymann PW, Longbottom JL, and Wilkins SR. Airborne allergens associated with asthma: particle sizes carrying dust mite and rat allergens measured with a cascade impactor. *J Allergy Clin Immunol* 1986; 77: 850–857.

109. Corn M, Koegel A, Hall T, Scott A, Newill A, and Evans R. Characteristics of airborne particles associated with animal allergy in laboratory workers. *Ann Occup Hyg* 1988; 32: 435–446.

110. Wood RA, Chapman MD, Adkinson NF, Jr, and Eggleston PA. The effect of cat removal on allergen content in household-dust samples. *J Allergy Clin Immunol* 1989; 83: 730–734.

111. van der Brempt X, Charpin D, Haddi E, da Mata P, and Vervloet D. Cat removal and Fel d I levels in mattresses. *J Allergy Clin Immunol* 1991; 87: 595–596.

112. Munir AK. Environmental factors influencing the levels of indoor allergens. *Pediatr Allergy Immunol* 1995; 6: 13–21.

113. Munir AKM, Einarsson R, and Dreborg SKG. Indirect contact with pets can confound the effect of cleaning procedures for reduction of animal allergen levels in house dust. *Pediatr Allergy Immunol* 1994; 5: 32–39.

114. van der Heide S, van Aalderen WM, Kauffman HF, Dubois AE, and de Monchy JG. Clinical effects of air cleaners in homes of asthmatic children sensitized to pet allergens. *J Allergy Clin Immunol* 1999; 104: 447–451.

115. Wood RA, Johnson EF, Van Natta ML, Chen PH, and Eggleston PA. A placebo-controlled trial of a HEPA air cleaner in the treatment of cat allergy. *Am J Respir Crit Care Med* 1998; 158: 115–120.

116. De Blay F, Chapman MD, and Platts-Mills TAE. Airborne cat allergen (Fel d 1): environmental control with the cat *in situ*. *Am Rev Respir Dis* 1991; 143: 1334–1339.

117. Klucka CV, Ownby DR, Green J, and Zoratti E. Cat shedding of Fel d 1 is not reduced by washings, Allerpet/c spray or acepromazine. *J Allergy Clin Immunol* 1995; 95: 1164–1171.

118. Perzanowkski MS, Wheatley LM, Avener DB, Woodfolk JA, and Platts-Mills TAE. The effectiveness of Allerpet/c in reducing the cat allergen Fel d 1. *J Allergy Clin Immunol* 1997; 100: 428–430.

119. Avner DB, Perzanowski MS, Platts-Mills TAE, and Woodfolk JA. Evaluation of different techniques for washing cats: quantitation of allrgen removed from the cat and the effect on airborne Fel d 1. *J Allergy Clin Immunol* 1997: 100: 307–312.

120. Hodson T, Custovic A, Simpson A, Chapman M, Woodcock A, and Green R. Washing the dog reduces dog allergen levels, but the dog needs to be washed twice a week. J *Allergy Clin Immunol* 1999; 103: 581–585.

121. Green R, Simpson A, Custovic A, Faragher B, Chapman M, and Woodcock A. The effect of air filtration on airborne dog allergen. *Allergy* 1999; 54: 484–488.

122. Green R, Simpson A, Custovic A, and Woodcock A. Vacuum cleaners and airborne dog allergen. *Allergy* 1999; 54: 403–405.

123. Eggleston PA, Newill CA, Ansari AA, Pustelnik A, Sheau-Rong L, Evans R III, Marsh DG, Longbottom JL, and Corn M. Task-related variation in airborne concentrations of laboratory animal allergens: studies with Rat n 1. *J Allergy Clin Immunol* 1989; 84: 347–352.

124. Bernstein DI and Bernstein IL. Occupational asthma, in *Allergy Principles and Practice*, Middleton E et al., Eds. St. Louis, MO: Mosby, 1998, pp. 963–980.

125. Bush RK and Portnoy JM. The role and abatement of fungal allergens in allergic diseases. *J Allergy Clin Immunol* 2001; 107: S430–S40.

126. Platts-Mills TA, Hayden ML, Chapman MD, and Wilkins SR. Seasonal variation in dust mite and grass-pollen allergens in dust from the houses of patients with asthma. *J Allergy Clin Immunol* 1987; 79: 781–791.

127. Dharmage S, Bailey M, Raven J, Mitakakis T, Thien F, Forbes A, Guest D, Abramson M, and Walters EH. Prevalence and residential determinants of fungi within homes in Melbourne, Australia. *Clin Exp Allergy* 1999; 29: 1481–1489.

128. Vijay H, Taker A, Banerjee B, and Kurup V. Mold allergens, in *Allergens and Allergen Immunotherapy*, 2nd ed., Lockey RF and Bukaniz S, Eds. New York: Marcel Dekker, 1999, pp. 133–154.

129. King N and Auger P. Indoor air quality, fungi, and health: how do we stand? *Can Family Phys* 2002; 48: 298–302.

130. Koster JAD and Thorne PS. Bioaerosol concentration in non-compliant, complaint and intervention homes in the Midwest. *Am Ind Hyg Assoc J*, 1995; 56: 573–580.

131. Dotterud LK, Vorland LH, and Falk ES. Viable fungi in indoor air in homes and schools in the Sor-Varanger community during winter. *Pediatr Allergy Immunol* 1995; 6: 181–186.

132. Verhoeff AP, van Wijnen JH, van Reenen-Hoekstra ES, Samson RA, van Strien RT, and Brunekreef B. Fungal propagules in house dust. II. Relation with residential characteristics and respiratory symptoms. *Allergy* 1994; 49: 540–547.

133. Douwes J, van der Sluis B, Doekes G, van Leusden F, Wijnands L, van Strien R, Verhoeff A, and Brunekreef B. Fungal extracellular polysaccharides in house dust as a marker for exposure to fungi: relations with culturable fungi, reported home dampness, and respiratory symptoms. *J Allergy Clin Immunol* 1999; 103: 494–500.

134. Garrett MH, Rayment PR, Hooper MA, Abramson MJ, and Hooper BM. Indoor airborne fungal spores, house dampness and associations with environmental factors and respiratory health in children. *Clin Exp Allergy* 1998; 28: 459–467.

135. Maloney MJ, Wray BB, DuRant RH, and Smith L. Effect of an electronic air cleaner and negative ionizer on the population of indoor mold spores. *Ann Allergy* 1987; 59: 192–194.

136. U.S. Environmental Protection Agency. Clear Your Home of Asthma Triggers: Your Children Will Breathe Easier. Washington, D.C. Report 402-F-99-005, 1999.

137. Burge HA, Solomon WR, and Muilenberg ML. Evaluation of indoor plantings as allergen exposure sources. *J Allergy Clin Immunol* 1982; 70: 101–108.

138. Solomon WR, Burge HA, and Boise JR. Exclusion of particulate allergens by window air conditioners. *J Allergy Clin Immunol* 1980; 65: 305–308.

139. Garrison RA, Robertson LD, Koehn RD, and Wynn SR. Effect of heating–ventilation–air conditioning system sanitation on airborne fungal populations in residential environments. *Ann Allergy* 1993; 71: 548–556.

140. Eggleston PA and Arruda LK. Ecology and elimination of cockroaches and allergens in the home. *J Allergy Clin Immunol* 2001; 107: S422–S429.

141. Arruda LK, Vailes LD, Ferriani VPL, Santos ABR, Pomes A, and Chapman MD. Cockroach allergens and asthma. *J Allergy Clin Immunol* 2001; 107: 419–428.

142. Gelber LE, Seltzer LH, Bouzoukis JK, Pollart SM, Chapman MD, and Platts-Mills TA. Sensitization and exposure to indoor allergens as risk factors for asthma among patients presenting to hospital. *Am Rev Respir Dis* 1993; 147: 573–578.

143. de Blay F, Sanchez J, Hedelin G, Perez-Infante A, Verot A, Chapman M, and Pauli G. Dust and airborne exposure to allergens derived from cockroach (*Blattella germanica*) in low-cost public housing in Strasbourg (France). *J Allergy Clin Immunol* 1997; 99: 107–112.

144. Rosenstreich DL, Eggleston P, Kattan M, Baker D, Slavin RG, Gergen P, Mitchell H, McNiff-Mortimer K, Lynn H, Ownby D, and Malveaux F. The role of cockroach allergy and exposure to cockroach allergen in causing morbidiy among inner-city children with asthma. *New Engl J Med* 1997; 335: 1356–1363.

145. Sarpong SB, Wood RA, and Eggleston PA. Short-term effects of extermination and cleaning on cockroach allergen Bla g 2 in settled dust. *Ann Allergy Asthma Immunol* 1996; 76: 257–260.

146. Sarpong SB, Wood RA, Karrison T, and Eggleston PA. Cockroach allergen (Bla g 1) in school dust. *J Allergy Clin Immunol* 1997; 99: 486–492.

147. Rullo VE, Rizzo MC, Arruda LK, Sole D, and Naspitz CK. Daycare centers and schools as sources of exposure to mites, cockroach, and endotoxin in the city of Sao Paulo, Brazil. *J Allergy Clin Immunol* 2002; 110: 582–588.

148. Hemingway J and Small GJ. Resistance mechanisms in cockroaches: key to control strategies, in *Proceedings of First International Conference on Insect Pests in the Urban Environment*, Wildey KB and Robinson WH, Eds. Exeter, UK: BPCC Wheatons Ltd., 1993; pp. 141–152.

149. Mollet JA, Vailes LD, Avner DB, Perzanowski MS, Arruda LK, Chapman MD, and Platts-Mills TA. Evaluation of German cockroach (Orthoptera: Blattellidae) allergen and seasonal variation in low-income housing. *J Med Entomol* 1997; 34: 307–311.

150. Eggleston PA, Wood RA, Rand C, Nixon WJ, Chen PH, and Lukk P. Removal of cockroach allergen from inner-city homes. *J Allergy Clin Immunol* 1999; 104: 842–846.

151. Williams LW, Reinfried P, and Brenner RJ. Cockroach extermination does not rapidly reduce allergen in settled dust. *J Allergy Clin Immunol* 1999; 104: 702–703.

152. Gergen PJ, Mortimer KM, Eggleston PA, Rosenstreich D, Mitchell H, Ownby D, Kattan M, Baker D, Wright EC, Slavin R, and Malveaux F. Results of the National Cooperative Inner-City Asthma Study (NCICAS) environmental intervention to reduce cockroach allergen exposure in inner-city homes. *J Allergy Clin Immunol* 1999; 103: 501–506.

153. Kinney PL, Northridge ME, Chew GL, Gronning E, Joseph E, Correa JC, Prakash S, and Goldstein I. On the front lines: an environmental asthma intervention in New York City. *Am J Public Health* 2002; 92: 24–26.

154. Sporik R, Holgate ST, Platts-Mills TAE, and Cogswell JJ. Exposure to house-dust mite allergen (Der p 1) and the development of asthma in childhood: a prospective study. *New Engl J Med* 1990; 323: 502–507.

155. Arshad SH, Matthews S, Gant C, and Hide DW. Effect of allergen avoidance on development of allergic disorders in infancy. *Lancet* 1992; 339: 1493–1497.

156. Hide DW, Matthews S, Matthews L, Stevens M, Ridout S, Twiselton R, Gant C, and Arshad SH. Effect of allergen avoidance in infancy on allergic manifestations at age two years. *J Allergy Clin Immunol* 1994; 93: 842–846.

157. Hide DW, Matthews S, Tariq S, and Arshad SH. Allergen avoidance in infancy and allergy at four years of age. *Allergy* 1996; 51: 89–93.

158. Custovic A, Simpson BM, Simpson A, Hallam C, Craven M, Brutsche M, and Woodcock A. Manchester Asthma and Allergy Study: low-allergen environment can be achieved and maintained during pregnancy and in early life. *J Allergy Clin Immunol* 2000; 105: 252–258.

159. Custovic A, Simpson BM, Simpson A, Kissen P, and Woodcock A. Effect of environmental manipulation in pregnancy and early life on respiratory symptoms and atopy during first year of life: a randomised trial. *Lancet* 2001; 358: 188–193.

160. Brunekreef B, Smit J, de Jongste J, Neijens H, Gerritsen J, Postma D, Aalberse R, Koopman L, Kerkhof M, Wijga A, and van Strien. The prevention and incidence of asthma and mite allergy (PIAMA) birth cohort study: design and first results. *Pediatr Allergy Immunol* 2002; 13: 55–60.

161. Van Strien RT, Koopman LP, Kerkhof M, Spithoven J, de Jonste JC, Gerritsen J, Neijens HJ, Aalberse RC, Smit HA, and Brunekreef B. Mite and pet allergen levels in homes of children born to allergic and nonallergic parents: the PIAMA Study. *Environ Health Perspect* 2002; 110: A693–A698.

162. Koopman LP, Van Strien RT, Kerkhof M, Wijga A, Smit HA, De Jongste J, Gerritsen J, Aalberse RC, Brunekreef B, and Neifens HJ. Placebo-controlled trial of house dust mite-impermeable mattress covers: effect on symptoms in early childhood. *Am J Respir Crit Care Med* 2002; 166: 307–313.

20

Immunotherapy and Asthma

MOISÉS A. CALDERÓN-ZAPATA and STEPHEN R. DURHAM

National Heart and Lung Institute, Imperial College School of Medicine
London, U.K.

I. Introduction

Allergen-specific immunotherapy (SIT) or allergen vaccination is a therapeutic practice in which the sensitized patient receives gradually increasing amounts of allergen vaccine in order to achieve hyposensitization and reduce symptoms during natural exposure to the allergen.[1] The idea of administering allergen extracts is not recent; allergen-specific immunotherapy has been widely used for more than 90 years to treat allergic disease.[2] However, only during the past few decades has our increased understanding of the mechanisms of allergic disease provided a framework for rational therapy of allergic disease based on the complex inflammatory reaction rather than on the symptoms alone.

Allergen injection immunotherapy is highly effective in carefully selected patients with IgE-mediated disease. During the past few decades, many double-blind, placebo-controlled studies have convincingly demonstrated the clinical efficacy of specific immunotherapy with standardized extracts of inhaled allergens such as grass pollen,[3–5] ragweed,[6] mites,[7–9] and cat dander.[10–11]

Despite an understanding of the physiopathology of asthma and the advances in its pharmacological treatment, the prevalence of asthma has increased worldwide during the past two decades.[12] IgE-mediated allergy is extremely common in asthma of both children and adults, and an allergen-based treatment is very important for the management of allergic asthma[13] to allow modification of the onset of the disease and the onset of its exacerbations.

The effectiveness of specific immunotherapy in allergic asthma has been controversial and its safety has also raised many ethical issues. However, it is clear that the appropriate use of specific immunotherapy in certain asthmatic patients can in the short term reduce the responses to allergic triggers that precipitate symptoms and may in the long term decrease bronchial inflammation and nonspecific bronchial hyperreactivity where bronchial remodeling is not prominent.[13]

II. Mechanisms of Immunotherapy

Recent studies have provided new information as to how immunotherapy may alter the inflammatory processes involved in allergic responses. The mechanisms implicated in specific immunotherapy are likely to be heterogeneous and complex and produce immunomodulatory effects on different inflammatory cells and their inflammatory mediators during early and late phase responses. These mechanisms may depend on the nature of the allergen, the target organ, the genetic status of the host, the route, the dose and duration of immunotherapy, and the uses of different adjuvants.

A. Antibody Responses

Conventional allergen immunotherapy is capable of blunting the typical rise in IgE antibody levels seen following allergen exposure.[14] The serum IgE concentration has also been shown to be inversely correlated with the rise in blocking IgG total and IgG4 antibodies within the first year of treatment with specific immunotherapy.[15–19] Studies by Peng et al. exploring the IgG subclasses have shown that IgG1 is the dominant immunoglobulin produced during the early phase of immunotherapy, whereas IgG4 begins to appear in significant quantities only after prolonged immunotherapy.[20] The rise in IgG antibodies led to the proposal that antibodies exert "blocking" activity by competing with IgE for allergen binding to inhibit the IgE-dependent activation of mast cells, basophils, and other IgE receptor-expressing cells.[21,22] This blocking activity is also able to suppress *in vitro* allergen-specific T cell responses by inhibiting IgE-mediated allergen presentation by B cells.[23] This may translate *in vivo* as greatly increasing the doses of allergen required to achieve T cell responses.

B. Cellular Responses

The effects of immunotherapy on the production of inflammatory mediators and their effects on immediate and late phase reactions have been evaluated extensively using both nasal and bronchial provocation tests. Creticos and colleagues demonstrated that after specific nasal allergen challenge with ragweed, concentrations of histamine, TAME-esterase, and PGD2 were significantly lower in nasal secretions of ragweed-sensitized patients who underwent 3 to 5 years of ragweed immunotherapy compared with controls.[24] Moreover, specific immunotherapy with ragweed attenuates both the early and late phase reactions in ragweed-allergic patients, with significant reductions in the generation of histamine, TAME-esterase, and kinins in nasal secretions collected at the late phase.[25] These findings may also explain the reductions in the migrations of eosinophils, basophils, and neutrophils into the inflammatory site by SIT.

It has also been shown that successful immunotherapy blunts the typical seasonal influx of eosinophils into the nasal mucosa in a dose-dependent manner.[26] Grass pollen-sensitive patients have shown a trend for decreased eosinophil recruitment accompanied by inhibition of the late cutaneous response.[27,28]

Under experimental and natural conditions, the effect of grass pollen immunotherapy on eosinophil numbers in the nasal mucosa has been studied. Nasal biopsies were collected from placebo and actively treated patients before and 24 hours after allergen provocation tests.[29] This study showed that the inhibition of the late nasal response was associated with a decrease in the numbers of eosinophils but not neutrophils. More recently, it has been demonstrated that seasonal increases in the numbers of eosinophils within the nasal epithelia and the lamina propria were reduced in patients who underwent 2 years of immunotherapy with grass pollen antigen compared with placebo-treated individuals.[30] The correlation observed between eosinophil numbers and overall symptoms, suggests that the inhibition of tissue eosinophilia that occurs during natural grass pollen exposure may contribute to the clinical efficacy of SIT.

Similarly, grass pollen immunotherapy in adults is associated with a decrease in the number of cutaneous tryptase-only positive mast cells.[31] Furthermore, the number of metachromatic cells is also reduced in the nasal mucosa surface after treatment with immunotherapy specific to house dust and Alternaria in patients with perennial allergic rhinitis.[32]

Specific immunotherapy has also been shown to prevent the priming of eosinophil adhesion to VCAM-1 and ICAM-1 during the pollen season in patients allergic to birch pollen who had asthma, but not in those without asthma.[33] In contrast, neutrophils from the immunotherapy-treated group, both with and without asthma, demonstrated priming of their adhesion to E-selectin and ICAM-1 during the season. The latter results indicate that specific immunotherapy induced a shift from the production of primarily eosinophil priming agents to neutrophil priming agents that may be caused by a shift from Th2 to Th1 lymphocytes.

C. Cytokine and T Cell Responses

T cells and the cytokines they produce are thought to play major roles in orchestrating the allergic inflammatory response. Following activation, Th1 cells produce interferon (IFN)-γ and interleukin (IL)-2, whereas Th2 cells produce mainly IL-4, IL-5, and IL-13. Both IL-12 and IFN-γ promote and sustain Th1 responses, whereas IL-4 is the major growth factor promoting the differentiation of Th2 cells.[34,35]

Factors that determine the evolution of Th1 and/or Th2 responses include (1) nature and dose of antigen, with the possibility that high doses of allergen may favor the induction of Th1 type responses;[36] (2) nature of the antigen-presenting cells, with macrophages favoring Th1 responses, possibly via production of IL-12, whereas antigen presentation by B cells, particularly at low antigen concentrations, favors the development of Th2 cells;[37] and (3) different dendritic cell subsets with varying concentrations of DC1 and DC2 cells implicated in the development of Th1 and Th2 responses.[38] DC2-type dendritic cells have been identified in atopic individuals, and their ability to drive Th2 responses appears to relate to low levels of IL-12 expression.[39]

After processing by antigen-presenting cells, specific peptides are presented via major histocompatibility complex (MHC) class II molecules to the antigen-specific T cell receptor. This activation requires the interactions of other molecules on antigen-presenting cells and T cells, respectively, including HLA-DR with CD4, CD80/CD86 with CD28/CTLA-4, and CD40 with CD40 ligand. A preferential costimulation via the CD86 molecule may favor Th2 responses.[40] Insufficient costimulation may result in a state of T cell unresponsiveness or anergy.[41]

Allergen immunotherapy alters the cytokine profiles of allergen-specific T cells and switches Th2-type immune responses in patients with atopy toward Th0- or Th1-type responses. The modification of Th2 cell responses occurs by immune deviation with an increase in Th0/Th1 and/or T cell anergy with a decrease in Th2/Th0[42] (Figure 20.1). These immunomodulatory effects have been correlated with the efficacy of specific immunotherapy, at least in grass pollen allergy.[43]

Varney et al. demonstrated that after 1 year of grass pollen immunotherapy, significant increases in IFN-γ and IL-2 mRNA-expressing cells are detected in skin biopsies taken 24 hours after intradermal allergen challenge.[27] Moreover, cutaneous biopsies showed an increase in the expression of mRNA encoding one of the subunits of IL-12, and this feature was also correlated positively with IFN-γ mRNA expression.[44] When patients were subsequently evaluated after 7 years of grass pollen immunotherapy, IL-4 mRNA expression in response to intradermal allergen challenge was decreased, suggesting that changes to cytokine responses after specific immunotherapy may evolve during prolonged treatment.

Similarly, specific immunotherapy for 1 year was associated with increased allergen-dependent IFN-γ mRNA expression within the nasal mucosal lamina propria when evaluated 24 hours after intranasal mucosal allergen provocation.

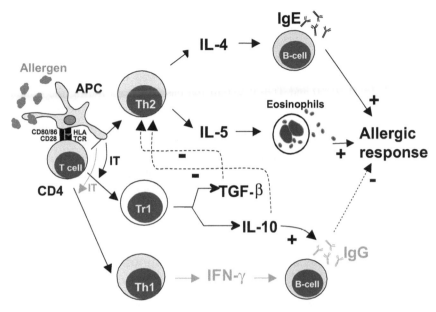

Figure 20.1 Mechanisms of allergen immunotherapy via immune deviation or anergy induction.

This was not accompanied by significant reductions in IL-4 and IL-5 mRNA.[43] Seasonal increases in nasal mucosal IFN-γ and IL-5 mRNA expression were observed only in immunotherapy and placebo patients, respectively. Following 2 years of immunotherapy, the ratio of IFN-γ to IL-5 expression within the mucosa was significantly higher in the immunotherapy patients.[45] Majori and colleagues demonstrated a down-regulation of peripheral blood CD4+ and CD8+ T cell activation in grass pollen-sensitive patients following 1 year of injection immunotherapy as shown by a reduction in surface expression of the activation markers, CD25 (p55 IL-2 receptor) and human leukocyte antigen HLA-DR.[46]

More recently, interest has focused on the potential role of so-called regulatory T cells that express the inhibitory cytokines IL-10 and/or transforming growth factor (TGF)-β. IL-10 may induce anergy in peripheral T cells.[47] Francis et al.[48] evaluated the role of IL-10 production and CD4+CD25+ by peripheral T cells in response to grass pollen immunotherapy. Subjects undergoing SIT produced significantly more IL-10 than atopic control individuals (p <0.001), and the number of peripheral CD4+CD25+ cells identified by flow cytometry after allergen stimulation was also greater in the immunotherapy group. Moreover, only T cells from patients receiving SIT were positive for intracellular IL-10. The authors concluded that SIT with grass pollen results in the generation of a population of circulating T cells that express the IL-10+CD4+CD25+ phenotype in response to allergen stimulation.

These processes have also been shown to follow immunotherapy treatment of house dust mite–sensitive patients in whom increases in both IL-10 and TGF-β by peripheral T-cells were observed.[49] Nouri-Aria and colleagues confirmed increases in local IL-10 and TGF-β within the nasal mucosa during the pollen season.[50] Both IL-10 and TGF-β may act to inhibit T cell proliferation and cytokine production following immunotherapy with a variety of antigens including insect venom, mite, and grass.[48,51] These cytokines may also be important in the modulation of allergen-specific antibody responses after immunotherapy because IL-10 is an important switch factor for B cell production of IgG4, whereas TGF-β preferentially induces IgA production. IgG4 has potential as a "blocking antibody," and increased mucosal IgA may play a role by allergen "exclusion" following successful immunotherapy.

III. Efficacy and Safety of Specific Immunotherapy

A. Clinical Efficacy

The effectiveness of allergen SIT has been highlighted in several well-controlled studies and recently in a World Health Organization position paper on allergen immunotherapy.[1] SIT should be considered in selected patients with specific IgE antibodies to clinically relevant allergens who have long durations of symptoms or in whom pharmacotherapy is partially or wholly ineffective or induces side effects. Therefore, the rationale for prescribing SIT depends on the degree to which symptoms can be alleviated by medication and whether effective avoidance of allergen is possible. The quality of allergen vaccines is also critical, and an optimal maintenance dose of 5 to 20 μg of major allergen per injection correlates with clinical efficacy. SIT is specific to the antigen administrated.

SIT with grass pollen is a highly effective treatment for patients with severe summer hay fever, who are unresponsive to conventional anti-allergic drugs including topical corticosteroids and antihistamines.[4] SIT has long-lasting clinical effects.[3] The efficacy of grass pollen SIT is suggested by the decrease of target organ sensitivity during nasal and/or conjunctival allergen challenge. This has been widely documented in optimally designed double-blind placebo-controlled trials.

The clinical efficacy of SIT in asthma has also been documented in a considerable number of placebo-controlled trials. Two systematic reviews and meta-analyses of clinical trials of SIT assessed the efficacy of subcutaneous immunotherapy in asthma.[52,53] Both reviews concluded that individuals randomized to receive SIT reported significantly fewer asthma symptoms, required significantly less asthma medication, and demonstrated both reduced nonspecific and reduced allergen-specific bronchial hyperreactivity (BHR) compared with those given placebo.

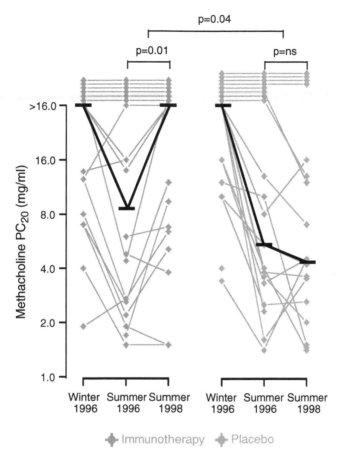

Figure 20.2 Seasonal changes in airway methacholine responsiveness before and after SIT to grass pollen. (From Walker SM et al. *J Allergy Clin Immunol* 2001; 107: 87–93. With permission.)

The efficacy of SIT in bronchial asthma has been demonstrated especially in patients with limited sensitization. In a 2-year study, subjects with mild asthma and sensitized only to grass pollen, grass pollen SIT significantly decreased seasonal chest symptoms (p <0.04) and prevented increases in airway methacholine PC_{20} (provocation concentration of methacholine that causes a 20% decrease in FEV_1; Figure 20.2). A doubling-dose enhancement in PC_{20} during the pollen season was observed in placebo-treated patients.[54]

Creticos et al. evaluated the efficacy of SIT for asthma exacerbated by seasonal ragweed exposure.[55] Patients who reported seasonal asthma symptoms, medication use, and decreased peak expiratory flow (PEF) were randomly assigned to receive placebo or ragweed extract SIT. The authors emphasized measurements of PEF as they provided objective day-to-day assessments of airflow obstruction and the severity of asthma. During treatment, the SIT group no longer had seasonal declines in PEF rates, whereas PEF rates in the placebo group continued to diminish. In contrast, both groups showed some improvement in asthma symptoms both in their preseasonal baseline assessments and during the ragweed season. This suggests that regular visits with a physician and careful adjustments of medication doses to alleviate symptoms provide clinical benefits.

The effect of subcutaneous SIT for *Dermatophagoides pteronyssinus* was recently assessed by Pifferi and colleagues.[56] Fifteen asthma subjects (aged 6 to 14 years) monosensitized to house dust mite received SIT during a 3-year treatment period; 14 asthmatic children were matched as controls and did not receive SIT. In the SIT group, significant improvements in asthmatic symptoms and marked reductions in drug use were observed. The SIT group also showed significant decreases in nonspecific bronchial reactivity. No new allergen sensitivities developed during the study period in the SIT-treated group (p = 0.01). Although patient numbers were small, this study suggests that SIT is effective in asthmatic children sensitive to mites and may reduce specific bronchial reactivity and prevent the onset of new sensitizations in monosensitized individuals.

In contrast to single allergen immunotherapy in patients with limited spectra of allergies, injections of mixtures of multiple allergens in polysensitized patients are highly controversial.[57] A double-blind, placebo-controlled trial of multiple-allergen immunotherapy was performed in 121 allergic children with moderate to severe, perennial (year-round) asthma. The children, who required daily medication for asthma control, were randomly assigned to receive subcutaneous injections of a mixture of up to seven aero-allergen extracts or placebo for more than 2 years. The principal outcome was the daily medication score in the 60 days preceding and during immunotherapy. No differences were noted between the groups in the use of medical care, symptoms, or PEF rates. One conclusion is that the use of multiple allergens in SIT showed no clinical efficacy in asthma. Another is that monosensitized patients or those with symptoms induced by a few selected seasonal or perennial allergens are more likely to respond to SIT than those with multiple sensitivities. Finally, patients with severe asthma requiring treatment with oral corticosteroids are unsuitable because of low efficacy and greatly increased risk of side effects that may occasionally be serious; several fatalities have been reported.

B. Safety of Specific Immunotherapy

Side effects after the administration of subcutaneous SIT include local or systemic reactions. Local reactions at injection sites may be immediate or delayed. In

Table 20.1 Adverse Events Arising from Allergen Immunotherapy — Grading of Systemic Reactions

Grade	Systemic Reactions
1	Nonspecific (not IgE-mediated): discomfort, headache, arthralgia, etc.
2	Mild: mild rhinitis and/or asthma (PEFR >60%)
3	Nonlife-threatening: urticaria, angioedema, severe asthma (PEFR <60%)
4	Anaphylactic reaction

general, the local reactions are minor and well tolerated and do not require treatment other than reassurance. Rarely, chronic administration may result in subcutaneous nodules, particularly with alum-containing vaccines; these nodules disappear over time.

Systemic reactions may occur in 10 to 15% of subjects although these adverse events generally are mild and involve rhinitis and/or wheezing that resolves with antihistamine treatment or use of a bronchodilator. Life-threatening reactions occur very rarely but deaths have been reported. Anaphylaxis is well recognized as a complication of allergen SIT but fatal reactions are rare (Table 20.1).

Hejjaoui et al. studied the occurrence of systemic reactions due to SIT in a group of 500 patients allergic to grass pollen.[58] The same rush SIT protocol and the same standardized extracts were used in all patients. The rate of systemic reactions increased in patients who had asthma (and allergic rhinitis) during the previous season compared with those with allergic rhinitis alone. The incidences of generalized urticaria and anaphylaxis were similar in both groups, but bronchial symptoms occurred mainly in asthmatic patients. This study indicates that asthmatic patients are at higher risk for adverse reactions during SIT. Rush SIT may expose patients to high risks of systemic reactions. With the use of premedications, exclusion of asthmatic patients with FEV_1 levels below 70% of predicted values at the time of the injection, and cessation of rush SIT if large local reactions were noticed, systemic reactions decreased to an acceptable rate and they were always of mild severity.

The risk of fatal reaction appears increased in patients with asthma and may be caused by bronchial hyperresponsiveness to mediators released by allergens. The annual fatality rate from the administration of SIT in the United States remains low: 1 fatality per 2 million doses.[59] The survey of United States fatalities due to SIT suggests that the risk of death was increased in asthma patients who were corticosteroid-dependent, required hospital or emergency room visits for treatment, experienced increased bronchospasm at the time of SIT administration, or had compromises of other vital systems such as the cardiovascular system.

In the United Kingdom, 26 patients died between 1957 and 1986 from anaphylaxis due to administration of SIT with house dust mite (HDM) or grass

Table 20.2 Adverse Events Arising
from Immunotherapy — Risk Factors

Errors in dosage
Presence of symptomatic asthma
High degree of hypersensitivity (SPT/RAST)
Use of blockers
Injections from new vials
Injections during periods of exacerbation of symptoms

SPT = Skin Prick test. RAST = Radioallergosorbent test

pollen. Most (16 of 17 for whom the indication for SIT was known) received IT for asthma, suggesting that asthma is a strong risk factor for fatal outcomes from systemic reactions.[60]

The Committee on Safety of Medicines found most of these cases occurred where adequate facilities for cardiorespiratory resuscitation were not available. Since then, the recommendation in the United Kingdom is that SIT should be performed only by experienced personnel in the presence of a trained physician and in a hospital-based specialist clinic with immediate access to adrenaline and resuscitative measures. Patients should be observed for at least 30 minutes following injection (60 minutes in the United Kingdom). Routine screening with peak flow before each injection and before the patient departs from the physician's office after injection should be performed for all patients undergoing SIT (Table 20.2).

IV. Long-Term Benefits Following Discontinuation of Immunotherapy

The long-term benefit after discontinuation of SIT has been shown in a number of well-documented, well-controlled studies. In patients with asthma caused by animal dander allergy, the effect of SIT using cat or dog allergen extracts was found to persist for at least 5 years after termination of SIT.[61] Similarly, Jacobsen et al.[62] studied the long-term effects of tree pollen SIT by following up the symptom scores and skin tests of 36 patients 6 years after a 3-year course of SIT. They showed that 86% of the patients with allergic rhinitis and 68% of the asthmatic patients maintained improvements after discontinuation of therapy. Skin sensitivity significantly decreased during treatment, and the skin test reactions evaluated 6 years after SIT treatment remained significantly lower than pretreatment levels.

Durham et al.[63] conducted a randomized, double-blind, placebo-controlled trial on the discontinuation of SIT for grass pollen allergy in patients in whom

3 to 4 years of this treatment had previously been shown to be effective. During the 3 years of this trial, primary outcome measures were scores for seasonal nasal and chest symptoms and the use of rescue medication. A matched control group of rhinitic subjects who had never received SIT were followed over the same period in order to control for the natural history of the disease during the prolonged follow-up period. The researchers found that both symptoms and rescue medication requirements remained low after the discontinuation of SIT and noted no significant differences between patients who continued SIT and those who discontinued it. Prolonged clinical benefit was accompanied by a persistent inhibition of the late cutaneous response and suppression of T cell and IL-4 synthesis at the site of the intradermal challenge with grass pollen.

More recently, a study of 60 children (mean age 8.5 years) who suffered from allergic asthma/rhinitis due to mites evaluated the long-lasting effect of sublingual SIT.[64] Thirty-five children underwent a 4- to 5-year course of sublingual SIT with standardized extract and 25 received only drug therapy. The immunotherapy-treated group showed a significant difference versus baseline for the presence of asthma (p <0.01) after treatment, whereas no difference was observed in the control group. The mean PEF results were significantly higher in the active group than in the control group after 10 years. This study shows that sublingual SIT is also effective in children and that it maintains its clinical efficacy at least 4 to 5 years after discontinuation of treatment.

V. Immunotherapy and Progression of Rhinitis to Asthma

One potential aspect of the long-term effect of SIT is the possibility of preventing the progression of allergic rhinitis to asthma. A link of these two allergic disorders was demonstrated in numerous epidemiological studies. Approximately 75% of patients with allergic asthma and 40% of patients with nonallergic asthma will have perennial rhinitis, while 20% of patients with perennial allergic rhinitis will have signs of asthma.[65] Twenty-five to 43% of patients with allergic rhinitis naturally develop asthma within 10 years.[66,67]

To evaluate disease progression after SIT, the recently published multicenter preventative allergy treatment (PAT) study involving 205 children (aged 6 to 14 years; mean age = 10.7 years) with grass or birch pollen allergies was performed. The children were recruited from six pediatric allergy clinics in Northern Europe[68] and randomly assigned to receive SIT for 3 years or served as controls. The children diagnosed with only allergic rhinitis underwent methacholine challenges at baseline evaluations. Twenty percent of children who had no diagnoses of asthma had abnormal methacholine challenge studies at inclusion. The children treated with SIT had significantly fewer asthma symptoms after 3 years of treatment, as evaluated by clinical diagnosis (odds ratio 2.52; p <0.05). Methacholine bronchial provocation test results also improved in the active group (p <0.05). It was concluded that patients treated with SIT for 3 years had significantly fewer asthma symptoms than the untreated control groups.

VI.   Immunotherapy and Onset of New Allergic Sensitivities

SIT also decreases the tendencies of allergic patients to develop additional allergen sensitivities. Encouraging data demonstrating the effects of SIT on the natural courses of allergies arose from a 3-year follow-up survey performed by Des Roches et al. They demonstrated prevention of the onset of new sensitivities in children receiving SIT.[69] The study consisted of 44 children monosensitized to HDM: 22 children who received SIT to HDM and 22 children who acted as a control group and did not receive SIT. All patients who did not receive SIT developed sensitization to other allergens such as animal dander, Alternaria species, or pollen, whereas 45% (10 of 22) of those in the actively treated group did not develop any new sensitivities (p <0.001). Those who did developed far fewer sensitivities than the untreated control group.

These results were confirmed in a 6-year follow-up study of children monosensitized to HDM who received SIT for 3 years.[70] The number of children with new sensitizations was significantly lower in the SIT-treated group compared with the control group. Collectively, these results indicate that SIT in monosensitized patients may prevent new sensitizations and thus raise with the question whether allergen immunotherapy should be considered earlier in the course of disease to prevent progression or the development of new allergies.

VII.   Allergen Immunotherapy: Future Strategies

Alternative approaches include the use of immunotherapy via the sublingual route. This has been shown to be effective, although probably less so than conventional injection immunotherapy. Whether long-term benefit will occur following discontinuation of sublingual immunotherapy has not yet been established. The use of adjuvants such as bacterial DNA (immunostimulatory sequences, CpG, MPL, or *M. vaccae*) has the potential to increase efficacy and reduce side effects.[71–73]

Peptide immunotherapy involves the use of short allergen peptides that retain immunostimulatory properties while avoiding allergen–IgE cross-linking that may otherwise result in systemic side affects associated with conventional immunotherapy. Preliminary results are encouraging for these different modalities, although substantial clinical trials have yet to be performed.

Table 20.3 Allergen Immunotherapy: WHO Recommendations

High dose standardized vaccines
    (5 to 20 µg major allergen per monthly maintenance injection)
Mixtures of allergens in polysensitized patients of no proven value
Optimum duration = 3 to 5 years
Administration in specialist clinics by trained persons with immediate access to adrenaline
Observation period after injection (30 minutes)
Risks increased in asthma

Table 20.4 Allergen Immunotherapy: Summary Points

SIT has been shown, through documentation of well-controlled studies, to be highly effective for the treatment of allergic rhinitis.
SIT is the only specific and curative approach for the treatment of IgE-mediated allergy.
SIT has the potential to influence the natural course of allergic disease and prevent new sensitizations.
SIT may be effective in preventing the onset of asthma in children with allergic rhinitis.
Although SIT has been shown to be highly effective in allergic asthma, asthma is a significant risk factor for systemic reactions during SIT; only patients with controlled asthma should receive SIT.
SIT induces prolonged clinical remission when the treatment is continued for several years.
The prophylactic effect, as shown by long-term benefit after discontinuation and a possible reduction in the onset of new allergen sensitivities, raises the question whether immunotherapy should be considered earlier and not be confined to use in patients in whom pharmacotherapy has failed.

VIII. Conclusions

Allergen immunotherapy is the only active treatment approach that has the potential to alter the natural courses of allergic disorders. SIT currently is an efficacious treatment for certain selected patients with allergic rhinitis and mild to moderate asthma. The optimal candidate for SIT is the patient with mild to moderate asthma that is induced by a few selected seasonal or perennial allergens.

    Although SIT is undoubtedly effective for asthma, the risk-to-benefit ratio is greatly increased and, at least in the United Kingdom, asthma is viewed as a relative contraindication to SIT. Possible exceptions to this are patients who develop periodic wheezing and are free of asthma for the rest of the year and the occasional symptomatic and monosensitive patients who find avoidance impossible, for example, veterinarian staff members subject to occupational exposures. The safety of SIT limits its use; however, the systemic reactions induced by SIT are usually mild when an appropriate protocol is used. SIT should not be used in patients with severe asthma or in patients with asthma who receive adequate pharmacotherapy and whose FEV_1 values are below 70% of predicted values (Table 20.3 and Table 20.4).

References

1. Bousquet J, Lockey RF, and Malling HJ. WHO position paper. Allergen immunotherapy: therapeutic vaccines for allergic diseases. *Allergy* 1998; 53: 1–42.
2. Noon L. Prophylactic inoculation against hay fever. *Lancet* 1911; 1: 1572–1573.
3. Durham SR, Walker SM, Varga EM, Jacobson MR, O'Brien F, Noble W, Till SJ, Hamid Q, and Nouri-Aria K. Long-term clinical efficacy of grass pollen immunotherapy. *New Engl J Med* 1999; 341: 468–475.
4. Varney VA, Gaga M, Frew AJ, Aber VR, Kay AB, and Durham SR. Usefulness of immunotherapy in patients with severe summer hay fever uncontrolled by anti-allergic drugs. *Br Med J* 1991; 302: 265–269.
5. Bousquet J, Hejjaoui A, Skassa-Brociek W, Guerin B, Maasch HJ, Dhivert H, and Michel FB. Double-blind, placebo-controlled immunotherapy with mixed grass pollen allergoids. I. Rush immunotherapy with allergoid and standardized orchard grass pollen extract. *J Allergy Clin Immunol* 1987; 80: 591–598.
6. Cockcroft D, Cuff M, Tarlo S, Dolovich J, and Hargreave F. Allergen-injection therapy with glutaraldehyde-modified ragweed pollen–tyrosine adsorbate: a double-blind trial. *J Allergy Clin Immunol* 1977; 60: 56–62.
7. Warner JO, Price JF, Soothill JF, and Hey EN. Controlled trial of hyposensitisation to *Dermatophagoides pteronyssinus* in children with asthma. *Lancet* 1978; 2: 912–915.
8. Olsen OT, Larsen KR, Jacobsen L, and Svendsen UG. A 1-year, placebo-controlled, double-blind, house dust mite immunotherapy study in asthmatic adults. *Allergy* 1997; 52: 853–859.
9. Pilcher CE, Marquardsen A, Sparholt S, Bircher A, and Bischof M. Specific immunotherapy with *Dermatophagoides pteronyssinus* and *D. farinae* results in decreased bronchial hyperreactivity. *Allergy* 1997; 52: 274–283.
10. Heddin G, Graff-Lonnevig V, Heilborn H, Lilja G, Norrlind K, and Pegelow K. Immunotherapy with cat and dog dander extracts. V. Effects of 3 years of treatment. *J Allergy Clin Immunol* 1991; 87: 955–964.
11. Varney VA, Edwards J, Tabbah K, Brewster H, Mavroleon G, and Frew AJ. Clinical efficacy of specific immunotherapy to cat dander: a double-blind placebo-controlled trial. *Clin Exp Allergy* 1997; 27: 860–867.
12. Weiss ST. Epidemiology and heterogeneity of asthma. *Ann Allergy Asthma Immunol* 2001; 87: 5–8.
13. Bousquet J. Immunotherapy is clinically indicated in the management of allergic asthma. *Am J Respir Crit Care Med* 2001; 164: 2139–2140.
14. Lichtenstein LM, Ishizaka K, Norman PS, Sobotka A, and Hill B. IgE antibody measurements in ragweed hay fever: relationship to clinical severity and the results of immunotherapy. *J Clin Invest* 1973; 52: 472–482.

15. Gehlhar K, Schlaak M, Becker, and Bufe A. Monitoring allergen immunotherapy of pollen-allergic patients: the ratio of allergen-specific IgG4 to IgG1 correlates with clinical outcome. *Clin Exp Allergy* 1999; 29: 497–506.

16. McHugh SM, Lavelle B, Kemeny DM, Patel S, and Ewan PW. A placebo-controlled trial of immunotherapy with two extracts of *Dermatophagoides pteronissinus* in allergic rhinitis, comparing clinical outcome with changes in antigen-specific IgE, IgG, and IgG subclasses. *J Allergy Clin Immunol* 1990; 86: 521–531.

17. Creticos PS, Reed CE, Norman PS, Khoury J, Adkinson NF Jr, Buncher CR, Busse WW, Bush RK, Gadde J, Li JT, Richerson HB, Rosenthal RP, Solomon WR, Steinberg P, and Yunginger JW. Ragweed immunotherapy in adult asthma. *New Engl J Med* 1996; 334: 501–506.

18. Creticos PS. The consideration of immunotherapy in the treatment of allergic asthma. *Ann Allergy Asthma Immunol* 2002; 87; 13–27.

19. Maggi E, Romagnani S, and Ricci M. Regulatory mechanisms of IgE synthesis and their regulation in atopy. *Allergol Immunopathol* 1992; 20: 165–169.

20. Peng Z, Naclerio RM, and Norman PS. Quantitative IgE and IgG subclass responses during and after long-term ragweed immunotherapy. *J Allergy Clin Immunol* 1992; 9: 519–529.

21. Garcia BE, Sanz ML, Gato JJ, Fernandez J, and Oehling A. IgG4 blocking effect on the release of antigen-specific histamine. *J Invest Allergol Clin Immunol* 1993; 3: 26–33.

22. Lambin P, Bouzoumou A, Murrieta M, Debbia M, Rouger P, Leynadier F, and Levy DA. Purification of human IgG4 subclass with allergen-specific blocking activity. *J Immunol Methods* 1993; 165: 99–111.

23. van Neerven RJ, Wikborg T, Lund G, Jacobsen B, Brinch-Nielsen A, Arnved J, and Ipsen H. Blocking antibodies induced by specific allergy vaccination prevent the activation of CD4+ T cells by inhibiting serum-IgE-facilitated allergen presentation. *J Immunol* 1999; 163: 2944–2952.

24. Creticos PS, Adkinson NF, Jr, Kagey-Sobotka A, Proud D, Meier HL, Naclerio RM, Lichtenstein LM, and Norman PS. Nasal challenge with ragweed in hay fever patients: effect of immunotherapy. *J Clin Invest* 1985; 76: 2247–2253.

25. Iliopoulos O, Proud D, Adkinson NF, Jr, Creticos PS, Norman PS, Kagey-Sobotka A, Lichtenstein LM, and Naclerio RM. Effects of immunotherapy on the early, late and rechallenge nasal reaction to provocation with allergen: changes in inflammatory mediators and cells. *J Allergy Clin Immunol* 1991; 87: 855–866.

26. Furin MJ, Norman PS, Creticos PS, Kagey-Sobotka A, Lichtenstein LM, and Naclerio RM. Immunotherapy decreases antigen-induced eosinophil migration into the nasal cavity. *J Allergy Clin Immunol* 1991; 88: 27–32.

27. Varney VA, Hamid QA, Gaga M, Ying S, Jacobson M, Frew AJ, Hay AB, and Durham SR. Influence of grass pollen immunotherapy on cellular infiltration and cytokine mRNA expression during allergen-induced late-phase cutaneous responses. *J Clin Invest* 1993; 92; 644–651.

28. Nish WA, Charlesworth EN, Davis TL, Whisman BA, Valtier S, Charlesworth MG, and Leiferman KM. The effect of immunotherapy on the cutaneous late phase response to antigen. *J Allergy Clin Immunol* 1994; 93: 484–493.

29. Durham SR, Ying S, Varney VA, Jacobson MR, Sudderick RM, Mackay IS, Kay AB, and Hamid QA. Grass pollen immunotherapy inhibits allergen-induced infiltration of CD4+ T cells and eosinophils in the nasal mucosa and increases the number of cells expressing messenger RNA for interferon-gamma. *J Allergy Clin Immunol* 1996; 97: 1356–1365.

30. Wilson DR, Nouri-Aria KT, Walker SM, Pajno GB, O'Brien F, Jacobson MR, Mackay IS, and Durham SR. Grass pollen immunotherapy: symptomatic improvement correlates with reductions in eosinophils and IL-5 mRNA expression in the nasal mucosa during the pollen season. *J Allergy Clin Immunol* 2001; 107: 971–976.

31. Durham SR and Till SJ. Immunologic changes associated with allergen immunotherapy. *J Allergy Clin Immunol* 1998; 102: 157–164.

32. Otsuka H, Mezawa A, Ohnishi M, Okubo K, Seki H, and Okuda M. Changes in nasal metachromatic cells during allergen immunotherapy. *Clin Exp Allergy* 1991; 21: 115–119.

33. Hakansson L, Heinrich C, Rak S, and Venge P. Priming of eosinophil adhesion in patients with birch pollen allergy during pollen season: effect of immunotherapy. *J Allergy Clin Immunol* 1997; 99: 551–562.

34. Maggi E, Parronchi P, Manetti R, Somonelli C, Piccinni MP, De Carli M, Ricci M, and Romagnani S. Reciprocal regulatory effects on IFN-gamma and IL-4 on the in vitro development of human Th1 and Th2 clones. *J Immunol* 1992, 148: 2142–2147.

35. Maggi E. The Th1/Th2 paradigm in allergy. *Immunotechnology* 1998; 3: 233–244.

36. Hosken NA, Shibuya K, Heath AW, Murphy KM, and O'Garra A. The effect of antigen dose on CD4+ T-helper cell phenotype development in a T cell receptor-alpha beta-transgenic mode. *J Exp Med* 1995; 182: 1579–1584.

37. Secrist H, De Kruyff RH, and Umetsu DT. Interleukin-4 production by CD4+ T cells from allergic individuals is modulated by antigen concentration and antigen-presenting cell type. *J Exp Med* 1995; 181: 1081–1089.

38. Kapsenberg ML, Hilkens CM, Wierenga EA, and Kalinski P. The paradigm of type 2 antigen-presenting cells: implications for atopic allergy. *Clin Exp Allergy* 1999; 29: 33–36.

39. Reider N, Reider D, Ebner S, Holzmann S, Herold M, Fritsch P, and Romani N. Dendritic cells contribute to the development of atopy by an insufficiency in IL-12 production. *J Allergy Clin Immunol* 2002; 109: 89–95.

40. Freeman GJ, Boussiotis VA, Anumanthan A, Bernstein GM, Ke XY, Rennert PD, Gribben JG, and Nadler LM. B7-1 and B7-2 do not deliver identical costimulatory signals since B7-2 but not B7-1 preferentially costimulates the initial production of IL-4. *Immunity* 1995; 2: 523–532.

41. Harding FA, MacArthur JA, Gross JA, Raulet DH, and Allison JP. CD28-mediated signalling co-stimulates murine T-cells and prevents induction of anergy in T-cell clones. *Nature* 1992; 356: 607–609.

42. Varga EM, Nouri-Aria KT, Till SJ, and Durham SR. Immunomodulatory treatment strategies for allergic diseases. *Curr Drug Targets Inflammation Allergy* 2003; 2: 31–46.

43. Wilson DR, Nouri-Aria KT, Walker SM, Pajno GB, O'Brien F, Jacobson MR, Mackay IS, and Durham SR. Grass pollen immunotherapy: symptomatic improvement correlates with reduction in eosinophils and IL-5 mRNA expression in the nasal mucosa during the pollen season. *J Allergy Clin Immunol* 2001; 107: 971–976.

44. Varga EM, Walchholz P, Nouri-Aria KT, Verhoef A, Corrigan CJ, Till SJ, and Durham SR. T-cells from human allergen-induced late asthmatic responses express IL-12 receptor B2 subunit mRNA and respond to IL-12 *in vitro*. *J Immunol* 2000; 165: 2877–2885.

45. Wachholz P, Nouri-Aria KT, Verhoef A, Walker SM, Till SJ, and Durham SR. Grass pollen immunotherapy for hay fever is associated with increases in local mucosal but not peripheral Th1/Th2 ratios. *Immunology* 2002; 105: 56–62.

46. Majori M, Bertacco S, Piccoli ML et al. Specific immunotherapy downregulates peripherial blood CD4 and CD8 T-lymphocyte activation in grass pollen-sensitive asthma. *Eur Respir J* 1998; 11: 1263–1267.

47. Akdis CA, Blesken T, Akdis M, Wuthrich B, and Blaser K. Role of interleukin 10 in specific immunotherapy. *J Clin Invest* 1998; 102: 98–106.

48. Francis J, Till SJ, and Durham SR. Induction of IL-10+CD4+CD25+ T cells by grass pollen immunotherapy. *J Allergy Clin Immunol* 2003; 111: 1255–1261.

49. Adkis CA, Kussebi F, Pulendram B, Akdis M, Lauener RP, Schidt-Weber CB, Klunker S, Isitmangil G, Hansjee N, Wynn TA, Dillon S, Erb P, Baschang K, and Alkan SS. Inhibition of T-helper 2-type responses, IgE production and eosinophilia by synthetic lipopeptides. *Eur J Immunol* 2003; 33: 2717–2726.

50. Nouri-Aria KT, Jacobson MR and Durham SR. Grass pollen immunotherapy increases IL-10 and TGB-beta mRNA expression in the nasal mucosa during the pollen season. *J Allergy Clin Immunol* 2002; 109: S171.

51. Akdis CA, Blesken T, Akdis M, Wuthrich B, and Blaser K. Role of interleukin 10 in specific immunotherapy. *J Clin Invest* 1998; 102: 98–106.

52. Abramson M, Puy R, and Weiner J. Is allergen immunotherapy effective in asthma? A meta-analysis of randomised controlled trials. *Am J Respir Crit Care Med* 1995; 151: 969–974.

53. Abramson M, Puy R, and Weiner J. Immunotherapy in asthma: an updated systematic review. *Allergy* 1999; 54: 1022–1041.

54. Walker SM, Pajno GB, Torres-Lima M, Wilson DR, and Durham SR. Grass pollen immunotherapy for seasonal rhinitis and asthma: a randomized, controlled trial. *J Allergy Clin Immunol* 2001; 107: 87–93.

55. Creticos PS, Reed CE, Norman PS, Khoury J, Adkinson NF, Jr, Buncher CR, Busse WW, Bush RK, Gadde J, Li JT, Richerson HB, Rosenthal RR, Solomon WR, Stienberg P, and Yunginger JW. Ragweed immunotherapy in adult asthma. *New Engl J Med* 1996; 334: 501–506.

56. Pifferi M, Baldini G, Marrazini G, Baldini M, Ragazzo V, Pietrobelli A, and Boner AL. Benefits of immunotherapy with standardized *Dermatophagoides pteronyssinus* extract in asthmatic children: a three-year prospective study. *Allergy* 2002; 57: 785–790.

57. Adkinson NF, Eggleston PA, Eney D, Goldstein EO, Schuberth KC, Bacon JR, Hamilton RG, Weiss ME, Arshad H, Meinert CL, Tonascia J, and Wheeler B. A controlled trial of immunotherapy for asthma in allergic children. *New Engl J Med* 1997; 336: 324–31.

58. Hejjaoui A, Ferrando R, Dhivert H, Michel FB, and Bousquet J. Systemic reactions occurring during immunotherapy with standardized pollen extracts. *J Allergy Clin Immunol* 1992; 89: 925–933.

59. Reid MJ, Lockey RF, Turkeltaub PC, and Platts-Mills TAE. Survey of fatalities from skin testing and immunotherapy, 1985–1998. *J Allergy Clin Immunol* 1993; 92: 6–15.

60. Committee on Safety of Medicines. Desensitisation vaccines. *Br Med J* 1986; 293: 949.

61. Hedlin G, Heilborn H, Lilja G, Norrlind K, Pegelow K, Sundin B, and Lowenstein H. Long-term follow-up of patients treated with a three-year course of cat or dog immunotherapy. *J Allergy Clin Immunol* 1995; 96: 879–885.

62. Jacobsen L, Nuchel B, Wihl JA, Lowenstein H, and Ipsen H. Immunotherapy with partially purified and standardized tree-pollen extracts. IV. Results from long-term (6-year) follow-up. *Allergy* 1997; 52: 914–920.

63. Durham SR, Walker SM, Varga EM, Jacobson MR, O'Brien F, Noble W, Till SJ, Hamid Q, and Nouri-Aria K. Long-term clinical efficacy of grass pollen immuno-therapy. *New Engl J Med* 1999; 341: 468–475.

64. Di Rienzo V, Marcucci F, Puccinelli P, Parmiani S, Frati S, Sense L, Canonica GW, and Passalacqua G. Long-lasting effect of sublingual immunotherapy in children with asthma due to house dust mite: a 10-year prospective study. *Clin Exp Allergy* 2003; 33: 206–210.

65. Rowe-Jones JM. The link between the nose and lung, perennial rhinitis and asthma: is it the same disease? *Allergy* 1997; 52: 20–28.

66. Settipane RJ, Hagy GW, and Settipane GA. Long-term risk factors for developing asthma and allergic rhinitis: a 23-year follow-up study of college students. *Allergy Proc* 1994; 15: 21–25.

67. Corren J. Allergic rhinitis and asthma: how important is the link? *J Allergy Clin Immunol* 1997; 99: 781–786.

68. Möller C, Dreborg S, Ferdousi HA, Halken S, Høst A, Jacobsen L, Koivikko A, Koller DY, Niggemann B, Norberg LA, Urbanek R, Valovirta E, and Wahn U. Pollen immunotherapy reduces the development of asthma in children with seasonal rhi-noconjunctivitis (the PAT study). *J Allergy Clin Immunol* 2002; 109: 251–256.

69. Des Roches A, Paradis L, Menardo JL, Bouges S, Daures JP, and Bousquet J. Immunotherapy with a standardized dermatophagoides pterohyssinus extract. VI. Specific immunotherapy prevents the onset of new sensitizations in children. *J Allergy Clin Immunol* 1997; 99: 450–453.

70. Pajno GB, Barberio G, De Luca F, Morabito L, and Parmiani S. Prevention of new sensitizations in asthmatic children monosensitized to house dust mite by specific immunotherapy: six-year follow-up study. *Clin Exp Allergy* 2001; 31: 1392–1397

71. Valenta R and Kraft D. From allergen structure to new form of allergen-specific immunotherapy. *Curr Opin Immunol* 2002; 14: 718–727

72. Valenta R. Recombinant allergen-based concepts for diagnosis and therapy of type I allergy. *Allergy* 2002; 57: 66–77.

73. Oldfield WL, Larche M, and Kay AB. Effect of T-cell peptides derived from Fel d 1 on allergic reactions and cytokine production in patients sensitive to cats: a randomized controlled trial. *Lancet* 2002; 360: 47–53.

21

Anti-Cytokine Therapy

LARRY BORISH

Beirne Carter Center for Immunology Research
University of Virginia Health System
Charlottesville, Virginia, U.S.A.

I. Introduction

Cytokines are secreted proteins with growth, differentiation, and activation functions that regulate and determine the natures of immune responses. Which cytokines are produced in response to an immune insult determines initially whether an immune response develops and subsequently whether that response is cytotoxic, humoral, cell-mediated, or allergic. This recognition of the importance of cytokines to allergic inflammation and asthma has led to the development of means to modulate cytokine activity as potential pharmacological agents in the treatment of allergic diseases. Inhibition of cytokine production is among the most important anti-inflammatory mechanisms for corticosteroids and calcineurin antagonists such as cyclosporine A, tacrolimus (FK506), and pimecrolimus. However, numerous agents currently in various stages of development specifically target inflammation produced by cytokines in allergic disorders. These include the use of cytokines that are themselves anti-inflammatory or have activities that may inhibit allergic inflammation. Alternatively, novel methods under development target the activities of allergenic cytokines.

II. Mechanisms of Cytokine Inhibition

A. Neutralizing Antibodies

Neutralizing antibodies have long been recognized as potentially useful thera-peutic agents. However, neither monoclonal antibodies nor heterologous antisera will have roles in human allergic diseases secondary to their immunogenicity. Allergic diseases such as asthma will require prolonged therapy with any phar-macological agent. Ongoing treatment with foreign antibodies will rapidly result in the development of serum sickness and loss of efficacy of the antibody sec-ondary to the development of neutralizing antibodies. Several approaches are avail-able to lessen the tendency to develop antibodies against these foreign antibodies.

Chimeric antibodies consist of fusion proteins that combine the human Fc fragments of immunoglobulin molecules with animal Fab fragments. Such an approach was used in the development of anti-tumor necrosis factor (TNF) anti-bodies (infliximab, Centocor). While less immunogenic than completely foreign antibodies, chimeric antibodies still retain some immunogenicity that may lead to their inexorable loss of function. Interestingly, the use of infliximab is associ-ated with a dose-dependent inhibition of the tendency to produce these harmful neutralizing antibodies, suggesting that the immunosuppressive properties of infliximab inhibit immune responses against itself.[1]

An improvement upon chimeric antibodies was the development of human-ized antibodies. These antibodies retain the murine DNA coding sequence for the antigen-binding component of the antibody, yet use human DNA for the structural framework sequences of the Fab portion and the Fc sequence of the antibody. These antibodies bind and neutralize their target cytokines but greatly reduce the immunogenicity of the mouse molecule. Humanized antibodies to IgE are currently available in some parts of the world[2] (omalizumab, Genentech) and humanized antibodies to interleukin (IL)-4 and IL-5 have been developed. Humanized antibodies still retain some potential for the development of neutral-izing antibodies and may be associated with reduced affinity for their target.

A final approach that has the potential to completely eliminate the immu-nogenicity of neutralizing antibodies is the development of fully human mono-clonal antibodies. This technology involves the generation of monoclonal antibodies in mice that are genetically engineered to have human (B and T lymphocyte) immune systems. For example, a human anti-IL-4 receptor that would have the ability to inhibit binding of both IL-4 and IL-13 to their shared receptor has been developed.

B. Soluble Receptors

Cytokines function through their ability to bind to specific receptors with high affinity. Most receptors represent multimers of several identical proteins

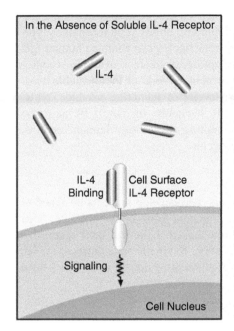
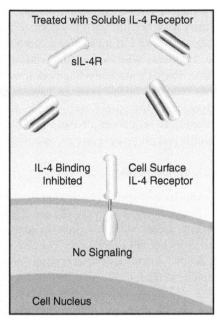

Figure 21.1 Inhibition of cytokines with soluble receptors: Soluble IL-4 receptor represents the extracellular region of the IL-4 receptor α chain. It retains the ability to bind IL-4 with high affinity and high specificity. Because IL-4R binds and sequesters IL-4 and does not induce cellular activation, it serves as an anti-inflammatory mechanism that may counter the effects of IL-4 in asthma.

(homodimers or even homotrimers) or, alternatively, two or three distinct proteins (heterodimers or heterotrimers). These receptor proteins have critical roles in contributing to the avidity of cytokine binding and to signaling. Secreted (or soluble) forms of many of these receptors occur naturally and are produced via alternative RNA splicing of the nascent receptor gene transcript, leading to a protein product that lacks transmembrane and cytoplasmic domains but is instead exported from cells.

Alternatively, naturally occurring soluble receptors may develop through protease cleavage from the surface membrane. Depending on the affinity of these naturally occurring monomeric soluble receptors, they may retain their ability to interact with ligands. Because they lack cytoplasmic sequences, they cannot induce cellular activation but they can bind and sequester the cytokine, resulting in a naturally occurring anti-inflammatory mechanism (Figure 21.1).

Soluble receptors can also be cloned and developed in an appropriate expression system as pharmacologic agents, for example, soluble human interleukin-4 receptor (Immunex). Because many soluble monomeric cytokine receptors have insufficient affinity to bind and sequester their targets, several molecular techniques have been devised to optimize their binding ability. The techniques typically involve use of molecular recombination technology to combine human IgG Fc fragments with two of the soluble receptors to create a cytokine receptor homodimer–Fc antibody fragment fusion protein. Several of these soluble cytokine receptor fusion proteins have been developed including soluble TNFR[3] (etanercept, Immunex) and soluble IL-13R (Genetics Institute). Because the amino acid sequences of these soluble receptors are entirely human proteins, soluble receptors are generally nonimmunogenic.

C. Muteins

Molecular biology has been used in other ways to develop reagents designed to modulate cytokine activity. The generation of mutant forms of cytokines has been used to create synthetic proteins termed muteins that bind to their respective receptors but fail to transduce cellular activation. Synthetic antagonists to IL-1β, IL-4, and granulocyte macrophage colony-stimulating factor (GM-CSF) have been described.

D. Antisense Oligonucleotides

Antisense oligonucleotides represent small DNA sequences complementary to mRNA transcripts specific to cytokines. These DNA sequences are taken up by cells where they will generate DNA:RNA double stranded nucleic acids. These DNA:RNA fragments are deleted by specific enzymes, thereby preventing translation of the mRNA transcript.

E. Signaling Inhibitors

Alternatively, small molecules capable of blocking cytokine signaling have the potential to block cytokine activity. For example, specific inhibitors of p38 MAP kinase, an important signaling protein involved in functional responses to IL-4, IL-5, tumor necrosis factor (TNF)-α, and CCL11 (eotaxin) are under development (SB 203580, GlaxoSmithKline) and have been shown to inhibit eosinophil chemotaxis, degranulation, adhesion, and survival.[4,5]

III. Inhibitors of Cytokines Associated with Innate Immunity

Cytokines primarily derived from mononuclear phagocytic cells and other antigen-presenting cells (APCs) such as dendritic cells are particularly effective in promoting the cellular infiltrate and damage to resident tissue characteristic of inflammation. The processing of antigens as they are taken up by APCs, metabolized, and presented to T helper (Th) lymphocytes provides one pathway for this class of cytokine production.

Alternatively, monocytes, dendritic cells, and many other cells are triggered to produce cytokines through the innate immune system using pattern recognition receptors that recognize stereotypic components of pathogens that do not occur on mammalian cells. These receptors, such as lipopolysaccharide (LPS) receptors (CD14) acting through toll-like receptors (TLRs) e.g., TLR2 and TLR4, contribute to the ability of the immune system to distinguish pathogens from nonpathogenic proteins to which the immune system may become exposed. The cytokines predominantly produced by these innate immune responses include TNF, IL-1, IL-6, CXCL8 (IL-8), CXCL10 (IP10), and other members of the chemokine family, IL-12, IL-15, IL-18, and IL-23. The potent pro-inflammatory cascades initiated by TNF and IL-1 make these cytokines uniquely important potential targets in diminishing immune and inflammatory diseases. The use of IL-12 (and potentially 1L-18 and IL-23) to inhibit Th2 immune deviation will be discussed later.

A. Tumor Necrosis Factor

TNF represents two homologous proteins primarily derived from mononuclear phagocytes (TNF-α) and lymphocytes (TNF-β).[6] The active forms of both cytokines are homotrimers. In addition to mononuclear phagocytes, TNF-α may be produced by neutrophils activated lymphocytes, natural killer (NK) cells, endothelial cells, and mast cells. The most potent inducers of TNF by monocytes are LPSs and other ligands acting through toll-like receptors. TNF-α is processed as a membrane-bound protein from which the soluble active factor is derived via cleavage using the TNF-α converting enzyme (TACE).[7]

TNF-β can be synthesized and processed as a typical secretory protein but is usually linked to the cell surface by forming heterotrimers with a third membrane-associated member of this family designated lymphotoxin-β. TNF-α and TNF-β bind to the same two distinct cell surface receptors — TNFR I (p75) and TNFR II (p55) — with similar affinities, and produce similar, although not identical, effects.[8] TNF is expressed in asthmatic lungs, and inhalation of TNF-α can increase airway hyperresponsiveness.[9]

TNF has many biological effects that may contribute to asthma. TNF interacts with endothelial cells to induce intercellular adhesion molecule-1 (ICAM-1), vascular cell adhesion molecule-1 (VCAM-1), and E-selectin, permitting the egress of granulocytes into inflammatory loci. It is a potent activator of neutrophils, mediating adherence, chemotaxis, degranulation, and the respiratory burst. In asthma, TNF-α has the potential to enhance the chemotaxis of eosinophils, activate T lymphocytes, and promote growth of fibroblasts.

Two TNF antagonists have been approved in the United States. Etanercept (Immunex) is a soluble TNF receptor fusion protein consisting of two p75 receptors bound to the human Fc portion of human IgG1. Infliximab (Centocor) is a chimeric antihuman TNF antibody. These drugs have important distinct features that may influence their ranges of therapeutic efficacy. Soluble receptors bind and sequester only soluble TNF. In contrast, the antibody is capable of binding both soluble TNF and membrane-bound TNF. This extends to infliximab the potential for opsonizing and eliminating the activities of cells expressing membrane TNF, including disease-specific T lymphocytes. Etanercept has been demonstrated to be a safe and highly effective treatment of rheumatoid arthritis, psoriatic arthritis, juvenile rheumatoid arthritis, and psoriasis. Infliximab is safe and highly effective in the treatment of Crohn's disease, rheumatoid arthritis, and psoriasis. The utility of both of these agents in asthma is currently under investigation. A recent uncontrolled study reported beneficial effects of etanercept in asthmatics.[10]

B. Interleukin-1

The IL-1 family represents four peptides (IL-1α, IL-1β, the IL-1 receptor antagonist (ra), and IL-18).[11,12] IL-1α and IL-1β have similar biologic activities and both proteins along with IL-1ra interact with similar affinities to the two IL-1 receptors. Type I receptors transduce the biologic effects attributed to IL-1.[13] These are in contrast to type II receptors that have minimal intracellular domains. The capture and sequestration of IL-1 by these inactive type II receptors serve an anti-inflammatory function similar to the functions of soluble receptors. The capacity of IL-1ra to bind to the type I (pro-inflammatory) IL-1R without transducing biologic activities is the basis for its capacity to function as a cytokine antagonist.[11] IL-1ra is secreted naturally in inflammatory processes and is thought to modulate the potentially deleterious effects of IL-1 in the natural course of inflammation.

Its production is up-regulated by many cytokines including IL-4, IL-6, IL-13, and transforming growth factor (TGF)-β. One of the most important biologic activities of IL-1 is its ability to activate T lymphocytes by enhancing the production of IL-2 and expression of IL-2 receptors. In the absence of IL-1, a diminished immune response or a state of tolerance develops. IL-1 augments B cell proliferation and increases immunoglobulin synthesis. IL-1 stimulates endothelial cell adherence of leukocytes through the up-regulation of ICAM-1, VCAM-1, and E-selectin.

IL-1 is readily identified in an asthmatic lung[14] where it is likely to contribute to inflammation through its ability to induce adhesion molecule expression, activate and recruit granulocytes, and co-activate T helper lymphocytes. Both soluble IL-1 receptors and the IL-1 receptor antagonist have been proposed as

Table 21.1 T Helper Cell Subtypes

Th1	Th2	Both	Tr1 Cells
IFN-γ	IL-4	TNF-α	TGF-β
TNF-β	IL-5	GM-CSF	IL-10
	IL-9	IL-2	
	IL-25	IL-3	
		IL-10	
		IL-13	

therapeutic agents in asthma. No studies of IL-1 antagonists have been performed in human asthmatics. However, IL-1ra has been shown to eliminate the late phase response in a guinea pig model of asthma.[15]

IV. Immune Deviation: Stimulation of Th1-Like Responses

Subclasses of T helper lymphocytes have been characterized on the basis of their repertoires of cytokines (Table 21.1).[16] Naive Th0 cells produce primarily IL-2 but may also synthesize cytokines characteristic of both Th1 and Th2 lymphocytes. In humans, type 1 helper cells produce interferon (IFN)-γ and TNF-β but not IL-4 and IL-5. Type 2 helper cells produce IL-4, IL-5, IL-9, and IL-25 but not IFN-γ or TNF-β. Both classes produce GM-CSF, TNF-α, IL-2, IL-3, IL-10, and IL-13.

Although distinct Th1 and Th2 cytokine profiles may not be apparent in human cells, there remains an inverse relationship between the tendency of T lymphocytes to produce IFN-γ as opposed to IL-4 or IL-5. Type 1 T helper lymphocytes activate T cells and monocytes, promote cell-mediated immune responses, and are important in antibody-dependent immunity. Type 2 T helper lymphocytes that produce IL-4, IL-5, and IL-13 and function in the relative absence of IFN-γ induce allergic immune responses. A third class of T helper lymphocytes termed T regulatory (Tr1) lymphocytes[17] are characterized by their production of the immunosuppressive cytokines TGF-β and IL-10 and may be important in actively preventing or terminating immune responses.

The use of immune modulators capable of stimulating immune deviation from Th2 to Th1 responses has been proposed as a therapeutic modality in asthma. This is based on the reported observations that nonatopic individuals generate Th1-like responses to allergens and immunotherapy functions to convert Th2- into Th1-like responses.[18,19] However, functional Th1 responses stimulate the recruitment and activation of mononuclear phagocytes and are associated with cellular immunity and granuloma formation — features not present in healthy subjects or in subjects who have successfully responded to immunotherapy. If present *in vivo*, these Th1-like cells must, therefore, be present in a milieu that prevents cellular inflammation from developing. The absence of inflammation in normal subjects is maintained by influences that promote the development of tolerance.

The cytokine milieu of the nonasthmatic respiratory tract is characterized by elevated concentrations of IL-10 and TGF-β that, as will be discussed later, may help mitigate inflammatory responses. Immunotherapy and CpG peptide therapies are associated with the generation of IL-10-producing T regulatory lymphocytes, and these may serve to prevent the development of cellular inflammation that could otherwise be associated with immune deviation toward Th1-like lymphocytes.[20,21] Th1-like lymphocytes also induce humoral immune responses; Th2-to-Th1 immune deviations that promote humoral antibody and not cellular immune responses to allergens are also not likely to be harmful.

Th1 differentiation is mediated by IL-12, IL-18, and IL-23.[22] Insofar as mononuclear phagocytes are the major sources of IL-12, this suggests a mechanism whereby antigens more likely to be processed by macrophages, including bacterial antigens and intracellular parasites, produce Th1 responses. In addition, innate immune reactions mediated through pattern recognition receptors such as TLRs are important stimuli of these Th1 immune deviating responses. For example, in addition to the actions of LPSs on TLR4, an important stimulus for Th1 immune deviation is the use of CpG-containing immune stimulatory DNA sequences that function through their ability to interact with TLR9. Similar to IL-12, IL-18 also induces the differentiation of Th1-like cells and IL-18 is a growth factor for these cells. IL-18 receptor expression is up-regulated by IL-12, and thereby, these two cytokines synergize to stimulate IFN-γ release.

IL-23 is a heterodimer that uses one protein of the IL-12 heterodimer and is homologous to the other subunit of IL-12. IL-23 uses the IL-12Rβ1 chain for its receptor. It is a potent inducer of IFN-γ and is therefore also likely to contribute to Th1 differentiation. In addition to CpG sequences discussed elsewhere in this volume, several cytokines associated with Th1 immunity have been proposed as therapeutic agents in asthma.

A. Interferon-γ

IFN-γ is primarily made by T cells and natural killer cells and is the most important cytokine responsible for cell-mediated immunity.[23] IFN-γ stimulates antigen presentation and cytokine production by monocytes and also stimulates monocyte effector functions, including adherence, phagocytosis, secretion, the respiratory burst, and nitric oxide production. The net result is the accumulation of monocytes at the sites of cellular immune responses, with their activation into macrophages capable of killing intracellular pathogens.

In addition to its effects on mononuclear phagocytes, IFN-γ stimulates killing by NK cells and neutrophils. It stimulates adherence of granulocytes to endothelial cells through the induction of ICAM-1, an activity shared with IL-1 and TNF. IFN-γ functions as an inhibitor of allergic responses through its capacity to inhibit IL-4-mediated expression of low-affinity IgE receptors and the isotype switch to IgE. The pro-inflammatory potency of IFN-γ precludes its usefulness in allergic airway disease. In murine models, the infusion of IFN-γ-producing T lymphocytes is associated with exacerbations of asthmatic inflammation.

Nebulized IFN-γ did not produce clinical benefit or reduce eosinophilic inflammation in asthmatic subjects.[24] Even so, IFN-γ may have a role in the treatment of atopic dermatitis. This condition is characterized by a mild immunodeficiency with diminished phagocytic cell function, and therefore, stimulation of mononuclear phagocytes and neutrophils along with the neutralization of IL-4 justifies the therapeutic use of IFN-γ. Clinical studies with IFN-γ have established its usefulness in both lowering serum IgE concentrations and mitigating the severity of the atopic dermatitis.

B. Interleukin-12

IL-12 is primarily derived from mononuclear phagocytic cells and dendritic cells.[25] The biologically active form is a heterodimer consisting of a larger subunit that is homologous to the soluble receptor for IL-6 and a smaller subunit that is homologous to IL-6. IL-12 activates and induces proliferation, cytotoxicity, and cytokine production of NK cells. Other activities attributed to IL-12 include proliferation of T helper and cytotoxic lymphocytes.

The ability of IL-12 to inhibit the differentiation of Th2-like cells forms the basis for its proposed utility in asthma. In murine models of asthma, administration of IL-12 inhibited bronchial hyperreactivity, bronchoalveolar lavage (BAL), and tissue eosinophilia and reduced specific IgE concentrations.[26] Similarly, as might be predicted from their synergistic influences on Th1 immune deviation, co-administration of IL-12 and IL-18 was also effective in murine models of asthma.[27]

A trial of weekly administration of IL-12 to subjects with mild asthma, however, showed no effects on either the early or late phase response to allergen challenge and did not attenuate bronchial hyperreactivity.[28] However, evidence for an influence on immune deviation was shown by the ability of IL-12 therapy to reduce circulating and sputum eosinophils and Th2-associated cytokines. Unfortunately, IL-12 therapy elicited several adverse side effects including flu-like symptoms and transient elevations of hepatic transaminases. These effects raised some concerns regarding the ultimate utility of agents designed to potentiate Th1-like immune responses.

V. Inhibition of Th2 Cytokines

A. Interleukin-4

IL-4 has shown numerous activities critical to the development of asthma and allergic inflammation. IL-4 induces transcription of ε heavy chain transcripts leading to the immunoglobulin isotype switch from IgM to IgE.[29,30] It further contributes to IgE-mediated responses through its ability to up-regulate both low affinity IgE receptor (FcεRII, CD23) expression on B lymphocytes and monocytes and high affinity (FcεRI) receptor expression on mast cells. Another important activity of IL-4 in allergic inflammation is its ability to induce expression of VCAM-1. This produces enhanced adhesiveness of endothelium for T cells, eosinophils, basophils, and monocytes, but not neutrophils, as is characteristic of allergic reactions.[31] IL-4 receptors, but not IL-13 receptors, are present on mast cells where they function to induce expression of the LTC_4 synthase enzyme, thereby determining the capacities of mast cells to produce cysteinyl leuko-trienes.[32] IL-4 stimulates mucin production and contributes to the excessive mucus production in the asthmatic airways.

Probably the most important activity of IL-4 in asthma and allergies is derived from its ability to drive the initial differentiation of naïve Th0 lymphocytes toward a Th2 phenotype.[33] The original source of the IL-4 responsible for Th2 differentiation is unclear but is likely to be provided by the naïve Th0 lymphocytes themselves. IL-4 is also important in maintaining allergic immune responses by preventing apoptosis of T lymphocytes.[34] The production of IL-4 by Th2 lym-phocytes renders these cells refractory to the anti-inflammatory influences of corticosteroids. Functional IL-4 receptors are heterodimers consisting of the IL-4Rα chain interacting with the shared γ chain or the IL-13Rα1 chain.[35] The shared use of the IL-4Rα chain by IL-13 and IL-4 and the activation by this chain of the signaling protein Stat6 explain many of the common biological activities of these two cytokines (Table 21.2). However, in addition to mast cells, IL-13 receptors are not expressed on T lymphocytes, and IL-13 does not share the ability of IL-4 to induce Th2-like immune deviation.

Table 21.2 Biological Properties of IL-4 and IL-13

Property	IL-4	IL-13
Th2 induction	+	−
IgE switch	+	+
FcεRII (CD23)	+	+
FcεRI/LTC4 synthase induction	++	−
VCAM-1/eosinophil transmigration	+	+
Mucus production	+	++
Bronchial hyperresponsiveness	+	++
Subepithelial fibrosis	−	+

Table 21.3 Pharmacological Agents with IL-4 or IL-13 Inhibitory Activity

	Soluble human IL-4 receptor	IL-13 receptor: Fc fusion protein	IL-4 double mutein	IL-4/ IL-13 trap	Humanized anti-IL-4 antibody	Human anti-IL-4 receptor antibody
Inhibition of IL-4	Yes	No	Yes	Yes	Yes	Yes
Inhibition of IL-13	No	Yes	Yes	Yes	Yes	Yes
Half-life	5 days	1 week?	4 to 6 hours	5 days?	18 to 21 days	18 to 21 days
Route of administration	Inhaled	Systemic	Systemic	Systemic	Systemic	Systemic

IL-4 has been identified in sera, bronchoalveolar lavage fluids, and lung tissues of asthmatic subjects, and in nasal polyp tissues and the nasal mucosa of subjects with allergic rhinitis. Numerous agents have been developed to antagonize IL-4 as potential therapeutic agents in asthma (Table 21.3) including soluble IL-4 receptors (Immunex), a genetically engineered double soluble receptor ("trap") for both IL-4 and IL-13 (Regeneron), humanized anti-IL-4 antibodies (Protein Design Labs), an IL-4 mutein (Bayer), and human anti-IL-4 receptor antibodies (Immunex).

In two separate studies, soluble IL-4 receptors were shown to have clinical efficacy in asthma. In a phase I study, subjects with mild or moderate persistent asthma were withdrawn from inhaled corticosteroids and randomly assigned to receive placebo or soluble IL-4R by nebulizer.[36] Treatment with IL-4R was associated with significantly better FEV_1 and asthma symptom scores, and reduced β_2 agonist use. Exhaled nitric oxide scores were significantly improved among patients receiving IL-4R, consistent with an anti-inflammatory effect. In a phase I and II study, subjects with moderate persistent asthma discontinued inhaled corticosteroids and were randomized to 12 weekly nebulizations of IL-4R or placebo.[37] In the absence of inhaled corticosteroids, patients receiving IL-4R had stable FEV_1 values (–0.09 L, –2% predicted) compared with a significant decline observed in the placebo group (–0.35 L, –13% predicted).

Efficacy was demonstrated by a nearly stable daily FEV_1 measured at home by a hand-held device (–0.1 L, –4% predicted) compared with a significant decline in the placebo group (–0.5 L, –18% predicted). Unfortunately, two more recent studies did not demonstrate the clinical efficacy of soluble IL-4R in asthma. Nebulized soluble IL-4R may not adequately deliver therapy to bronchial-associated lymphatic tissues and therefore may not influence Th2-like lymphocyte differentiation or survival. It remains plausible, therefore, that systemic IL-4 antagonists such as the humanized anti-IL-4 antibody may still prove effective in asthma. A phase I trial of this agent demonstrated its safety in asthma; however, larger phase II studies failed to confirm efficacy.

B. Interleukin-13

IL-13 is homologous to IL-4 and shares many of its biologic activities (Table 21.2). Thus, IL-13 also induces the IgE isotype switch and VCAM-1 expression.[38] IL-13 receptors are heterodimers containing IL-4Rα chains and unique IL-13Rα chains. IL-13Rα expression is more limited than IL-4 receptors and includes endothelial cells, B cells, mononuclear phagocytes, and basophils, but not mast or T cells. This more limited distribution of IL-13Rα explains the unique ability of IL-4 to induce Th2 lymphocyte differentiation and mast cell activation. However, IL-13 is more widely produced than IL-4, including by Th1-like lymphocytes, and is more readily identified in allergic inflammatory tissue.[39]

In murine models, IL-13 seems more important than IL-4 in inducing the asthma phenotype insofar as mice over-expressing IL-13 demonstrate eosinophilic inflammation, mucus hypersecretion, airway fibrosis, and nonspecific airway hyperreactivity (AHR).[40] Arguably, IL-4 may be more important in inducing the asthmatic phenotype through its influences on Th2 lymphocyte differentiation, whereas IL-13 appears more important in maintaining the asthmatic state. In a murine model, soluble IL-13 receptors were effective in reducing bronchial hyperreactivity, pulmonary eosinophilia, and IgE production,[40] and these soluble receptors and other IL-13 antagonists are in clinical development for humans (Table 21.3).

C. Interleukin-5

IL-5 is the most important eosinophilopoietin, and mice transgenic for constitutive IL-5 expression develop eosinophilia.[41] In addition to stimulating eosinophil production, IL-5 is chemotactic for eosinophils and activates mature eosinophils, inducing eosinophil secretion and enhanced cytotoxicity. Another mechanism by which IL-5 promotes accumulation of eosinophils is through its ability to up-regulate αdβ2 integrins on eosinophils, thereby promoting their adherence to VCAM-1-expressing endothelial cells. IL-5 prolongs eosinophil survival by blocking apoptosis.[42]

A final important contribution of IL-5 to asthmatic inflammation is its ability to activate basophils. Administration of IL-5 to humans causes mucosal eosinophilia and an increase in bronchial hyperreactivity. IL-5 interacts with specific IL-5 receptors that consist of a heterodimer containing IL-5Rα and a β chain (CD131) shared with GM-CSFR and IL-3R.[43] All three of these cytokines contribute to the activity of eosinophils in allergic inflammation through their capacities to prolong eosinophil survival and activate mature eosinophils. Therapeutic agents directed against their shared β chain may be particularly potent inhibitors of eosinophilic inflammation.

A role for anti-IL-5 therapy in asthma is supported by the capacity of this antibody to prevent the development of airway hyperreactivity and eosinophil inflammation in a guinea pig model of asthma.[44] However, human trials with two different humanized anti-interleukin-5 antibodies have been disappointing. A single intravenous injection of a humanized monoclonal anti-IL-5 antibody in moderate asthma significantly reduced sputum and blood eosinophilia but had no effect on either the late asthmatic response to an allergen challenge or bronchial hyperreactivity.[45] Similar results have been observed in subsequent studies including those of longer duration. Lung biopsy studies have shown that anti-IL-5 (mepolizumab) was associated with only a 55% reduction of lung tissue eosinophils and no reduction in staining for major basic protein. This failure to eradicate eosinophils adequately from the lungs may have been the basis for the disappointing clinical results.[46]

Residual eosinophilia may relate to constitutive IL-5-independent eosinophil production by the bone marrow, the local differentiation of eosinophils from tissue precursors in the airways, or to the differentiation of lung eosinophils from IL-5 to GM-CSF dependence. Further studies of IL-5 antagonism addressing the ability of this agent to synergize either with GM-CSF antagonists or chemokines or adhesion molecule antagonists that might block eosinophil trafficking into the asthmatic lung are therefore warranted.

D. Interleukin-9

IL-9 was originally described as a mast cell growth factor[47] and contributes to mast cell–mediated allergic responses through its ability to stimulate the production of mast cell proteases and IgE high affinity receptor α chains. IL-9 is derived from eosinophils, mast cells, and Th2-like lymphocytes, and it supports the growth and survival of antigen-specific T lymphocytes. Its selective production by Th2 cells suggests a role in allergic inflammation and, in human T lymphocytes, this is a feature shared only with IL-4, IL-5, and IL-25. IL-9 has other important activities in allergic inflammation including inducing expression of CCL11 (eotaxin), IL-5 receptors, and chemokine receptor 4. It synergizes with IL-4 to enhance the production of IgE and with IL-5 to enhance the production of eosinophils. Anti-IL-9 antibodies inhibit eosinophilia, Th2 cytokine production, and airway hyperreactivity in murine models of asthma.[48]

E. Chemokines

Chemokines are a group of small molecules able to induce chemotaxis of a variety of cells including neutrophils, monocytes, lymphocytes, eosinophils, basophils, and fibroblasts. These molecules mediate their activities through interactions with members of the seven-transmembrane, G protein-coupled receptor superfamily. To date, 47 chemokines and 18 chemokine receptors have been described. Many of the chemokine receptors can bind more than one ligand, allowing extensive overlap and redundancy of chemokine function.

The chemokines recruit and activate leukocytes to mount immune responses and initiate wound healing. While chemotaxis stands as the hallmark feature of chemokines, their physiological role is more complex than originally described. Other functions of chemokines include lymphocyte trafficking, endothelial cell adhesion, hematopoiesis, antigen processing in lymphoid tissue, and immune surveillance.[49] The carefully ordered expression of chemokines is essential to the function and appropriate structural development of immune tissue. For example, chemokines are necessary in lymph nodes for their architectural arrangement and interactions of B, T, and dendritic cells in their appropriate regions.

The chemokines can be subdivided into four families based on the positioning of their N terminal cysteine residues. The CXC subfamily (CXCL1 through CXCL16) is characterized by the separation of the first two cysteines by a variable amino acid. In the CC subfamily (CC1 through CC28), the cysteine residues are adjacent to each other. In addition, these groups may be distinguished by their primary target cells. The CXC subfamily primarily targets neutrophils and the CC family targets monocytes, T cells, and eosinophils. Most of the known chemokines are contained in these two families.

Chemokines have important roles specific to the development of allergic inflammation and asthma. CCL3 (MIP-1α), CCL5 (RANTES), CCL7 (MCP-3), CCL11 (eotaxin-1), CCL24 (eotaxin-2), and CCL26 (eotaxin-3) contribute to eosinophil recruitment and activation. Unlike other eosinophil chemoattractants such as LTB$_4$, platelet-activating factor, and C5a, these chemokines are more selective for eosinophils. Injection with CCL5 or CCL11 results in an eosinophilic and mononuclear cell infiltrate in the absence of neutrophils. CCL5 and CCL11 acting in synergy with IL-5 are the most important eosinophil chemoattractants in allergic inflammation.[50]

In addition to eosinophils, macrophages, mast cells, and T cells, CCL11 production has been described in structural cells of the airway including airway smooth muscles and fibroblasts. Several chemokines, including CCL2 (MCP-1), CCL3 (MIP-1α), CCL5 (RANTES), CCL7 (MCP-3), and CCL13 (MCP-4), may contribute to the allergic response by inducing recruitment and histamine release from basophils. Chemokines are also relevant to allergic inflammation through their effects on T cell differentiation and cytokine secretion. Th1-like lymphocytes tend to express CCR5 and CXCR3 receptors, whereas Th2-like lymphocytes are more characterized by their expression of CCR3, CCR4, and CCR8.

Functioning through the CCR5 receptor, CCL3 (MIP-1α), CCL4 (MIP-1β), and CCL5 (RANTES) or through the CXCR3 receptor, CXCL9 (Mig), CXCL10 (IP-10), and CXCL11 (I-TAC) can promote the development of IFN-γ–producing Th1-like cells. In contrast, CCL1 (I-309) interacting with CCR8, CCL7 (MCP-3), CCL8 (MCP-2), CCL11 (eotaxin-1), CCL13 (MCP-4), CCL24 (eotaxin-2), and CCL26 (eotaxin-3) interacting with CCR3 or CCL17 (TARC) and CCL22 (MDC) interacting with CCR4 can all contribute to a Th2-like phenotype.[51] IL-4 and IL-13 stimulate CCL17 (TARC) expression, thereby promoting Th2 responses.[52] Up-regulated CCL17 (TARC) has been described in allergic inflammation.

Increased levels of the chemokines CCL2 (MCP-1), CCL3 (MIP-1α), CCL5 (RANTES), CCL7 (MCP-3), CCL11 (eotaxin-1), CCL13 (MCP-4), CCL24 (eotaxin-2), CXCL8 (IL-8), and CXCL10 (IP-10) have been demonstrated in bronchoalveolar lavage and biopsy samples of asthmatics.[53] In murine models of asthma, CCL2 (MCP-1), CCL5 (RANTES), CCL11 (eotaxin-1), CXCL10 (IP-10), and CXCL12 (SDF-1α/β) all contribute to AHR and inflammation.

Several compounds are currently in development to antagonize chemokine receptor function. However, while the current focus has been to develop antagonists for specific receptors, the pleiotropy of the chemokines and their receptors may necessitate the use of multiple antagonists targeting multiple receptors in order to achieve full inhibition of function.

Instillation of CCL2 (MCP-1) in the lungs of mice induced prolonged AHR associated with mast cell degranulation. Neutralization of CCL2 blocked the development of AHR in response to antigen. Several potential antagonists to CCL2 or its receptor (CCR2) are currently being developed.[54] Probably the most intriguing target in asthma is the CCR3 receptor. Many of the chemokines implicated in the asthmatic response including CCL5 (RANTES), CCL7 (MCP-3), CCL8 (MCP-2), CCL11 (eotaxin-1), CCL13 (MCP-4), CCL24 (eotaxin-2), and CCL26 (eotaxin-3) function through the CCR3 receptor. Both CCR3 and CCL11 are over-expressed in asthmatics and correlate with disease severity.[55]

Using a mouse model, a neutralizing antibody to CCL11 reduced eosinophil recruitment into the lung after allergen challenge and reduced associated AHR.[56] Both a nonpeptide antagonist of CCR3 (SB-328437) and an amino piperidine derivative of CCL11 (UCB-35625) also blocked eosinophil recruitment in allergen models of asthma and are currently undergoing clinical trials.[57] A different CCR3 antagonist in development (F-1322) also inhibits thromboxane A_2 synthase and 5-lipoxygenase and is a histamine antagonist. *In vitro*, F-1322 inhibited CCL11-induced chemotaxis of eosinophils, and *in vivo* it suppressed eosinophil migration into airways in response to IL-5 and CCL11 infusion in guinea pigs.[58]

VI. Anti-Inflammatory Cytokines

Anti-inflammatory cytokines include TGF-β, IL-10, and as previously discussed, IL-1ra. The T helper lymphocyte that primarily produces TGF-β and IL-10 has been proposed to represent a distinct family of regulatory T cells (Tregs) including the T repressor (Tr1) or type 3 T helper (Th3) cell. TGF-β represents a family of peptides that regulate cell growth and have both stimulatory and inhibitory effects on different cell types.[59] TGF-β is an important stimulant of fibrosis and promotes wound healing and scar formation. In immunity, it inhibits B lymphocytes, T helper lymphocytes, and cytotoxicity of mononuclear phagocytes, CD8 T cells, and NK cells. TGF-β is constitutively produced in the healthy lung and may contribute to the maintenance of immune nonresponsiveness to otherwise benign inhaled bioaerosols and allergens. TGF-β may lessen allergic inflammation through a capacity to inhibit IgE synthesis and mast cell proliferation. In contrast to these anti-inflammatory effects, TGF-β is a chemoattractant for macrophages and supports the α isotype switch to IgA by B cells.[60] In allergic inflammation, the expression of TGF-β may be associated with the fibrosis observed in asthma. The too numerous pleiotropic activities of TGF-β preclude its consideration as a target for pharmacologic manipulation in asthma.

A. Interleukin-10

Although produced by both Th1- and Th2-like lymphocytes, the regulatory T lymphocytes are the primary source of IL-10. IL-10 inhibits production of IFN-γ and IL-2 by Th1 lymphocytes; IL-4 and IL-5 by Th2 lymphocytes[61]; IL-1β, IL-6, IL-8, IL-12, and TNF-α by mononuclear phagocytes; and IFN-γ and TNF-α by NK cells. In addition, IL-10 inhibits monocyte MHC class II, CD23, ICAM-1, iNOS, and B7 expression. Inhibition of B7 expression results in the inability of the APC to provide the accessory signal necessary for T helper activation.[62] This inhibition of accessory function is primarily responsible for the inhibition of Th1 and Th2 cytokine production.

Constitutive expression of IL-10 by APC and regulatory Tregs in the respiratory tract of normal subjects has a critical role in the induction and maintenance of tolerance to allergens and otherwise benign bioaerosols. In contrast, asthma and allergic rhinitis are associated with diminished IL-10 expression in the allergic airway that contributes to the development of an inflammatory milieu.[63,64] Support for a modulating role for IL-10 in human allergic disease is further derived from observations that IL-10 inhibits eosinophil survival and IL-4-induced IgE synthesis.

In murine studies, the administration of IL-10 is associated with diminished eosinophilic inflammation, mediated in part by inhibition of IL-5 expression.[65] The concept that IL-10 may be useful in humans is supported by observations that virtually all therapies currently in use to treat allergies and asthma are associated with increased production of IL-10 including theophylline,[66] leukotriene modifiers,[67] and corticosteroids.[68] In addition, immunotherapy is associated with dramatic up-regulation of IL-10.[20,69] *In vitro*, the addition of neutralizing anti-IL-10 antibodies to T lymphocytes rendered tolerant to allergen during a course of immunotherapy was associated with restoration of their ability to proliferate and secrete cytokines.[20] Similarly, the efficacy of CpG-containing

DNA immunostimulatory sequences has recently been shown to stimulate IL-10 production.[21] This IL-10 may serve both to suppress allergic inflammation and to ameliorate the potential for pro-inflammatory effects that might otherwise be associated with induction of Th1-like allergen-specific lymphocytes.

VII. Summary

Numerous facets of the asthmatic phenotype are mediated by cytokines, and manipulation of cytokines has exciting therapeutic potential for this disorder. Several cytokine antagonists such as soluble TNF receptors and anti-TNF antibodies have established their efficacy in the treatment of immune inflammatory diseases, and studies are in progress to extend these observations to asthma. Similarly, Th2-to-Th1 immune deviation may form an important basis for the efficacy of immunotherapy, and the ability to accomplish this objective with either Th1-inducing cytokines or stimulants of innate immunity such as CpG oligonucleotides has obvious potential in asthma. Finally, numerous cytokine antagonists, including those directed against IL-4, IL-5, IL-9, IL-13, and chemokines such as CCL11 (eotaxin) are being evaluated in asthma.

The record to date of single cytokine antagonists in asthma trials has been disappointing. This may reflect the sheer number of cytokines involved in producing asthma and the tremendous redundancy of the cytokine network. Several agents currently used in the treatment of asthma and other atopic disorders such as corticosteroids and calcineurin inhibitors use cytokine inhibition as one of the more important mechanisms for their efficacy. These agents are effective, however, because of their ability to block numerous cytokines. Arguably, therefore, it may become essential to use several cytokine antagonists to optimize their synergistic influences. For example, inhibition of eosinophilopoiesis with an IL-5 antagonist may need to synergize with an antagonist of eosinophil trafficking such as a CCL11/CCR3 or VCAM-1 inhibitor. Blockage of IL-4's induction of the asthmatic phenotype may synergize with blocking IL-13's effects on maintaining that phenotype. Multidrug therapy has become the mainstay of the treatment of complex disorders such as neoplasia and infectious diseases such as tuberculosis and HIV, and it is plausible that such approaches will similarly be required for asthma.

References

1. Maini RN, Breedveld FC, Kalden JR et al. Therapeutic efficacy of multiple intravenous infusions of anti-tumor necrosis factor alpha monoclonal antibody combined with low-dose weekly methotrexate in rheumatoid arthritis. *Arthritis Rheum* 1998; 41: 1552–1563.

2. Milgrom H, Fick RB, Jr, Su JQ et al. Treatment of allergic asthma with monoclonal anti-IgE antibody. *New Engl J Med* 1999; 341: 1966–1973.

3. Weinblatt ME, Kremer JM, Bankhurst AD et al. A trial of etanercept, a recombinant tumor necrosis factor receptor:Fc fusion protein, in patients with rheumatoid arthritis receiving methotrexate. *New Engl J Med* 1999; 340: 253–259.

4. Underwood DC, Osborn RR, Kotzer CJ et al. SB 239063, a potent p38 MAP kinase inhibitor, reduces inflammatory cytokine production, airways eosinophil infiltration, and persistence. *J Pharmacol Exp Ther* 2000; 293: 281–288.

5. Wong CK, Zhang JP, Ip WK, and Lam CW. Activation of p38 mitogen-activated protein kinase and nuclear factor kappa-B in tumour necrosis factor-induced eotaxin release of human eosinophils. *Clin Exp Immunol* 2002; 128: 483–489.

6. Beutler B and Cerami A. The biology of cachectin/TNF: a primary mediator of the host response. *Annu Rev Immunol* 1989; 7: 625–655.

7. Perez C, Albert I, DeFay K, Zachariades N, Gooding L, and Kriegler M. A non-secretable cell surface mutant of tumor necrosis factor (TNF) kills by cell-to-cell contact. *Cell* 1990; 63: 251–258.

8. Tartaglia LA and Goeddel DV. Two TNF receptors. *Immunol Today* 1992; 13: 151–153.

9. Obase Y, Shimoda T, Mitsuta K, Matsuo N, Matsuse H, and Kohno S. Correlation between airway hyperresponsiveness and airway inflammation in a young adult population: eosinophil, ECP, and cytokine levels in induced sputum. *Ann Allergy Asthma Immunol* 2001; 86: 304–310.

10. Babu S, Hasan A, Bell E et al. Etanercept for the treatment of patients with chronic severe asthma. *Chest* 2002; 122: S179.

11. Arend WP. Interleukin-1 receptor antagonist. *Adv Immunol* 1993; 54: 167–227.

12. Dinarello CA and Wolff SM. The role of interleukin-1 in disease. *New Engl J Med* 1993; 328: 106–113.

13. Sims JE, Gayle MA, Slack JL et al. Interleukin 1 signaling occurs exclusively via the type I receptor. *Proc Natl Acad Sci USA* 1993; 90: 6155–6159.

14. Borish L, Mascali JJ, Dishuck J, Beam WR, Martin RJ, and Rosenwasser LJ. Detection of alveolar macrophage-derived IL-1 beta in asthma. Inhibition with corticosteroids. *J Immunol* 1992; 149: 3078–3082.

15. Okada S, Inoue H, Yamauchi K et al. Potential role of interleukin-1 in allergen-induced late asthmatic reactions in guinea pigs: suppressive effect of interleukin-1 receptor antagonist on late asthmatic reaction. *J Allergy Clin Immunol* 1995; 95: 1236–1245.

16. Mosmann TR and Coffman RL. TH1 and TH2 cells: different patterns of lympho-kine secretion lead to different functional properties. *Annu Rev Immunol* 1989; 7: 145–173.

17. Sakaguchi S. Regulatory T cells: key controllers of immunologic self-tolerance. *Cell* 2000; 101: 455–458.

18. Wierenga EA, Snoek M, de Groot C et al. Evidence for compartmentalization of functional subsets of CD2+ T lymphocytes in atopic patients. *J Immunol* 1990; 144: 4651–4666.

19. Hamid QA, Schotman E, Jacobson MR, Walker SM, and Durham SR. Increases in IL-12 messenger RNA+ cells accompany inhibition of allergen-induced late skin responses after successful grass pollen immunotherapy. *J Allergy Clin Immunol* 1997; 99: 254–260.

20. Akdis CA, Blesken T, Akdis M, Wuthrich B, and Blaser K. Role of interleukin 10 in specific immunotherapy. *J Clin Invest* 1998; 102: 98–106.
21. Yi AK, Yoon JG, Yeo SJ, Hong SC, English BK, and Krieg AM. Role of mitogen-activated protein kinases in CpG DNA-mediated IL-10 and IL-12 production: central role of extracellular signal-regulated kinase in the negative feedback loop of the CpG DNA-mediated Th1 response. *J Immunol* 2002; 168: 4711–4720.
22. Manetti R, Parronchi P, Giudizi MG et al. Natural killer cell stimulatory factor (interleukin 12 [IL-12]) induces T helper type 1 (Th1)-specific immune responses and inhibits the development of IL-4-producing Th cells. *J Exp Med* 1993; 177: 1199–1204.
23. Farrar MA and Schreiber RD. The molecular cell biology of interferon-gamma and its receptor. *Annu Rev Immunol* 1993; 11: 571–611.
24. Boguniewicz M, Martin RJ, Martin D et al. The effects of nebulized recombinant interferon-gamma in asthmatic airways. *J Allergy Clin Immunol* 1995; 95: 133–135.
25. Brunda MJ. Interleukin-12. *J Leukoc Biol* 1994; 55: 280–288.
26. Gavett SH, O'Hearn DJ, Li X, Huang SK, Finkelman FD, and Wills-Karp M. Interleukin 12 inhibits antigen-induced airway hyperresponsiveness, inflammation, and Th2 cytokine expression in mice. *J Exp Med* 1995; 182: 1527–1536.
27. Hofstra CL, Van Ark I, Hofman G, Kool M, Nijkamp FP, and Van Oosterhout AJ. Prevention of Th2-like cell responses by coadministration of IL-12 and IL-18 is associated with inhibition of antigen-induced airway hyperresponsiveness, eosinophilia, and serum IgE levels. *J Immunol* 1998; 161: 5054–5060.
28. Bryan SA, O'Connor BJ, Matti S et al. Effects of recombinant human interleukin-12 on eosinophils, airway hyper-responsiveness, and the late asthmatic response. *Lancet* 2000; 356: 2149–2153.
29. Coffman RL, Ohara J, Bond MW, Carty J, Zlotnik A, and Paul WE. B cell stimulatory factor-1 enhances the IgE response of lipopolysaccharide-activated B cells. *J Immunol* 1986; 136: 4538–4541.
30. Romagnani S. Regulation and deregulation of human IgE synthesis. *Immunol Today* 1990; 11: 316–321.
31. Schleimer RP, Sterbinsky SA, Kaiser J et al. IL-4 induces adherence of human eosinophils and basophils but not neutrophils to endothelium: association with expression of VCAM-1. *J Immunol* 1992; 148: 1086–1092.
32. Hsieh FH, Lam BK, Penrose JF, Austen KF, and Boyce JA. T helper cell type 2 cytokines coordinately regulate immunoglobulin E-dependent cysteinyl leukotriene production by human cord blood-derived mast cells: profound induction of leukotriene C(4) synthase expression by interleukin-4. *J Exp Med* 2001; 193: 123–133.
33. Seder RA, Paul WE, Davis MM, and Fazekas de St. Groth B. The presence of interleukin-4 during *in vitro* priming determines the lymphokine-producing potential of CD4+ T cells from T cell receptor transgenic mice. *J Exp Med* 1992; 176: 1091–1098.
34. Vella A, Teague TK, Ihle J, Kappler J, and Marrack P. Interleukin 4 (IL-4) or IL-7 prevents death of resting T cells: Stat-6 is probably not required for the effect of IL-4. *J Exp Med* 1997; 186: 325–330.
35. Izuhara K and Shirakawa T. Signal transduction via the interleukin-4 receptor and its correlation with atopy. *Int. J Mol Med* 1999; 3: 3–10.

36. Borish L, Nelson H, Lanz M et al. Interleukin-4 receptor in moderate atopic asthma, a phase I/II randomized, placebo-controlled trial. *Am J Respir Crit Care Med* 1999; 160: 1816–1823.
37. Borish LC, Nelson HS, Corren J et al. Efficacy of soluble IL-4 receptor for the treatment of adults with asthma. *J Allergy Clin Immunol* 2001; 107: 963–970.
38. Zurawski G and de Vries JE. Interleukin 13, an interleukin 4-like cytokine that acts on monocytes and B cells, but not on T cells. *Immunol Today* 1994; 15: 19–26.
39. Zhu Z, Homer RJ, Wang Z et al. Pulmonary expression of interleukin-13 causes inflammation, mucus hypersecretion, subepithelial fibrosis, physiologic abnormalities, and eotaxin production. *J Clin Invest* 1999; 103: 779–788.
40. Wills-Karp M, Luyimbazi J, Xu X et al. Interleukin-13: central mediator of allergic asthma. *Science* 1998; 282: 2258–2261.
41. Clutterbuck EJ, Hirst EM, and Sanderson CJ. Human interleukin-5 (IL-5) regulates the production of eosinophils in human bone marrow cultures: comparison and interaction with IL-1, IL-3, IL-6, and GMCSF. *Blood* 1989; 73: 1504–1512.
42. Rothenberg ME, Petersen J, Stevens RL et al. IL-5-dependent conversion of nor-modense human eosinophils to the hypodense phenotype uses 3T3 fibroblasts for enhanced viability, accelerated hypodensity, and sustained antibody-dependent cytotoxicity. *J Immunol* 1989; 143: 2311–2316.
43. Kitamura T, Sato N, Arai K, and Miyajima A. Expression cloning of the human IL-3 receptor cDNA reveals a shared beta subunit for the human IL-3 and GM-CSF receptors. *Cell* 1991; 66: 1165–1174.
44. Mauser PJ, Pitman A, Witt A et al. Inhibitory effect of the TRFK-5 anti-IL-5 antibody in a guinea pig model of asthma. *Am Rev Respir Dis* 1993; 148: 1623–1627.
45. Leckie MJ, ten Brinke A, Khan J et al. Effects of an interleukin-5 blocking monoclonal antibody on eosinophils, airway hyper-responsiveness, and the late asthmatic response. *Lancet* 2000; 356: 2144–2148.
46. Flood-Page PT, Menzies-Gow AN, Kay AB, and Robinson DS. Eosinophil's role remains uncertain as anti-interleukin-5 only partially depletes numbers in asthmatic airway. *Am J Respir Crit Care Med* 2003; 167: 199–204.
47. Hultner L, Druez C, Moeller J et al. Mast cell growth-enhancing activity (MEA) is structurally related and functionally identical to the novel mouse T cell growth factor P40/TCGFIII (interleukin-9). *Eur J Immunol* 1990; 20: 1413–1416.
48. Cheng G, Arima M, Honda K et al. Anti-interleukin-9 antibody treatment inhibits airway inflammation and hyperreactivity in mouse asthma model. *Am J Respir Crit Care Med* 2002; 166: 409–416.
49. Moser B and Loetscher P. Lymphocyte traffic control by chemokines. *Nat Immunol* 2001; 2: 123–128.
50. Venge J, Lampinen M, Hakansson L, Rak S, and Venge P. Identification of IL-5 and RANTES as the major eosinophil chemoattractants in the asthmatic lung. *J Allergy Clin Immunol* 1996; 97: 1110–1115.
51. Luther SA and Cyster JG. Chemokines as regulators of T cell differentiation. *Nat Immunol* 2001; 2:102–107.
52. Terada N, Nomura T, Kim WJ et al. Expression of C-C chemokine TARC in human nasal mucosa and its regulation by cytokines. *Clin Exp Allergy* 2001; 31: 1923–1931.

53. Miotto D, Christodoulopoulos P, Olivenstein R et al. Expression of IFN-gamma-inducible protein; monocyte chemotactic proteins 1, 3, and 4; and eotaxin in TH1- and TH2-mediated lung diseases. *J Allergy Clin Immunol* 2001; 107: 664–670.

54. Witherington J, Bordas V, Cooper DG et al. Conformationally restricted indolopiperidine derivatives as potent CCR2B receptor antagonists. *Bioorg Med Chem Lett* 2001; 11: 2177–2180.

55. Ying S, Robinson DS, Meng Q et al. Enhanced expression of eotaxin and CCR3 mRNA and protein in atopic asthma: association with airway hyperresponsiveness and predominant co-localization of eotaxin mRNA to bronchial epithelial and endothelial cells. *Eur J Immunol* 1997; 27: 3507–3516.

56. Gonzalo JA, Lloyd CM, Wen D et al. The coordinated action of CC chemokines in the lung orchestrates allergic inflammation and airway hyperresponsiveness. *J Exp Med* 1998; 188: 157–167.

57. White JR, Lee JM, Dede K et al. Identification of potent, selective non-peptide CC chemokine receptor-3 antagonist that inhibits eotaxin-, eotaxin-2-, and monocyte chemotactic protein-4-induced eosinophil migration. *J Biol Chem* 2000; 275: 36626–36631.

58. Mochizuki A, Tamura N, Yatabe Y et al. Suppressive effects of F-1322 on the antigen-induced late asthmatic response and pulmonary eosinophilia in guinea pigs. *Eur J Pharmacol* 2001; 430: 123–133.

59. Sporn MB and Roberts AB. Transforming growth factor-beta: recent progress and new challenges. *J Cell Biol* 1992; 119: 1017–1021.

60. Sonoda E, Matsumoto R, Hitoshi Y et al. Transforming growth factor beta induces IgA production and acts additively with interleukin 5 for IgA production. *J Exp Med* 1989; 170: 1415–1420.

61. Del Prete G, De Carli M, Almerigogna F, Giudizi MG, Biagiotti R, and Romagnani S. Human IL-10 is produced by both type 1 helper (Th1) and type 2 helper (Th2) T cell clones and inhibits their antigen-specific proliferation and cytokine production. *J Immunol* 1993; 150: 353–360.

62. Ding L, Linsley PS, Huang LY, Germain RN, and Shevach EM. IL-10 inhibits macrophage costimulatory activity by selectively inhibiting the up-regulation of B7 expression. *J Immunol* 1993; 151: 1224–1234.

63. Borish L, Aarons A, Rumbyrt J, Cvietusa P, Negri J, and Wenzel S. Interleukin-10 regulation in normal subjects and patients with asthma. *J Allergy Clin Immunol* 1996; 97: 1288–1296.

64. Borish L. IL-10: evolving concepts. *J Allergy Clin Immunol* 1998; 101: 293–297.

65. Zuany-Amorim C, Creminon C, Nevers MC, Nahori MA, Vargaftig BB, and Pretolani M. Modulation by IL-10 of antigen-induced IL-5 generation, and CD4+ T lymphocyte and eosinophil infiltration into the mouse peritoneal cavity. *J Immunol* 1996; 157: 377–384.

66. Mascali JJ, Cvietusa P, Negri J, and Borish L. Anti-inflammatory effects of theophylline: modulation of cytokine production. *Ann Allergy Asthma Immunol* 1996; 77: 34–38.

67. Stelmach I, Jerzynska J, and Kuna P. A randomized, double-blind trial of the effect of glucocorticoid, antileukotriene and beta-agonist treatment on IL-10 serum levels in children with asthma. *Clin Exp Allergy* 2002; 32: 264–269.

68. John M, Lim S, Seybold J et al. Inhaled corticosteroids increase interleukin-10 but reduce macrophage inflammatory protein-1alpha, granulocyte-macrophage colony-stimulating factor, and interferon-gamma release from alveolar macrophages in asthma. *Am J Respir Crit Care Med* 1998; 157: 256–262.
69. Gaglani B, Borish L, Bartelson BL, Buchmeier A, Keller L, and Nelson HS. Nasal immunotherapy in weed-induced allergic rhinitis. *Ann Allergy Asthma Immunol* 1997; 79: 259–265.

22

IgE and Anti-IgE Therapy in Allergic Asthma and Rhinitis

E.M. SALAGEAN, P.H. HOWARTH, and S.T. HOLGATE

University of Southampton School of Medicine
and Southampton General Hospital
Southampton, U.K.

I. Introduction

The first description of an immediate allergic reaction probably appeared 5000 years ago when King Menes, who then ruled Egypt, was described in 3000 B.C. as dying from a hornet sting.[1] Between 400 B.C. and 200 A.D., the writings of Greek physicians such as Hippocrates, Aretaeus, and Galen described individuals who suffered sudden attacks of shortness of breath that the physicians called asthma. The link between a reaction to environmental exposure and asthma was implicated in 1552, when Dr. Carden, an Italian physician, cured the archbishop of St. Andrew's of asthma by getting rid of the archbishop's feather quilt and pillows. Later, during the 17th century, German authors described weakness, fainting, and asthma in subjects exposed to cats, mice, dogs, and horses.

The mechanistic nature of this environmental link to asthma was undefined until 1906 when Von Pirquet introduced *allergy* as a term meaning *changed reactivity* to describe the altered capacity of the body to react to foreign substances. The relationship between a serum factor and allergic disease was recognized in the early 1920s when Otto Carl W. Prausnitz and a colleague named Heinz Küstner identified a *reagin*. They took serum from Küstner, who was allergic to fish, and injected it into the skin of Prausnitz. When the fish antigen was subsequently injected into the sensitized site, an immediate wheal and flare reaction occurred. This reaction (designated the P-K reaction based on the initials of the researchers' surnames) was the first scientific description of the mechanism of the allergic reaction that showed that a serum factor (reagin) could passively transfer hypersensitivity reactions from an allergic individual to the skin of a nonallergic patient.

It was another 45 years before the seminal work of the Ishizakas and their colleagues[1-4] and the independent work of Johansson and Bennich[5] noted that reagin consisted of a novel class of serum antibody designated immunoglobulin E (IgE). In 1966 Ishizaka's group in Denver reported an antiserum that could precipitate reagin, producing a decrease in its activity. Furthermore, the antiserum was shown to bond to both a mixture of reaginic serum and by autoradiography to an allergen trace-labeled with an isotope. This factor did not belong to any of the four known immunoglobulin classes and was, therefore, postulated to represent a new immunoglobulin provisionally called gamma-E-globulin. One reason for the name was that the factor, when injected into the skin, caused erythema.

Independently of this work and for other reasons, Bennich and Johansson of Uppsala, Sweden, detected an atypical myeloma protein found to share the physicochemical properties characteristic of reagin. They provisionally named the factor IgND and it could be detected in sera of healthy individuals. Patients with allergic asthma had, on average, six-fold higher concentrations of IgND than normal individuals.

In 1967, the two laboratories exchanged reagents and found that antiserum to gamma-E-globulin reacted with isolated ND protein and that purified ND protein could block the reaction of anti-gamma-E-globulin in a biological test system for reaginic activity. At a workshop in Lausanne in February 1968, in which the main researchers from the two groups participated, it was finally agreed that sufficient data on the structure and antigenicity of the material were available to allow the declaration of a new immunoglobulin[6] they named IgE (erythema globulin).

The observations that E myeloma protein when injected into monkeys could be detected on mast cells in the skin, omentum, small intestine, and bronchi, and that treatment of these tissues with ^{125}I-labeled anti-IgE resulted in binding of the antibody to mast cells linked IgE with mast cells. Although work in the late 1960s indicated that reaginic activity, through reactions with inflammatory cells, stimulated the release of various vasoactive mediators of importance in development of clinical symptoms and signs, only access to IgE allowed *in vitro* experimental, immunochemical studies to be undertaken to explore these considerations.

Further research indicated that the Fc fragment of the IgE molecule bound with high affinity to specific cell surface receptors (ScERs) present on both basophils and mast cells and that cross-linking of ScERs by allergen-IgE antibody complexes, aggregated IgE, or anti-IgE receptor antibodies induced histamine and SRS-A release. Thus, both immunological and physiological investigations of the mechanisms of anaphylaxis and allergy showed that, almost 100 years after their identification, mast cells are crucial to immediate allergic reactions.

Specific antisera to IgE became available, and in 1967, Johansson and Bennich, in collaboration with Wide of Uppsala, developed the radioallergosorbent test (RAST), an *in vitro* test for measurement of IgE antibodies to allergens.[7] RAST results showed a very good correlation of the presence of IgE antibody in serum and positive skin and provocation tests and symptoms of allergy.[8]

This finding suggested that immunological interventions intended to eliminate or decrease symptoms of atopic disease could be effective only if IgE sensitization was present. In the mid-1960s, the diagnosis of allergy was based primarily on intradermal skin tests using allergen extracts, and results were far from standardized. With the availability of IgE and the development of tests for IgE antibodies for the first time it became possible to analyze and standardize allergen preparations. In addition, the ability to measure IgE serum allowed the evaluation of IgE within populations and enabled better understanding of the relationship of IgE measurement and the clinical expressions of differing diseases.

II. Serum IgE and Epidemiology

Several population-based studies examined the distribution of serum IgE levels in the general population.[9–16] The overall geometric mean levels of IgE ranged from approximately 20 to 40 IU/ml with variations according to age, sex, and geographic distribution. Other studies have shown that geometric mean levels of serum IgE are typically lower in studies of nonallergic subjects when compared with mixed pools of allergic and nonallergic subjects.[9,10,17–23] Serum IgE levels are age-related, with peak levels occurring during childhood, usually between the ages of 8 to 12 years, and decreasing thereafter.[9,13,17,18,24–26] Serum IgE levels of adults are higher in men than in women[9,10,12,13,15,19,24,27] although differences by gender are not as well established as in younger populations.

Serum IgE may vary by ethnicity: serum IgE levels are higher in blacks than in whites,[17,18,25] and one study indicates that serum IgE levels are higher in North American Indians.[26] It is not clear whether differences among these racial and ethnic groups are due to genetic differences, differences in environmental exposure, or modulating factors such as increased exposures to infections, attacks of gastroenteritis, upper respiratory tract infections, and bronchopneumonia in infancy. Other studies demonstrated that smokers had higher IgE levels than nonsmokers,[12,19,28–30] but the relationship between smoking and IgE levels has not been established clearly.[29,31]

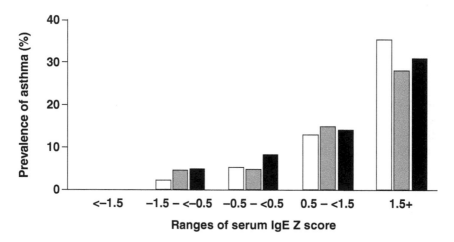

Figure 22.1 Increasing prevalence of asthma with increasing serum IgE Z scores. White bars = 6 to <35 years. Gray bars = 35 to <55 years. Black bars = 55+ years. Illustrating the increasing prevalence of asthma with increasing IgE Z scores irrespective of age. (From Burrows, B. et al., *New Engl J Med* 1989; 320: 271–277. With permission.)

On average, asthma patients have higher IgE levels than healthy controls,[11,17–19,22,32,33] but considerable overlap exists in the distribution of IgE among normal and asthmatic populations. In the Tucson Epidemiological Study, mean IgE levels were higher in all age groups of asthma patients when compared with individuals without asthma. Asthma was almost always associated with higher serum total IgE levels, thus challenging the concept that asthma has both allergic and nonallergic forms.[20] The higher the IgE, the greater the prevalence of asthma, regardless of age (Figure 22.1).

Studies of children with asthma confirm that serum IgE levels are higher (99–548 IU)[17,27,34] in those with asthma than in nonasthmatic children (16.2-51 IU).[9,17,35,36] Several studies found an association of serum IgE levels and bronchial responsiveness in both asymptomatic subjects and patients with histories of asthma.[24,34,37–41] In one study,[24] the relationship between bronchial responsiveness measured by methacholine challenge and serum IgE levels was strongest for patients with active asthma as compared with those without symptoms. In a population-based study in Italy, IgE levels and atopy were found to predict bronchial responsiveness.[40]

The relationship between serum IgE levels and lung function has also been explored. In a French study,[42] total serum IgE was found to be related inversely to age and height-adjusted FEV_1 score, particularly in subjects who had never smoked. Several other studies examined the predictive value of serum IgE levels on lung function in subjects followed longitudinally. The French study[42] noted a significant inverse relationship between serum IgE levels and 5-year FEV$_1$ declines observed in nonsmokers and former smokers, but not in current smokers.[43] In the Normative Aging Study, no relationship between log IgE level and annual change in measures of pulmonary function was found in smokers or nonsmokers. Thus, IgE levels were not predictive of accelerated rates of decline in pulmonary function for middle-aged and older men in this study.[43]

Other studies explored the relationship between serum IgE and clinical severity of asthma in pediatric populations. One important study, The Childhood Asthma Management Program (CAMP), based on 1028 children with mild to moderate asthma, found that log serum IgE positively correlated with duration of asthma and with the mean daily albuterol puffs used to treat symptoms during the month preceding study enrollment.[44] Two studies from Australia[45,46] found that mean serum IgE increased as the severity of asthma increased, although wide variation and overlap in IgE distribution in the asthmatic and control groups of children were observed.[46] Other studies reported no relationships between serum IgE levels and frequency and severity of asthma attacks or physician-diagnosed asthma severity.[47,48] There is some suggestion that IgE levels in children may predict those in whom asthma will persist. In a longitudinal study of 540 children by Sherrill et al., higher mean serum IgE levels in those younger than 1 year of age were associated with higher mean serum IgE levels at ages 6 and 11 and persistent wheezing.[49]

In conclusion, IgE levels may correlate with severity of asthma but cannot be used as markers to distinguish between patients with or without asthma. A number of factors influence the clinical phenotype. It is also apparent not only that expression clinical disease is regulated by a genetic predisposition to produce IgE toward allergens, but that the level of chronic exposure to environmental allergens is also an important variable.

III. IgE Structure, Synthesis and Cell Interactions

The production of IgE is tightly regulated and involves a complex network of cellular and molecular signals. Immunoglobulins are synthesized and secreted by end cells of the B cell lineage (plasma cells) in the bone marrow or regional lymph nodes and reach various tissues by diffusion through the blood or by way of migrating cells. IgE, similar to other immunoglobulins, is composed of two heavy and two light chains. The combined amino terminal ends of these two chains create the two antigen-combining sites of the molecule that have the same specificities for the antigen (Figure 22.2).

Different parts of the molecule have different functional activities, as revealed using proteolytic enzymes. Digestion with papain cleaves the amino

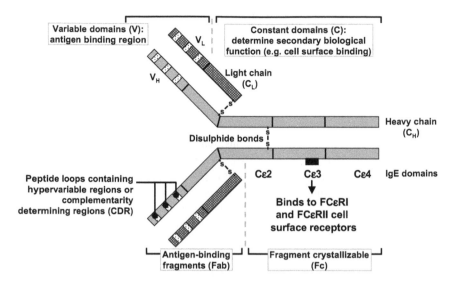

Figure 22.2   Human IgE. Fab, Fc, variable, and constant domains as well as the C3 binding site for FcRI and FcRII cell surface receptors are shown.

terminal side of the inter-heavy chain disulfide bonds, producing two Fab (fragment-antigen-binding) fragments that recognize the antigen. The other fragment can be crystallized and is thus termed Fc (fragment crystallisable). Pepsin digestion cleaves the molecule to the carboxy terminal side of the inter-heavy chain disulfide bonds and generates a Fab dimer to leave a rather smaller Fc fragment designated p Fc'.

Both the light and heavy polypeptide chains consist of a series of similar globular subunits or domains. Although the various light and heavy chain domains have considerable overall similarities, the amino terminal domain shows a marked degree of variation in many of its amino acid residues and is considered *variable* in contrast to the other domains that vary little from each other and are termed *constant*. Immunoglobulin variable domains are encoded by numerous V, D, and J exons whose diversity of selection, junctional variation, V_H/V_L combination, and somatic mutation among different B cells generates the enormous repertoire of antigen-combining sites.

IgE production is mainly under the control of T cells and T cell cytokines. In the case of allergic immune reactions, naïve T cells develop toward the so-called Th-2 type defined by the predominant production of Th-2 cytokines, especially IL-4, IL-5, and IL-13.[50] Differentiation of B cells to IgE-producing plasma cells requires two distinct signals, the first provided by IL-4 and IL-13[51] and the second by interaction between the costimulatory CD40 antigen on the surfaces of B cells and its CD40L ligand on T cell surfaces.[52] Without this interaction, B cells will undergo apoptosis. The IL-4 cytokine is a crucial factor for isotype switching to IgE and alone is sufficient for the initiation of germline transcription, but additional stimuli are required for the expression of mature mRNA and IgE synthesis.[53] When compared with IL-4, IL-13 is produced by activated T cells in larger quantities and for longer periods of time. Effector T cells exist which induce IgE isotype switching of human B cells exclusively via IL-13.

Both IL-4 and IL-13 are involved in IgE-related diseases. Increased expression of IL-13 mRNA has been demonstrated in the nasal mucosa of allergic rhinitis patients and at the sites of allergen challenges in asthmatics. Although IL-4 and IL-13 share many of their effects on the immune system, they may modulate B cell proliferation in costimulation via surface IgM or CD40 antigen differentially. Human B cells proliferate well upon costimulation by IL-13 and anti-CD40 monoclonal antibodies, but not upon costimulation by IL-13 and anti-IgM antibodies.[54] In contrast, IL-4 stimulates proliferation with either anti-IgM or anti-CD40 costimulation.[54,55] It has been suggested that the common gamma chain shared by IL-2R and IL-4R may contribute preferentially to signals generated via surface Ig, whereas IL-13R may costimulate more efficiently with CD40-generated signals.[54] The facts that surface Ig functions as the specific antigen receptor for B cells and stimulation via CD40 provides a polyclonal signal for B cell activation, and IgE switching may have consequences for the roles of IL-4 and IL-13 in the production of antigen-specific versus polyclonal IgE.[56]

Biological activities of IgE are mediated through specific receptors, of which the high affinity receptor (FcεRI) is expressed on mast cells, basophils, dendritic cells, Langherhans cells, monocytes, and epithelial cells. The low affinity receptor (FcεRII, CD23) is expressed on B lymphocytes and eosinophils. FcεRI is composed of four subunits designated $\alpha\beta\gamma_2$. Studies identified the 11 N-terminal amino acid residues [329 through 340] of the C3 domain of IgE as essential for high affinity binding to the α chain of the FcεRI complex. They demonstrated that the essential structural determinant for IgE/FcεRI recognition depends on a consecutive sequence of 11 amino acids [343 through 353] in Cε3 computed to form a loop structure [A–B] at the interface of the Cε4 domain and comprising a ridge with further interactions involving the C–D and D–E loop structures. CD23 seems to be the most important receptor affecting IgE production, at least in rodents.

IgE binds FcεRI via its Fc region (constant domains $C\varepsilon_2$, $C\varepsilon_3$, and $C\varepsilon_4$)[57] and multivalent antigen binding by the IgE Fab domains to result in cross-linking and aggregation of FcεRI–IgE complexes and dimerization of FcεRI, the principal activating signal for mast cells and basophils. FcεRI binds IgE at a very low concentration ($K_A = 10^9$ M^{-1}), greatly prolonging the *in vivo* half-life of IgE.

FcεRI cross-linking initiates a cascade of intracellular signaling events regulated by FcεRI α and β subunits and triggers the release of inflammatory mediators, cytokines, and chemokines.[58] Thus, allergen exposures in sensitized patients lead to binding of specific allergens to IgE–FcεRI complexes on mast cells, which activates the allergic cascade characteristic of the early IgE-mediated reaction.[59,60] The cross-linking of receptors immediately triggers the release and production of preformed and newly synthesized mediators such as histamine, tryptase, cysteinyl leukotrienes, and prosfanoids, in addition to the release of pro-inflammatory cytokines and chemokines. Depending on the site of allergen exposure, the pro-inflammatory mediators cause immediate reactions such as airway smooth muscle contraction, mucus hypersecretion, mucosal edema of upper or lower airways, neural responses such as pruritis and sneezing and conjunctivitis.[61] Released cytokines and chemokines may amplify the cellular immune responses that regulate the pathophysiology of allergic disease[62] and suggest that IgE may contribute to both subsequent inflammatory reactions such as the airway eosinophilia associated with late allergic response and the development of airway remodeling.

In addition to initiating immediate-type hypersensitivity reactions and facilitating antigen focusing, IgE was shown to have the ability to modulate the expression of its own receptors, FcεRI and CD23. FcεRI numbers are four- to five-fold greater on peritoneal mast cells and bone marrow basophils from wild-type animals than on those from IgE$^{-/-}$mice.[63] Similarly, wild-type mice express approximately four- to six-fold more CD23 on their B cells than do IgE$^{-/-}$animals.[64] Both receptors can be up-regulated *in vivo* in the IgE$^{-/-}$mice by intravenous injection of IgE. There is a direct correlation between FcεRI density and excitability of mast cells. IgE-mediated up-regulation of FcεRI significantly enhances the ability of mast cells sensitized with IgE to degranulate in response to allergen challenge. Thus, IgE affects a positive feedback mechanism that enhances immediate hypersensitivity responses. Up-regulation of CD23 by IgE may enhance allergic responses in the bronchial mucosa by stimulating antigen uptake and presentation.

An unusual family of F cell–derived IgE binding factors may significantly influence the IgE response.[65] The family is divided into either IgE-potentiating or IgE-suppressive factors based on their ability to augment or inhibit IgE responses, respectively. Although derived from the same gene, two additional T cell products determine different modifications: glycosylation inhibitory factor (GIF) and glycosylation enhancing factor (GEF). Administration of GIF to allergen-challenged mice suppresses IgE responses. The regulatory effects of GIF and GEF in human atopic diseases in comparison with other IgE-regulating factors are currently unknown. Consequently, the importance of IgE-potentiating and IgE-suppressive factors still remains to be established.[66]

Other factors determine elimination of IgE, but they are not as well understood. Human IgE binds to additional immunoglobulin receptors including FcεRII and FcεRIII, and this may mediate phagocytosis (and degradation) of IgE complexed with antigen. Although this route may aid in the elimination of antigen–

antibody complexes, it probably does not participate in the maintenance of basal IgE serum levels consisting primarily of uncomplexed antibodies.

Loss or degradation of serum IgE occurs through extravascular and intra-vascular catabolic pathways. Most IgE synthesis occurring in response to *Trichinella spiralis* helminth exposure occurs within the wall of the rodent gut by differentiated B cells–plasma cells. Antibody synthesized in this location is transported into the lumen of the gut as a result of an IL-4 inducible mechanism. A similar mechanism may operate in atopic syndromes as IgE is found consistently in the airways of atopic patients. IgE is classified as a secreted immunoglobulin. It does not bind the poly-IgE transporter required for luminal transport of the other secreted antibody, IgA, indicating that the IgE transport mechanism involves distinct receptors or binding factors. The data strongly support IgE as a secreted immunoglobulin instead of a factor undergoing elimination through catabolism. Most IgE is secreted from the body at mucosal sites through a specific transport mechanism controlled by IL-4.

IV. Anti-IgE and Its Development as Therapy

Current drugs for allergic diseases, such as antihistamines, bronchodilators (β-adrenergic receptor antagonists), leukotriene receptor antagonists, and corticosteroids treat allergic symptoms and concomitant inflammatory reactions, but produce few or no fundamental long-term effects on the disease process. Desensitization immunization (immunotherapy) with allergens is mainly used for allergic rhinitis and is less effective for asthma. Therefore, a treatment that targets the allergic process to inhibit the cascade and produces fewer side effects than current drugs is clearly desirable.

Because IgE is the central macromolecular effector responsible for the progression of allergic reactions, neutralizing it and inhibiting its synthesis appear to be rational approaches for the treatment of allergic diseases such as allergic asthma, seasonal allergic rhinitis (SAR), insect venom allergies, and food allergies. The serum levels of IgE antibodies to cow milk and hen eggs predict the probability of a positive outcome of an allergic reaction upon food challenge in children. In contrast to asthmatics with IgE directed against specific allergens, patients with nonallergic asthma have negative skin tests to common allergens and tend to have more severe disease. They do, however, have Th2-type inflammatory responses in the airways similar to those observed in patients with allergic asthma, and indications suggest that their disease may also be IgE-directed. Many nonspecific factors such as infection and air pollutants are known to exert mitogenic effects and stimulate polyclonal IgE production.[67] Significant local IgE production has been described in the airways of some patients, indicating that IgE may also play a role in nonallergic asthma pathogenesis.[68,69] It is thus possible that anti-IgE therapy in asthma may be useful as a treatment for the classical allergic form of the disease and may also play a role in the management of nonallergic disease.

Because of the pivotal role of IgE, directly antagonizing or inhibiting IgE responses by anti-IgE antibodies was identified as a novel and promising approach to treat allergic diseases and allows intervention early in the inflammatory cascade.[70,71] The concept that allergen-specific IgE initiates acute allergic airway symptoms and promotes ongoing allergic responses has driven the development of therapeutics such as blockers of the interaction of IgE with its high-affinity FcεRI receptor. The aim was to develop an inhibitor of IgE that would bind to FcεRI and lack the ability to trigger the degranulation of IgE-sensitized cells. It was achieved by the generation of a monoclonal antibody (MAb) that bound IgE to the same site as the α chain of the high-affinity FcεR1 receptor interacted with the third domain of the heavy chain Cε3[72] and, therefore, did not cause activation or anaphylaxis.[73] This development resulted in a humanized MAb (Rhu-MAb E25), termed Omalizumab.

Several main features are required of an anti-IgE for it to be therapeutically useful. It must

- Recognize and bind tightly to human serum IgE, but not to IgG or IgA, with affinity comparable to the interaction between IgE and its high-affinity IgE Fc receptor (FcεRI).
- Inhibit the binding of IgE to FcεRI.
- Not bind to IgE bound to mast cells or basophils and thus not cause degranulation (nonanaphylactic antibody).
- Block mast cell degranulation following passive sensitization *in vitro* or challenge with allergen *in vivo*.
- Be unspecific for allergen specificity of the IgE antibody; it must bind to any IgE molecule.

The chimerized or humanized anti-IgE antibodies with a set of unique binding properties could be used for isotype-specific control of IgE and, thus, would seem to represent a logical therapeutic approach to IgE-mediated diseases. The intended pharmacological aims of the anti-IgEs are two-fold: (1) to inhibit or neutralize free IgE and (2) to down-regulate IgE production by B cells.[74–76]

If these aims are achieved, the levels of IgE in blood and interstitial fluids for binding to FcεRI will be greatly reduced, and the sensitivity of mast cells and basophils to allergens should be gradually alleviated. On the other hand, because anti-IgE does not bind to IgE bound by FcεRI, they do not cross link FcεRI-bound IgE on sensitized mast cells and basophils in contrast to most anti-IgE antibodies that do not possess these unique epitope specific-binding properties.[77] Also, because the anti-IgEs do not bind to IgE bound by FcεRII which is expressed broadly on lymphocytes, macrophages, platelet, and many other cell types, they are not expected to cause adverse effects associated with such binding.

In 1991, Hook et al.[78] first described a MAb to human IgE that failed to elicit histamine release, and they correctly concluded that the determinant recognized on IgE was excluded by the FcεRI interaction. It was subsequently shown that similar antibodies to mouse IgE could effectively inhibit IgE binding to its receptors.[79] However, these antibodies also induced receptor cross-linking. Later, antibodies to mouse IgE were isolated; this inhibited IgE binding without producing IgE receptor dimerization because the antibodies reacted to a single determinant within the region of IgE recognized by the α chain of FcεRI. However, they could interact with IgE expressed on the surfaces of B hybridoma cells.

Naturally occurring anti-IgE autoantibodies had been recognized since 1989. Such antibodies, depending upon their sites of binding to IgE, could amplify or inhibit IgE-mediated responses. Anti-IgE autoantibodies have been reported in atopic dermatitis, Hymenoptera sting allergy, and asthma.[80] Most recently, a high proportion (60%) of patients with chronic idiopathic urticaria were shown to have antibodies against the α chain of FcεRI; up to 10% had anti-IgE antibodies.

Fractionation and characterization of these different anti-IgE auto antibodies show that most belong to the IgG class and may inhibit or enhance IgE-FcεRI binding.[81] A nonanaphylactogenic antibody to human IgE was generated by virtue of its inability to trigger histamine release from IgE-sensitized basophils.[82] Two other approaches were followed. The first was to select a MAb specific for the region of membrane IgE exposed on switched B cells.[83] A second approach was to use homology scanning mutagenesis to generate a murine antibody (MAE-11) that identified the same key amino acids in the C3 domain of IgE as did the chain of FcεRI.[73] The target structures of these nonanaphylactic murine antibodies were studied by site-directed mutagenesis of IgE and shown to comprise six key residues: Arg 465, Ser 411, Lys 414, Glu 452, Arg 465, and Met 469, localized in three loops with Cε3 to form a ridge on the most exposed portion of human IgE.[73] The binding site of IgE for FcεR2 (CD23) lies within the same region that binds to FcR1.[62] Therefore, antibodies selected for the latter also inhibit binding to CD23.3 to form a ridge on the most exposed portion of human IgE.[73]

The use of anti-IgE to inhibit IgE responses was described first in 1982 by Bozelka et al.[84] who showed that treatment of mice from birth with rabbit-derived polyclonal anti-IgE antibodies reduced serum IgE levels — an observation later extended to adult mice.[85] Of particular interest in these studies was the effect that anti-IgE treatment had on reducing the number of IgE secreting B cells; moreover, when the antibody was given during immunization, the secondary IgE response was attenuated but did not prevent induction of memory.[86]

The total and antigen-directed IgE in the serum fell by over 90% and this was paralleled by a similar decrease in IgE-secreting cells. This latter effect required bivalent recognition of surface IgE and the absence of appropriate costimulatory signals, but it did not require T cell help.[87,88] Treatment of mice with a single injection of an anaphylactogenic anti-IgE MAb during primary immunization reduced serum IgE (but not IgG) to undetectable levels for over 2 months, even when the animals were exposed to antigen on a weekly basis.

With the production and characterization of non-anaphylactogenic rat IgG1 against mouse Ig, it has been possible to analyse responses on mice immunity.[74,89–91] Treatment of preimmunized mice reduced specific IgE by over 80% without altering IgG secondary responses. Three months after treatment, IgE responsiveness had returned to normal. With the development of techniques to produce MAbs, more monogenous populations of antibodies directed specifically against the high-affinity murine receptor were created. Not surprisingly, while some MAbs prevented IgE binding and mast cell degranulation, others stimulated these responses, presumably by cross-linking cell-bound IgE in a manner similar to an antigen. MAbs that attached to free IgE by binding only to the domain by which IgE associates to its receptor sites were selected. Thus, the MAbs did not attach to cell-bound IgE and the anti-IgE/IgE complex blocked the binding of the IgE to its receptors.

However, the xenobiotic molecules still had the potential to trigger a host reaction and they were "humanized" for this reason. The process removed the immunogenic position of the murine IgG antibody and spliced in its place a corresponding human IgG framework. In principle, a humanized anti-IgE retains the antigen-binding domain of murine origin but attains human homology for the remainder of the molecule. In practice, this problem was negotiated by generating both chimeric and reshaped "humanized" mouse nonanaphylactogenic anti-human IgE antibodies in the form of CGP 51901 (chimeric)[74] and CGP 56901 (humanized)[92] derived from the parental mouse antibody TES-C21 and Rhu MAb E25 (humanized) derived from the MAE-11 mouse clone.[72]

The humanization technology pioneered by Gregory Winter and colleagues[93] involved the grafting of the murine antigen-binding loops (complementarity-determining regions [CDRs]) onto the human antibody framework. Selected nonhuman framework residues also had to be incorporated into the humanized antibody to maintain proper CDR conformation.[92] Both TES-C21 and MAE-11 were humanized with a human Ig framework derived from consensus sequences of human V_L and V_H subgroups[94] that allowed use of the most common framework found in human IgG antibodies. On this basis, CGP 51901 and E25 (containing fewer than 5% mouse sequences) were selected for further study because their activities were most comparable with those of the parent murine antibodies.

When studied *in vitro*, these antibodies blocked the passive sensitization of human basophils and mast cells. Importantly, they failed to bind to IgE bound to

FcεRI and FcεRII and trigger mediator release.[95,96] Like the parent MAbs, CGP 511901 and E25 recognized IgE expressed on the surfaces of B cells but not IgE-sensitizer FcεRII-bearing cells.[74] They were shown to inhibit IgE production by human B cells *in vitro*.[74] Despite these similarities, the two humanized antibodies were directed to separate epitopes on the Cε3 region of IgE. A series of safety studies showed that both antibodies bound only to B cells and not mast cells in various tissues.[97] E25 bound with comparable affinity to cynomolgus monkey (3×10^{10} M) and human IgE (1.7×10^{10} M).[98] This reaction was explored *in vivo*. Twice-weekly intramuscular injections of E25 in animals presensitized with 27 μg of human ragweed–specific IgE resulted in reduced skin wheal responses to ragweed antigens in five of six animals, with a 100% response rate after the second dose of E25 that persisted for 1 month.[74,91]

The clear inhibitory effect of anti-IgE MAb E25 on mast cell-dependent skin whealing suggests that it may also inhibit late-phase inflammatory responses produced by mast cell cytokine release. Antigen challenge of mice lungs induced an eosinophilic response linked to IL-4 and IL-5 production by Th-2 polarized T cells.[99,100] Systemic administration of MAb E25 totally suppressed antigen-induced eosinophil recruitment. This depended upon an FcεR2 mechanism because the protective effect of MAb E-25 on the eosinophilia was lost in CD23-deficient mice or in the presence of CD23-blocking antibodies.

At least in the mouse system, the suggestion was that anti-IgE inhibited antigen-induced eosinophilia by reducing IgE-facilitated antigen presentation for T cell stimulation. Administration of anti-IgE MAb to rats before or shortly after passive sensitization with antigen-specific IgE inhibited immediate bronchoconstriction by over 90%[91,101] and caused about 70% inhibition of the antigen-acquired bronchial hyperresponsiveness to 5-HT challenge.[101] Similar results were reported for the ability of a nonanaphylactogenic anti-IgE MAbs to inhibit sensitization of both monkey and human bronchi *in vitro*.[102,103]

The demonstration that MAbs that bound to the FcεRIα-binding region of IgE could influence immediate and late-phase allergic-type responses in animals and did not induce histamine release set the stage for exploration of the effects of Rhu-MAb E25 (omalizumab) in humans and in allergic disease. One concern remained outstanding: would anti-IgE interfere with protection against parasites? It, thus, came as a surprise that anti-IgE treatment of mice infected with *Nippostrongylus brasiliensis*[104] or *Schistosoma mansoni*[105] resulted in effective elimination of parasites, decreased worm burden, and reduced the number of parasite eggs; this paralleled the fall in serum IgE. Thus, high levels of serum IgE induced by parasites may be peripheral consequences of strong Th-2 cell parasite induction and increased IL-4 production and may not be centrally involved in parasite-immune defenses as previously thought.

Helminths are likely to contain factors that stimulate polyclonal nonparasite-specific IgE responses in the same way as the "superantigens" from *Staphylococcus*

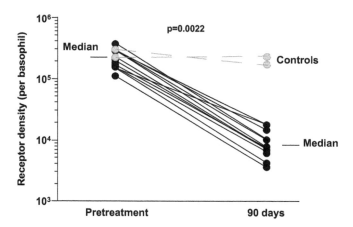

Figure 22.3 Down-regulation of FcRI expression on human basophils during *in vivo* treatment of atopic patients with anti-IgE antibody over a 90-day period. Solid lines represent patients; dashed lines represent controls. (From McGlashan, D.W., Jr. et al., *J Immunol* 1997; 158: 1438–1445. With permission.)

aureus are known to do. Increased serum IgE levels may also be attributable to cleavage of FcεRII by the parasite-derived proteolytic enzymes. It appeared unlikely that anti-IgE therapy would prevent parasite elimination, and the exploration of the potential of omalizumab became focused on humans.

V. Therapeutic Potential of Omalizumab

In addition to the inhibition of the mast cell mechanism, a reduction of free IgE can be expected to suppress the effects of IgE at high-affinity receptors on other cells.[106] For example, high affinity receptors have been localized on mast cells, basophils, various APCs of the skin, and circulating monocytes. IgE binding to these cells appears to enhance their ability to stimulate T lymphocyte activation. Interference with IgE binding may further diminish allergen-mediated inflammation.

The experimental use of anti-IgE antibodies has provided evidence for other allergy-associated actions of IgE and its receptors. A marked down-regulation in high affinity receptors on basophils from allergic subjects was noted after 3 months of intravenous E25 treatment (two biweekly doses of 0.015 or 0.03 mg/kg/ IU/ml; Figure 22.3).[107] Additionally, experiments with mice sensitized to house dust mites and treated with anti-IgE antibody showed significantly reduced lung eosinophilia following allergen challenge and diminished production of IL-5 by airway Th-2 cells. Because IL-5 is associated with chemotaxis and longevity of eosinophils, an IgE-mediated Th-2 response (by yet undefined mechanisms) that

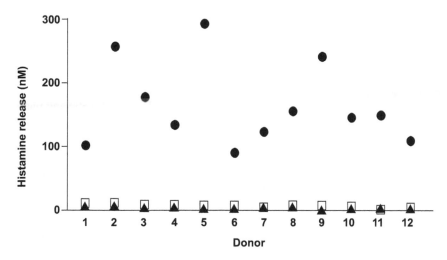

Figure 22.4   Effects of omalizumab [Rhu MAb-E25; (□) on ragweed (●) and spontaneous histamine (▲) release from lung parenchyma. No effect on spontaneous histamine
release; inhibition of ragweed-induced histamine release. (From Shields, R.L. et al., *Int
Arch Allergy Immunol* 1995; 107: 308–312. With permission.)

could be blocked by anti-IgE therapy offers a way to directly reduce late phases
of allergic reactions. Thus, the anti-IgE approach exerts multiple effects through
all reactions linked to IgE-dependent mechanisms and move the debate about
actions beyond the well-recognized mast cell- or basophil-mediated histamine
release.

A. Pharmacology

E25 (omalizumab) has been shown to bind human IgE with equally high affinity
and specificity as bound cynomolgus monkey IgE, supporting the selection of
this species for further nonclinical pharmacology and toxicology studies.[98] It
reduced high-affinity receptor expression *in vitro* and *in vivo* by decreasing free
IgE. Omalizumab treatment reduced FcεRI on human basophils, such that histamine *in vitro* release was reduced or eliminated in response to antigen challenge.[96]
E25 does not bind to IgE attached to receptors on mast cells and basophils.
Furthermore, it does not stimulate histamine release when administered alone,
but inhibits allergen-induced release (Figure 22.4). The antibody has been shown
to lack the ability to bind to IgA and IgG, indicating its specificity for IgE.[108]

Consistent with preclinical data, E25 has been shown to decrease levels of
both free IgE and FcεRI after each dose (0.15 to 0.03 mg/kg/IU/mL) in atopic
individuals. No data suggest that administration of E25 and the resultant decrease

in levels of free IgE caused a positive feedback signal to induce synthesis (IgE) rebound. Serum IgE levels returned to baseline when omalizumab therapy was withdrawn.

B. Pharmacokinetics and Pharmacodynamics

In preclinical analyses, the binding characteristics and pharmacokinetic and pharmacodynamic properties of E25 were evaluated in mice and monkeys. In cynomolgus monkeys, IgE binds to immobilized E25 with similar affinity to human IgE (K_d = 0.19 nM and 0.06 nM, respectively).[98] E25–IgE complexes were detected in the sera of primates after IV administration and were characterized as small (MW <10^6 daltons), similar in size to those formed *in vitro* with molar excesses of human IgE.[108] The antibody does not combine with cell-bound IgE; no association was found between ^{125}I-labeled E25 and blood cells. Tissue distribution studies using ^{125}I-labeled E25 indicated no specific uptake of radioactivity in cynomolgus monkey tissue at 1 hour and at 96 hours after IV bolus doses.

Although some radioactivity was observed in the thyroid at 96 hours, it is believed to have resulted from free ^{125}I uptake by the gland. The uptake of E25 appeared restricted to the plasma compartment, with an initial $t_{1/2}$ of approximately 5.5 hours and a terminal half-life of 1 to 4 weeks after SC or IV administration.[109,110] Both ^{125}I-E25 and its complexes with IgE appear to be cleared slowly from the blood. Urinary excretion was the major route of elimination and accounted for the removal of more than 50% of the administered dose at 96 hours.[109,110]

Excretion was found to be linear during this period. Serum clearance was greater in animals with higher baseline values of IgE — a property with potential clinical relevance for atopic patients with high circulating levels of IgE.[109,110] When all serum IgE was complexed by sufficient doses of omalizumab, free IgE levels were reduced and maintained at undetectable levels. The PK characteristics in children and adolescents were consistent with those seen in adults after weight normalization.

Although the clearance of E25–IgE complexes appeared slow, the limited size of the complexes (trimers and lexamers) and the lack of any specific uptake by the kidneys indicated an absence of deposition of these complexes in this organ and other tissues. Clearance of free IgE was greater than that of the complex which, in turn, was greater than that of omalizumab alone. Decreases in free IgE and increases in total IgE were reversible after drug washout.

C. Toxicology and Animal Safety Studies

Animal studies have not shown any evidence of toxicity with administration of up to 100 mg/kg in mice and 50 mg/ml in monkeys — doses much higher than the proposed clinical doses of 2 to 4 mg/kg.[111] Multiple doses (up to 5 mg/kg) three times a week for 4 weeks were well tolerated by monkeys. In September 2000, the U.S. Food and Drug Administration (FDA) requested Genentech and Novartis to suspend new trials of omalizumab; long-term trials in progress could continue. The hold on new trials arose from concerns about the preclinical toxicity of omalizumab and, more specifically, the follow-up antibody designated E26. Thrombocytopenia was reported in juvenile cynomolgus monkeys (aged 8 to 10 months) given 5 to 27 times the maximum clinical dose of omalizumab for 26 weeks and E26 at 3 to 15 times the maximum dose.

The decreased platelet counts were accompanied by prolongations in bleeding time in the high-dose group and moderate increases in megakaryocyte counts in the bone marrow. All effects were reversible upon cessation of anti-IgE treatment. In response to FDA requests, Novartis and Genentech carried out additional preclinical trials to determine a specific explanation of the toxicity. Novartis suspected a species specificity for the adverse events because no thrombocytopenic events had occurred in studies with adult cynomolgus monkeys at doses as high as 75mg/kg/wee k. Phase III clinical trials were completed and the supplementary data were submitted to the FDA. The hold on clinical trials was lifted in November 2000. No anaphylaxis was reported following systemic administration of doses as high as 50 mg/kg.

These data demonstrate that relevant animal models can tolerate single and multiple doses of E25 and high doses of the antibody. None of the animal studies revealed clinical or pathological signs of toxicity including onset of immune complex–mediated diseases. Antibodies to omalizumab were detected in 14% of treated juvenile monkeys. No antibodies were detected in adult animals treated with omalizumab. The presence of anti-omalizumab antibodies did not affect its serum concentrations or alter platelet profiles when test animals were compared with animals without anti-omalizumab antibodies.

Administration of anti-IgE resulted in the formation of immune complexes. The complexes formed *in vitro* by E25 with IgE were shown to be small by gel filtration chromatography and analytic ultracentrifugation.[97,108] A molar equivalence, the largest complex of approximately 1×10^6 daltons in size, predominated. The complex is best described as a cyclic hexamer consisting of three molecules of each immunoglobulin. E25–IgE complexes *in vivo* were again small but were similar to the complexes formed *in vitro* when IgE was in excess. These experiments conducted in cynomolgus monkeys showed no specific uptake in any particular tissue 1 hour and 96 hours after administration.

D. Clinical Study Experience

1. Dose Justification

The doses and dosing regimens necessary to achieve the targeted free IgE suppression were estimated based upon

Baseline IgE (IU/mL)	Bodyweight (kg)							
	20–30	>30–40	>40–50	>50–60	>60–70	>70–80	>80–90	>90–150
>30–100	150	150	150	150	150	150	150	300
>100–200	150	150	300	300	300	300	300	450
>200–300	150	300	300	300	450	450	450	600
>300–400	300	300	450	450	450	600	600	
>400–500	300	450	450	600	600	750	750	
>500–600	300	450	600	600	750			
>600–700	450	450	600	750				
>700–800	450	600	750					
>800–900	450	600	750					
>900–1,000	600	750						
>1,000–1,100	600	750						
>1,100–1,200	600							
>1,200–1,300	750							

- Doses ≤ 300mg per 4-week interval are administered once/4 weeks
- Doses > 300mg/4-week interval are split into two equal doses administered every 2 weeks (i.e. 600mg total = 300mg every 2 weeks)

Figure 22.5 Dosing schedule for anti-IgE therapy with omalizumab based on IgE measurement and body weight.

- The ratio of serum omalizumab (nM) to serum IgE (nM) necessary to maintain suppression, i.e., 16–21 to 1[112]
- The dose of antibody necessary to maintain an average serum concentration at or above the minimum drug-to-IgE ratio
- The dosing frequency necessary to ensure adequate serum concentrations with an acceptable number of visits and injections

Early phase I and II studies used dosing adjusted only for body weight (mg/kg). That ensured that serum levels of omalizumab were comparable across all body weights, but did not ensure that the serum IgE levels would be suppressed to a comparable extent in every subject because allergic subjects have wide ranges of baseline serum IgE concentrations. Therefore, adjustments of doses based upon baseline serum IgE would ensure consistent omalizumab-to-IgE ratios. Doses had to be adjusted for body weight because the target populations included both children and adults and the subjects' weights ranged from 20 to 150 kg (Figure 22.5).

Individualized dosing via intravenous bolus administration was used for the phase II study of allergic asthma.[113] The route of administration for the phase III asthma studies was changed from IV to SC, and the dosing interval was extended from every 2 weeks to every 4 weeks. The minimal effective IV dose from phase II (0.006 mg/kg/IU/ml) was increased to an SC equivalent dose of 0.008 mg/kg/IU/ml. Doses were doubled for the 4-week dosing intervals to ensure the same steady state, average total omalizumab serum concentration as the 2-week doses. Doses in excess of 300 mg/month were split into two equal doses administered every 2 weeks. The split doses were required to reduce injection volumes and numbers of injections and to ensure that single dose administrations were within the dose limits.

2. Initial Clinical Experience

The first study investigated the tolerability and pharmacokinetic and pharmaco-dynamic profiles of increasing single doses of omalizumab in 59 healthy individuals and patients with allergies.[114] The concentration of free IgE in serum decreased rapidly after administration of omalizumab and gradually returned to baseline over a period of several weeks after the last dose.[115] Omalizumab was well tolerated by the patients and no anaphylactic reactions were observed during the study. Similar results were obtained in two subsequent multiple-dose studies; the first enrolled 24 adult patients with either allergic rhinitis or mild asthma[116] and the second enrolled 34 children and adolescents with moderate to severe allergic asthma.[117] In these multiple dose studies, free IgE in serum decreased with increasing doses of omalizumab, gradually returned to baseline after the last omalizumab treatment, and was not associated with any allergic reactions or medication-related adverse events.

On the basis of these encouraging initial findings, a single-blind Phase I clinical trial was initiated to examine the safety and tolerability of omalizumab in comparison with a placebo among 12 adult patients with moderate to severe asthma.[118] Patients were treated weekly with a placebo or omalizumab (0.15 mg/kg SC or 0.50 mg/kg IV) for 3 weeks; clinical evaluations were performed for a total of 6 weeks. No adverse responses to treatment or changes in physiologic or laboratory values were observed during the study. At the end of 3 weeks of treatment, the concentration of free IgE in serum had decreased to an average of 60% of its baseline value among patients who received the lower dose of omalizumab and to 20% of its baseline value among patients who received the higher dose.

Among the first clinical trials investigating the efficacy and safety of E25 was one evaluating the protective effects of pretreatment on the allergen-induced early asthmatic response.[119] The study investigated the effects of E25 on the provocation dose of allergen causing a 15% reduction in FEV_1 from baseline (PC_{15} allergen) during the early asthmatic response. In this multicenter, randomized, double-blind, parallel-group study, E25 was well tolerated and only one patient was withdrawn because of a generalized urticarial rash after the first dose. When compared with baseline values, the median PC_{15} allergen values on days 27, 55, and 77 were increased by 2.3, 2.2, and 2.7 doubling doses, respectively, with E25 and –0.3, +0.1, and –0.8 doubling doses with placebo ($p < 0.002$). The methacholine PC_{20} value improved slightly after E25, becoming significant on day 76 ($p < 0.05$).

Table 22.1 and Table 22.2 summarize data from ten completed phase IIb, III, and IIIb studies of 3047 patients, of whom 1865 were treated with omalizumab;

Table 22.1 Summary of Omalizumab (E25) Clinical Trials in Asthma

Study Number	Design	Total Number of Patients	Number Receiving E25	Ages of Allergic Asthma Patients	Dose of E25 (mg SQ)	Results
008	R, DB, PC	525	268	12–74	150, 300 every 4 wk; 225, 300, 375 every 2 wk × 52wk	Decrease of asthma exacerbation; reduction in dose of BDP; improved asthma symptoms and respiratory function; improved asthma-related QOL
009	R, DB, PC	546	274	12–76	150, 300 every 4 wk; 225, 300, 375 every 2 wk × 52wk	Decrease of asthma exacerbation; reduction in dose of BDP; improved asthma symptoms and respiratory function; improved asthma-related QOL
010	R, DB, PC	334	225	6–12	150, 300 every 4 wk; 225, 300, 375 every 2 wk × 28 wk	Reduction in BDP dose; decrease of asthma exacerbations
010 Extension	OL, UC	309	309	6–12	150, 300 every 4 wk; 225, 300, 375 every 2 wk × 28 wk	
011	R, DB, PC	341	176	12–75	150, 300 every 4 wk; 225, 300, 375 every 2 wk × 32 wk	Reduction of inhaled CS dose; reduced asthma symptoms scores; improved QOL scores

DB = double blind. OL = open label. PC = placebo controlled. R = randomized. UC = uncontrolled. QOL = quality of life. BDP = beclamethasone dipropionate. CS = corticosteroid.

Table 22.2 Summary of Omalizumab (E25) Clinical Trials in Allergic Rhinitis

Study Number	Design	Total Patient Number	Number Receiving E25	Ages of Patients; Diseases	Dose of E25 (mg SQ)	Results
006	R, DB, PC	536	400	12–75 SAR	50, 150, 300 every 3–4 wk × 12 wk	Improved average daily nasal symptoms severity score; improved daily rescue medication use; improved daily ocular symptoms score
006ext	OL, UC	287	287	12–75 SAR	300 every 3–4 wk × 12 wk	Improved average daily nasal symptoms severity score; improved daily rescue medication use; improved daily ocular symptoms score
007	R, DB, PC	251	165	17–66 SAR	300 every 3–4 wk × 12 wk	Improved average daily nasal symptoms severity score; improved daily rescue medication use; improved daily ocular symptoms score
014	R, DB, PC	289	144	12–75 PAR	150 to 300 every 4 wk; 225, 300, 375 every 2 wk × 16 wk	Reduced mean daily nasal severity scores; decreased use of rescue antihistamines; better RQLQ scores; superior global evaluation for investigators and patients
D01 (1A11)	R, DB, PC	225	114	6–17 SAR	150, 300 every 4 wk; 225, 300, 375 every 2 wk × 6 mo	Better symptoms load scores over entire pollen season; reduced use of rescue medication

DB = double blind. OL = open label. PC = placebo controlled. R = randomized. UC = uncontrolled. PAR = perennial allergic rhinitis. SAR = seasonal allergic rhinitis. QOL = quality of life. RQLQ = rhinoconjunctivitis quality of life questionnaire.

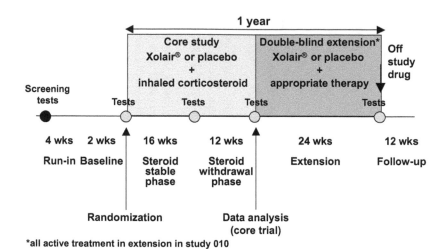

Figure 22.6 Common protocol for phase III studies. (From Busse, W.W. et al., *J Allergy Clin Immunol* 2001; 108: 184–190; Soler, M. et al., *Eur Respir J* 2001; 18: 254–261; Milgrom, H. et al., *Paediatrics* 2001; 108: E36. With permission.)

1746 patients, of whom 1042 received omalizumab, completed studies of allergic asthma. For seasonal allergic rhinitis (SAR), 679 patients (of 1012 participants) received omalizumab. Active treatments were received by 144 subjects with perennial allergic rhinitis (PAR) in a study involving 289 participants.

The phase III program included three large studies in patients with moderate to severe allergic asthma treated conventionally with the inhaled beclomethasone dipropionate (BDP) corticosteroid and short-acting inhaled β_2 agonists. Phase III studies (protocols 008, 009, and 010)[120–122] provided the primary evidence of the efficacy of SC omalizumab in the treatment of patients with allergic asthma and are considered the pivotal studies for demonstration of efficacy for this indication.

A U.S. study (protocol 008) and an international study (protocol 009) were conducted in 1071 adults and adolescents aged 12 to 75 years who were symptomatic on entry to the study. A third study (protocol 010) was conducted in the U.S. in 334 pediatric patients 6 to 12 years of age. Compared with the adults, a larger proportion of the pediatric patients had asthma that was milder in severity. This population was well controlled on current therapy and asymptomatic at study entry.[122]

The BDP dosages were adjusted during the run-in period to the lowest optimal doses required to maintain control (as judged by symptoms and peak expiratory flow [PEF]). The adjusted dose was continued for 4 weeks prior to randomization to active or placebo treatment. All studies had similar designs (Figure 22.6). During the first 16 weeks of double-blind treatment (the add-on phase), patients were maintained on baseline doses of BDP without adjustment unless an exacerbation of asthma occurred. In the following 12 weeks, controlled attempts were made to reduce the doses of BDP at regular intervals (steroid reduction phase). These two phases constituted the core treatment phase. In an extension phase, treatment was continued for a total of 1 year with double-blind treatment of adults and adolescents or open treatment of the children. The extension phases were designed to accumulate data for safety analysis.

Omalizumab was administered as an SC injection. Doses were calculated on the basis of patients' levels of serum-free IgE and body weights (Figure 22.5). Doses of 300 mg and lower could be administered every 4 weeks. Higher doses were given every 2 weeks because of the larger volume of injection required. In the phase III program, 60% of patients were treated with four weekly injections.

The numbers of exacerbations per patient and degrees of reduction in doses of BDP were separate and important efficacy variables. An exacerbation of asthma was defined as a worsening that required treatment with oral or intravenous corticosteroids or doubling of a patient's baseline BDP dose. In the two studies in adults and adolescents, the mean numbers of asthma exacerbations per patient were significantly lower in the omalizumab treatment group during both study phases.

Pooled results showed means of 0.28 and 0.60 exacerbations per patient in the active and placebo groups, respectively, during the add-on phase (p <0.001) and 0.38 and 0.71 (p <0.001) during the steroid reduction phase. In the less severely affected pediatric population, the number of asthma exacerbations was significantly lower with active treatment in the steroid reduction phase only (0.42 with omalizumab versus 0.72 with placebo; p <0.001). The median percentage reduction in BDP dose achieved was 50% in the placebo treatment groups in the studies in adults and adolescents compared with 75% and 83% in the active treatment groups in the two studies, respectively (p <0.001 for both). In the pediatric study, patients achieved median BDP dose reductions of 100% with omalizumab and 67% with placebo (p = 0.001). Approximately 20% of placebo-treated patients and 40% of omalizumab-treated patients in studies 008 and 009 were able to withdraw from BDP completely; the respective figures in the pediatric study were 39% and 55%.

In studies 008 and 009, significant differences in favor of active treatment were observed for total asthma symptom score, daily number of puffs of rescue medication, PEF levels, and FEV_1 (in study 009; see Figure 22.7). These variables remained significantly different in favor of omalizumab during the steroid reduction phase, suggesting that control of asthma was maintained. During the 1-year treatment period across all three studies, 19 patients in the placebo groups required hospitalization for asthma exacerbations compared with two omalizumab-treated patients.

In all studies, the asthma-specific quality of life (QOL) was assessed using the instruments developed by Juniper and colleagues.[123–125] In comparison with placebo, QOL was significantly better in patients treated with omalizumab, and

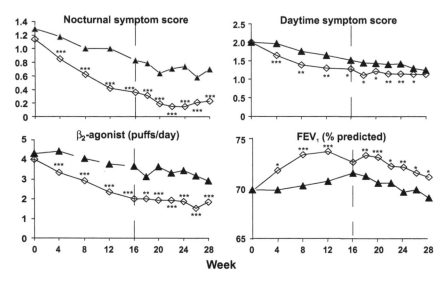

*p<0.05, **p<0.001 vs placebo

Figure 22.7 Improvement in standard control measures in patients with severe asthma randomized to receive omalizumab (n = 268) or placebo (n = 272). (From Sears, M.R. et al., *Clin Allergy* 1980; 10: 423–431. With permission.)

more patients achieved clinically meaningful improvements in QOL scores. Global evaluation of treatment effectiveness also favored active treatment based on patients' and investigators' opinions.

3. Responder Profiling

The pooled results of the key phase III studies were analyzed in an effort to see whether some patients experienced better responses to treatment than others. The patients were stratified according to disease severity and efficacy was judged on the basis of median percentage BDP reduction. Responders could not be identified and efficacy did not appear to differ in patients whose disease was categorized as mild, moderate, or severe. Further studies are investigating whether in all its pooled trials responders can be differentiated in any way from non-responders.

4. Severe Asthma

Studies 008[120] and 009[121] focused on patients with more severe asthma and further data were obtained from this group because anti-IgE therapy is likely to be most cost effective in this population. Study 011 evaluated the effects of omalizumab on patients with severe allergic asthma, including patients on high doses of inhaled corticosteroids and a subset that also took oral corticosteroids.[126] Patients received omalizumab during a 16-week steroid stabilization phase followed by a 16-week steroid reduction phase. Patients received at least 0.016 mg/kg omalizumab administered SC every 2 to 4 weeks. A comparison of omalizumab- and placebo-treated patients showed the following:

- Reduced inhaled corticosteroid dose by percentage as measured by fluticasone dose (61.3% versus 46.4%, p = 0.004) in the inhaled corticosteroid subpopulation
- Reduced absolute fluticasone dose in the inhaled group (750 versus 500 µg/day, p = 0.003)
- Reduced corticosteroid dose in patients overall (inhaled plus oral, 62.5% versus 50%, p = 0.017)
- Reduced asthma symptoms scores in patients overall (p <0.05) and improved QOL scores during the steroid stabilization (p = 0.043) and steroid reduction phases (p = 0.003)

Omalizumab also improved QOL in severe asthma patients.[127] A separate study confirmed the beneficial effects of omalizumab in improving QOL in patients with severe allergic asthma in a year-long study.[128] Pooled analyses of double-blind, placebo-controlled, randomized phase III studies with omalizumab revealed that this treatment reduces the likelihood of severe disease and produces significant reductions in the rates of unscheduled asthma-related outpatient visits, asthma-related emergency room visits, and hospitalizations (Figure 22.8).[129,130] These studies and other extension studies have shown the long-term benefit of omalizumab in the control of severe allergic asthma.[131]

E. Omalizumab and Allergic Rhinitis

A large multicenter study compared three SC doses of omalizumab (50, 150, and 300 mg) and a placebo.[132] The dose–response relationships to symptoms, QOL, and reductions in the use of rescue medications were studied in 536 patients with moderate to severe ragweed-induced allergic rhinitis of at least 2-years' duration. Because baseline IgE levels are important in the dosing strategy, the patients were treated as follows. Those with serum IgE levels of 30 to 150 IU/ml received the assigned treatment at 0, 4, and 8 weeks. Those with IgE levels of 151 to 700 IU/ml received treatments at 0, 3, 6, and 9 weeks. Patients were followed for 12 weeks and an additional 12-week observation period was included in the study design.[132]

The difference between the placebo and the 300 mg omalizumab groups was statistically significant throughout the pollen season and the peak season (p = 0.001, one-sided Student's t-test) comparing the mean daily nasal symptom severity scores (sneezing or itchy, runny, or stuffy nose). Patients receiving the

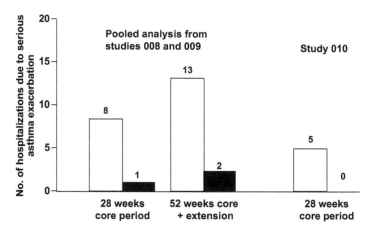

Figure 22.8 Hospital admissions during phase III studies comparing omalizumab with placebo, relating to studies 008,[120] 009,[121] and 010,[122] illustrating the protective effects of subcutaneous therapy with omalizumab in preventing hospital admissions and the development of severe and potentially fatal asthma.

150 mg dose of omalizumab had lower mean symptom scores, but the difference from the scores in the placebo group was not statistically significant. In the placebo group, increases in pollen count correlated with a deterioration of QOL as manifested by higher RQLQ scores. At the highest dose of omalizumab, RQLQ scores during the peak pollen season were lower.[133] The proportion of days on which rescue medications were taken and the number of tablets ingested was reduced by 50% in the 300-mg omalizumab group, significantly reduced in the 150-mg omalizumab group, but not in the 50-mg omalizumab and placebo groups.

The relationship between the dose of omalizumab and free IgE in serum was linear. At the 300-mg dose of omalizumab, the percentage of patients with serum IgE levels below the detectable level of 25 ng/ml was approximately 65% (Figure 22.9). A similar relationship existed between the reduction in IgE levels and nasal symptom severity scores and changes in the use of rescue medication.[132] Thus, if treatment is to be effective in SAR, a condition that may involve monosensitization, and all the IgE is directed toward the same allergen, a major reduction in IgE is necessary to translate this into clinical benefit.

A Scandinavian group studied the efficacy of omalizumab in treating SAR caused by birch pollen (study 007).[134] Two hundred fifty-one patients were randomized to receive omalizumab at 300 mg SC — the maximum effective dose determined by the previous study — or placebo in a two-to-one ratio. The study design was similar to that of the earlier trial. In all parameters of efficacy (daily nasal symptom severity score, average number of rescue antihistamine tablets

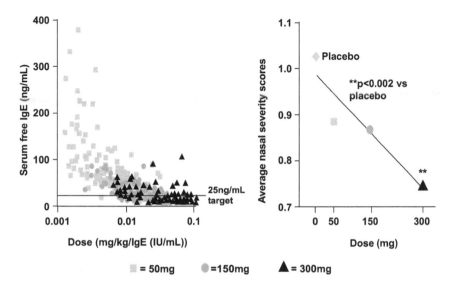

Figure 22.9 Relationship between reduction in serum IgE (left) and improvement in nasal symptom scores (right) in patients with ragweed-sensitive SAR receiving one of three doses of omalizumab (50, 150, or 300 mg) versus placebo. (From Casale, T.B. et al., *JAMA* 2001; 286: 2956–2967. With permission.)

taken per day, proportion of days on which any medication for seasonal allergic rhinoconjunctivitis was used, and responses to the RQLQ), omalizumab was superior to placebo (Figure 22.10).

In both studies, omalizumab was well tolerated and no significant differences were found between the treated and placebo groups in the overall incidence of adverse events or in the incidence of drug-related adverse events. Three patients reported a total of four episodes of urticaria after administration of omalizumab, but these were mild and required no treatment. No drug-related adverse events were noted and no anaphylactic reactions or serum sickness occurred.

No anti-omalizumab antibodies were detected. One concern about omalizumab treatment that remained unresolved after these trials was whether it could be re-administered safely after treatment was discontinued for a prolonged period. This was the reason for adding an extension to the 006 study involving patients with ragweed-induced seasonal allergic rhinitis. Of the 364 patients treated with omalizumab in study protocol 006, 287 participated in the 12-week open-label extension trial.[135] Subjects with baseline serum IgE levels above 150 IU/ml (37%) received 300 mg SC every 3 weeks. Subjects with baseline IgE levels of 150 IU/ml or lower (63%) were treated every 4 weeks. No placebo arm was involved and no efficacy parameters were studied. The incidence of drug-related adverse

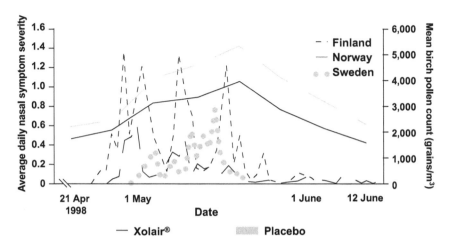

Figure 22.10   Average daily nasal symptom scores in patients receiving 300 mg subcutaneous omalizumab or placebo in a Scandinavian study of birch pollen SAR showing significant prevention of symptom development in the active treatment group. (From Adelroth, E. et al., *J Allergy Clin Immunol* 2000; 106: 253–259. With permission.)

events was similar in both treated groups; most frequent events were headaches, upper respiratory tract infections, and rashes. No antibodies against omalizumab were detected.

Two additional supportive studies [014 and D01] evaluated the efficacy and safety of omalizumab in the treatment of allergic rhinitis. Study 014 was a phase IIIB, conducted in PAR patients 12 to 75 years of age.[136] Patients received 0.016 mg/kg/IgE (IU/ml) omalizumab administered SC every 2 to 4 weeks for 16 weeks in an open-label study design. The results, compared with placebo, are all statistically significant:

- Reduced mean daily nasal severity scores (p ≤0.001)
- Decreased use of rescue antihistamine medications (p = 0.005)
- Better RQLQ scores
- Superior global evaluations compared with placebo from investigators (p ≤0.001) and patients (p ≤0.001) at the end of the treatment phase

A more recent placebo-controlled study on 289 patients with moderate to severe PAR substantiated these findings. Improvements in nasal symptoms, postnasal discharges, ocular symptoms, and rescue medication usage were significant in the omalizumab treatment group as compared with the placebo group.[137] Forty percent of the omalizumab trial patients showed large improvements in QOL as compared with 25% receiving placebo (p = 0.0001) at 8 weeks. By 16 weeks, the improvements were 51% and 27%, respectively (p = 0.001). The active treatment was well tolerated. No differences in adverse event profiles were noted between treated and placebo groups.[138]

Study D01 (IA11) was a phase IIIb investigation of the efficacy, safety and tolerability of omalizumab as an adjunct to specific immunotherapy (SIT) in children 6 to 17 years old with birch pollen– and grass pollen–induced SAR. Omalizumab 0.016 mg/kg/IgE (IU/ml) was administered every 2 to 4 weeks for 24 weeks. Patients treated with omalizumab plus immunotherapy in a placebo-controlled study design produced better symptom load scores over the entire pollen season (p ≤0.001) and showed reduced need for rescue medications (p ≤0.001) than those receiving placebo plus immunotherapy.[139,140] An even more interesting approach would be to use omalizumab as a protective umbrella during the initial phase of SIT in the hope that it would allow faster dose increases and higher maintenance doses with lower risks of adverse reactions. Omalizumab may open a therapeutic avenue for patients who are not adequately treated with SIT, especially those with multiple organ involvement. Using anti-IgE to provide a period during which SIT could be given more safely could serve as another approach to using SIT for other conditions such as food hypersensitivity and latex allergy.

1. Safety and Tolerability

The overall profile of adverse events showed little difference between the two treatment groups; the injections of omalizumab were well tolerated. The safety database of this drug includes approximately 2000 patients, of whom 1331 were treated with SC omalizumab following recommended dosing regimens for allergic asthma and SAR. Six hundred sixty patients were treated for a minimum of 6 months and 410 for 1 year. All patients in the key phase III studies (allergic asthma and SAR) were tested for anti-omalizumab antibodies at baseline and at follow up; none developed measurable anti-omalizumab titers.

No evidence of immune complex disease or similar syndromes was found. One omalizumab-treated patient experienced an anaphylactoid reaction attributed to the consumption of an antibiotic to which the patient had an established history of adverse reactions. Systemic urticaria, reported for 3.4% of children and 1.4% of adults, was the only adverse event considered to have a potential relationship with omalizumab treatment. The urticaria was mild to moderate in severity and appeared to be more common in children receiving the highest doses (750 mg every 4 weeks). No dose relationship was evident in adults.

If IgE is involved in host defenses against parasitic infections, one potential side effect of anti-IgE treatment may be an increased incidence of such infections. In the pivotal studies on omalizumab, only a few cases of parasitic infestation were observed. Patients treated with omalizumab experienced no more infestation than subjects on placebo. Most other infections such as herpes zoster occurred with comparable frequency in omalizumab- and placebo-treated patients. Therefore, it seems that treatment with omalizumab is unlikely to produce deleterious effects on the risks or courses of parasitic or other infections. However, more prolonged follow-up periods are required to verify the conclusions of the initial studies.

The relevance of IgE to neoplasia is still controversial, in contrast to the involvement of other immune system components such as cytokines and T (cytotoxic) cells. A large survey in the United States found that after adjustment for age, sex, race, and smoking history, a history of allergy, but not of asthma, seemed to increase the risk of subsequent malignancy. According to Cockcroft et al.,[141] patients with atopy, hay fever, and asthma seemed to have some degree of protection against lung, gut, bladder, and prostate cancers but not against other cancers. If IgE is involved in defense mechanisms against cancer, reducing free IgE levels via anti-IgE treatment may exert adverse effects on these immune defenses. However, this risk has not been borne out by early toxicology studies or clinical trials to date. Because the incidence of malignancy in the patient population under study is very low, surveillance for this potential effect of therapeutic intervention continues, and so far is reassuring.

2. Effects on Allergic Skin Reactivity

An open-label study was conducted to test the hypothesis that treatment with omalizumab would prevent allergic skin reactivity to a skin prick test with dust mite antigen.[136] A total of 47 patients with PAR and positive skin prick tests to dust mite antigen were randomly assigned to receive one of two dosages of omalizumab, with the amount adjusted on the basis of baseline serum concentrations of IgE (0.015 to 0.030 mg/kg/IU/ml IgE every other week).

Skin reactivity was tested after 6 months of treatment, at which time the skin wheal area in response to injections of several different dilutions of dust mite extract was significantly deceased from baseline by omalizumab treatment (p $\leq$0.001). At baseline, the mean summed wheal area of all dilutions of dust mite extract tested was 155 mm^2 (with an SEM of ±31 mm^2) for the low-dose omalizumab group and 181 ± 43 mm^2 for the high-dose group. After 6 months of treatment, the summed wheal area in response to dust mite extract was 61 ± 15 mm^2 for the low-dose group and 34 ± 11 mm^2 for the high-dose group. Urticarial reactions were noted after the first dose of omalizumab in four patients; three elected to remain in the study, and no further reactions were noted with subsequent omalizumab injections.

3. Anti-Inflammatory Effects

A phase III, placebo-controlled, multicenter clinical study investigated whether anti-IgE antibody in addition to SIT affected the leukotriene pathway.[142] Ninety-two children (age range of 6 to 17 years) with sensitization to birch and grass pollen and SAR were randomized to one of four treatment groups. Two groups received birch SIT and two groups received grass SIT for at least 14 weeks before the start of the birch pollen season. After 12 weeks of SIT titration, anti-IgE or a placebo was added for 24 weeks. Anti-IgE was administered SC on the basis of body weight and serum total IgE levels, providing a dose of at least 0.016 mg/kg/IU/ml IgE every 4 weeks.

A recent placebo-controlled, randomized endobronchial biopsy study investigated the effects of omalizumab therapy on tissue cell numbers and activation status in mild persistent asthma.[143] Treatment for 16 weeks was associated with significant reductions in tissue eosinophils, FcϵRI$^+$ cells, CD$_3$$^+$, CD$_4$$^+$, and CD$_8$$^+$ T lymphocytes, B lymphocytes, and cells staining positive for the secretory form of IL-4 (antibody 3H4) that serves as an index of cytokine generation by mast cells. Numbers of mast cells and basophils did not change and, surprisingly, no changes were noted in resting lung function (FEV$_1$) or bronchial responsiveness (PC$_{20}$) despite baseline levels that allowed room for improvement. The striking findings of reduced inflammatory cells within the biopsies, including a 90% reduction in IL-4 sensory mast cells, a near-90% reduction in FcϵRI-positive mast cells, and an 80% reduction in tissue eosinophils are thus difficult to put into perspective in view of the lack of any observable effect on bronchial hyperresponsiveness.

VI. Other Approaches to Neutralizing IgE

The administration of a nonanaphylactogenic humanized monoclonal antibody against IgE to improve IgE-mediated disease is a process of passive immunization. The dose must be adjusted for each individual based on baseline total IgE and weight. Despite this individualization, treatment has not been as effective as would have been anticipated based on animal studies. In this respect, species differences may be important. Human studies involving treatment up to 1 year have so far failed to demonstrate any effect of omalizumab on serum total IgE levels.[113,119,120] Thus, in contrast to the animal studies, the present levels of anti-IgE administration have not appeared to produce any effects on IgE synthesis. Whether this can be achieved through greater inhibition of IgE levels or alternative approaches is unknown, but other strategies of IgE regulation are under consideration.

One such approach is designing an immunotherapeutic vaccine that can induce the host's own generation of anti-IgE antibodies by active immunization. To be successful, the same criterion applied to omalizumab, namely that induced antibodies inhibit IgE-binding to FcϵR1, should apply. The vaccine should inhibit IgE-dependent histamine release but not induce degranulation. Initial development, based on an appreciation of the IgE-binding domains on the heavy chain of IgE, focused on a Cε4 peptide complexed with a carrier protein[144] and a bacterially expressed, recombinant antigen comprising IgE domains Cε2 and Cε3 coupled to a carrier protein.[145] The large immunogens were able to inhibit IgE-mediated skin reactions in sensitized rats. They were, however, limited by low immunogenicity and the potential that a large IgE fragment was likely to be anaphylactogenic.

This led to the concept that an appropriately selected short-chain peptide that would not be anaphylactogenic and could be modified to promote its immunogenicity might fill the desired role. One such synthetic peptide, modified from positions 413 through 435 of a loop region of Cε3, subjected to conformational constraint, and immunopotentiated by linkage to a promiscuous T helper site to produce a chimeric immunogen was shown in animal studies to elicit anti-IgE antibodies and block IgE-mediated histamine release.[146] This immunogen was shown to induce polyclonal site-specific anti-IgE antibodies that do not signal for degranulation. Vaccination of dogs led to significant reductions in serum total IgE.[146] Unlike classical desensitization, this peptide vaccine is not allergen-specific and would thus be effective for all IgE-mediated reactions. Whether it can achieve the desired clinical benefits in humans remains to be evaluated. If this approach proves effective in humans, it will produce significant cost advantages over monoclonal antibody therapy, and effects would be achievable with far fewer injections.

Other approaches under development include a monoclonal antibody to soluble CD23. The soluble form of this receptor augments IgE production by B cells, and the MAb against sCD23 has been shown to reduce circulating total IgE levels although not to a degree that results in clinical efficacy in naturally occurring SAR.[147]

VII. Conclusions

Targeting IgE with a neutralizing monoclonal antibody has provided the first example of a biologically targeted therapy in asthma if one excludes allergen immunotherapy. The results of the asthma and rhinitis trials with omalizumab clearly place IgE as one of the principal portals for the manifestations of these allergic disorders and emphasize the complex interactions that must occur between multiple effector cells in the allergic cascade. Having now set the stage, the challenge for the future is the design of small molecular weight drugs or peptide vaccines that produce longer lasting suspensions of IgE pathways and may serve to prevent the development or progression of allergic diseases and asthma.

References

1. Ishizaka K and Ishizaka T. Physicochemical properties of reaginic antibody. 1. Association of reaginic activity with an immunoglobulin other than gamma A or gamma G globulin. *J Allergy* 1966; 37: 169–185.
2. Ishizaka K, Ishizaka T, and Hornbrook MM. Physicochemical properties of reaginic antibody. V. Correlation of reaginic activity with gamma E globulin antibody. *J Immunol* 1966; 97: 840–853.
3. Ishizaka K and Ishizaka T. Identification of gamma E antibodies as a carrier of reaginic activity. *J Immunol* 1967; 99: 1187–1198.
4. Ishizaka K, Ishizaka T, and Terry WD. Antigenic structure of gamma E globulin and reaginic antibody. *J Immunol* 1967; 99: 849–858.
5. Johansson SG and Bennich H. Immunological studies of an atypical (myeloma) immunoglobulin. *Immunology* 1967; 13: 381–394.
6. Bennich HH, Ishizaka K, Johansson SGD, Rowe DS, Stanwolfe DR, and Terry WD. Immunoglobulin E: a new class of human immunoglobulin. *Bull WHO* 1968; 38: 151–152.
7. Wide L, Bennich H, and Johansson, SGD. Diagnosis of allergy by an *in vitro* test for allergen antibodies. *Lancet* 1967; ii: 1105–1107.
8. Stenius B and Wide L. Reaginic antibody (IgE), skin, and provocation tests to *Dermatophagoides culinae* and house dust in respiratory allergy. *Lancet* 1969; 2: 455–458.
9. Barbee RA, Halonen M, Lebowitz M, and Burrows B. Distribution of IgE in a community population sample: correlations with age, sex, and allergen skin test reactivity. *J Allergy Clin Immunol* 1981; 68: 106–111.
10. Holford-Strevens V, Warren P, Wong C, and Manfreda J. Serum total immunoglobulin E levels in Canadian adults. *J Allergy Clin Immunol* 1984; 73: 516–522.
11. Gerrard JW, Geddes CA, Reggin PL, Gerrard CD, and Horne S. Serum IgE levels in white and metis communities in Saskatchewan. *Ann Allergy* 1976; 37: 91–100.
12. Omenaas E, Bakke P, Elsayed S, Hanoa R, and Gulsvik A. Total and specific serum IgE levels in adults: relationship to sex, age, and environmental factors. *Clin Exp Allergy* 1994; 24: 530–539.
13. Meretey K, Jakab A, Szilassy K, and Medgyesi GA. IgE levels in normal human sera and IgG preparations. *Haematologia* (Budapest) 1989; 22: 151–159.
14. Oryszczyn MP, Annesi I, Neukirch F, Dore MF, and Kauffmann F. Longitudinal observations of serum IgE and skin prick test response. *Am J Respir Crit Care Med* 1995; 151: 663–668.
15. Nielsen M and Menne T. The relationship between IgE-mediated and cell-mediated hypersensitivities in an unselected Danish population: Glostrup Allergy Study, Denmark. *Br J Dermatol* 1996; 134: 669–672.
16. D'Souza W, Lewis S, Cheng S, McMillan D, Pearce N, Town I, Rigby S, Skidmore C, Armstrong R, and Rutherford R. The prevalence of asthma symptoms, bronchial hyperresponsiveness and atopy in New Zealand adults. *NZ Med J* 1999; 112: 198–202.

17. Wittig HJ, Belloit J, De Fillippi I, and Royal G. Age-related serum immunoglobulin E levels in healthy subjects and in patients with allergic disease. *J Allergy Clin Immunol* 1980; 66: 305–313.
18. Grundbacher FJ and Massie FS. Levels of immunoglobulin G, M, A, and E at various ages in allergic and nonallergic black and white individuals. *J Allergy Clin Immunol* 1985; 75: 651–658.
19. Criqui MH, Seibles JA, Hamburger RN, Coughlin SS, and Gabriel S. Epidemiology of immunoglobulin E levels in a defined population. *Ann Allergy* 1990; 64: 308–313.
20. Burrows B, Martinez FD, Halonen M, Barbee RA, and Cline MG. Association of asthma with serum IgE levels and skin-test reactivity to allergens. *New Engl J Med* 1989; 320: 271–277.
21. Sears MR, Chow CM, and Morseth DJ. Serum total IgE in normal subjects and the influence of a family history of allergy. *Clin Allergy* 1980; 10: 423–431.
22. Mygind N, Dirksen A, Johnsen NJ, and Weeke B. Perennial rhinitis: an analysis of skin testing, serum IgE, and blood and smear eosinophilia in 201 patients. *Clin Otolaryngol* 1978; 3: 189–196.
23. Wuthrich B. Serum IgE in atopic dermatitis: relationship to severity of cutaneous involvement and course of disease as well as coexistence of atopic respiratory diseases. *Clin Allergy* 1978; 8: 241–248.
24. Sunyer J, Anto JM, Sabria J, Roca J, Morell F, Rodriguez-Roisin R, and Rodrigo MJ. Relationship between serum IgE and airway responsiveness in adults with asthma. *J Allergy Clin Immunol* 1995; 95: 699–706.
25. Grundbacher FJ. Causes of variation in serum IgE levels in normal populations. *J Allergy Clin Immunol* 1975; 56: 104–111.
26. Gerrard JW, Ko CG, Dalgleish R, and Tan LK. Immunoglobulin levels in white and metis communities in Saskatchewan. *Clin Exp Immunol* 1977; 29: 447–456.
27. Sears MR, Burrows B. Flannery EM. Herbison GP. Hewitt CJ. and Holdaway MD. Relation between airway responsiveness and serum IgE in children with asthma and in apparently normal children. *New Engl J Med* 1991; 325: 1067–1071.
28. Tollerud DJ, O'Connor GT, Sparrow D, and Weiss ST. Asthma, hay fever, and phlegm production associated with distinct patterns of allergy skin test reactivity, eosinophilia, and serum IgE levels: the Normative Aging Study. *Am Rev Respir Dis* 1991; 144: 7767–7781.
29. Vollmer WM, Buist AS, Johnson LR, McCamant LE, and Halonen M. Relationship between serum IgE and cross-sectional and longitudinal FEV$_1$ in two cohort studies. *Chest* 1986; 90: 416–423.
30. Warren CP, Holford-Strevens V, Wong C, and Manfreda J. The relationship between smoking and total immunoglobulin E levels. *J Allergy Clin Immunol* 1982; 69: 370–375.
31. Oryszczyn MP, Annesi I, Neukirch F, Dore MF, and Kauffmann F. Relationships of total IgE level, skin prick test response, and smoking habits. *Ann Allergy* 1991; 67: 355–358.
32. Annesi I, Oryszczyn MP, Frette C, Neukirch F, Orvoen-Frija E, and Kauffmann F. Total circulating IgE and FEV$_1$ in adult men: an epidemiologic longitudinal study. *Chest* 1992; 101: 642–648.

33. Salkie ML, Weimer N, and Herbert FA. Serum total IgE and allergen specific IgE in an adult asthmatic population. *Diagn Immunol* 1983; 1: 72–74.
34. Zeiger R and Heller S. The development and prediction of atopy in high-risk children: follow-up at age seven years in a prospective randomised study of combined maternal and infant food allergen avoidance. *J Allergy Clin Immunol* 1999; 95: 1179–1190.
35. Wright AL, Holberg CJ, Martinez FD, Halonen M, Morgan W, and Taussig LM. Epidemiology of physician-diagnosed allergic rhinitis in childhood. *Pediatrics* 1994; 94: 895–901.
36. Hansen LG, Halken S, Host A, Moller K, and Osterballe O. Prediction of allergy from family history and cord blood IgE levels: follow-up at the age of 5 years. IV. Cord blood IgE. *Pediatr Allergy Immunol* 1993; 4: 34–40.
37. Inouye T, Tarlo S, Broder I, Corey P, Davies G, Leznoff A, Mintz S, and Thomas P. Severity of asthma in skin test-negative and skin test-positive patients. *J Allergy Clin Immunol* 1985; 75: 313–319.
38. Bousquet J, Coulomb Y, Arrendal H, Robinet-Levy M, and Michel FB. Total serum IgE concentrations in adolescents and adults using the phadebas IgE PRIST technique. *Allergy* 1982; 37: 397–406.
39. Lebowitz MD, Bronnimann S, and Camilli AE. Asthmatic risk factors and bronchial reactivity in non-diagnosed asthmatic adults. *Eur J Epidemiol* 1995; 11: 541–548.
40. European Community Respiratory Health Survey. Determinants of bronchial responsiveness in the European Community Respiratory Health Survey in Italy: evidence of an independent role of atopy, total serum IgE levels, and asthma symptoms. *Allergy* 1998; 53: 673–681.
41. Grol MH, Postma DS, Vonk JM, Schouten JP, Rijcken B, Koeter GH, and Gerritsen J. Risk factors from childhood to adulthood for bronchial responsiveness at age 32–42 years. *Am J Respir Crit Care Med* 1999; 160: 150–156.
42. Scalabrin DM, Bavbek S, Perzanowski MS, Wilson BB, Platts-Mills TA, and Wheatley LM. Use of specific IgE in assessing the relevance of fungal and dust mite allergens to atopic dermatitis: a comparison with asthmatic and nonasthmatic control subjects. *J Allergy Clin Immunol* 1999; 104: 1273–1279.
43. Shadick NA, Sparrow D, O'Connor GT, DeMolles D, and Weiss ST. Relationship of serum IgE concentration to level and rate of decline of pulmonary function: Normative Aging Study. *Thorax* 1996; 51: 787–792.
44. Laprise C and Boulet LP. Asymptomatic airway hyperresponsiveness: a three-year follow-up. *Am J Respir Crit Care Med* 1997; 156: 403–409.
45. Hogarth-Scott RS, Howlett BJ, McNicol KN, Simons MJ, and Williams HE. IgE levels in the sera of asthmatic children. *Clin Exp Immunol* 1971; 9: 571–576.
46. McNichol KN and Williams HE. Spectrum of asthma in children. II. Allergic components. *Br Med J* 1973; 4: 12–16.
47. Spittle BJ and Sears MR. Bronchial asthma: lack of relationships between allergic factors, illness severity and psychosocial variables in adult patients attending an asthma clinic. *Psychol Med* 1984; 14: 847–852.
48. Wilson NM, Dore CJ, and Silverman M. Factors relating to the severity of symptoms at 5 years in children with severe wheeze in the first 2 years of life. *Eur Respir J* 1997; 10: 346–353.

49. Sherrill DL, Stein R, Halonen M, Holberg CJ, Wright A, and Martinez FD. Total serum IgE and its association with asthma symptoms and allergic sensitization among children. *J Allergy Clin Immunol* 1999; 104: 28–36.

50. Mosmann TR, Cherwinski H, Bond MW, Giedlin MA, and Coffman RL. Two types of murine helper T cell clone. I. Definition according to profiles of lymphokine activities and secreted proteins. *J Immunol* 1986; 136: 2348–2357.

51. Lebman DA and Coffman RL. Interleukin-4 causes isotype switching to IgE in T cell-stimulated clonal B cell cultures. *J Exp Med* 1988; 168: 853–862.

52. Vercelli D, Jabara HH, Arai K, and Geha RS. Induction of human IgE synthesis requires interleukin-4 and T/B cell interactions involving the T cell receptor/CD3 complex and MHC class II antigens. *J Exp Med* 1989; 169: 1295–1307.

53. Vercelli D, Raif S, and Geha. RS. Regulation of IgE Synthesis in humans: a tale of two signals. *J Allergy Clin Immunol* 1991; 8: 285–295.

54. Callard RE, Matthews DJ, and Hibbert L. IL-4 and IL-13 receptors: are they one and the same? *Immunol Today* 1996; 17; 108–110.

55. McKenzie ANJ, Culpepper JA, DeWaal-Malefyt R, Briere F, Punnonen J, Aversa G, Sato A, Dang W, Cocks BG, Menon S, Vries JED, Banchereau J, and Zurawski G. Interleukin-13, a T cell-derived cytokine that regulates human monocyte and B cell function. *Proc Nat Acad Sci USA* 90: 1993; 3735–3739.

56. Brinkman V and Kinzel B. IL-4 and IL-13 in atopy: regulation of production and effects, in *IgE Regulation: Molecular Mechanisms*, Vercelli D, Ed, Chichester: John Wiley & Sons. 1997, pp. 75–101.

57. Ishizako K, Ishizaka T, and Lee EH. Biologic function of the Fe fragments of E-myeloma. *Protein Immunochem* 1970; 7: 687–702.

58. Plant M, Pilice JH, Watson CJ, Hauley-Hyde J, Nordau RP, and Paul W. Mast cell lines produce lymphokines in response to cross-linkage of FcRW$_I$ or to calcium ionophore. *Nature* 1989; 339: 64–67.

59. Holgate ST, Robinson C, Church MK, and Howarth PH. The release and role of inflammatory mediators in asthma. *Clin Immunol Rev* 1985; 4: 241–288.

60. Holgate ST. Contribution of inflammatory mediators to the immediate asthmatic reaction. *Am Rev Respir Dis* 1987; 135: S57–S62.

61. Howarth PH, Salagean M, and Dokic D. Allergic rhinitis: not purely a histamine-related disease. *Allergy* 2000; 55: 7–16.

62. Sutton BJ and Gould HJ. The human IgE network. *Nature* 1993, 366: 421–428.

63. Yamaguchi M, Lantz CS, Oettgen HC, Katona IM, Fleming T, Miyajima I, Kinet JP, and Galli SJ. IgE enhances mouse mast cell FcRI expression *in vitro* and *in vivo*: evidence for a novel amplification mechanism in IgE-dependent reactions. *J Exp Med* 1997; 185: 663–672.

64. Kisselgof AB and Oettgen HC. The expression of murine B cell CD23 *in vivo* is regulated by its ligand, IgE. *Int Immunol* 1998; 10: 1377–1384.

65. Ishizaka K. IgE binding factors and regulation of IgE antibody response. *Annu Rev Immunol* 1988; 6: 513–534.

66. Corry DB and Kheradmand F. Induction and regulation of the IgE response. *Nature* 1999; 402: B18–B23.

67. Johansson SG, Hourihane JO, Bousquet J, Bruijnzeel-Koomen C, Dreborg S, Haahtela T, Kowalski ML, Mygind N, Ring J, van Cauwenberge P, van Hage-Hamsten M, and Wuthrich B. European Academy of Allergology and Clinical Immunology Nomenclature Task Force: revised nomenclature for allergy. *Allergy* 2001; 56: 813–824.

68. Humbert M, Grant JA, Taborda-Barata L, Durham SR, Pfister R, Menz G, Barkans J, Ying S, and Kay AB. High-affinity IgE receptor (Fc$_\varepsilon$RI)-bearing cells in bronchial biopsies from atopic and nonatopic asthma. *Am J Respir Crit Care Med* 1996; 153: 1931–1937.

69. Humbert M, Menz G, Ying S, Corrigan CJ, Robinson DS, Durham SR, and Kay AB. The immunopathology of extrinsic (atopic) and intrinsic (non-atopic) asthma: more similarities than differences. *Immunol Today* 1999; 20: 528–533.

70. Fick RB Jr, Fox JA, and Jardieu PM. Immunotherapy approach to allergic disease. *Immunopharmacology* 2000; 48: 307–310.

71. Bryan SA, Leckie MJ, Hansel TT, and Barnes PJ. Novel therapy for asthma. *Expert Opin Invest Drugs* 2000; 9: 25–42.

72. Presta L, Shields R, O'Connell L, Lahr S, Porter J, Gorman C, and Jardieu P. The binding site on human immunoglobulin-E for its high-affinity receptor. *J Biol Chem* 1994; 269: 26368–26373.

73. Presta LG, Lahr SJ, Shields RL, Porter JP, Gorman CM, Fendly BM, and Jardieu PM. Humanization of an antibody directed against IgE. *J Immunol* 1993; 151: 2623–2632.

74. Davis FM, Gossett LA, Pinkston KL, Liou RS, Sun LK, Kim YW, Chang NT, Chang TW, Wagner K, Bews J et al. Can anti-IgE be used to treat allergy? *Springer Sem Immunopathol* 1993; 15: 51–73.

75. Chang TW. Treating hypersensitiveness with anti-IgE monoclonal antibodies that bind to IgE-expressing B cells but not to basophils. U.S. Patent 5,543, 634, 1996.

76. Chang TW, Davis FM, Sun NC, Sun CR, MacGlashan DW, Jr, and Hamilton RG. Monoclonal antibodies specific for human IgE-producing B cells: a potential therapeutic for IgE-mediated allergic diseases. *Biotechnology* 1990; 8: 122–126.

77. Hook WA, Zinsser FU, Berenstein EH, and Siraganian RP. Monoclonal antibodies defining epitopes on human IgE. *Mol Immunol* 1991; 28: 631–639.

78. Hook WA, Berenstein EH, Zinsser FU, Fischler C, and Siraganian RP. Monoclonal antibodies to the leukocyte common antigen (CD45) inhibit IgE-mediated histamine release from human basophils. *J Immunol* 1991; 147: 2670–2676.

79. Baniyash M and Eshhar Z. Inhibition of IgE binding to mast cells and basophils by monoclonal antibodies to murine IgE. *Eur J Immunol* 1984; 14: 799–807.

80. Magnusson CG and Johansson SG. Clinical significance of anti-IgE autoantibodies and immune complexes containing IgE. *Clin Rev Allergy* 1989; 7: 73–103.

81. Stadler BM, Rudolf MP, Zurcher AW, Miescher S, and Vogel M. Anti-IgE in allergic sensitization. *Immunol Cell Biol* 1996; 74: 195–200.

82. Chang TW, Davis FM, Suncry-MacGlashan DW, and Hamilton RG. Monoclonal antibodies specific for human IgE producing B cells: a potential therapeutic for IgE-mediated allergic diseases. *Biol Technnol* 1990; 8: 122–126.

83. Peng C, Davis FM, Sun LK, Liou RS, Kim YW, and Chang TW. A new isoform of human membrane-bound IgE. *J Immunol* 1992; 148: 129–136.

84. Bozelka BE, McCants ML, Salvaggio JE, and Lehrer SB. IgE isotype suppression in anti-epsilon-treated mice. *Immunology* 1982; 46: 527–532.

85. Bozelka BE, McCants ML, Salvaggio JE, and Lehrer SB. Effects of anti-epsilon on total and specific IgE levels in adult mice. *Int Arch Allergy Appl Immunol* 1985; 78: 51–56.

86. Haba S and Nisonoff A. Effects of syngeneic anti-IgE antibodies on the development of IgE memory and on the secondary IgE response. *J Immunol* 1994; 152: 51–57.

87. Haba S and Nisonoff A. Role of antibody and T cells in the long-term inhibition of IgE synthesis. *Proc Natl Acad Sci USA* 1994; 91: 604–608.

88. Haak-Frendscho M, Robbins K, Lyon R, Shields R, Hooley J, Schoenhoff M, and Jardieu P. Administration of an anti-IgE antibody inhibits CD23 expression and IgE production *in vivo*. *Immunology* 1994; 82: 306–313.

89. Heusser C and Jardieu P. Therapeutic potential of anti-IgE antibodies. *Curr Opin Immunol* 1997; 9: 805–813.

90. Heusser CH, Bews J, Brinkmann V, Delespesse G, Kilchherr E, Ledermann F, Le Gros G, and Wagner K. New concepts of IgE regulation. *Int Arch Allergy Appl Immunol* 1991; 94: 87–90.

91. Heusser CH, Wagner K, Bews JPA, Coyle A, Bertrand C, Einsle K, Kips J, Eum SY, Lefort J, and Vargaftig BB. Demonstration of the therapeutic potential of non-anaphylactogenic anti-IgE antibodies in murine models of skin reaction, lung function and inflammation. *Int Arch Allergy Immunol* 1997; 113: 231–235.

92. Kolbinger F, Saldanha J, Hardman N, and Bendig MM. Humanization of a mouse anti-human IgE antibody: a potential therapeutic for IgE-mediated allergies. *Protein Eng* 1993; 6: 971–980.

93. Riechmann L, Clark M, Waldmann H, and Winter G. Reshaping human antibodies for therapy. *Nature* 1988; 332: 323–327.

94. Carter P, Presta L, Gorman CM, Ridgway JB, Henner D, Wong WL, Rowland AM, Kotts C, Carver ME, and Shepard HM. Humanization of an anti-p185HER2 antibody for human cancer therapy. *Proc Nat Acad Sci USA* 1992; 89: 4285–4289.

95. Haak-Frendscho M, Ridgway J, Shields R, Robbins K, Gorman C, and Jardieu P. Human IgE receptor alpha-chain IgG chimera blocks passive cutaneous anaphylaxis reaction *in vivo*. *J Immunol* 1993; 151: 351–358.

96. Shields RL, Whether WR, Zioncheck K, O'Connell L, Fendly B, Presta LG, Thomas D, Saban R, and Jardieu P. Inhibition of allergic reactions with antibodies to IgE. *Int Arch Allergy Immunol* 1995; 107: 308–312.

97. Fox JA, Hotaling TE, Struble C, Ruppel J, Bates DJ, and Schoenhoff MB. Tissue distribution and complex formation with IgE of an anti-IgE antibody after intravenous administration in cynomolgus monkeys. *J Pharmacol Exp Ther* 1996; 279: 1000–1008.

98. Meng YG, Singh N, and Wong WL. Binding of cynomolgus monkey IgE to a humanized anti-human IgE antibody and human high affinity IgE receptor. *Mol Immunol* 1996; 33: 635–642.

99. Coyle AJ, Le Gros G, Bertrand C, Tsuyuki S, Heusser CH, Kopf M, and Anderson GP. Interleukin-4 is required for the induction of lung Th-2 mucosal immunity. *Am J Respir Cell Mol Biol* 1995; 13: 54–59.

100. Nakajima H, Iwamoto I, Tomoe S, Matsumura R, Tomioka H, Takatsu K, and Yoshida S. CD4+ T lymphocytes and interleukin-5 mediate antigen-induced eosinophil infiltration into the mouse trachea. *Am Rev Respir Dis* 1992; 146: 374–377.

101. Coyle AJ, Eurmsy Lefort J, Heusser C, and Vargaflig B. Central role of IgE to antigen induced bronchoconstriction: eosinophil accumulation and airway hypereactivity: inhibition by a non-aphylactogenic anti IgE monoclonal antibody. *Am J Respir Crit Care Med* 1996; 153; A217.

102. Saban R, Haak-Frendscho M, Zine M, Ridgway J, Gorman C, Presta LG, Bjorling D, Saban M, and Jardieu P. Human FcERI-IgG and humanized anti-IgE monoclonal antibody MaE11 block passive sensitization of human and rhesus monkey lung. *J Allergy Clin Immunol* 1994; 94: 836–843.

103. Rabe KF, Watson N, Dent G, Morton BE, Wagner K, Magnussen H, and Heusser CH. Inhibition of human airway sensitization by a novel monoclonal anti-IgE antibody 17-9. *Am J Respir Crit Care Med* 1998; 157: 1429–1435.

104. Marshall JS, Wells PD, and Bell EB. Accelerated elimination of *N. brasiliensis* from the small intestine after auto-anti-IgE induction. *Immunology* 1987; 60: 303–308.

105. Amiri P, Haak-Frendscho M, Robbins K, McKerrow JH, Stewart T, and Jardieu P. Anti-immunoglobulin E treatment decreases worm burden and egg production in *Schistosoma mansoni*-infected normal and interferon gamma knockout mice. *J Exp Med* 1994; 180: 43–51.

106. Milgrom H. Is there a role for treatment of asthma with omalizumab? *Arch Dis Child* 2003; 88: 71–74.

107. MacGlashan DW, Jr, Bochner BS, Adelman DC, Jardieu PM, Togias A, McKenzie-White J, Sterbinsky SA, Hamilton RG, and Lichtenstein LM. Down-regulation of $Fc_{e}RI$ expression on human basophils during *in vivo* treatment of atopic patients with anti-IgE antibody. *J Immunol* 1997; 158: 1438–1445.

108. Liu J, Lester P, Builder S, and Shire SJ. Characterization of complex formation by humanized anti-IgE monoclonal antibody and monoclonal human IgE. *Biochemistry* 1995; 34: 10474–10482.

109. Schoernhoff M, Lim Y, Frochlich J, Fick RB, and Bates D. A pharmacodynamic model describing free IgE concentrations following administration of a recombinant humanised monoclonal anti-IgE antibody in humans (abstract). *Pharm Res* 1995; 12: S411.

110. Schoernhoff M, Bates D, Ruppel J, Fei D, Fox JA, Thomas D et al. Pharmacokinetics/pharmacodynamics following administration of a humanised recombinant monoclonal anti IgE antibody in the cynomolgus monkey (abstract). *Allergy Clin J* 1995; 95: 356.

111. Novartis Pharmaceutical Corporation, Basel, Switzerland. Data on file.

112. Fox JA. Binding of MAb-E25 to Serum IgE in Atopic Individuals, Report FR99. Genentech Corporation, South San Francisco, CA, 2000, pp. 510–560.

113. Milgrom H, Fick RB, Su JQ et al. Treatment of allergic asthma with monoclonal anti-IgE antibody. *New Engl J Med* 1999; 341: 1966–1923.

114. Froehlich J, Schorenhoff M, Tremblay T, Ruppel J, and Jardieu P. Initial human study with a humanised recombinant anti-IgE monoclonal antibody: safety, tolerance and pharmacokinetic (PK) dynamic profile. *Clin Pharmacol Ther* 1995; 57: 162.

115. Schulman ES. Development of a monoclonal anti IgE antibody (malizumab) for the treatment of allergic respiratory disorders. *Am J Respir Crit Care Med* 2001; 164: S6–S11.

116. Froehlich J, Schoenhoff M, Jardieu P, Ruppel J, Fei D, Buckeley P, and Bush R, Multiple doses of recombinant humanised monoclonal anti-IgE antibodies are safely tolerated and disease-free serum IgE to undetectable levels *J Allergy Clin Immunol* 1995; 95: 356 (abstract).

117. Buisberg D, Froehlich J, Schoenhoff M, and Mendelson J. Multiple administration of the anti-IgE recombinant humanised monoclonal antibody E25 (rhu MAb-E25) reduced free IgE levels in a dose-dependent manner in adolescents and children with moderate to severe allergic asthma. Presented at American College of Chest Physicians 25th Annual Meeting, Chicago, 1999.

118. Correy J, Froehlich J, Schoenhoff M, Spedal S, Rachelefsky G, Schauker H, Patnaik M, and Siegal S. Phase I study of anti-IgE recombinant humanised monoclonal antibody rhu MAb-E25 (E25) in adults with moderate to severe asthma. *J Allergy Clin Immunol* 1996; 97: 245.

119. Boulet LP, Chapman KR, Cote J. et al. Inhibitory effects of an anti-IgE antibody E25 on allergen-induced early asthmatic response. *Am J Respir Crit Care Med* 1997; 115: 1835–1840.

120. Busse WW, Correy J, Lanier BQ et al. Omalizumab, anti-IgE recombinant humanised monoclonal antibody for the treatment of severe allergic asthma. *J Allergy Clin Immunol* 2001; 108: 184–190.

121. Soler M, Matz J, Townley RG et al. The anti-IgE antibody, omalizumab reduced exacerbations and steroid requirements in allergic asthmatics. *Eur Respir J* 2001; 18: 254–261.

122. Milgrom H, Berger W, Nayak A et al. Treatment of childhood asthma with anti-immunoglobulin E antibody (omalizumab). *Paediatrics* 2001; 108: E36.

123. Juniper EF, Guya HGH, Feeny DH et al. Measuring quality of life in children with asthma. *Qual Life Res* 1996; 5: 35–46.

124. Juniper EF, Guya HGH, Ferrie PJ et al. Measuring quality of life in asthma. *Am Rev Respir Dis* 1993; 147: 832–838.

125. Juniper EF, Guya HGH, William A, and Griffith LE. Determining a minimal important change in a disease-specific quality of life questionnaire. *J Clin Epidemiol* 1999; 47: 81–87.

126. Holgate ST, Chachalin A, Herbert J et al. Omalizumab, a novel therapy for severe allergic asthma. *Eur Respir J* 2001, 18: S37.

127. Holgate ST, Chachalin A, Herbert J et al. Omalizumab improves quality of life in patients with severe allergic asthma. *Eur Respir J* 2001, 18: S37.

128. Finn A, Gross G, van Bavel J, Lee T, Windom H, Everhard F, Fowler-Taylor A, Liu J, and Gupta N. Omalizumab improves asthma-related quality of life in patients with severe allergic asthma. *J Allergy Clin Immunol* 2003; 111: 278–284.

129. Corren J, Casale T, Deniz Y, and Ashby M. Omalizumab, a recombinant humanised anti-IgE antibody, reduced asthma-related emergency room visits and hospitalisations in patients with allergic asthma. *J Allergy Clin Immunol* 2003, 111: 87–90.

130. Holgate ST, Bousquet J, Wenzel S, Fox H, Liu J, and Castellsague J. Efficacy of omalizumab, an anti-immunoglobulin E antibody, in patients with allergic asthma at high risk of serious asthma-related morbidity and mortality. *Curr Med Res Opin* 2001; 17: 233–240.

131. Lanier BQ, Corren J, Lumry W, Liu J, Fowler-Taylor A, and Gupta N. Omalizumab is effective in the long-term control of severe allergic asthma. *Ann Allergy Asthma Immunol* 2003; 91: 154–159.

132. Casale TB, Condemi J, La Force C et al. Effects of omalizumab on symptoms of rhinitis. *JAMA* 2001; 286: 2956–2967.

133. Nayak A, LaForce CF, Rowe M, Waltnous M, Fick R, McCaulry M et al. Rhu MAb-E25 improves quality of life in patients with seasonal allergic rhinitis (abstract). *J Allergy Clin Immunol* 1999; 103: 549.

134. Adelroth E, Rak S, Haahtela T, Assaud G, Rosenhall L, Zetterstrom O, Byrne A, Champion K, Thistlewell J, Cioppa GD et al. Recombinant humanized MAb-E25, an anti-IgE MAb, in birch pollen induced seasonal allergic rhinitis. *J Allergy Clin Immunol* 2000; 106: 253–259.

135. Casale TB, Condemi J, Bernstein JA, Busse WW, Nayak A, Fick R, Fowler-Taylor A, Gupta N. and Rohane PW. Safety of administration of rhu MAb-E25 in seasonal allergic rhinitis (abstract). *J Allergy Asthma Immunol* 2000; 84: A70.

136. Togias A, Corren J, Shapiro G et al. Anti-IgE treatment reduces skin test reactivity. *J Allergy Clin Immunol* 1998; 101: S171.

137. Chervinsky P. Busse W, Casale T et al. Xolair® in the treatment of perennial allergic rhinitis. *J Allergy Clin Immunol* 2001; 107: 513.

138. Casale T, Chervinsky P, Busse W et al. Omalizumab in the treatment of perennial allergic rhinitis. *Eur Resp J* 2001; 18: S37.

139. Kuehr J, Zielen S, Schauer U et al. Omalizumab (Xolair®, rhu MAb-E25) in children with seasonal allergic rhinitis to birch and grass pollen: superior efficacy of Xolair® plus specific immunotherapy alone during grass pollen season. *Allergy* 2001; 56: 93–94.

140. Wahn U, Zielen S, Schauer U et al. Omalizumab (Xolair®, rhu mAB-E25) plus specific immunotherapy in children with allergic rhinitis is superior to specific immunotherapy alone. *Allergy* 2001; 56: 61.

141. Cockcroft DW, Klein GJ, Donovan RE, and Copland GM. Is there a negative correlation between malignancy and respiratory atopy? *Ann Allergy* 1979; 43: 345–347.

142. Kopp MV, Riedinger F, Beischerd D et al. Combined effect of omalizumab (rhuMAb-25, Xolair®) and specific immunotherapy on *in vitro* leukotrine release. *Allergy* 2001; 56: 93.

143. Djukanovic R, Wilson SJ, Kraft M, Jarjour NN, Steel M, Chung KF, Bao W, Fowler-Taylor A, Matthews J, Busse WW, Holgate ST, and Fahy JV. The effects of recombinant, humanized anti-IgE antibody (omalizumab) treatment on airway inflammation in allergic asthma. *Am J Respir Crit Care Med* Dec. 2004.

144. Stanworth DR, Jones VM, Lewin IV, and Nayyar S. Allergy treatment with a peptide vaccine. *Lancet* 1990; 336: 1279–1281.
145. Hellman L. Profound reduction in allergen sensitivity following treatment with a novel allergy vaccine. *Eur J Immunol* 1994; 24: 415–420.
146. Wang CY, Walfield AM, Fang X et al. Synthetic IgE peptide vaccine for immunotherapy of allergy. *Vaccine* 2003; 21: 1580–1590.
147. Holgate ST and Brodie D. New targets for allergic rhinitis: a disease of civilisation. *Nature Rev Drug Dis* 2003; 2: 903–914.

23

DNA Vaccination for Asthma

DAVID H. BROIDE

University of California San Diego
La Jolla, California, U.S.A.

I. Introduction

Asthma is an inflammatory disease of the airways characterized by infiltration of the airways with lymphocytes expressing several Th2-type cytokines including interleukin (IL)-4 (a switch factor for IgE synthesis), IL-5 (an eosinophil growth factor), IL-9 (an inducer of mucus expression), and IL-13 (a cytokine that can induce airway hyperreactivity).[1,2] A variety of novel therapeutic strategies for asthma are currently under investigation to determine whether interruption of the cascade of pro-inflammatory cytokines can reduce levels of airway inflammation and associated airway hyperreactivity. In general, therapeutic strategies for asthma have focused on antagonizing single downstream cytokines and mediators (IL-5, LTC_4) or alternatively targeting an upstream cell (Th2 lymphocyte) that regulates the expression of multiple downstream cytokines and mediators.[3]

The advantage of targeting a downstream mediator is its probable greater safety margin compared with targeting an upstream cell that regulates the expression of multiple mediators and cytokines, some of which may be important to host defense. However, therapies that target a single cytokine or mediator may be less likely to beneficially impact a disease such as asthma in which multiple cells, cytokines, and mediators play important roles in disease expression.

Thus, one novel approach to down-regulating the complex inflammatory response in asthma is to use DNA-based vaccines to target the Th2 cells that express several cytokines important to the pathogenesis of asthma. In this chapter we will review results of studies investigating the therapeutic potentials of several DNA-based vaccine strategies including the use of immunostimulatory DNA sequences containing a CpG DNA motif (also known as ISS), cyrosine phosphorotheate guanosone (CpG) DNA conjugated to an allergen protein, and DNA allergen gene vaccines in animal models of asthma, and discuss results of preliminary studies in humans.

II. Immunostimulatory DNA

A. Identification of CpG DNA as an Immunostimulatory DNA Sequence

In the 1980s, Japanese investigators attempted to identify the components of *Mycobacterium bovis* bacillus Calmette–Guerin (BCG) responsible for its antitumor activity.[4] Although BCG is a complex of proteins, DNA, RNA, lipids, and carbohydrates, investigators found that its antitumor activity was contained in its DNA fraction.[4] To determine whether the immunostimulatory activity of DNA derived from BCG was dependent on the sequence of DNA bases, different base pair sequences of single-stranded oligoDNAs were synthesized and the ability of these oligoDNAs to augment natural killer (NK) cell function in mouse spleen cells evaluated. The immunostimulatory activity of the DNA was noted to be contained in a 6-base pair DNA sequence that followed the 5′–purine–purine–CpG–pyrimidine–pyrimidine–3′ formula.[5]

The identification of this key immunostimulatory DNA sequence allowed further studies to characterize its receptor binding, signal transduction, immune modulation, and anti-inflammatory effects in animal models and in human disease. Although the immunomodulatory properties of CpG DNA were initially identified based on its antitumor activity, CpG DNA was subsequently shown to inhibit and reverse asthmatic responses precipitated by allergen or viruses in mouse models of asthma.[6–8]

B. Th1 Immune Response to CpG DNA

CpG DNA induces a strong Th1 immune response to antigen stimulation *in vitro* and *in vivo*. The immune response to CpG DNA is characterized by the expression of Th1 cytokines including interferon (IFN)-γ, IL-6, IL-10, IL-12, IL-18, IFN-α, and IFN-β.[9–15] CpG DNA also up-regulates the expression of Th1 cytokine receptors such as the IFN-γ receptor.[15] In addition to inducing Th1 responses, CpG DNA inhibits expression of Th2 cytokines including IL-4,[7] IL-5,[6] IL-9,[16] and IL-13[17] in the lungs, while also reducing levels of expression of Th2 cytokine receptors such as the IL-4 receptor.[15] This inhibitory effect of CpG DNA on Th2 cells is the rationale for investigating its effectiveness as a novel therapy in asthma. Although CpG DNA exerts marked immunomodulatory effects on T lymphocytes, this effect is not due to its direct effect on T lymphocytes because T lymphocytes do not express receptors for CpG DNA. Rather, the immunomodulatory effect of CpG DNA is due to its effect on cells that express Toll-like receptor (TLR)-9, the receptor for CpG DNA, in particular dendritic cells and B cells.

C. TLR-9: Receptor for CpG

The TLR family consists of type I transmembrane proteins with leucine-rich repeats in the extracellular domains and Toll/IL-1 receptor (TIR) homology domains in the cytoplasm.[18,19] At least ten members of the TLR family have been identified and are phylogenetically conserved from insects to mammals.

Studies with TLR-9-deficient mice have demonstrated that TLR-9 receptors are important in mediating the immunostimulatory activity of CpG DNA.[20] In contrast, TLR-2- or TLR-4-deficient cells respond normally to CpG DNA.[20] In *in vitro* studies, wild-type splenocytes, but not TLR-9-deficient splenocytes, proliferated in response to stimulation with CpG DNA.[20] Similarly, peritoneal macrophages from wild-type, but not TLR-9-deficient, mice expressed cytokines (IL-12, IL-6) when stimulated with CpG DNA.[20] Stimulation with CpG DNA induced activation of mitogen-activated protein kinases (MAPKs) such as c-Jun N terminal kinase (JNK) and the NF-κB transcription factor (Figure 23.1).

NF-κB is activated in wild-type macrophages stimulated with CpG DNA, but not in TLR-9-deficient macrophages stimulated with CpG DNA,[20] demonstrating the importance of TLR-9 to CpG DNA-mediated activation of NF-κB. CpG DNA-mediated activation of NF-κB and MAPKs is required for all downstream events induced by CpG DNA. Endosomal acidification of CpG DNA[23] and CpG DNA-induced reactive oxygen species generation[24] precede activation of NF-κB and MAPKs (Figure 23.1).

In vivo studies in TLR-9-deficient mice demonstrated the important role TLR-9 plays in mediating the Th1 immune response to antigens in the presence of CpG DNA.[20] Lymph node cells from wild-type mice injected *in vivo* with OVA antigen and CpG DNA generated the Th1 cytokine IFN-γ, whereas lymph node cells derived from TLR-9-deficient mice injected *in vivo* with OVA and CpG DNA did not produce IFN-γ.[20] These studies underscore the *in vivo* importance of TLR-9 to the Th1 immune responses induced by CpG DNA *in vivo*.

While several members of the TLR family are expressed on plasma membranes, signaling through TLR-2 involves the redistribution of this receptor from the membrane into phagosomal vesicles.[18,19,25] Whether CpG DNA interacts with TLR-9 on the cell surface or in the cytoplasm (as is the case with other TLR family members) is not yet known. Although TLR-9 has a transmembrane domain

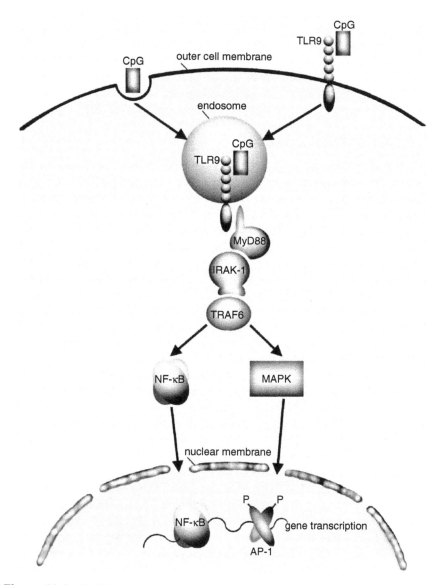

Figure 23.1 CpG DNA activation of TLR-9 intracellular signaling cascade. Studies suggest that CpG DNA is endocytosed into an endosomal vesicle where it binds to TLR-9[26] or that CpG DNA binds to TLR-9 at the cell surface.[22] After CpG DNA binds to TLR-9, it initiates a signaling cascade with recruitment of MyD88, IRAK-1, and TRAF6. Oligomerization of TRAF6 leads to activation of downstream kinases including IKK (which activates the transcription factor NF-κB) and MAPK (which activates the transcription factor AP-1).

and signal peptides, it is thought to be expressed on the cell surface.[20] TLR-9 may be internalized with its ligand CpG DNA into endosomes via nonspecific endocytosis and activated intracellularly after endosomal maturation. Studies support cell surface expression of TLR-9[22] and also support localization of TLR-9 to an intracellular cytoplasmic compartment.[26]

D. Human TLR-9

Human and mouse TLR-9 are 76% identical at the amino acid level.[20] The function of human TLR-9 has been studied in cell lines that do not express TLR-9. They were transiently co-transfected with human TLR-9 and a NF-κB-dependent luciferase reporter.[22] CpG DNA significantly increased NF-κB-dependent luciferase activity in cell lines transfected with human TLR-9 and this response was abrogated by CpG methylation. These studies support the role of human TLR-9 in mediating signaling responses to CpG DNA *in vitro*.

Human dendritic cells express high levels of TLR-9 and mediate many of the biologic effects of CpG DNA.[27–30] The levels of expression of human TLR-9 and other Toll receptors differ in subsets of human dendritic cells. The CD11c negative subset (plasmacytoid dendritic cells) is TLR-9-positive and the CD11c positive subset (myeloid dendritic cells) is TLR-9-negative.[30] As a consequence, plasmacytoid dendritic cells that express TLR-9 can be stimulated with CpG DNA, while myeloid dendritic cells do not respond to CpG DNA. CpG DNA induces human plasmacytoid dendritic cells to express IFN-α that subsequently can stimulate NK cells and T cells to produce IFN-γ and thus promote Th1 immune responses.

E. Signaling through TLR-9

Upon recognition of CpG DNA, TLR-9 recruits the myeloid differentiation factor 88 (MyD88) adaptor molecule via the interactions of their C terminal Toll/IL-1R domains.[31] This recruitment of MyD88 to TLR-9 initiates a signaling pathway that sequentially involves IL-1R-associated kinase 1 (IRAK1) and TNF receptor-associated factor 6 (TRAF6).[32] Oligomerization of TRAF6 leads to activation of downstream kinases such as MAPK and the IKK complex.[31] This in turn results in activation of transcription factors including AP-1 and NF-κB. The TLR-9 MyD88-mediated signaling pathway is important for the CpG DNA-induced activation of MAPK (e.g., JNK), NF-κB, and subsequent production of cytokines in monocytic cells.[31]

F. CpG DNA in Mouse Models of Allergy and Asthma Prevention

Several studies have demonstrated that CpG DNA (also known as ISS) can inhibit Th2 cytokine responses as well as eosinophilic inflammation and airway hyper-reactivity to methacholine in mouse models of asthma.[6,7,33,34] CpG DNA does not reduce eosinophilic inflammation by inducing eosinophilic apoptosis, but rather inhibits generation of IL-5, resulting in decreased production and release of eosinophils from the bone marrow.[6] It has a relatively rapid onset of action, reducing the number of tissue eosinophils within 1 day of administration *in vivo*,[6] and is effective in inhibiting eosinophilic airway inflammation via systemic or mucosal (intranasal or intratracheal) administration.[6]

While a single systemic dose is very effective in inhibiting IL-5, eosinophilic airway inflammation, and bronchial hyperresponsiveness, the inhibition of Th2 responses is not sustained permanently.[35] Th2 responses to inhaled antigen recur at 4 weeks following a single systemic dose of CpG DNA. This suggests that it may be necessary to administer CpG DNA repeatedly at monthly intervals to maintain inhibition of Th2 responses, airway inflammation, and airway hyperreactivity.[35] However, studies of mucosal delivery of two doses demonstrated a prolonged inhibition of eosinophilic airway inflammation for 2 months.[33]

The mechanism by which CpG DNA inhibits allergic inflammatory responses *in vivo* may be more complex than that initially hypothesized based on results of studies in which it induced a strong Th1 immune response. Despite its induction of a strong Th1 response, the anti-allergic effect of CpG DNA may not be mediated by this mechanism *in vivo*. Studies using IFN-γ- and IL-12-deficient mice demonstrated that CpG DNA can mediate its anti-allergic effect *in vivo* independent of the IFN-γ and IL-12 Th1 cytokines.[36] It can also inhibit eosinophilic inflammation and airway hyperreactivity in mice depleted of NK cells, a major source of IFN-γ induced by CpG DNA.[37] Thus, the ability of CpG DNA to induce a Th1 response and IFN-γ expression may not be essential to its inhibitory effect on allergic inflammation *in vivo*. However, some studies suggest that the induction of IFN-γ and a Th1 response is essential to the anti-allergic effect of CpG DNA.[33]

G. Role of MAP Kinase in Mediating Anti-Allergic Effects of CpG DNA *in Vivo*

Studies using pharmacologic inhibitors of mitogen-activated protein kinase (MAPK) suggest an important role for MAP kinase in mediating the anti-allergic effects of CpG DNA *in vivo*.[38] Intrapulmonary administration of CpG DNA results in its rapid localization to alveolar macrophages, triggering the phosphorylation of p38 MAPK.[38] *In vitro* CpG DNA up-regulates IL-12 p40 expression by alveolar macrophages, and these effects are blocked by a pharmacologic inhibitor of p38 MAPK.[38] Intrapulmonary administration of a pharmacologic inhibitor of MAPK blocks the ability of CpG DNA to induce IL-12 expression in the lungs and its ability to inhibit allergic lung inflammation. These findings suggest that MAPK plays an important role *in vivo* in mediating the anti-inflammatory effect of CpG DNA.

H. CpG DNA in Mouse Models of Established Airway Inflammation

Initial studies evaluated whether CpG DNA could prevent eosinophilic inflammation and airway hyperreactivity when administered prior to allergen inhalation challenge.[6,7] Subsequent studies also investigated whether CpG DNA could be administered after allergen inhalation challenge to reverse rather than prevent eosinophilic airway inflammation and airway hyperreactivity.[39,40] CpG DNA was administered 24 hours after allergen challenge at a time when significant eosinophilic airway inflammation already was present.[39]

The effects of the CpG DNA therapy on the resolution of eosinophilic airway inflammation were assessed 6 days after therapy was instituted — a time point when untreated mice sensitized and challenged with allergen still have significant levels (approximately 40 to 50%) of bronchoalveolar lavage fluid eosinophilia. Administration of CpG DNA post-allergen challenge significantly reduced airway eosinophilia, airway hyperreactivity, and mucus expression.[39] These studies suggest that CpG DNA, like corticosteroids, can be used to reverse an episode of allergen-induced airway inflammation.

I. Comparison of CpG DNA and Corticosteroids in Mouse Models of Asthma

Because corticosteroids currently represent the best available anti-inflammatory therapy in asthma, studies have compared the effectiveness of CpG DNA and corticosteroids in inhibiting allergic inflammatory responses in mouse models of asthma.[6,39] Interestingly, in preventive mouse models of asthma, a single dose of CpG DNA was shown to reduce airway eosinophilia as effectively as daily injections of corticosteroids administered for 7 days.[6] In mouse models in which therapy was administered after the induction of airway hyperreactivity, CpG DNA decreased airway hyperreactivity as effectively as dexamethasone[39] (see Figure 23.2).

The combination of CpG DNA and dexamethasone therapy is more effective than monotherapy with either agent alone in reducing airway hyperreactivity (Figure 23.2).[39] Both CpG DNA and corticosteroids inhibit the generation of the Th2 cytokine IL-5 and both therapies inhibit bone marrow generation of eosinophils and the resultant influx of eosinophils into the lungs (Figure 23.3). However, CpG DNA and corticosteroids differ in their mechanisms of eosinophil clearance from the lungs to regional lymph nodes and induction of cellular apoptosis in peribronchial regions. Corticosteroids increase apoptosis and clearance of airway eosinophils; CpG DNA does not.[39] In addition, CpG DNA induces the expression of IFN-γ, a Th1 cytokine that has anti-eosinophilic effects,[41] whereas corticosteroids do not induce IFN-γ (Figure 23.4). CpG DNA and corticosteroids both inhibit

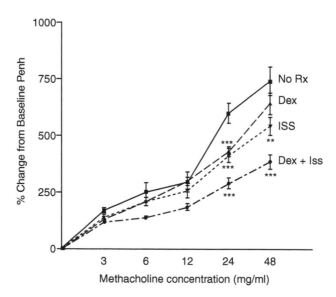

Figure 23.2 Inhibition of allergen-induced airway reactivity to methacholine by ISS, dexamethasone, and combined treatment. Treatment with ISS 1 day after the inhaled allergen challenge inhibited the methacholine (Mch)-induced increase in Penh (n = 24; p = 0.001 at 24 mg/ml Mch and p = 0.008 at 48 mg/ml Mch compared with untreated mice). Treatment with dexamethasone significantly inhibited allergen-induced airway reactivity to Mch compared with untreated mice at 24 mg/ml Mch only (n = 23; *p = 0.004 at 24 mg/ml Mch and p = 0.11 at 48 mg/ml Mch). Combined treatment with ISS and dexamethasone significantly inhibited airway responsiveness to Mch compared with ISS alone (Mch 24 mg/ml, p = 0.002; Mch 48 mg/ml, p = 0.0001) or dexamethasone alone (Mch 24 mg/ml, p = 0.0001; Mch 48 mg/ml, p <0.0001). Results are expressed as mean ± SEM. (From Ikeda R et al., *Am J Respir Cell Mol Biol* 2003; 28: 655–663. With permission.)

mucus production to a similar degree (Figure 23.5). The combination of the shared and distinct anti-inflammatory pathways may account for the additive effects of CpG DNA and corticosteroids on inhibiting airway hyperreactivity.

J. CpG DNA and Mouse Models of Respiratory Syncytial Virus-Induced Asthma

Because CpG DNA activates the innate immune system to generate antiviral cytokines such as IFN-γ,[5,42] its ability to inhibit viral-induced asthma was examined in a mouse model of respiratory syncytial virus (RSV)-induced airway inflammation. Mice pretreated with CpG DNA expressed the antiviral cytokine IFN-γ in the lungs and this was associated with significantly reduced RSV viral titers, peribronchial inflammation, and mucus secretion.[8]

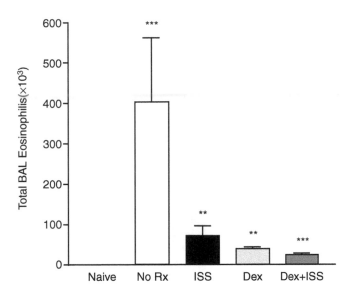

Figure 23.3 Inhibition of bronchoalveolar lavage (BAL) eosinophilia by ISS and dexamethasone. OVA challenge induced significant BAL eosinophilia in untreated mice compared with nonchallenged naïve mice (***$p < 0.0001$). Treatment with ISS 1 day after the inhaled allergen challenge significantly reduced BAL fluid eosinophilia compared with untreated mice (**$p = 0.001$), as did treatment with dexamethasone (**$p = 0.0002$). Combined treatment with ISS and dexamethasone significantly decreased BAL fluid eosinophilia compared with untreated mice (***$p < 0.0001$). Results are expressed as mean ± SEM. (From Ikeda R et al., *Am J Respir Cell Mol Biol* 2003; 28: 655–663. With permission.)

CpG DNA stimulated NK cells to generate IFN-γ via an indirect mechanism[12] mediated by CpG DNA's activation of macrophage generation of IL-12 that subsequently stimulated NK cells to generate IFN-γ.[43] CpG DNA induced expression of several IFNs, including IFN-γ, IFN-α, and IFN-β, all of which inhibit RSV replication *in vitro*.[8] Administration of CpG DNA to mice inhibited RSV replication within days of RSV infection *in vivo*, suggesting that its effect is primarily due to activation of innate immunity as opposed to adaptive immunity. The importance of IFNs to the control of viral infections is further suggested from studies of viral infections in mice deficient in IFN-α receptors or IFNs.[44,45]

The mechanisms by which CpG DNA induces these antiviral effects *in vivo* are not known but may involve the induction by CpG DNA of antiviral cytokines such as IFN-γ, IFN-α, and IFN-β and its activation of other innate immune system cells (macrophages, dendritic cells, NK cells, B cells) whose functions may be

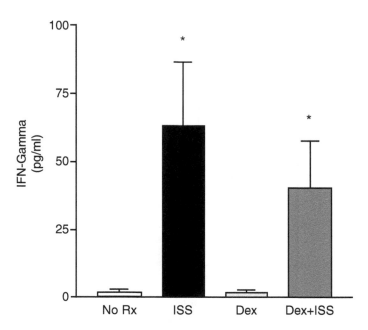

Figure 23.4   BAL IFN-γ levels were below the sensitivity of the IFN-γ assay in OVA-challenged untreated and OVA-challenged dexamethasone-treated mice. In OVA challenged mice, ISS significantly induced BAL IFN-γ (*p = 0.03; untreated versus ISS), as did the combination of ISS and dexamethasone (*p = 0.03; untreated versus ISS + dexamethasone). Dexamethasone in combination with ISS slightly reduced levels of BAL IFN-γ compared with ISS therapy alone but this was not statistically significant (p = ns; dexamethasone + ISS versus ISS monotherapy). (From Ikeda R et al., *Am J Respir Cell Mol Biol* 2003; 28: 655–663. With permission.)

important in viral clearance. Thus, CpG DNA therapy administered to prevent allergen-induced airway inflammation and airway hyperreactivity may provide additional potential benefits in reducing the severity of RSV infections that are known precipitants of asthma.[46]

K.   Inhibition by CpG DNA of TGF-β Expression and Airway Remodeling in Mice

While initial studies demonstrated that CpG DNA could inhibit and reverse eosinophilic inflammation and airway hyperreactivity in mouse models of acute allergen challenge, more recent studies demonstrated that CpG DNA can prevent airway remodeling in mice exposed to repetitive airway challenges with allergens.[17,47] Mice chronically exposed to OVA for 1 to 6 months developed sustained

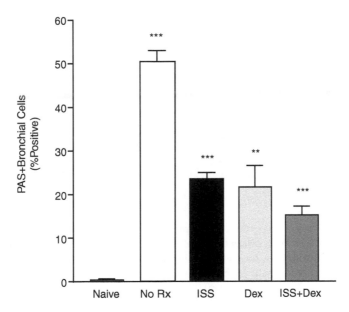

Figure 23.5 Reduction in the percentage of PAS-positive airway cells induced by ISS and dexamethasone. OVA-challenged untreated mice had significantly more PAS-positive airway cells compared with naïve unchallenged mice (***p <0.0001). ISS significantly reduced the percentage of PAS-positive airway cells (*** p <0.0001 compared with untreated OVA-challenged mice), while dexamethasone similarly decreased the percentage of PAS-positive airway cells (**p = 0.0008). Combined treatment decreased the percentage of PAS-positive airway cells further (***p <0.0001 compared with no treatment). (From Ikeda R et al., *Am J Respir Cell Mol Biol* 2003; 28: 655–663. With permission.)

eosinophilic airway inflammation and sustained airway hyperresponsiveness to methacholine compared with control mice. They also developed features of airway remodeling including thickening of the peribronchial smooth muscle layer, peribronchial myofibroblast accumulation, expression of the TGF-β profibrotic growth factor, TGF-β and subepithelial collagen deposition.[17]

Administration of CpG DNA systemically every other week starting prior to the first airway allergen challenge significantly inhibited the development of airway hyperresponsiveness (Figure 23.6), eosinophilic inflammation, Th2 cytokine expression, airway mucus production, and importantly, airway remodeling in mice chronically exposed to OVA for 3 to 6 months.[17] Features of airway remodeling reduced by therapy with CpG DNA included reduction of the increased thickness of the peribronchial smooth muscle layer and inhibition of peribronchial myofibroblast accumulation and peribronchial fibrosis. In particular, CpG DNA

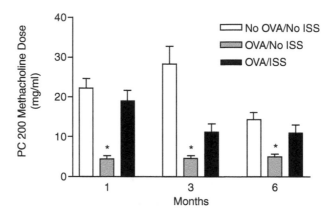

Figure 23.6 Chronic airway OVA exposure induces airway hyperreactivity: Modulation by ISS treatment. The PC_{200} concentration of methacholine was calculated in mice repetitively challenged with OVA for up to 6 months. Mice repetitively challenged with OVA (OVA/No ISS) had significantly lower PC_{200} values compared to age-matched control mice at 1 month (p = 0.0005), 3 months (p <0.0001), and 6 months (p <0.0001; control versus OVA/No ISS). ISS-treated mice repetitively challenged with OVA (OVA/ISS) had significantly higher PC_{200} values at 1 month (p <0.0001), 3 months (p = 0.004), and 6 months (p = 0.001; OVA/No ISS versus OVA/ISS), indicating that ISS treatment reduced the increased airway hyperreactivity to methacholine induced by chronic airway antigen challenge. (From Ikeda R et al., *J Immunol* 2003; 171: 4860–4867. With permission. Copyright 2003. The American Association of Immunologists).

reduced levels of peribronchial collagen V deposition as assessed by immuno-histochemistry.[17] It also significantly reduced bronchoalveolar lavage and lung levels of TGF-β,[17] suggesting that inhibition of TGF-β expression may account for the reduction in airway remodeling.

TGF-β stimulates fibroblasts to produce extracellular matrix proteins (collagen, fibronectin), decreases the production of enzymes that degrade the extracellular matrix (collagenase), and increases the production of proteins inhibiting enzymes that degrade the extracellular matrix (tissue inhibitor of metalloprotease or TIMP).[48] The net effect is to increase the production of extracellular matrix proteins. In subjects with asthma, increased levels of TGF-β have been reported in bronchoalveolar lavage and biopsy specimens.[49,50] TGF-β expression correlates with the degree of subepithelial fibrosis, and levels of TGF-β are significantly increased in patients with severe asthma who have prominent airway eosinophilic inflammation.[49,50] Overall, these studies suggest that CpG DNA prevents Th2-mediated airway inflammation in response to acute allergen challenge and also TGF-β expression and airway remodeling associated with chronic allergen challenge.

L. Effect of CpG DNA on Peribronchial Accumulation of Mast Cells in Mice

The demonstration that mast cells express TLR-9,[16] the receptor for CpG DNA, led to studies directed at determining whether CpG DNA modulates mast cell proliferation or mediator release. Several studies demonstrated increased numbers of mast cells in the airways of asthmatic humans[51,52] and this correlates significantly with airway hyperreactivity and the severity of asthma. Recent studies also demonstrated increased numbers of mast cells in airway smooth muscles in asthmatics compared with controls,[53] suggesting a potential direct interaction of mast cells and smooth muscle cells in inducing airway hyperreactivity as well as smooth muscle remodeling (hypertrophy, hyperplasia, and differentiation into myofibroblasts).

Because few peribronchial mast cells were noted in the lungs of naïve mice or in the lungs of OVA-sensitized mice challenged acutely with OVA by inhalation, the effect of CpG DNA on the functions of mast cells in mouse models of asthma has been difficult to study. OVA-sensitized mice exposed to repetitive OVA inhalation for 1 to 6 months showed significant accumulations of peribronchial mast cells.[16] This chronic allergen challenge model allowed investigation of the effects of CpG DNA on mast cell accumulation in the lungs and on mast cell function.

Repetitive OVA allergen inhalation induced accumulation of peribronchial mast cells in the large, medium, and small sized airways of OVA-sensitized mice.[16] This increased peribronchial accumulation of mast cells in the lungs was associated with increased expression of the Th2 cell-derived mast cell growth factors including IL-4 and IL-9, but not of the non-Th2 cell-derived stem cell factor.[16] The accumulation of peribronchial mast cells may be due to recruitment and/or local proliferation of mast cell precursors or mature mast cells.

The lack of accumulation of peribronchial mast cells following an acute OVA challenge and the peak accumulation of peribronchial mast cells after 1 month of repetitive OVA challenge are consistent with a model in which time is needed for resident or recruited mast cell precursors in the lungs to differentiate under local cytokine stimulation into mast cells. Additional evidence against recruitment of circulating mast cells to the airways is derived from the histologic analysis of the lung distribution of mast cells in repetitively OVA-challenged mice in which no gradients of mast cells were detected in lung sections from pulmonary blood vessels to the airway.

Pretreating mice with CpG DNA prior to repetitive allergen challenge for 1 to 6 months significantly inhibited the accumulation of peribronchial mast cells (Figure 23.7) and the lung expression of the IL-4 and IL-9 mast cell growth factors (Figure 23.8).[16] *In vitro* studies demonstrated that mouse bone marrow-derived mast cells (MBMMCs) strongly expressed TLR-9 (Figure 23.9) and

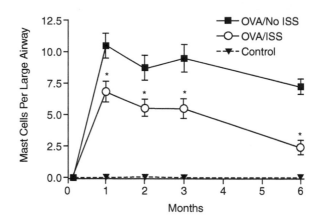

Figure 23.7 Chronic airway OVA exposure induces accumulation of peribronchial mast cells. Modulation by ISS treatment. Repetitive OVA antigen challenge (OVA/No ISS) induced a significant accumulation of mast cells in large airways at 1 month (p= 0.0001, vs control), 2 months, (p= 0.0001, vs control), 3 months (p= 0.0002, vs control), and 6 months (p= 0.0001, vs control). ISS treatment (OVA/ISS) significantly reduced the number of mast cells in large airways at 1 month (p=0.006, vs OVA/No ISS), 2 months (p=0.006, vs OVA/No ISS), 3 months (p=0.02, vs OVA/No ISS), and 6 months (p<0.0001, vs OVA/No ISS). (From Ikeda R et al., *J Immunol* 2003; 171: 4860–4867. With permission. Copyright 2003. The American Association of Immunologists).

bound rhodamine-labeled CpG DNA.[16] However, incubation of MBMMCs with CpG DNA *in vitro* did not inhibit MBMMC proliferation or antigen/IgE-mediated MBMMC degranulation.[16] Thus, although mast cells express TLR-9, CpG DNA does not directly inhibit mast cell proliferation *in vitro*. It does induce mast cells to express significant levels of IL-6.[16]

The generation of IL-6 in response to CpG DNA stimulation is likely to be a beneficial effect of CpG DNA in allergic inflammation. Studies with IL-6 transgenic mice demonstrated an important anti-inflammatory role for IL-6 in mouse models of asthma.[54] These studies demonstrated that mice exposed to repetitive (but not acute) OVA challenges had accumulations of peribronchial mast cells and expressed increased levels of mast cell growth factors in the lungs. Although mast cells express TLR-9, CpG DNA does not directly inhibit mast cell proliferation *in vitro*, suggesting that it inhibits accumulation of peribronchial mast cells *in vivo* by indirect mechanisms that include inhibiting the lung expression of Th2 cell-derived mast cell growth factors.

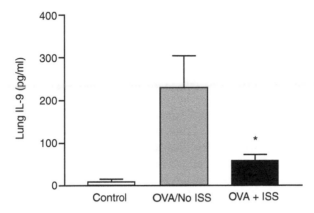

Figure 23.8 Chronic airway OVA exposure induces expression of IL-9. Modulation by ISS treatment. Levels of IL-9 were measured in the lungs of mice by ELISA. Mice challenged with OVA for 3 months had significantly higher levels of lung IL-9 compared with control mice ($p < 0.0001$, OVA/No ISS versus control). ISS treatment for 3 months significantly reduced lung IL-9 levels ($p = 0.02$, OVA + ISS versus OVA/No ISS). (From Ikeda R et al., *J Immunol* 2003; 171: 4860–4867. With permission. Copyright 2003. The American Association of Immunologists).

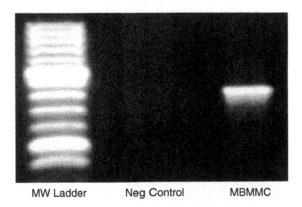

Figure 23.9 RT-PCR demonstrates that MBMMCs express the TLR-9 receptor. Lane 1 is the MW ladder (TLR-9 PCR product band is 600 bp). Lane 2 is the negative control (PCR reagents alone; no MBMMC)s. Lane 3 represents MBMMCs. (From Ikeda R et al., *J Immunol* 2003; 171: 4860–4867. With permission. Copyright 2003. The American Association of Immunologists).

M. Potential for CpG DNA-Based Therapy in Human Allergy and Asthma

In humans, as in mice, TLR-9 is the receptor for CpG DNA, and thus cell types that express TLR-9 (dendritic cells) respond to CpG DNA stimulation.[27] In contrast, human monocytes and NK cells that do not express TLR-9 cannot respond directly to CpG DNA, but can respond in mixed cell populations through stimulation of a contaminating TLR-9 expressing cells in the mixed cell population.[27]

CpG DNA directly activates human dendritic cells (plasmacytoid dendritic cell subset) to express increased levels of co-stimulatory molecules and cytokines. In particular, it stimulates such cells to express increased levels of major histocompatibility complex (MHC) class II, ICAM-1, co-stimulatory molecules (CD40, CD54, CD80, CD86), cytokines (IL-6, IFN-α), and chemokines (IL-8, IP-10). In studies of mononuclear cells derived from dust mite–allergic individuals, CpG DNA inhibited Der p 1–induced IL-4 production and induced Der p 1 IFN-γ production.[55] The current literature contains no published results of studies investigating the safety and efficacy of CpG DNA *in vivo* in human allergy and asthma.

III. Conjugation of CpG DNA and Protein Antigen

A. Inhibition of Allergic Responses

The activation of T cells by dendritic cells is the result of a sequence of steps including antigen uptake, peptide presentation, expression of co-stimulatory molecules, and IL-12 secretion. Studies have been performed to determine whether CpG DNA conjugated to a protein antigen is more effective than CpG DNA alone in mediating dendritic cell activation of T cells. CpG DNA is known to increase the expression of co-stimulatory molecules[56] and enhance IL-12 expression by dendritic cells.[14]

Because antigen is required for CpG DNA to mediate its effect, studies have been performed to determine whether a conjugation of CpG DNA and protein antigen has a stronger ability to induce Th1 immune responses to antigen compared with co-injection of both CpG DNA and protein antigen. The ability of CpG DNA conjugated to a protein antigen to induce Th1 cells is 100-fold higher than that induced by a mixture of equivalent amounts of CpG DNA and antigen.[57] A similar efficacy of CpG DNA–antigen conjugate was noted in the activation of CD8$^+$ cytotoxic lymphocytes. The enhanced immunomodulatory activity of the CpG–antigen conjugate is hypothesized to be the result of the uptake of the conjugated CpG and antigen by the same antigen presenting cell. When the CpG and antigen are not conjugated, they will not always end up in the same antigen-presenting cell.

The presence of CpG DNA and antigen in the same antigen-presenting cell is likely to enhance the antigen-presenting properties of the cell. Studies of CpG DNA tagged with phycoerythrin revealed that dendritic cells bound >100-fold more CpG DNA conjugated to antigen compared with phycoerythrin mixed with CpG DNA.[58] CpG DNA conjugated to antigen, therefore, potentiates the ability of dendritic cells to promote Th1 cellular immune responses.[58] Low doses of antigen and CpG DNA that are below the threshold for T cell activation are also able to induce Th1 cells when covalently conjugated.

B. Immune Response to CpG DNA–Allergen Protein Conjugate

The use of CpG DNA conjugated to allergen protein for the treatment of allergic disease has been investigated in animal models and humans. The primary advantage of the conjugate is that the physical link of CpG DNA to protein allergens increases the likelihood of their delivery to the same antigen-presenting cell, resulting in an amplified, antigen-specific Th1 immune response.[57,58]

Theoretically the conjugate may also be less allergenic than the mixture because steric hindrance or electrostatic blockade of IgE-binding epitopes could occur when CpG DNA coats the allergen.[57] Thus, the CpG DNA component of the conjugate may prevent the allergen component from cross-linking IgE attached to high affinity IgE receptors on mast cells or basophils. This is suggested from *in vitro* studies in which the conjugate inhibited allergen-induced histamine release from human basophils.[57]

A CpG DNA–allergen protein conjugate was studied *in vivo* in a mouse model of ragweed allergy. Injection of Amb a 1, the major short ragweed allergen protein, induced a Th2 response characterized by high IL-5 production and low levels of IFN-γ. The CpG DNA–Amb a 1 conjugate was much more effective than a mixture of Amb a 1 and CpG DNA in generating a Th1 immune response.[57] The CpG DNA–Amb a 1 conjugate can also reverse a preexisting Th2-biased immune response in mice primed to develop Th2 responses to antigen.[57] These results demonstrate that allergen conjugated to CpG DNA can enhance the Th1 immune response, reverse a preexisting Th2 immune bias, and potentially reduce the allergenicity of allergen protein immunotherapy.

C. CpG DNA–Allergen Protein Conjugate Therapy and Mouse Models of Allergy and Asthma

In mouse models of asthma, either airway mucosal delivery or intradermal administration of a CpG DNA–allergen protein conjugate significantly reduced airway hyperreactivity to methacholine for at least 2 months.[59,60] The conjugate was 100-fold more efficient than the unconjugated mixture in reducing airway eosinophilia and bronchial hyperreactivity.[59]

D. Potential for CpG DNA–Allergen Protein Conjugate-Based Therapy in Human Allergy and Asthma

In studies of human mononuclear cells, a CpG DNA–ragweed protein conjugate was more effective at enhancing IFN-γ production and inhibiting IL-4 production compared with CpG DNA alone.[61] The CpG DNA–Amb a 1 conjugate induced significantly less basophil histamine release compared to ragweed alone.[62] Preliminary studies suggest that a CpG DNA–Amb a 1 conjugate is less allergenic than the allergen protein based on immediate hypersensitivity skin test reactivity.[62] and that a six injection regimen of the conjugate reduces symptoms of allergic rhinitis in ragweed-sensitized human subjects followed through the ragweed season.[63] Further studies are needed to demonstrate whether this approach is safe and effective in treating human allergy and asthma.

IV. Allergen Gene Vaccines and Asthma

A number of terms (e.g. genetic vaccination, genetic immunization, pDNA immunization, pDNA vaccination, DNA vaccination, and gene vaccination) have been used to describe the injection of a plasmid DNA (pDNA) encoding a protein antigen. Gene vaccines have been investigated in infectious diseases, cancer, allergies, and asthma. Gene vaccines encoding an allergen can inhibit IgE and Th2 immune responses and airway hyperreactivity in animal models of asthma.[64–66] CpG DNA sequences in the noncoding plasmid backbone of the pDNA act as Th1 adjuvants and promote Th1 rather than Th2 responses to the encoded allergen. Mice pretreated with intradermal injections of pDNA encoding OVA protein developed significantly less bronchoalveolar lavage fluid eosinophils and lung eosinophils after inhalation of OVA protein compared with mice injected with a control pDNA construct.[65]

In a rat model of asthma, immunization with a pDNA encoding the Der p 5 allergen inhibited the IgE response, histamine release into bronchoalveolar lavage fluid, and bronchial hyperreactivity following challenge with aerosolized dust mite allergen Der p5.[66] The response to the gene vaccine appeared antigen-specific becausse the rats immunized with pDNA encoding the Der p 5 allergen were protected against Der p 5 allergen challenge but not against a different challenge such as ovalbumin.[66] No published studies cover the safety or efficacy of DNA vaccines encoding allergens in humans with allergy or asthma.

V. Conclusion

A variety of DNA-based vaccine strategies (CpG DNA, CpG DNA–allergen protein conjugate, allergen gene vaccine) have demonstrated the potential to prevent or reverse allergen-induced airway inflammation, Th2 cytokine responses, mucus production, and airway hyperreactivity in animal models of asthma. Additional ongoing studies in humans will determine whether these strategies are safe and effective for treating patients with asthma.

Acknowledgment

DHB's work was supported by National Institutes of Health grants AI 33977 and AI38425.

References

1. Busse WW and Lemanske RF Jr. Asthma. *New Engl J Med* 2001; 344: 350–362.
2. Larche M, Robinson DS, and Kay AB. The role of T lymphocytes in the pathogenesis of asthma. *J Allergy Clin Immunol* 2003; 111: 450–463.
3. Barnes PJ. Cytokine modulators for allergic diseases. *Curr Opin Allergy Clin Immunol* 2001; 1: 555–560.
4. Tokunaga T, Yamamoto H, Shimada S, Abe H, Fukuda T, Fujisawa Y, Furutani Y, Yano O, Kataoka T, Sudo T. Antitumor activity of deoxyribonucleic acid fraction from *Mycobacterium bovis* BCG. I. Isolation, physico-chemical characterization, and antitumor activity. *J Natl Cancer Inst* 1984; 72: 955–962.
5. Yamamoto S, Yamamoto T, Kataoka T, Kuramoto E, Yano O, and Tokunaga T. Unique palindromic sequences in synthetic oligonucleotides are required to induce IFN and augment IFN-mediated natural killer cell activity. *J Immunol* 1992; 148: 4072–4076.
6. Broide D, Schwarze J, Tighe H, Gifford T, Nguyen MD, Malek S, Van Uden J, Martin-Orozco E, Gelfand EW, and Raz, E. Immunostimulatory DNA sequences inhibit IL-5, eosinophilic inflammation, and airway hyperresponsiveness in mice. *J Immunol* 1998; 161: 7054–7062.
7. Kline JN, Waldschmidt TJ, Businga TR, Lemish JE, Weinstock JV, Thorne PS, and Krieg AM. Modulation of airway inflammation by CpG oligodeoxynucleotides in a murine model of asthma. *J Immunol* 1998; 160: 2555–2559.
8. Cho J, Miller M, Baek K, Castaneda D, Nayar J, Roman M, Raz E, and Broide D. Immunostimulatory DNA sequences inhibit respiratory syncytial viral load, airway inflammation, and mucus secretion. *J Allergy Clin Immunol* 2001; 108: 697–702.
9. Roman M, Martin-Orozco E, Goodman JS, Nguyen MD, Sato Y, Ronaghy A, Kornbluth, RS; Richman, DD; Carson, DA; and Raz, E. Immunostimulatory DNA sequences function as T helper-1-promoting adjuvants. *Nat Med* 1997; 3: 849–854.
10. Klinman DM, Yi AK, Beaucage SL, Conover J, and Krieg AM. CpG motifs present in bacteria DNA rapidly induce lymphocytes to secrete interleukin 6, interleukin 12, and interferon gamma. *Proc Natl Acad Sci USA* 1996; 93: 2879–2883.
11. Krieg AM, Yi AK, Matson S, Waldschmidt TJ, Bishop GA, Teasdale R, Koretzky GA, and Klinman DM. CpG motifs in bacterial DNA trigger direct B-cell activation. *Nature* 1995; 374: 546–549.

12. Ballas ZK, Rasmussen WL, and Krieg AM. Induction of natural killer activity in murine and human cells by CpG motifs in oligodeoxynucleotides and bacterial DNA. *J Immunol* 1996; 157: 1840–1845.
13. Liang H, Nishioka Y, Reich CF, Pisetsky, DS, and Lipsky PE. Activation of human B cells by phosphorothioate oligodeoxynucleotides. *J Clin Invest* 1996; 98: 1119–1129.
14. Hartmann G, Weiner GJ, and Krieg AM. CpG DNA: a potent signal for growth, activation, and maturation of human dendritic cells. *Proc Natl Acad Sci USA* 1999; 96: 9305–9310.
15. Horner AA, Widhopf GF, Burger J, Takabayashi K, Cinman N, Ronaghy A, Spiegelberg H, and Raz E. Immunostimulatory DNA mediated inhibition of IL-4 dependent IgE synthesis from human B cells. *J Allergy Clin Immunol* 2001; 108: 417–423.
16. Ikeda R, Miller M, Nayar J, Walker L, Cho JY, McElwain K, McElwain S, Raz E, and Broide DH. Accumulation of peribronchial mast cells in a mouse model of OVA allergen-induced chronic airway inflammation: modulation by immuno-stimulatory DNA sequences. *J Immunol* 2003; 171: 4860–4867.
17. Cho JY, Miller M, Baek KJ, Han JW, Nayar J, Rodriguez M, Lee SY, McElwain K, McElwain S, Raz E, and Broide DH. Immunostimulatory DNA inhibits TGF-β expression and airway remodeling. *Am J Resp Cell Mol Biol* 2004; 30: 651–661.
18. Gordon S. Pattern recognition receptors: doubling up for the innate immune response. *Cell* 2002; 111: 927–930.
19. Medzhitov R. Toll-like receptors and innate immunity. *Nat Rev Immunol* 2001; 1: 135–145.
20. Hemmi H, Takeuchi O, Kawai T, Kalsho T, Sato S, Snajo H, Matsumato M, Hoshino K, Wagner H, Takeda K, and Akira S. A Toll-like receptor recognizes bacterial DNA. *Nature* 2000; 408: 740–745.
21. Bauer S, Kirschning CJ, Hacker H, Redecke V, Hausmann S, Akira S, Wagner H, and Lipford GB. Human TLR9 confers responsiveness to bacterial DNA via species-specific CpG motif recognition. *Proc Natl Acad Sci USA* 2001; 98: 9237–9242.
22. Takeshiata F, Leifar CA, Gursel I, Ishii KJ, Takeshita S, Gursel M, and Klinman DM. Role of TLR9 in CpG DNA-induced activation of human cells. *J Immunol* 2001; 167: 3555–3558.
23. Macfarlane DE and Manzel L. Antagonism of immunostimulatory CpG oligode-oxynucleotides by quinacrine, chloroquine, and structurally related compounds. *J Immunol* 1998; 160: 1122–1131.
24. Yi AK, Tuetken R, Redford T, Waldschmidt M, Kirsch J, and Krieg AM. CpG motifs in bacterial DNA activate leukocytes through the pH-dependent generation of reactive oxygen species. *J Immunol* 1998; 160: 4755–4761.
25. Aderem A and Ulevitch RJ. Toll like receptors in the induction of the innate immune response. *Nature* 2000; 406: 782–787.
26. Ahmad-Nejad P, Hacker H, Rutz M, Bauer S, Vabulas RM, and Wagner H. Bacterial CpG-DNA and lipopolysaccharides activate Toll-like receptors at distinct cellular compartments. *Eur J Immunol* 2002; 32: 1958–1968.

27. Hornung V, Rothenfusser S, Britsch S, Krug A, Jahrsdorfer B, Giese T, Endres S, and Hartmann G. Quantitative expression of Toll-like receptor 1–10 mRNA in cellular subsets of human peripheral blood mononuclear and sensitivity to CpG oligodeoxynucleotides. *J Immunol* 2002; 168: 4531–4537

28. Kadowaki N, Ho S, Antonenko S, Malefyt RW, Kastelein RA, Bazan F, and Liu YJ. Subsets of human dendritic cell precursors express different toll-like receptors and respond to different microbial antigens. *J Exp Med* 2001; 194: 863–869.

29. Boonstra A, Asselin-Paturel C, Gilliet M, Crain C, Trinchieri G, Liu YJ, and O'Garra A. Flexibility of mouse classical and plasmacytoid-derived dendritic cells in directing T helper type 1 and 2 cell development: dependency on antigen dose and differential toll-like receptor ligation. *J Exp Med* 2003; 197: 101–109.

30. Rothenfusser S, Tuma E, Endres S, and Hartmann G. Plasmacytoid dendritic cells: the key to CpG. *Hum Immunol* 2002; 63: 1111–1119.

31. Hacker H, Vabulas RM, Takeuchi O, Hoshino K, Akira S, and Wagner H. Immune cell activation by bacterial CpG DNA through myeloid differentiation marker 88 and tumor necrosis factor receptor-associated factor (TRAF)-6. *J Exp Med* 2000; 192: 595–600.

32. Chuang TH, Lee J, Kline L, Mathison JC, and Ulevitch RJ. Toll-like receptor 9 mediates CpG DNA signaling. *J Leukoc Biol* 2002; 71: 538–544.

33. Sur S, Wild JS, Choudhury BK, Sur N, Alam R, and Klinman DM. Long-term prevention of allergic lung inflammation in a mouse model of asthma by CpG oligodeoxynucleotides. *J Immunol* 1999; 162: 6284–6293.

34. Serebrisky D, Teper AA, Huang CK, Lee SY, Zhang TF, Schofield BH, Kattan M, Sampson HA, and Li XM. CpG oligonucleotides can reverse Th2-associated allergic airway responses and alter the B7.1/B7.2 expression in a murine model of asthma. *J Immunol* 2000; 165: 5906–5912.

35. Broide D, Stachnick G, Castaneda D, Nayar J, Miller M, Cho JY, Roman M, Zubeldia J, Hayashi T, and Raz E. Systemic administration of immunostimulatory DNA sequences mediate reversible inhibition of Th2 responses in a mouse model of asthma *J Clin Immunol* 2001; 21: 163–170.

36. Kline JN, Krieg AM, Waldschmidt TJ, Ballas ZK, Jain V, and Businga TR. CpG oligodeoxynucleotides do not require Th1 cytokines to prevent eosinophilic airway inflammation in a murine model of asthma. *J Allergy Clin Immunol* 1999; 104: 1258–1264.

37. Broide DH, Stachnick G, Castaneda D, Nayar J, Miller M, Cho JY, Rodriguez M, Roman M, and Raz E. Immunostimulatory DNA mediates inhibition of eosinophilic inflammation and airway hyperreactivity independent of natural killer cells *in vivo*. *J Allergy Clin Immunol* 2001; 108: 759–763.

38. Choudhury BK, Wild JS, Alam R, Klinman DM, Boldogh I, Dharajiya N, Mileski WJ, and Sur S. *In vivo* role of p38 mitogen-activated protein kinase in mediating the anti-inflammatory effects of CpG oligodeoxynucleotide in murine asthma. *J Immunol* 2002; 169: 5955–5961.

39. Ikeda RK, Nayar J, Cho JY, Miller M, Rodriguez M, Raz E, and Broide DH. Resolution of airway inflammation following OVA inhalation: comparison of ISS DNA and corticosteroids. *Am J Respir Cell Mol Biol* 2003; 28: 655–663.

40. Kline JN, Kitagaki K, Businga TR, and Jain VV. Treatment of established asthma in a murine model using CpG oligodeoxynucleotides. *Am J Physiol Lung Cell Mol Physiol* 2002; 283: L170–L179.

41. Li XM, Chopra RK, Chou TY, Schofield BH, Wills-Karp M, and Huang SK. Mucosal IFN-γ gene transfer inhibits pulmonary allergic responses in mice. *J Immunol* 1996; 157: 3216–3219.

42. Katze MG, He Y, and Gale M, Jr. Viruses and interferon: a fight for supremacy. *Nat Rev Immunol* 2002; 2: 675–687.

43. Chace JH, Hooker NA, Mildenstein KL, Krieg AM, and Cowdery JS. Bacterial DNA-induced NK cell IFN-γ production is dependent on macrophage secretion of IL-12. *Clin Immunol Immunopathol* 1997; 84: 185–193.

44. van den Broek MF, Muller U, Huang S, Zinkernagel RM, and Aguet M. Immune defence in mice lacking type I and/or type II interferon receptors. *Immunol Rev* 1995; 148: 5–18.

45. Bogdan C. The function of type I interferons in antimicrobial immunity. *Curr Opin Immunol* 2000; 12: 419–424.

46. Holt PG and Sly PD. Interactions between RSV infection, asthma, and atopy: unraveling the complexities. *J Exp Med* 2002; 196: 1271–1275.

47. Jain VV, Kitagaki K, Businga T, Hussain I, George C, O'Shaughnessy P, and Kline JN. CpG-oligodeoxynucleotides inhibit airway remodeling in a murine model of chronic asthma. *J Allergy Clin Immunol* 2002; 110: 867–872.

48. Blobe GC, Schiemann WP, and Lodish HF. Role of transforming growth factor beta in human disease. *New Engl J Med* 2000; 342: 1350–1358.

49. Vignola AM, Chanez P, Chiappara G, Merendino A, Pace E, Rizzo A, la Rocca AM, Bellia V, Bonsignore G, and Bousquet J. Transforming growth factor-beta expression in mucosal biopsies in asthma and chronic bronchitis. *Am J Respir Crit Care Med* 1997; 156: 591–599.

50. Redington AE, Madden J, Frew AJ, Djukanovic R, Roche WR, Holgate ST, and Howarth PH. Transforming growth factor-beta 1 in asthma: measurement in bronchoalveolar lavage fluid. *Am J Respir Crit Care Med* 1997; 156: 642–647.

51. Pesci A, Foresi A, Bertorelli G, Chetta A, and Oliveri D. Histochemical characteristics and degranulation of mast cells in epithelium and lamina propria of bronchial biopsies from asthmatic and normal subjects. *Am Rev Respir Dis* 1993; 147: 684.

52. Gauvreau GM, Lee J, Watson RM, Irani AA, Schwartz LB, and O'Byrne PM. Increased numbers of both airway basophils and mast cells in sputum after allergen inhalation challenge of atopic asthmatics. *Am J Respir Crit Care Med* 2000; 161: 1473.

53. Brightling CE, Bradding P, Symon FA, Holgate ST, Wardlaw AJ, and Pavord ID. Mast cell infiltration of airway smooth muscle in asthma. *New Engl J Med* 2002; 346: 1699.

54. Wang J, Homer RJ, Chen Q, and Elias JA. Endogenous and exogenous IL-6 inhibit aeroallergen-induced Th2 inflammation. *J Immunol* 2000; 165: 4051.

55. Bohle B, Jahn-Schmid B, Maurer D, Kraft D, and Ebner C. Oligodeoxynucleotides containing CpG motifs induce IL-12, IL-18, and IFN-gamma production in cells from allergic individuals and inhibit IgE synthesis *in vitro*. *Eur J Immunol* 1999; 29: 2344–2353.

56. Martin-Orozco E, Kobayashi H, Van Uden J, Nguyen MD, Kornbluth RS, and Raz E. Enhancement of antigen-presenting cell surface molecules involved in cognate interactions by immunostimulatory DNA sequences. *Int Immunol* 1999; 11: 1111–1118.

57. Tighe H, Takabayashi K, Schwartz D, Van Nest G, Tuck S, Eiden JJ, Kagey-Sobotka A, Creticos PS, Lichtenstein LM, Spiegelberg HL, and Raz E. Conjugation of immunostimulatory DNA to the short ragweed allergen amb a 1 enhances its immunogenicity and reduces its allergenicity. *J Allergy Clin Immunol* 2000; 106: 124–134.

58. Shirota H, Sano K, Hirasawa K, Terui T, Ohuchi K, Hattori T, Shirato K, and Tamura, G. Novel roles of CpG oligodeoxynucleotides as a leader for the sampling and presentation of CpG tagged antigen by dendritic cells. *J Immunol* 2001; 167: 66–74.

59. Shirota H, Sano K, Kikuchi T, Tamura G, and Shirato K. Regulation of murine airway eosinophilia and Th2 cells by antigen-conjugated CpG oligodeoxynucleotides as a novel antigen specific modulator *J Immunol* 2000; 164: 5575–5582.

60. Santeliz JV, Van Nest G, Traquina P, Larsen E, and Wills-Karp M. Amb a 1-linked CpG oligodeoxynucleotides reverse established airway hyperresponsiveness in a murine model of asthma. *J Allergy Clin Immunol* 2002; 109: 455–462.

61. Marshall JD, Abtahi S, Eiden J, Tuck S, Milley R, Haycock F, Reid MJ, Kagey-Sobotka A, Creticos PS, Lichtenstein LM, and Van Nest G. Immunostimulatory sequence DNA linked to the Amb a 1 allergen promotes Th1 cytokine expression while downregulating Th2 cytokine expression in PBMCs from human patients with ragweed allergy. *J Allergy Clin Immunol* 2001; 108: 191–197.

62. Creticos PS, Eiden JJ, Balcer SL, Van Nest G, Kagey-Sobotka A, Tuck SF, Norman PS, and Lichtenstein LM. Immunostimulatory oligodeoxynucleotides conjugated to Amb a 1: safety, skin test reactivity, and basophil histamine release. *J Allergy Clin Immunol* 2000; 105: S70.

63. Creticos PS, Eiden JJ, Broide DH, Balcer-Whaley SL, Schroeder JT, Khattignavong A, Li H, Norman P, and Hamilton R. Immunotherapy with immunostimulatory oligonucleotides linked to purified ragweed Amb a 1 allergen: effects on antibody production, nasal allergen provocation, and ragweed seasonal rhinitis. *J Allergy Clin Immunol* 2002; 109: 743.

64. Raz E, Tighe H, Sato Y, Corr M, Dudler JA, Roman M, Swain SL, Spiegelberg HL, and Carson DA. Preferential induction of a Th1 immune response and inhibition of specific IgE antibody formation by plasmid DNA immunization. *Proc Natl Acad Sci USA* 1996; 93: 5141–5145.

65. Broide D, Orozco EM, Roman M, Carson DA, and Raz E. Intradermal gene vaccination down-regulates both arms of the allergic response. *J Allergy Clin Immunol* 1997; 99: S129.

66. Hsu CH, Chua KY, Tao MH, Lai YL, Wu HD, Huang SK, and Hsieh KH. Immunoprophylaxis of allergen-induced immunoglobulin E synthesis and airway hyperresponsiveness *in vivo* by genetic immunization. *Nat Med* 1996; 2: 540–544.

24

DNA Vaccination for Asthma and Atopic Disorders

KUNIHIKO KITAGAKI and JOEL N. KLINE

University of Iowa
Iowa City, Iowa, U.S.A.

I. Introduction

DNA vaccination has generated great interest as a potential disease-modifying or curative treatment for atopic disorders, in part, because of its promotion of antigen (Ag)-specific type I CD4+ effector T cells (Th1).[1] Ag-encoding plasmid DNA has been shown in murine models to inhibit the induction of Ag-specific immunoglobulin (Ig) E and other aspects of atopic asthma.[2,3] Substantial evidence suggests that the induction of Th1 responses by DNA vaccination is largely due to the influence of "CpG motifs" within the coding sequences.[4,5]

II. Epidemiology of Asthma: Are Microbial Infections Naturally Protective?

Asthma is an inflammatory disease of the airways characterized by eosinophilic inflammation, bronchial hyperresponsiveness, and elevated IgE levels. Recent epidemiological studies demonstrated that the prevalence and morbidity of asthma and other allergic diseases are increasing worldwide, more prominently in industrialized than in developing countries. Additionally, the prevalence of asthma increases in developing countries as they become more westernized.

These data have been interpreted as suggesting that Western lifestyles may increase risk factors or reduce preventive factors for the development of asthma. Although increasing air pollution has been blamed by some, von Mutius et al. reported lower rates of asthma and allergic disorders in children from Munich than in those from Leipzig despite substantially worse air pollution in Leipzig.[6] In a follow-up study, this group found a particularly high rate of atopy among children without older siblings.[7]

The fact that older siblings expose their younger brothers and sisters at home to infections common in school or daycare at an earlier age has been interpreted as supporting the possibility that early life infections prevent later development of atopy. Indeed, children from Leipzig were more likely to be enrolled in out-of-home daycare than those from Munich.

Other studies identified an inverse relationship between early life infection and atopy. Martinez et al. found a lower incidence of atopy in children with histories of nonwheezing viral infection in early life.[8] Shaheen et al. also demonstrated that the risk of atopy was significantly reduced among children who had histories of measles in Guinea-Bissau.[9] Moreover, the presence of positive tuberculin responses has been associated with a reduced risk of asthma and atopy in Japanese schoolchildren.[10] These data support that a bias toward atopic or allergic response against environmental allergens may become dominant in the absence of microbial exposure during childhood.

Skeptics of the hygiene hypothesis note that a more prominent tuberculin response may result from a tendency toward antiatopic Th1 responses rather than responsibility for their generation, and that survival during the measles epidemic in Guinea-Bissau likewise may be influenced by a preexisting Th1 bias. It has also been suggested that pathogenesis of asthma is related to poor control of airway infections.[11] In particular, common cold viruses such as rhinovirus induce asthma exacerbations.[12] Therefore, the timing and specific nature of infections and exposure to microbial products may be important factors in determining whether microbial stimuli induce a naïve immune system to generate benign or nonatopic responses to common aeroallergens.

III.   Pathogenesis of Asthma: Imbalance of Th1 and Th2?

CD4[+] T cells play a central regulatory role in the pathogenesis of atopic conditions.[13] A current understanding of allergic diseases suggests that their pathogenesis derives from Th2-type immune deviation against otherwise benign specific antigens (allergens). CD4[+] T cells can be divided into type 1 helper T (Th1) and type 2 helper T (Th2) cells on the basis of their cytokine production.[14] Th1 cells produce interleukin (IL)-2 and interferon γ(IFN)-γ but not IL-4 or IL-5. Th2 cells produce IL-4, IL-5, and IL-13 but not IL-2 or IFN-γ. These lymphocyte groups

Table 24.1 Important Effects of Th1 and Th2 Cytokines in Asthma

Cytokine	Source	Effects in Asthma
IL-4	Th2 cells	↑ Th2 cell and ↓Th1 cell development[15,16]
	Mast cells	↑ IgE class switching[19]
	Eosinophils	↑ Growth of mast cells[20]
		↑ VCAM-1 expression on endothelium (eosinophil recruitment)[87]
IL-5	Th2 cells	↑ Eosinophil terminal differentiation,[21] chemotaxis,[22]
	Mast cells	activation[23] and survival[24]
	Eosinophils	↑ Airway eosinophilia and hyperresponsiveness[88]
IL-13	Th2	↑ IgE synthesis[25]
		↑ Airway hyperresponsiveness[26,27]
IFN-γ	Th1 cells	↑ Th1 cell and ↓Th2 cell development[16,18]
	NK cells	↓ Airway eosinophilia[89]
IL-12	Macrophage	↑ Th1 cell development[90]
	DCs	↑ IFN-γ production from T cells and NK cells[91]

DCs = dendritic cells.

are counter-regulatory. IL-4 promotes Th2 development[15] and inhibits Th1 development and cytokine production.[16] IFN-γ promotes Th1[15] development and inhibits the proliferation and cytokine synthesis of Th2 cells.[17,18]

Th2 cytokines (IL-4, IL-5, and IL-13) are implicated in the inflammation of asthma. IL-4 amplifies the asthmatic response by inducing IgE class switching by B cells[19] and stimulating growth of mast cells.[20] IL-5 is a terminal differentiation,[21] chemotactic,[22] activation,[23] and survival[24] factor for eosinophils. IL-13, independently from IL-4, induces IgE synthesis[25] and promotes airway hyperresponsiveness.[26, 27] Although Th2 cytokines are secreted by mast cells and eosinophils, they are considered central to the pathogenesis of atopic asthma because they produce these cytokines in an Ag-specific manner.[13] Table 24.1 summarizes their important effects.

IV. Immunostimulatory DNA: What Is CpG?

Following the observation that metastatic malignancies regressed during septic episodes, W.B. Coley reported in 1894 that repeated inoculations of erysipelas induced substantial reductions in otherwise untreatable malignant tumors.[28] These studies were ignored or forgotten until almost a century later when Tokunaga et al. found that bacterial DNA exerted strong antitumor activity.[29] They further reported that bacterial but not vertebrate DNA activated natural killer (NK) cells and B cells and induced IFN-γ.[30]

In 1995, Krieg et al. reported that the DNA motif containing a central unmethylated CpG dinucleotide in a specific base sequence (CpG motif) played a central role in determining the immunomodulatory effects of bacterial DNA.[31] CpG motifs in bacterial DNA are observed at the expected frequency of 1:16 and are generally unmethylated; in contrast, in mammalian DNA, these motifs are present at about one fourth of the expected frequency (1:64) and the cytosine residues are typically methylated.[32]

V. Signal Transduction of CpG DNA: TLR-9

Toll-like receptors (TLRs) are so-called "pattern recognition receptors" that identify molecular patterns of pathogens.[33] They are thought to have evolved as "danger signals" for the innate immune system and can respond rapidly to pathogens. Mice deficient in TLR-9 do not respond to CpG DNA;[34] only human cells that express TLR-9 mRNA can respond to CpG DNA.[35]

These findings suggest that TLR-9 is a key ligand for CpG-DNA. Cells transfected to express TLR-9 show significantly enhanced uptakes of CpG DNA into endocytic vesicles — a necessary step in signal transduction.[36] Downstream signaling cascades following binding of CpG DNA by TLR-9 involve myeloid differentiation marker 88 (MyD88), IL-1 receptor-associated kinase (IRAK), tumor necrosis factor receptor-associated factor 6 (TRAF6), NK-B, and mitogen-activated protein kinase (MAPK).[33,37] CpG DNA degrades I-κB, resulting in NF-κB translocation and activates JNK and p38 triggered by MAPK,[36,38,39] leading to phosphorylation and activation of c-Jun and ATF2, components of transcription factor AP-1.[36] These events lead to the up-regulation of genes involved in host defense (Figure 24.1).

VI. CpG DNA Induces Th1-Type Immune Responses

Oligodeoxynucleotides (ODNs) containing CpG motifs (CpG-ODNs) directly activate B cells, macrophages, and DCs and exert indirect effects on NK cells and T cells. The net result of these actions is the induction of Th1-type cytokine responses (summarized in Table 24.2). CpG-ODNs induce the activation of Ag-presenting cells (APCs) and enhance production of IL-12 and IL-18,[40,41] factors critical for the development of Th1 cells. Finally, induction of IgG2a (a Th1-associated isotype), but not IgE and IgG1 (Th2-associated isotypes), by CpG-ODNs support their role as adjuvants for Th1-specific vaccines.[42–44] *Leishmania major* infection in BALB/c mice induces pathogenic Th2 responses.[45] Administration of CpG-ODNs at the time of infection prevented mortality and inflammation[46] and was associated with the induction of Th1 cytokines.[47]

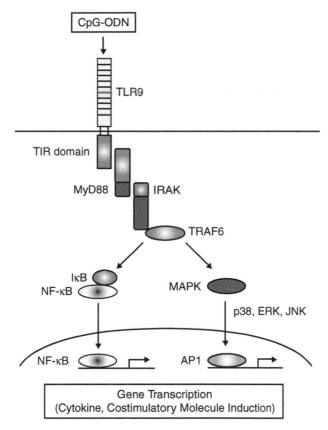

Figure 24.1 CpG-ODN-induced signal pathways. TLR-9 features leucine-rich repeats (LRRs). Intracytoplasmic Toll/IL-1 receptor homology (TIR) domains of TLR-9 initiate signaling cascades that can lead to activation of nuclear factor KB (NF-κB) and mitogen-activated protein kinase (MAPK). IRAK = IL-1 receptor-associated kinase. MyD88 = myeloid differentiation factor 88. TRAF = tumor necrosis factor receptor-associated factor.[86]

VII. CpG-ODN in Prevention of Asthma

Based on these findings, it was hypothesized that CpG-ODN may prevent Th2-driven asthmatic inflammation by inducing Th1-type responses. Initially, the effects of a synthetic CpG-ODN (No. 1826; TCCATGA**CG**TTCCTGA**CG**TT) were explored on a murine model of atopic asthma induced by antigens from *Schistosoma mansoni* eggs.[48] Co-administration of CpG-ODN with *Schistosoma mansoni* eggs was almost sufficient to prevent the development of airway eosinophilia, bronchial hyperreactivity, and Th2-type immune responses (serum IgE,

Table 24.2 Effects of CpG-ODNs on B Cells, Macrophages, DCs, NK Cells, and T Cells

Cell Type	Effects of CpG-ODNs
B cells	↓ Spontaneous apoptosis[92]
	↑ Proliferation,[31,93]
	↑ Cytokine production: IL-6,[31,93]
	↑ MHC class I and II, co-stimulatory molecules (CD80, 86, etc.), adhesion molecules, Fc receptor[94]
Macrophages	↑ Cytokine production: TNF-α,[95] IL-12[41]
	↑ MHC class I and II, co-stimulatory molecules (CD80, 86), adhesion molecules, Fc receptor[94]
DCs	↑ Cytokine production: IL-12, IL-6, IFN-α, IFN-β, TNF-α[40,65,96]
	↑ MHC class I and II, co-stimulatory molecules (CD80, 86), adhesion molecules, Fc receptor[94]
NK cells	Activation of NK cells by CpG-ODN requires IL-12 and IFN-γ from macrophages[41,59]
	↑ Cytokine production: IFN-γ [97,98]
	↑ Cytotoxic activity[97,98]
T cells	T cells do not respond to CpG-ODN directly[60]
	↑ Cytotoxic activity[96]

Th2 cytokine in bronchoalveolar lavage [BAL] fluid), and induced Th1-type immune responses (BAL IFN-γ). The effectiveness of CpG-ODN was further evaluated using a variety of mouse strains (BALB/c, DBA) and antigens.[49]

The effects of CpG-ODN in murine models of asthma were neither mouse-strain nor model dependent; furthermore, the development of airway inflammation could be abrogated by co-administration of CpG-ODN and allergen, even following systemic sensitization.[48] Broide et al. found that CpG-ODNs were effective whether administered intraperitoneally or intranasally,[50,51] and confirmed that a single administration produced long-lasting effects. Other studies also demonstrated the beneficial responses of CpG-ODN administered in the airway or enterally[52,53] (see Table 24.3).

To examine the duration of protection offered by CpG-ODN, Sur et al. used a ragweed-induced murine model of asthma.[52] Mice treated with CpG-ODN prior to airway challenge demonstrated significant reductions in eosinophilic airway inflammation following rechallenge 6 weeks later. Similarly, CpG ODN administered at the time of sensitization was effective in preventing inflammatory responses to inhaled allergen in the same time frame.[49]

Divergent results have been reported regarding the need for Ag along with CpG-ODN in preventing an asthmatic airway response. Co-administration of Ag with CpG-ODN was required, but Sur et al. described no additional benefit following co-administration of CpG-ODN with Ag.[52] Shirota et al. also found

Table 24.3 Summary of Studies of Effects of CpG-ODN on Murine Models of Asthma

Parameter	Kline et al.[48]	Broide et al.[50]	Sur et al.[52]	Shirota et al.[55]
Sequences of CpG-ODNs	TCCATGACG TTCCTGACG TT	TGACTGTGA ACGTTCGAG ATGA	GCTAGACGT TAGCGT and TCAACGTT	TCCATGACG TTCCTGACG TT
Allergen	Schistosome	OVA	Ragweed	OVA
Mouse strain	C57BL/6	BALB/c	BALB/c	BALB/c
Administration route	IP	IP/IN	IT	IT
CpG timing	At time of sensitization	Before challenge	Before challenge	Before challenge
CpG dose/mouse	30 μg	100 / 50 μg	35 μg	5 μg
Co-administration with Ag	Yes	No	No	Yes

IP = intraperitoneal. IN = intranasally. IT = intratracheal. OVA = ovalbumin. Ag = Antigen

that co-administration of CpG-ODN and Ag, but not CpG-ODN alone, prior to inhalation challenge prevented airway eosinophilia[54] and reported that conjugation of CpG-ODN to the Ag was more potent in preventing Ag-induced airway eosinophilia.[55]

Tighe et al. also showed that conjugation of CpG-ODN to the dominant peptide of ragweed induced stronger Th1 responses than a mixture of ODN and Amb a 1.[56] These data suggest that the effects of CpG-ODNs in preventing asthma are at least partly Ag-related. The mechanisms of CpG-ODNs in preventing asthma have not been determined conclusively. The original hypothesis that CpG-ODN-induced Th1 cytokines inhibit Th2 responses was supported by Sur's observation that CpG-ODNs failed to prevent Ag-induced airway eosinophilia in IFN-γ knockout (KO) mice.[52] We found that CpG-ODNs are effective in preventing Ag-induced airway eosinophilia and hyperreactivity in IFN-γ, IL-12, and even IFN-γ/IL-12 double KO mice.[57] We noted, however, a reduced responsiveness to CpG-ODNs in the absence of these Th1-type cytokines, leading to a shift in the dose–response curve, suggesting that IFN-γ and IL-12 can at least modulate the responses to CpG-ODNs. These data show that CpG-ODN-induced Th1-type cytokines are not the sole factors that prevent Ag-induced airway inflammation.

Broide et al. reported that CpG-ODNs inhibited Ag-induced airway eosinophilia and airway hyperreactivity in mice depleted of NK cells before challenge by specific antibodies.[58] These data further support the notion that IFN-γ is not a critical factor for the down-regulation of Th2 responses by CpG-ODNs because NK cells represent one of the main sources of IFN-γ induced by CpG-ODNs.[59]

In order to identify alternative factors responsible for the protection offered by CpG-ODNs, type I IFN (IFN-α and IFN-β) receptor KO mice[57] were studied

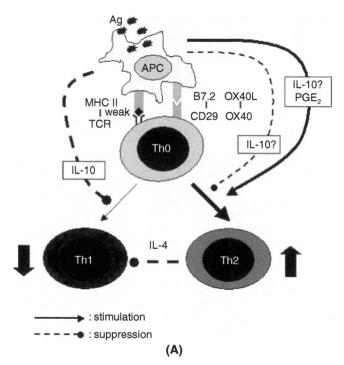

Figure 24.2 Regulation of Th2 responses by CpG-ODN. (A) Presentation of Ag by APC to a naïve T cell in the appropriate inflammatory milieu may lead to a Th2-committed response. (B) In contrast, Ag encountered and presented in the setting of CpG-ODN results in induction of IL-12 and suppresses development of a Th2 response associated with, but not necessarily requiring, induction of a Th1 response.

because CpG-ODNs are powerful inducers of IFN-α,[60] and IFN-α can inhibit Ag-induced airway eosinophilia.[61] CpG-ODNs effectively prevent eosinophilic airway inflammation and airway hyperreactivity in type I IFN receptor KO mice. IL-10 appears to play a role in the effects of CpG-ODNs, but, like the Th1-type cytokines, this may be more modulatory than central. Higher concentrations of CpG-ODNs are required in the absence of IL-10. IL-10 is induced by CpG-ODNs from multiple cell types including B cells, macrophages, and DCs.[62–64]

Although other soluble factors induced by CpG-ODNs may prevent Th2 responses, an interaction between T cells and APCs is also important in Th2 development. CpG-ODNs have many effects on APCs, including (1) up-regulation of MHC class II expression;[65,66] (2) IL-12/IL-10-independent up-regulation of the co-stimulatory molecule B7.1 but not B7.2;[40,63,67] (3) up-regulation of CD40, an important co-factor in IL-12-induced Th1 responses;[40,63] and (4) enhanced expression

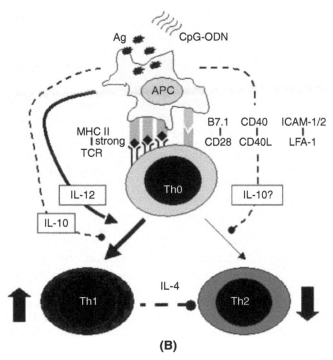

(B)

Figure 24.2 (continued)

of ICAM-1[68,69] thought to promote Th1 and suppress Th2 development. Figure 24.2 shows currently proposed mechanisms by which CpG-ODNs regulate Th2 responses.

VIII. CpG-ODNs in Immunotherapy of Established Asthma

Although controlled studies support the efficacy of standard allergen immunotherapy for many cases of allergic asthma,[70] it is underutilized at present. Its mechanisms remain uncertain, but it is thought to act, at least in part, through alternation of Th2-type to Th1-type immune responses against specific allergens. In the past, bacterial vaccines of heat-killed organisms that presumably contained CpG motif in the DNA were used as adjuvants with allergen immunotherapy.[71] It was hypothesized that CpG-ODN could overcome established asthma, especially in the context of allergen-specific immunotherapy. This was evaluated in a protocol in which mice were treated with allergen and/or ODNs after the establishment of Ag-induced asthma (Figure 24.3).[72] In contrast to the marked

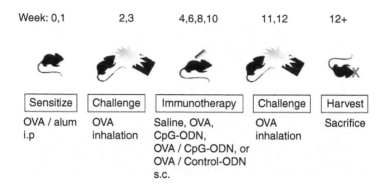

Figure 24.3 CpG-based immunotherapy in a murine model of asthma. Eosinophilic airway inflammation and airway hyperreactivity were induced by repeated inhalation of OVA by sensitized mice. After the asthma model was established, the mice received four biweekly subcutaneous injections of OVA (10 μg/mouse) alone or in the presence of control or CpG-ODNs (30 μg/mouse) prior to rechallenge with OVA.

airway eosinophilia, bronchial hyperreactivity, and elevated Ag-specific IgE seen in untreated mice, mice that received CpG-ODNs and Ag were significantly protected (Figure 23.4). This protection was not seen in mice treated with Ag or CpG-ODN alone.

The findings regarding the benefit of CpG-ODN alone are not consistent. Serebrisky et al. reported that administration of CpG-ODN without Ag was beneficial, at least when the ODNs were administered within 24 hours of Ag challenge.[67] Although the effects of co-administration of CpG-ODN and Ag were not examined, these data suggest that therapeutic effects of CpG-ODN on atopic asthma may be both Ag-specific and Ag-unrelated.

Santeliz et al. used conjugation of CpG-ODNs to Amb a 1 for the treatment of established ragweed-induced asthma in mice.[73] When the conjugated product was administered twice after a single airway challenge, significantly reduced levels of airway eosinophilia and hyperreactivity were seen. These observations suggest that CpG-ODN may prove to be an effective adjuvant for Ag-specific immunotherapy.

The mechanisms of therapeutic effects by CpG-ODN may differ from those responsible for prevention of atopic inflammation. Santeliz et al. suggest that the therapeutic effects of Ag-conjugated CpG-ODN are independent of Th2 suppression because the splenocytes of mice treated with Ag-conjugated CpG-ODNs still produced high levels of IL-5 after Ag stimulation *in vitro* and failed to suppress Ag-specific IgG1 production. They concluded that promoting Ag-specific Th1 responses, including Ag-specific IgG2a, was central to the therapeutic effects of CpG-ODNs. In contrast, Serebrisky et al. and our group reported that therapeutic treatment with CpG-ODNs suppressed serum Ag-specific IgE levels in murine

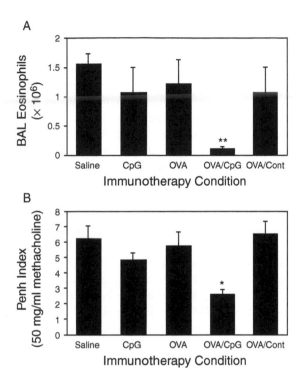

Figure 24.4 Effect of CpG-based immunotherapy on murine model of asthma. Immunotherapy using OVA plus CpG-ODNs resulted in significantly lower numbers of eosinophils in BAL fluid (A) and bronchial hyperreactivity to methacholine (B) compared with untreated mice. N = 8 mice/group; * p <0.05 and ** p <0.01 versus control group.

models of asthma.[67,72] These data suggest that the reversal of established atopic airway disease is at least partly mediated by the down-regulation of Ag-specific Th2 responses. Importantly, Parronchi et al. reported that CpG-ODNs inhibited Ag-induced IL-4 production from allergen-specific human CD4+ cells of atopic donors, suggesting a shift in the differentiation of a Th0/Th2-like response to a Th1-like profile of cytokine production.[74]

In order to evaluate the therapeutic effects of CpG-ODNs, we used splenocytes isolated from OVA-sensitized mice and analyzed the cytokine production pattern after stimulation with OVA and/or CpG-ODNs *in vitro*. The splenocytes were committed to Ag-specific Th2-type responses although the unsorted population certainly contained naïve T cells and likely some Th1-type cells. CpG-ODNs inhibited Ag-induced IL-5 production in a concentration-dependent manner.[72] Although Ag stimulation induced IFN-γ, CpG-ODNs exerted significantly synergistic induction of IFN-γ in the presence of Ag compared with induction in the absence of Ag. Interestingly, the induction pattern of IFN-γ by CpG-ODNs showed a bell-shaped pattern that was maximal at CpG-ODN of 0.1 μg/ml; this suggests that CpG-ODN suppresses Th2 and/or a switch from Th0/Th2 to Th1.

Questions remain regarding the role of Th1 cytokines in CpG-ODN-induced suppression of Th2 cytokines. Parronchi et al. found that suppression of IL-5 by CpG-ODN was completely blocked by the neutralization of IL-12 and IFNs.[74] In contrast, we found discordance between the maximal induction of IFN-γ and suppression of IL-5 production by CpG-ODN,[75] Although depletion of NK cells and CD8+ cells from splenocytes of sensitized mice reduced the level of IFN-γ production by CpG-ODNs, suppression of IL-5 by CpG-ODNs was not changed. Neutralizing antibodies against IFN-γ and IL-12 did not block suppression of IL-5 production by CpG-ODNs, and splenocytes isolated from IFN-γ/IL-12 double-KO mice likewise demonstrated suppression of IL-5 production when stimulated with CpG-ODN.

We next focused on IL-10 as a potential suppressive factor because CpG-ODNs can induce IL-10[62,76] and IL-10 is recognized as an immune suppressive cytokine.[77,78] First, we found a good correlation between the induction of IL-10 and suppression of IL-5 by CpG-ODNs. Elimination of IL-10 by either neutralizing antibody or KO mice reduced the suppressive effects of CpG-ODNs on IL-5 production although the cancellation was not complete. This was partly explained by overproduction of IFN-γ in the absence of IL-10; in wild-type mice, the reduced induction of IFN-γ seen in the settings of high concentrations of CpG-ODNs is explained by the concomitant induction of IL-10 that suppresses both Th1 and Th2 cytokine production. We concluded that CpG-ODN inhibits established Th2 immune responses partially through IFN-γ and IL-10 production, the latter serving to regulate excessive Th1 bias. This observation is important for clinical development of CpG-ODNs as immunotherapy adjuvants because excessive Th1 responses may be harmful. However, elimination of IFN-γ, IL-12, and IL-10 did not completely abrogate the suppressive effects of CpG-ODNs. Other suppressive mechanisms, perhaps involving altered expression of cell surface markers on APC or on T cells, may also be involved.

IX. Future Directions

DCs are the most potent APCs for the induction of a primary immune responses to exogenous Ag[79] and, in the lungs, a network of airway DCs exists to rapidly encounter environmental Ag.[80] It is postulated that pulmonary DCs are central in deviating the responses of naïve T cells, resulting in Ag-specific Th2 cells in the case of atopic asthma.[81] Transfer of Ag-pulsed DCs into the lungs of naïve mice led to the induction of eosinophilic airway inflammation by Ag inhalation,[82, 83] raising the possibility that local priming of DCs is crucial for the induction of allergic asthma. This suggests that targeting airway DCs may be beneficial in the prevention or treatment of asthma. Ag-pulsed DCs have been used as cellular vaccines and showed preventive or protective effects against certain tumors, partly though successful priming of Th1 and CD8+ cells.[84]

A new concept for immune deviation proposes that DCs determine the direction of immune deviation toward Th1 or Th2 from naïve T cells.[85] DCs that induce Th1 and Th2 responses are called DC1 and DC2, respectively. It has postulated that pathogen and pathogen-derived factors polarize immature DCs to mature DCs (DC1 or DC2), and DC1-produced IL-12 determines the initial immune deviation toward a Th1 type.

Because CpG-ODNs direct immature DCs to DC1 type,[66] DCs pulsed with Ag plus CpG-ODNs may serve as an effective vaccine for the treatment of asthma. Mucosal delivery may be an approach for priming airway DCs. Vaccination against allergic diseases including asthma has not been attempted, and allergen-specific immunotherapy is more commonly used for allergic rhinitis and conjunctivitis than for asthma. The use of CpG-ODNs as an adjuvant for immunotherapy may enhance both the safety and efficacy of this treatment. It is important to continue to evaluate both mechanisms of action and safety issues of this approach.

Acknowledgment

This work was supported by National Institutes of Health grants HL59324 and ES05605.

References

1. Sato Y, Roman M, Tighe H, Lee D, Corr M, Nguyen MD, Silverman GJ, Lotz M, Carson DA, and Raz E. Immunostimulatory DNA sequences necessary for effective intradermal gene immunization. *Science* 1996; 273: 352–354.
2. Raz E, Tighe H, Sato Y, Corr M, Dudler JA, Roman M, Swain SL, Spiegelberg HL, and Carson DA. Preferential induction of a Th1 immune response and inhibition of specific IgE antibody formation by plasmid DNA immunization. *Proc Natl Acad Sci USA* 1996; 93: 5141–5145.
3. Hsu CH, Chua KY, Tao MH, Huang SK, and Hsieh KH. Inhibition of specific IgE response *in vivo* by allergen–gene transfer. *Int Immunol* 1996; 8: 1405–1411.
4. Krieg AM, Yi AK, Schorr J, and Davis HL. The role of CpG dinucleotides in DNA vaccines. *Trends Microbiol* 1998; 6: 23–27.
5. Klinman DM, Yamshchikov G, and Ishigatsubo Y. Contribution of CpG motifs to the immunogenicity of DNA vaccines. *J Immunol* 1997; 158: 3635–3639.
6. von Mutius E, Fritzsch C, Weiland SK, Roll G, and Magnussen H. Prevalence of asthma and allergic disorders among children in united Germany: a descriptive comparison. *Br Med J* 1992; 305: 1395–1399.

7. von Mutius E, Martinez FD, Fritzsch C, Nicolai T, Reitmeir P, and Thiemann HH. Skin test reactivity and number of siblings. *Br Med J* 1994; 308: 692–695.
8. Martinez FD, Stern DA, Wright AL, Taussig LM, and Halonen M. Association of non-wheezing lower respiratory tract illnesses in early life with persistently diminished serum IgE levels. *Thorax* 1995; 50: 1067–1072.
9. Shaheen SO, Aaby P, Hall AJ, Barker DJ, Heyes CB, Shiell AW, and Goudiaby A. Measles and atopy in Guinea-Bissau. *Lancet* 1996; 347: 1792–1796.
10. Shirakawa T, Enomoto T, Shimazu S, and Hopkin JM. The inverse association between tuberculin responses and atopic disorder. *Science* 1997; 275: 77–79.
11. Gern JE. Viral and bacterial infections in the development and progression of asthma. *J Allergy Clin Immunol* 2000; 105: S497–S502.
12. Gern JE, Calhoun W, Swenson C, Shen G, and Busse WW. Rhinovirus infection preferentially increases lower airway responsiveness in allergic subjects. *Am J Respir Crit Care Med* 1997; 155: 1872–1876.
13. Kay AB. TH2-type cytokines in asthma. *Ann NY Acad Sci* 1996; 796: 1–8.
14. Mosmann TR, Cherwinski H, Bond MW, Giedlin MA, and Coffman RL. Two types of murine helper T cell clone. I. Definition according to profiles of lymphokine activities and secreted proteins. *J Immunol* 1986; 136: 2348–2357.
15. Swain SL, Weinberg AD, English M, and Huston G. IL-4 directs the development of Th2-like helper effectors. *J Immunol* 1990; 145: 3796–3806.
16. Parronchi P, De Carli M, Manetti R, Simonelli C, Sampognaro S, Piccinni MP, Macchia D, Maggi E, Del Prete G, and Romagnani S. IL-4 and IFN (alpha and gamma) exert opposite regulatory effects on the development of cytolytic potential by Th1 or Th2 human T cell clones. *J Immunol* 1992; 149: 2977–2983.
17. Gajewski TF and Fitch FW. Anti-proliferative effect of IFN-gamma in immune regulation. I. IFN-gamma inhibits the proliferation of Th2 but not Th1 murine helper T lymphocyte clones. *J Immunol* 1988; 140: 4245–4252.
18. Gajewski TF, Joyce J, and Fitch FW. Antiproliferative effect of IFN-gamma in immune regulation. III. Differential selection of TH1 and TH2 murine helper T lymphocyte clones using recombinant IL-2 and recombinant IFN-gamma. *J Immunol* 1989; 143: 15–22.
19. Del Prete G, Maggi E, Parronchi P, Chretien I, Tiri A, Macchia D, Ricci M, Banchereau J, De Vries J, and Romagnani S. IL-4 is an essential factor for the IgE synthesis induced in vitro by human T cell clones and their supernatants. *J Immunol* 1988; 140: 4193–4198.
20. Saito H, Hatake K, Dvorak AM, Leiferman KM, Donnenberg AD, Arai N, Ishizaka K, Ishizaka T. Selective differentiation and proliferation of hematopoietic cells induced by recombinant human interleukins. *Proc Natl Acad Sci USA* 1988; 85: 2288–2292.
21. Yamaguchi Y, Suda T, Suda J, Eguchi M, Miura Y, Harada N, Tominaga A, and Takatsu K. Purified interleukin 5 supports the terminal differentiation and proliferation of murine eosinophilic precursors. *J Exp Med* 1988; 167: 43–56.
22. Yamaguchi Y, Hayashi Y, Sugama Y, Miura Y, Kasahara T, Kitamura S, Torisu M, Mita S, Tominaga A, and Takatsu K. Highly purified murine interleukin 5 (IL-5) stimulates eosinophil function and prolongs *in vitro* survival: IL-5 as an eosinophil chemotactic factor. *J Exp Med* 1988; 167: 1737–1742.

23. Lopez AF, Sanderson CJ, Gamble JR, Campbell HD, Young IG, and Vadas MA. Recombinant human interleukin 5 is a selective activator of human eosinophil function. *J Exp Med* 1988; 167: 219–224.
24. Yamaguchi Y, Suda T, Ohta S, Tominaga K, Miura Y, and Kasahara T. Analysis of the survival of mature human eosinophils: interleukin-5 prevents apoptosis in mature human eosinophils. *Blood* 1991; 78: 2542–2547.
25. Punnonen J, Aversa G, Cocks BG, McKenzie AN, Menon S, Zurawski G, de Waal Malefyt R, and de Vries JE. Interleukin 13 induces interleukin 4-independent IgG4 and IgE synthesis and CD23 expression by human B cells. *Proc Natl Acad Sci USA* 1993; 90: 3730–3734.
26. Grunig G, Warnock M, Wakil AE, Venkayya R, Brombacher F, Rennick DM, Sheppard D, Mohrs M, Donaldson DD, Locksley RM, and Corry DB. Requirement for IL-13 independently of IL-4 in experimental asthma. *Science* 1998; 282: 2261–2263.
27. Wills-Karp M, Luyimbazi J, Xu X, Schofield B, Neben TY, Karp CL, and Donaldson DD. Interleukin-13: central mediator of allergic asthma. *Science* 1998; 282: 2258–2261.
28. Coley WB. Treatment of inoperable malignant tumors with toxins of erysipelas and *Bacillus prodigiosus*. *Trans Am Surg Assoc* 1894; 12: 183–212.
29. Tokunaga T, Yamamoto H, Shimada S, Abe H, Fukuda T, Fujisawa Y, Furutani Y, Yano O, Kataoka T, and Sudo T. Antitumor activity of deoxyribonucleic acid fraction from *Mycobacterium bovis* BCG. I. Isolation, physicochemical characterization, and antitumor activity. *J Natl Cancer Inst* 1984; 72: 955–962.
30. Yamamoto S, Kuramoto E, Shimada S, and Tokunaga T. *In vitro* augmentation of natural killer cell activity and production of interferon-alpha/beta and -gamma with deoxyribonucleic acid fraction from *Mycobacterium bovis* BCG. *Jpn J Cancer Res* 1988; 79: 866–873.
31. Krieg AM, Yi AK, Matson S, Waldschmidt TJ, Bishop GA, Teasdale R, Koretzky GA, and Klinman DM. CpG motifs in bacterial DNA trigger direct B-cell activation. *Nature* 1995; 374: 546–549.
32. Bird AP. CpG-rich islands and the function of DNA methylation. *Nature* 1986; 321: 209–213.
33. Medzhitov R and Janeway CA, Jr. Innate immunity: the virtues of a nonclonal system of recognition. *Cell* 1997; 91: 295–298.
34. Hemmi H, Takeuchi O, Kawai T, Kaisho T, Sato S, Sanjo H, Matsumoto M, Hoshino K, Wagner H, Takeda K, and Akira S. A Toll-like receptor recognizes bacterial DNA. *Nature* 2000; 408: 740–745.
35. Takeshita F, Leifer CA, Gursel I, Ishii KJ, Takeshita S, Gursel M, and Klinman DM. Cutting edge: role of Toll-like receptor 9 in CpG DNA-induced activation of human cells. *J Immunol* 2001; 167: 3555–3558.
36. Hacker H, Mischak H, Miethke T, Liptay S, Schmid R, Sparwasser T, Heeg K, Lipford GB, and Wagner H. CpG-DNA-specific activation of antigen-presenting cells requires stress kinase activity and is preceded by non-specific endocytosis and endosomal maturation. *EMBO J* 1998; 17: 6230–6240.
37. Hacker H, Vabulas RM, Takeuchi O, Hoshino K, Akira S, and Wagner H. Immune cell activation by bacterial CpG-DNA through myeloid differentiation marker 88 and tumor necrosis factor receptor-associated factor (TRAF)-6. *J Exp Med* 2000; 192: 595–600.

38. Yi AK and Krieg AM. CpG DNA rescue from anti-IgM-induced WEHI-231 B lymphoma apoptosis via modulation of I kappa B alpha and I kappa B beta and sustained activation of nuclear factor-kappa B/c-Rel. *J Immunol* 1998; 160: 1240–1245.

39. Yi AK and Krieg AM. Rapid induction of mitogen-activated protein kinases by immune stimulatory CpG DNA. *J Immunol* 1998; 161: 4493–4497.

40. Sparwasser T, Koch ES, Vabulas RM, Heeg K, Lipford GB, Ellwart JW, and Wagner H. Bacterial DNA and immunostimulatory CpG oligonucleotides trigger maturation and activation of murine dendritic cells. *Eur J Immunol* 1998; 28: 2045–2054.

41. Halpern MD, Kurlander RJ, and Pisetsky DS. Bacterial DNA induces murine interferon-gamma production by stimulation of interleukin-12 and tumor necrosis factor-alpha. *Cell Immunol* 1996; 167: 72–78.

42. Chu RS, Targoni OS, Krieg AM, Lehmann PV, and Harding CV. CpG oligodeoxynucleotides act as adjuvants that switch on T helper 1 (Th1) immunity. *J Exp Med* 1997; 186: 1623–1631.

43. Lipford GB, Bauer M, Blank C, Reiter R, Wagner H, and Heeg K. CpG-containing synthetic oligonucleotides promote B and cytotoxic T cell responses to protein antigen: a new class of vaccine adjuvants. *Eur J Immunol* 1997; 27: 2340–2344.

44. Roman M, Martin-Orozco E, Goodman JS, Nguyen MD, Sato Y, Ronaghy A, Kornbluth RS, Richman DD, Carson DA, and Raz E. Immunostimulatory DNA sequences function as T helper-1-promoting adjuvants. *Nat Med* 1997; 3: 849–854.

45. Locksley RM and Louis JA. Immunology of leishmaniasis. *Curr Opin Immunol* 1992; 4: 413–418.

46. Zimmermann S, Egeter O, Hausmann S, Lipford GB, Rocken M, Wagner H, and Heeg K. CpG oligodeoxynucleotides trigger protective and curative Th1 responses in lethal murine leishmaniasis. *J Immunol* 1998; 160: 3627-3630.

47. Walker PS, Scharton-Kersten T, Krieg AM, Love-Homan L, Rowton ED, Udey MC, and Vogel JC. Immunostimulatory oligodeoxynucleotides promote protective immunity and provide systemic therapy for leishmaniasis via IL-12- and IFN-gamma-dependent mechanisms. *Proc Natl Acad Sci USA* 1999; 96: 6970–6975.

48. Kline JN, Waldschmidt TJ, Businga TR, Lemish JE, Weinstock JV, Thorne PS, Krieg AM. Modulation of airway inflammation by CpG oligodeoxynucleotides in a murine model of asthma. *J Immunol* 1998; 160: 2555–2559.

49. Kline JN. Effects of CpG DNA on Th1/Th2 balance in asthma. *Curr Top Microbiol Immunol* 2000; 247: 211–225.

50. Broide D, Schwarze J, Tighe H, Gifford T, Nguyen MD, Malek S, Van Uden J, Martin-Orozco E, Gelfand EW, and Raz E. Immunostimulatory DNA sequences inhibit IL-5, eosinophilic inflammation, and airway hyperresponsiveness in mice. *J Immunol* 1998; 161: 7054–7062.

51. Broide D and Raz E. DNA-Based immunization for asthma. *Int Arch Allergy Immunol* 1999; 118: 453–456.

52. Sur S, Wild JS, Choudhury BK, Sur N, Alam R, and Klinman DM. Long term prevention of allergic lung inflammation in a mouse model of asthma by CpG oligodeoxynucleotides. *J Immunol* 1999; 162: 6284–6293.

53. Kline JN, Businga TR, VV J, and Hussain I. Oral administration of CpG oligodeoxynucleotides provide protection against inflammation in asthma (abstr.). *J Respir Clin Care Med* 2000; 161: A21.

54. Shirota H, Sano K, Kikuchi T, Tamura G, and Shirato K. Regulation of T-helper type 2 cell and airway eosinophilia by transmucosal coadministration of antigen and oligodeoxynucleotides containing CpG motifs. *Am J Respir Cell Mol Biol* 2000; 22: 176–182.

55. Shirota H, Sano K, Kikuchi T, Tamura G, and Shirato K. Regulation of murine airway eosinophilia and Th2 cells by antigen-conjugated CpG oligodeoxynucleotides as a novel antigen-specific immunomodulator. *J Immunol* 2000; 164: 5575–5582.

56. Tighe H, Takabayashi K, Schwartz D, Van Nest G, Tuck S, Eiden JJ, Kagey-Sobotka A, Creticos PS, Lichtenstein LM, Spiegelberg HL, and Raz E. Conjugation of immunostimulatory DNA to the short ragweed allergen amb a 1 enhances its immunogenicity and reduces its allergenicity. *J Allergy Clin Immunol* 2000; 106: 124–134.

57. Kline JN, Krieg AM, Waldschmidt TJ, Ballas ZK, Jain V, and Businga TR. CpG oligodeoxynucleotides do not require TH1 cytokines to prevent eosinophilic airway inflammation in a murine model of asthma. *J Allergy Clin Immunol* 1999; 104: 1258–1264.

58. Broide DH, Stachnick G, Castaneda D, Nayar J, Miller M, Cho J, Rodriquez M, Roman M, Raz E. Immunostimulatory DNA mediates inhibition of eosinophilic inflammation and airway hyperreactivity independent of natural killer cells *in vivo*. *J Allergy Clin Immunol* 2001; 108: 759–763.

59. Chace JH, Hooker NA, Mildenstein KL, Krieg AM, and Cowdery JS. Bacterial DNA-induced NK cell IFN-gamma production is dependent on macrophage secretion of IL-12. *Clin Immunol Immunopathol* 1997; 84: 185–193.

60. Sun S, Zhang X, Tough DF, and Sprent J. Type I interferon-mediated stimulation of T cells by CpG DNA. *J Exp Med* 1998; 188: 2335–2342.

61. Nakajima H, Nakao A, Watanabe Y, Yoshida S, and Iwamoto I. IFN-alpha inhibits antigen-induced eosinophil and CD4+ T cell recruitment into tissue. *J Immunol* 1994; 153: 1264–1270.

62. Redford TW, Yi AK, Ward CT, and Krieg AM. Cyclosporin A enhances IL-12 production by CpG motifs in bacterial DNA and synthetic oligodeoxynucleotides. *J Immunol* 1998; 161: 3930–3935.

63. Chiaramonte MG, Hesse M, Cheever AW, and Wynn TA. CpG oligonucleotides can prophylactically immunize against Th2-mediated schistosome egg-induced pathology by an IL-12-independent mechanism. *J Immunol* 2000; 164: 973–985.

64. Bauer M, Redecke V, Ellwart JW, Scherer B, Kremer JP, Wagner H, Lipford GB. Bacterial CpG-DNA triggers activation and maturation of human CD11c⁻, CD123⁺ dendritic cells. *J Immunol* 2001; 166: 5000–5007.

65. Jakob T, Walker PS, Krieg AM, Udey MC, and Vogel JC. Activation of cutaneous dendritic cells by CpG-containing oligodeoxynucleotides: a role for dendritic cells in the augmentation of Th1 responses by immunostimulatory DNA. *J Immunol* 1998; 161: 3042–3049.

66. Hartmann G, Weiner GJ, and Krieg AM. CpG DNA: a potent signal for growth, activation, and maturation of human dendritic cells. *Proc Natl Acad Sci USA* 1999; 96: 9305–9310.

67. Serebrisky D, Teper AA, Huang CK, Lee SY, Zhang TF, Schofield BH, Kattan M, Sampson HA, and Li XM. CpG oligodeoxynucleotides can reverse Th2-associated allergic airway responses and alter the B7.1/B7.2 expression in a murine model of asthma. *J Immunol* 2000; 165: 5906–5912.

68. Hartmann G and Krieg AM. CpG DNA and LPS induce distinct patterns of activation in human monocytes. *Gene Ther* 1999; 6: 893–903.
69. Chen W, Yu Y, Shao C, Zhang M, Wang W, Zhang L, and Cao X. Enhancement of antigen-presenting ability of B lymphoma cells by immunostimulatory CpG-oligonucleotides and anti-CD40 antibody. *Immunol Lett* 2001; 77: 17–23.
70. Creticos PS, Reed CE, Norman PS, Khoury J, Adkinson NF Jr, Buncher CR, Busse WW, Bush RK, Gadde J, and Li JT. Ragweed immunotherapy in adult asthma. *New Engl J Med* 1996; 334: 501–506.
71. Mueller HL and Lanz M. Hyposensitization with bacterial vaccine in infectious asthma: a double-blind study and a longitudinal study. *JAMA* 1969; 208: 1379–1383.
72. Kline JN, Kitagaki K, Businga TR, and Jain VV. Treatment of established asthma in a murine model using CpG oligodeoxynucleotides. *Am J Physiol Lung Cell Mol Physiol* 2002; 283: L170–L179.
73. Santeliz JV, Nest GV, Traquina P, Larsen E, and Wills-Karp M. Amb a 1-linked CpG oligodeoxynucleotides reverse established airway hyperresponsiveness in a murine model of asthma. *J Allergy Clin Immunol* 2002; 109: 455–462.
74. Parronchi P, Brugnolo F, Annunziato F, Manuelli C, Sampognaro S, Mavilia C, Romagnani S, and Maggi E. Phosphorothioate oligodeoxynucleotides promote the *in vitro* development of human allergen-specific CD4+ T cells into Th1 effectors. *J Immunol* 1999; 163: 5946–5953.
75. Kitagaki K, Jain VV, Businga TR, and Hussain I, Kline JN. Immunomodulatory effects of CpG oligodeoxynucleotides on established Th2 responses. *Clin Diagn Lab Immunol* 2002; 9: 1260–1269.
76. Schwartz DA, Wohlford-Lenane CL, Quinn TJ, and Krieg AM. Bacterial DNA or oligonucleotides containing unmethylated CpG motifs can minimize lipopolysaccharide-induced inflammation in the lower respiratory tract through an IL-12-dependent pathway. *J Immunol* 1999; 163: 224–231.
77. Fiorentino DF, Zlotnik A, Mosmann TR, Howard M, and O'Garra A. IL-10 inhibits cytokine production by activated macrophages. *J Immunol* 1991; 147: 3815–3822.
78. Zuany-Amorim C, Haile S, Leduc D, Dumarey C, Huerre M, Vargaftig BB, and Pretolani M. Interleukin-10 inhibits antigen-induced cellular recruitment into the airways of sensitized mice. *J Clin Invest* 1995; 95: 2644–2651.
79. Banchereau J, Briere F, Caux C, Davoust J, Lebecque S, Liu YJ, Pulendran B, and Palucka K. Immunobiology of dendritic cells. *Annu Rev Immunol* 2000; 18: 767–811.
80. Holt PG, Schon-Hegrad MA, Oliver J, Holt BJ, and McMenamin PG. A contiguous network of dendritic antigen-presenting cells within the respiratory epithelium. *Int Arch Allergy Appl Immunol* 1990; 91: 155–159.
81. Lambrecht BN. The dendritic cell in allergic airway diseases: a new player to the game. *Clin Exp Allergy* 2001; 31: 206–218.
82. Lambrecht BN, De Veerman M, Coyle AJ, Gutierrez-Ramos JC, Thielemans K, and Pauwels RA. Myeloid dendritic cells induce Th2 responses to inhaled antigen, leading to eosinophilic airway inflammation. *J Clin Invest* 2000; 106: 551–559.
83. Lambrecht BN, Pauwels RA, Fazekas De St Groth B. Induction of rapid T cell activation, division, and recirculation by intratracheal injection of dendritic cells in a TCR transgenic model. *J Immunol* 2000; 164: 2937–2946.

84. Flamand V, Sornasse T, Thielemans K, Demanet C, Bakkus M, Bazin H, Tielemans F, Leo O, Urbain J, and Moser M. Murine dendritic cells pulsed *in vitro* with tumor antigen induced tumor resistance *in vivo. Eur J Immunol* 1994; 24: 605–610.

85. Moser M and Murphy KM. Dendritic cell regulation of TH1-TH2 development. *Nat Immunol* 2000; 1: 199–205.

86. Kaisho T and Akira S. Dendritic-cell function in Toll-like receptor- and MyD88-knockout mice. *Trends Immunol* 2001; 22: 78–83.

87. Schleimer RP, Sterbinsky SA, Kaiser J, Bickel CA, Klunk DA, Tomioka K, Newman W, Luscinskas FW, Gimbrone MA Jr, and McIntyre BW, IL-4 induces adherence of human eosinophils and basophils but not neutrophils to endothelium: association with expression of VCAM-1. *J Immunol* 1992; 148: 1086–1092.

88. Van Oosterhout AJ, Ladenius AR, Savelkoul HF, Van Ark I, Delsman KC, and Nijkamp FP. Effect of anti-IL-5 and IL-5 on airway hyperreactivity and eosinophils in guinea pigs. *Am Rev Respir Dis* 1993; 147: 548–552.

89. Iwamoto I, Nakajima H, Endo H, and Yoshida S. Interferon gamma regulates antigen-induced eosinophil recruitment into the mouse airways by inhibiting the infiltration of CD4+ T cells. *J Exp Med* 1993; 177: 573–576.

90. Bliss J, Van Cleave V, Murray K, Wiencis A, Ketchum M, Maylor R, Haire T, Resmini C, Abbas AK, and Wolf SF. IL-12, as an adjuvant, promotes a T helper 1 cell, but does not suppress a T helper 2 cell recall response. *J Immunol* 1996; 156: 887–894.

91. Schoenhaut DS, Chua AO, Wolitzky AG, Quinn PM, Dwyer CM, McComas W, Familletti PC, Gately MK, and Gubler U. Cloning and expression of murine IL-12. *J Immunol* 1992; 148: 3433–3440.

92. Yi AK, Chang M, Peckham DW, Krieg AM, and Ashman RF. CpG oligodeoxyribonucleotides rescue mature spleen B cells from spontaneous apoptosis and promote cell cycle entry. *J Immunol* 1998; 160: 5898–5906.

93. Sun S, Beard C, Jaenisch R, Jones P, and Sprent J. Mitogenicity of DNA from different organisms for murine B cells. *J Immunol* 1997; 159: 3119–3125.

94. Martin-Orozco E, Kobayashi H, Van Uden J, Nguyen MD, Kornbluth RS, and Raz E. Enhancement of antigen-presenting cell surface molecules involved in cognate interactions by immunostimulatory DNA sequences. *Int Immunol* 1999; 11: 1111–1118.

95. Sparwasser T, Miethke T, Lipford G, Erdmann A, Hacker H, Heeg K, and Wagner H. Macrophages sense pathogens via DNA motifs: induction of tumor necrosis factor-alpha-mediated shock. *Eur J Immunol* 1997; 27: 1671–1679.

96. Tascon RE, Ragno S, Lowrie DB, and Colston MJ. Immunostimulatory bacterial DNA sequences activate dendritic cells and promote priming and differentiation of CD8+ T cells. *Immunology* 2000; 99: 1–7.

97. Cowdery JS, Chace JH, Yi AK, and Krieg AM. Bacterial DNA induces NK cells to produce IFN-gamma in vivo and increases the toxicity of lipopolysaccharides. *J Immunol* 1996; 156: 4570–4575.

98. Ballas ZK, Rasmussen WL, and Krieg AM. Induction of NK activity in murine and human cells by CpG motifs in oligodeoxynucleotides and bacterial DNA. *J Immunol* 1996; 157: 1840–1845.

25

Future Therapies

JEFFREY STOKES, CHRISTOPHER CLARK, and THOMAS B. CASALE

Creighton University Medical Center
Omaha, Nebraska, U.S.A.

I. Introduction

Asthma is a chronic inflammatory disorder characterized by reversible airway obstruction, airway hyperresponsiveness, and airway inflammation. It is an extremely heterogeneous disorder, and a multitude of factors — genetic (e.g., atopy), environmental, psychosocial, and biological — contribute to the disease process.[1] Specific cells implicated in asthma include eosinophils, T lymphocytes (T_H2), macrophages, neutrophils, mast cells, and epithelial cells. These cells release cytokines that initiate and propagate the inflammatory process. Cytokines activate transcription factors that bind to the promoter regions on genes to induce the expression of additional cytokines, chemokines, or adhesion molecules.

New insights into the pathogenesis of asthma have sparked extensive research aimed at developing safer, more effective treatments. Potential therapies include preventing allergic inflammation by attenuating the development of T_H2 lymphocytes by vaccines such as bacille Calmette-Guérin (BCG) or inhibiting specific transcription factors. Specific therapies to inhibit T_H2 cytokine production, for example, suplatast tosilate, were evaluated in patients with asthma. Monoclonal antibodies such as anti-CD4 and anti-CD23 were developed to decrease inflammation and IgE-mediated responses. Strategies aimed at directly

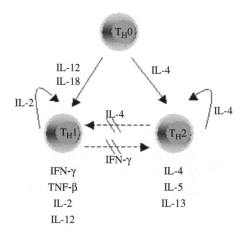

Figure 25.1 T_H1 and T_H2 lymphocyte cytokine profiles.

inhibiting the mediators of inflammation or preventing migration and chemotaxis of inflammatory cells to tissues also have roles in treating asthma. Dietary modification has been postulated to prevent allergic diseases such as asthma. Although many of these innovative treatments are in the early stages of development, they may ultimately reshape management strategies in the future.

II.   Immune-Modifying Therapies

A. TH_2-Directed Therapies

In genetically susceptible atopic individuals, aeroallergens may start a chain of events leading to airway inflammation. Allergen presentation to CD4 lymphocytes leads to the production and release of T_H2 cytokines (interleukins) designated IL-4, IL-5, and IL-13. IL-4 and IL-13 are required for IgE synthesis and mast cell growth and differentiation. IL-5 is important for eosinophil differentiation, recruitment, and activation. One strategy for treating allergic asthma is shifting from the T_H2 pattern to a T_H1-based pattern with increased production of interferon (IFN)-γ (Figure 25.1). The production of IFN-γ inhibits IL-4 and the development of T_H2 cells leading to decreases in IL-4, IL-5, and IL-13.

B.   Mycobacteria

Researchers have studied the therapeutic potentials of naturally occurring bacterial products such as BCG and mycobacteria infection. These agents lead to increases in IL-12, IL-18, and IFN-γ, swinging the pendulum away from the T_H2

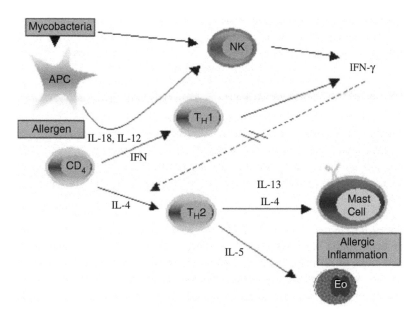

Figure 25.2 Proposed mechanism exhibited by mycobacteria on T_H2 cytokines.

paradigm and toward the T_H1 paradigm (Figure 25.2). In a mouse model of asthma, BCG vaccine and *Mycobacterium vaccae* administration prior to allergen exposure prevented the development of airway hyperresponsiveness. In addition, plasma levels of IL-12 were increased and IL-4 levels were decreased.[2] Other animal models demonstrated the ability of BCG administration prior to sensitization to attenuate airway hyperresponsiveness and airway eosinophilia.[3,4] In a mouse model, IL-4 levels were not increased after allergen administration while IFN-γ levels increased, thus preventing the typical T_H2 cytokine pattern seen with ovalbumin sensitization.[4]

The supporting evidence from human studies is not as clear. An early epidemiological study from Japan noted a significant association between positive tuberculin skin test responses and decreased atopy in humans (asthma, rhinitis, eczema, lower IgE levels).[5] This study seemed to suggest that early life exposure to mycobacterial antigens may decrease the incidence of atopy in children. Another possibility is that atopic children produce reduced responses to bacterial antigens due to decreases in interferon-γ.[6] Other studies have not reproduced this association with BCG vaccination and decreased atopy.[7,8] Thus, it is unclear whether BCG can impart protective immunity against the development of atopy and allergic diseases.

The effects of neonatal vaccination with BCG on children aged 7 to 14 years were evaluated. In children with family histories of atopy (rhinitis or eczema), BCG vaccination was associated with a lower prevalence of current asthma. In all children, BCG vaccination significantly reduced the levels of allergen-stimulated IL-10 production from lymphocytes *in vitro*, but levels of IL-4, IL-5, and IFN-γ were unaffected.[9]

Several pulmonary studies investigated whether BCG administered to allergic subjects would reverse or treat the disease process. When children and young adults with asthma were vaccinated with BCG, several improvements including increases in FEV_1 levels and morning and evening peak flow values were noted. Despite these improvements, no significant changes in symptom scores were noted.[10,11]

In 43 adults with moderate to severe asthma, treatment with BCG vaccination improved lung function 4, 8, and 12 weeks post-vaccination.[12] Additionally, sputum eosinophils were decreased and the sputum ratios of IFN-γ to IL-4 increased in the BCG-treated patients compared with those vaccinated with placebo. However, asthma symptom scores and weekly rescue medication use were not significantly different. At week 9, the inhaled corticosteroid usage was reduced in 22% of BCG-treated patients compared with 5% of placebo-treated patients.

Mycobacterium vaccae was evaluated as a treatment for asthma. Patients with asthma were treated with 0.5 mg heat-killed *M. vaccae* (HKMV), delipidated deglycolipidated *M. vaccae* (DDMV), or placebo via intradermal injection. No difference in asthma symptoms, peak expiratory flow (PEF), IgE, eosinophil levels, or the T cell proliferative and cytokine responses were noted with therapy.[13] Although initial data were promising, the practical and clinical uses of mycobacteria-based vaccines in preventing or treating allergic diseases appear limited.

C. Transcription Factors

Transciption factors, such as specific signal transducers and activators of transcription (STATs), GATA-3, and Janus kinases (JAKs), regulate T_H2 cytokine gene expression. Higher numbers of bronchial cells expressing GATA-3 were observed in atopic asthmatics compared with control subjects. In addition, more STAT-6 immunoreactive cells were present in asthmatic patients compared with controls.[14] By targeting these factors that may be up-regulated in atopic patients, several gene products important for allergic inflammation may be inhibited.

1. GATA-3

GATA-3 is a transcription factor noted to regulate the expression of IL-4, IL-5, and IL-13 and is key for T_H2 cell differentiation. Additionally, T_H2 cells express high levels of GATA-3, and GATA-3 levels in asthma correlate with expression of IL-5.[15] Expression of GATA-3 is increased in atopic asthma and allergic rhinitis. Moreover, GATA-3 and IL-5 mRNA levels are increased in nasal tissue of allergic rhinitics both before and after allergen challenge.[16] In GATA-3-deficient mouse models, decreased levels of IgE and eosinophil counts were noted following allergen challenge.[17] In another murine model of asthma, antagonizing GATA-3 function with GATA-3 antisense inhibited IL-4 production and the development of airway hyperresponsiveness after allergen challenge.[18]

2.   STAT-6

STAT-6 is also necessary for T_H2 cytokine gene production, especially IL-4. Atopic compared with nonatopic asthmatics showed higher densities of STAT-6-expressing cells in their airways.[14] An endogenous inhibitor of STAT-6, suppressor of cytokine signaling-1 (SOCS-1), inhibits IL-4 signaling.[19] STAT-6-deficient mice failed to develop airway hyperresponsiveness, elevations in IgE, goblet cell hyperplasia, and mucus production after allergen sensitization and challenge.[20]

3.   NF-κB, AP-1

Activation of NF-κB and activator protein (AP-1) transcription factors also contributes to the inflammatory pattern seen in asthma via the production of cytokines and their receptors. Glucocorticosteroids, potent anti-inflammatory compounds, inhibit this activation. One potential treatment is MOL-294, a selective inhibitor of the thioredoxin oxireductase. Thioredoxin regulates both AP-1 and NF-κB. In a murine model, MOL-294 reduced airway eosinophilia, mucus hypersecretion, airway hyperresponsiveness, and IL-13 and eotaxin release.[21] Another transcription factor inhibitor, SP100030, inhibits both NF-κB and AP-1. In a rat model, it reduced the expression of IL-2, IL-5, and IL-10 after allergen exposure, but airway eosinophilia and hyperresponsiveness were not affected.[22]

4.   Summary

Inhibition of transcription factors such as GATA-3, STAT-6, NF-κB, and AP-1 has shown promise in animal models of asthma. One potential drawback of this approach is that when an inflammatory response is required to combat infection, the body may not be able to respond effectively and appropriately. As unique targets of asthma inflammation, these factors, when inhibited, may selectively decrease cytokines critical for asthma development, but their risk-to-benefit ratio must be better defined.

D.   Suplatast Tosilate

Another treatment under investigation is suplatast tosilate, a relatively selective T_H2 cytokine inhibitor that suppresses the synthesis of both IL-4 and IL-5, thereby reducing the synthesis of IgE[23,24] (Figure 25.3). In a double-blind multicenter

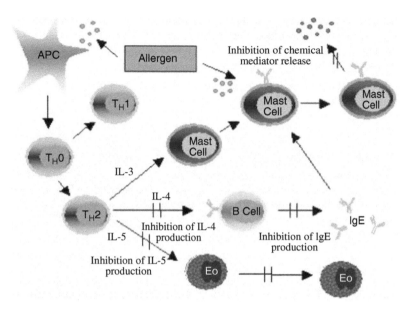

Figure 25.3 Mechanism of suplatast tosilate.

trial, 85 patients who had moderate to severe asthma and received high-dose inhaled corticosteroids were randomized to receive 100 mg oral suplatast tid or placebo for 8 weeks.[25] Suplatast significantly increased forced expiratory volume in 1 second (FEV_1) and PEF while also reducing symptom scores. After 4 weeks of therapy, an attempt was made to reduce the corticosteroid dosage by 50%. During the corticosteroid reduction phase, the placebo group demonstrated significantly greater decreases in PEF and asthma symptoms and significantly greater requirements for β_2 agonists. Concentrations of eosinophil cationic protein (ECP) and IgE were higher than baseline in the placebo group but decreased in the suplatast group during the study.

Another study examined 28 patients with asthma treated with 100 mg suplatast tosilate tid for 28 days. Suplatast treatment decreased serum and sputum eosinophils, exhaled nitric oxide levels, and airway responsiveness compared with the placebo group.[26] In cough-variant asthma patients, suplatast treatment improved cough thresholds for capsaicin and decreased percentages of sputum eosinophils.[27]

Sano and associates evaluated the effects of suplatast on airway inflammation in mild asthma.[28] Eosinophils and EG2+ cells were decreased in bronchial biopsies of mild asthma subjects treated with suplatast. Additionally, CD4+ and CD25+ cells decreased and CD8+ cells increased in bronchial mucosa of suplatast-treated patients. Symptom scores, PEF, and histamine-induced provocation all improved with suplatast treatment.

The further development of this therapy should prove interesting because early human trials have shown promise in decreasing inhaled corticosteroid use and airway inflammation while improving lung function and symptom scores.

E. Anti-CD23

The presence of IgE and eosinophils distinguishes the inflammatory responses associated with allergy and asthma compared with those of other respiratory diseases. IgE can bind to the low-affinity IgE receptor CD23 (FcϵRII) on B cells. The interaction of IgE with B cells via the CD23 receptor enhances antigen presentation and amplifies synthesis of IgE.[29] In a mouse model of allergic asthma, anti-CD23 treatment reduced allergen-induced airway bronchoconstriction.[30] In other mouse models of allergic sensitization, treatment with anti-CD23 significantly reduced IgE and IgG$_1$ levels, abolished bronchoalveolar lavage (BAL) eosinophilia, and normalized airway hyperresponsiveness. These changes were associated with increases in BAL IFN-γ and decreases in BAL IL-4.[31]

Human studies are currently underway. In allergic rhinitis, anti-CD23 antibody was well tolerated with no evidence of CD4$^+$ T cell depletion.[32] Anti-CD23 inhibited post-seasonal IgE rises in ragweed-allergic subjects. Early studies with monoclonal anti-CD23 antibody in asthma demonstrated substantial reductions in IgE levels with minimal side effects.[33] The reductions in IgE were dose-dependent and continued up to 85 days after administration. Despite this decrease in IgE, no clear effects on FEV$_1$ and asthma symptom-free days were noted. This pilot study was under-powered to discriminate these therapeutic benefits.

Thus, early studies have shown favorable tolerability but no clinical improvement in asthma. Despite this, the ability to decrease IgE levels may place anti-CD23 antibody in a unique position to treat allergic diseases. Further studies with adequate numbers of patients will be necessary before the clinical utility of this agent can be defined accurately.

F. Anti-CD4

CD4 is a critical marker for lymphocytes, especially T$_H$2 lymphocytes. Currently, two anti-CD4 monoclonal antibodies have been evaluated: keliximab (SB-210396) and clenoliximab (SB-217969). These are monkey–human chimeric anti-human antibodies of IgG4, and IgG1 subclasses, respectively.[34] In 22 patients with corticosteroid-dependent asthma (average FEV$_1$ was about 50% predicted) intravenous keliximab was evaluated. Only patients given high doses demonstrated improvements in morning PEF measurements. Keliximab significantly decreased CD4 lymphocytes at all doses and was not associated with any serious adverse events.[35] CD4 is present on both T$_H$1 and T$_H$2 cells and on other inflammatory cells. Thus, strategies aimed at this molecule must be carefully scrutinized for potential side effects in addition to benefits.

G. Anti-Tryptase

Tryptase is a protease released as a result of mast cell degranulation. It exerts a number of biologic effects that may contribute to the pathogenesis of asthma including increasing airway hyperresponsiveness, kinin production, eosinophil degranulation, and degrading vasoactive intestinal peptide (VIP). APC-366 is a tryptase inhibitor. In a pig model of allergic airway disease, APC-366 attenuated the increase in airway resistance and the decrease in dynamic lung compliance after allergen challenge.[36] In a sheep model of asthma, APC-366 treatment reduced both early and late phase asthmatic responses and airway hyperresponsiveness. Pretreatment with APC-366 decreased lung levels of eosinophils compared with levels in control sheep.[37] In humans, an early trial with inhaled APC-366 demonstrated a slight protective effect against the early and late antigen-induced airway responses. In addition, some protection against the increased airway hyperresponsiveness induced by antigen challenge was noted.[38] As more human studies are undertaken, the roles of APC-366 and other tryptase inhibitors in the treatment of asthma will become clearer.

H. Phosphodiesterase Inhibitors

Phosphodiesterase (PDE) inhibitors inhibit the PDE enzyme by specifically targeting one or a few of its 14 isoforms or by nonspecifically inhibiting all of them. The overall effect of this inhibition is an increase in cyclic 3'5-adenosine monophosphate (cAMP) and cyclic 3'5-guanosine monophosphate (cGMP) compounds that exert numerous biologic effects. Well-known examples of nonselective PDE inhibitors include theophylline (long employed in the treatment of asthma) and caffeine.

Nonselective PDE inhibitors have myriad possible mechanisms of action, but most mechanisms ascribed to asthma therapy have involved the ability to inhibit PDE 3 and PDE 4. Inflammatory cells of the immune system all contain PDE 3, PDE 4, or both, and some include additional PDE isoenzymes.[39] Inhibition of PDE 4 resulted in decreased release of mediators and inflammatory cytokines from basophils, eosinophils, monocytes lymphocytes, and neutrophils and decreased eosinophil chemotaxis and survival.[41] Other anti-inflammatory effects attributed to PDE 4 inhibition include down-regulation of endothelial cell adhesion molecules and up-regulation of IL-10 from T cells and monocytes. Inhibition of PDE 3 is synergistic with inhibition of PDE 4, but produces little in the way of independent effects on inflammatory cells.[39]

In several animal models, the *in vivo* effects of selective PDE inhibitors have been shown. In a guinea pig model of asthma, rolipram, a selective PDE 4 inhibitor, protected against histamine- and allergen-induced bronchoconstriction along with early and late asthmatic reactions. A dual PDE 3 and PDE 4 inhibitor,

Org 20241, reduced eosinophil influx into BAL fluid. Selective PDE 4 inhibitors have also been shown to attenuate allergen-induced eosinophilia and airway hyperreactivity in allergic guinea pigs, block ascaris-induced lung eosinophilia in allergic monkeys, and suppress hyperventilation-induced bronchospasm in nonallergic guinea pigs.[40,41]

Limited human data are available due to gastrointestinal side effects induced by first generation selective PDE inhibitors. A first-generation PDE 4 inhibitor, CP80,633, was used topically in 20 patients with atopic dermatitis and produced clinical improvements in all patients studied without adverse effects.[42] Zardaverine, a selective PDE 3–PDE 4 inhibitor was shown to exert modest bronchodilatory effects in patients with asthma, but was short acting and produced gastrointestinal side effects.[43]

Second generation PDE 4 inhibitors are better tolerated and more data exist on their efficacy. CDP840, an orally active, potent PDE 4 inhibitor, was studied in a double-blind, placebo-controlled trial of 54 patients. A significant attenuation of the late asthmatic response to allergen challenge was observed although no changes were seen in baseline FEV_1 values and no effects were noted on early asthmatic response, bronchodilation, or bronchial hyperresponsiveness to histamine. CDP840 was well tolerated.[44]

Cilomilast, another orally active second-generation PDE 4 inhibitor, improved lung functions and perceived quality of life in patients with chronic obstructive pulmonary disease (COPD); in asthma, only a trend in improved lung function was shown.[45]

In a randomized, double-blind, placebo-controlled crossover study, roflumilast, a new second-generation selective PDE 4 inhibitor was investigated in 16 patients with exercise-induced asthma.[46] The mean percentage FEV_1 decline after exercise was reduced by 41% with an improvement in lung function on days 1 and 14. Also, in an *ex-vivo* analysis of TNF in whole blood stimulated with LPS, a significant reduction in TNF secretion was observed in the treatment group. Roflumilast was well tolerated. Roflumilast was also recently studied in 25 subjects with allergic rhinitis in a randomized, double-blind, placebo-controlled crossover design revealing a significant improvement in nasal airflow, itching, obstruction, and rhinorrhea that reached significance by day 9 of therapy.[47]

The PDE 4 inhibitors have potential as novel treatments for allergic diseases. Studies in subjects with atopic dermatitis and allergic rhinitis have yielded promise, although results in asthma are conflicting. The newer second-generation PDE 4 inhibitors seem to be much better tolerated than their predecessors and demonstrate improved risk-to-benefit ratios. Because PDE 4 inhibitors have shown tremendous anti-inflammatory effects *in vitro* in animal models and in humans, additional large randomized placebo-controlled trials should be done, in particularly, to investigate their roles in the treatment of asthma.

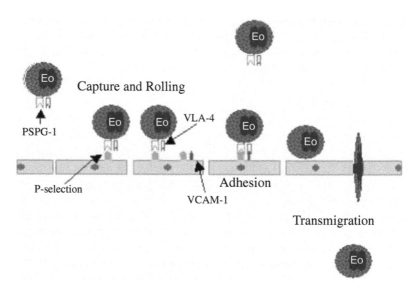

Figure 25.4   Eosinophil adhesion and migration.

I.   Anti-Adhesion Molecules

The development of airway inflammation involves the stimulated migration of inflammatory cells from the vasculature into the airways (Figure 25.4). This process requires the expression of adhesion molecules (selectins and integrins) on inflammatory cells, endothelium, and lung cells. Early studies with anti-endothelial leukocyte adhesion molecule (ELAM) monoclonal antibodies in a primate model of asthma demonstrated decreases in airway inflammatory cells and airway responsiveness.[48] These early data paved the way for further animal and human studies.

1.   P-selectin

Among the selectins, P-selectin appears the earliest after an inflammatory stimulus (e.g., histamine) and likely plays a significant role in allergic inflammation. P-selectin is involved in both eosinophil and neutrophil migration.[49] In P-selectin-deficient mice, eosinophil tissue recruitment into the lungs, eosinophil rolling, and firm adhesion to the endothelium were significantly reduced after allergen challenge.[50]

In vitro studies on human leukocytes demonstrated that P-selectin-based adhesion can be inhibited on neutrophils and eosinophils with glycomimetic compounds.[51] The inhibition of P-selectin by antagonists may inhibit human neutrophils more than eosinophils.[52] Monoclonal antibody compounds to P-selectin are under development currently.[54] It is hoped that by decreasing the effects of P-selectin, the ability of inflammatory cells to reach lung tissue and contribute to airway inflammation will be reduced.

2. VLA-4

Very late antigen-4 (VLA-4) is a critical adhesion molecule for eosinophil, basophil, and T-lymphocyte migration and may be a potential target for therapy. By blocking VLA-4, inflammatory cells may not reach the pulmonary tissues. Several animal models have demonstrated the effect of blocking VLA-4 on airway inflammation. In mouse models of asthma, treatment with an intranasal VLA-4 monoclonal antibody prior to allergen challenge inhibited IL-4 and IL-5 release. In addition, methacholine hyperresponsiveness and BAL levels of eosinophils and lymphocytes were reduced.[54]

Abraham and colleagues demonstrated the effectiveness of a VLA-4 inhibitor in a sheep model of asthma. Early work has shown that this VLA-4 inhibitor was capable of blunting early phase responses and almost completely abrogating late asthmatic responses. The likely mechanism was due to blocking increases in lymphocytes and eosinophils in the lungs after antigen challenge.[55] Furthermore, smaller doses that were ineffective singly exerted protective effects when given over 4 days. After allergen challenge, airway responsiveness increased in sheep given placebos or lower doses of VLA-4 inhibitor (1 mg via aerosol), but not in animals given higher doses (3 mg).[56]

Animal and human *in vitro* data on blocking the adhesion pathway appear promising. However, the effects of adhesion molecule antagonists in patients with asthma are only now being studied. Because adhesion molecules are important in the influx of inflammatory cells to fight pathogens, antagonists of these molecules must be carefully scrutinized for their risk-to-benefit ratios.

J. Chemokines

Chemokines are substances that mediate a range of inflammatory effects such as chemotaxis, degranulation, and integrin activation. The CCR3 and CCR8 chemokine receptors lend themselves to therapeutic intervention based on some of their specific characteristics apropos to allergic diseases such as asthma.

1. CCR3

Eosinophils express CCR3 receptors that bind with eotaxin and RANTES. This is important in eosinophil chemotaxis. CCR3 is also expressed on basophils and a subpopulation of T_H2 lymphocytes. Currently, an anti-CCR3 monoclonal antibody has demonstrated that more than 95% of the response of eosinophils to eotaxin and RANTES was mediated through CCR3.[57] In a primate model of inflammation, rhesus macaque anti-CCR3 antibodies were developed and demonstrated potent inhibition of eotaxin binding.[58]

2. CCR8

The CCR8 chemokine receptor may also demonstrate unique properties that make it a potential target for asthma treatment. In a mouse model of asthma, the expression of the CCR8 ligand is increased in inflamed lung tissue and CCR8 is selectively induced in antigen-activated eosinophils.[59] Despite this effect, the absence of CCR8 does not affect pulmonary eosinophilia after allergen challenge.[59] Additionally, no difference was noted between levels of IL-4, IL-5, and IL-13 in the BAL between CCR8-deficient mice and wild-type control mice.[61] A recent study demonstrated that no significant differences in BAL levels of IL-4, IL-5, IL-13, and IFN-γ were noted between CCR8-deficient mice and the wild-type controls after allergen challenge.[60]

Even though early data suggest that CCR8 may play a role in asthma, at least in the mouse model, the role appears to be limited and noncritical. CCR3 may be a better target for modulation, but no human clinical data are available.

III. Environmentally Based Therapies

A. Maternal and Fetal Diet Allergen Elimination

Allergen avoidance has long been a cornerstone of treatment for atopic disease. It is well established that early sensitization to foods begins the allergic march that often culminates in asthma. A direct correlation exists between the number of foods given before age 4 months and the risk of food allergy. Data suggest that a genetic tendency to develop atopy, in addition to some early, perhaps gestational, environmental exposures such as food allergens and tobacco smoke are responsible for setting the allergic march in motion. Infants with atopic family members are born with decreased abilities to produce IFN-γ by peripheral blood mononuclear cells (PBMCs) when compared with babies born to nonatopic families. This observation suggests that these infants are primed for developing allergy at birth.[61]

In a study involving 508 children, those who were persistently sensitized to food allergens for more than 1 year developed a 5.5-fold increased risk for developing asthma. If these children had atopic family histories, they faced a 67% risk of developing asthma by age 5.[62] It has also been shown that the introduction of wheat cereal into the diet before age 4 months is a risk factor for subsequent development of grass pollen asthma.[63] In addition, children exposed to four or more different types of food by 4 months of age had 2.9-fold increased risks of developing chronic eczema.[64,65]

A major question is whether the avoidance of allergen exposure helps in the prevention or treatment of asthma. In a position statement, the American Academy of Allergy, Asthma, and Immunology recommends that all patients with asthma be evaluated for allergy and to avoid substances to which they are allergic. Several studies have demonstrated benefits in prevention of asthma by avoidance of indoor allergens. Intense environmental manipulation resulting in decreased exposure to dust mites was shown to reduce nonviral respiratory symptoms in infants at high risk for atopy in the first year of life.[66]

In another study, 120 infants were chosen based on family histories of atopy and high cord-blood IgE levels and were randomly assigned to prophylactic or control groups.[67] In the prophylactic group, breast-feeding mothers avoided milk, eggs, fish, and nuts and avoided feeding their infants those foods plus soy, wheat, and oranges for the first 12 months of life. The living room and the infants' bedroom carpets were treated with acaricidal powder and foam every 3 months and Der p 1 dust concentrations were measured until the infants reached 12 months of age. The control group was not subjected to diet or environmental modifications. By age 12 months, allergic disorders had developed in 40% of the control infants and only 13% of those in the prophylactic group. The prevalences of asthma and eczema were also reduced statistically in the prophylactic group. By age 2 years, the incidence of allergy was still significantly lower than incidence in the control group, but rates of asthma and eczema, although lower, were no longer statistically significantly different.[68] By 4 years of age, the prophylactic group continued to show fewer positive skin prick tests (SPTs) to dietary and aeroallergens and less eczema than the control group.[69] The prophylactic group maintained less SPT positivity at age 8, but the reduction in current wheezing and rhinitis symptoms, although trending lower, did not reach significance.[70] Although asthma was not significantly reduced in this study after the subjects reached 1 year of age, it is quite interesting that a persistent trend toward fewer asthma symptoms persisted to age 8 years, and that this reduction was accompanied by significant decreases in SPT positivity. Had the number of subjects studied been larger, the significant reduction in asthma symptoms present at 1 year of age may have been shown to persist.

Because the incidence of asthma has dramatically risen in the recent past, intensive research has been done to determine the cause. All potential mechanisms are being thoroughly investigated and environmental factors are thought to play a large role in the upswing. At least in high-risk infants, environmental manipulation has been responsible for fewer allergies and fewer asthma symptoms. More prospective trials with larger numbers of subjects are needed to further elucidate the role of allergen exposure and avoidance in asthma development.

B. Dietary Fatty Acids and Asthma

Numerous studies focused on evaluating the effects of dietary fatty acid intake on immune modulation. Polyunsaturated fatty acid intake has been shown to produce beneficial effects in many disease states. Among polyunsaturated fats are the omega-3 (n-3) types, principally derived from fish oils, and omega-6 (n-6) fats such as arachadonic acid, so named due to the positions of their terminal double bonds. The principal role of arachadonic acid in atopic diseases is production of prostaglandins and leukotrienes (eicosanoids) that largely mediate inflammation and bronchoconstriction. If a diet rich in n-6 fatty acids, such as exists in western societies, is expected to result in more arachadonic acid available for inflammatory mediator synthesis, perhaps one rich in n-3 fatty acids would reduce this tendency. Indeed, consumption of n-3 fatty acids decreases the arachadonic acid contents in cell membranes, resulting in decreased eicosanoid production.[71–73]

Evidence also indicates that n-3 fatty acids decrease the activity of NF-κB.[72,74] Studies in healthy volunteers whose diets were supplemented with n-3 fatty acids revealed *ex vivo* decreases in IL-1, IL-6, TNF, and IL-12 produced by PBMCs.[75] In a multivariate analysis of 4366 children and 878 adults, eating fish more then once per week had a protective effect in children against developing bronchial hyperresponsiveness.[76]

Results of other studies of the effects of fish oil on established allergic diseases have largely been disappointing.[77–79] One such study found no significant differences in either the numbers of infiltrating inflammatory cells or the clinical manifestations resulting from the allergen-induced late-phase skin responses in adults before and after a 10-week trial of dietary fish oil supplementation.[77] In another study, fish oil supplementation failed to prevent pollen season–induced hay fever symptoms and bronchial hyperresponsiveness in adults with allergic rhinitis and asthma.[78]

In 39 asthmatic children aged 8 to 12 years randomized to receive either n-3 or n-6 fatty acids for 6 months, no clinical differences were noted in asthma severity, although a significant decrease in stimulated TNF production in the n-3 group compared with baseline levels was noted.[79] Measurements of plasma and cell membrane phospholipids indicated compliance with the treatment and, thus, would not be a reason for lack of effect. Large randomized placebo-controlled trials are needed to determine what benefit, if any, n-3 fatty acids can provide in treating asthma, but asthma prevention via supplementation looks more promising.

In terms of primary prevention, the Childhood Asthma Prevention Study (CAPS) was designed to examine the effects of n-3 fatty acid supplementation on asthma prevention in high risk children. The children were randomized before birth to receive n-3 fatty acid supplementation or a placebo beginning at 6 months of age. A total of 543 children completed the first 18 months of the study. Follow-up when they reached 18 months of age revealed a 9.8% absolute reduction in the prevalence of any wheeze and a 7.8% absolute reduction in the prevalence of wheeze longer than 1 week, although serum IgE, atopic status, and physician diagnosis of asthma factors were unaffected.[80] Follow-up at age 5 years is planned to further evaluate the treatment effects on asthma.

One recent trial investigated the cytokine profiles of cord blood taken from newborn babies whose atopic mothers were randomized to take supplementation with fish oil capsules high in n-3 fatty acids or placebos from 20 weeks gestation until birth.[81] Infants in the fish oil group had significantly lower plasma levels of IL-13 than controls. Whether this has clinical relevance in terms of prevention of allergic disease awaits follow-up as these children age.

C. Probiotics

A critical step in interactions between the immune system and exogenous antigen is the presentation of the antigen by antigen-presenting cells (APCs) to CD4+ T helper cells. Dendritic cells, potent APCs, are key to this process. Dendritic cells are distributed along epithelial barriers, including the entire intestinal epithelium, where they have been shown to penetrate the epithelial barrier in order to sample gut-associated bacteria without disrupting the barrier function.[82] This direct sampling of flora may produce different immunologic signals, depending on the type of bacteria present.

Probiotics are live microbial food supplements that beneficially affect the host animal by improving its intestinal microbial balance.[83] Probiotics tend to be bacteria or yeasts that are present as normal flora in varying concentrations in the human GI tract.

Different strains and doses of Lactobacilli induce production of different cytokines, and some strains can cancel out the effects elicited by others. For example, low levels of *L. casei* strongly induce IL-12, IL-6, and TNF, whereas higher levels result in a tremendous increase in IL-10 expression. The induction of inflammatory cytokines was blocked by combining *L. casei* with *L. reuteri*, although IL-10 levels remained elevated.[84] TGF-β, a regulatory cytokine that leads to down-regulation of the IL-12 receptor in mice, was strongly induced by *L. paracasei*. Lactobacilli have also been shown to induce IgA secretion and up-regulate dendritic cell surface markers such as B-7-2.[84,85]

Probiotics may be able to promote immune tolerance through a variety of effects including those on cytokines and dendritic cells.[86] In one study, neonatal germ-free BALB/c mice were susceptible only to oral tolerance induction after their GI flora were reconstituted with *Bifidobacteria infantis*, demonstrating the influence of GI flora on the immune system, in this case by down-regulating the T_H2 response.[86] IL-10 and TGF-β are now well established as regulatory cytokines and their induction by Lactobacillus has been demonstrated. In a study by Von Der Weid et al., *L. paracasei* added to mixed lymphocyte cultures from naïve BALB/c mice resulted in decreased CD4$^+$ T cell proliferation; marked increases of TGF-β; decreased production of IL-4, IL-5, and IFN-γ; and maintenance of IL-10 levels.[87] Induction of TGF-β$_2$ was also demonstrated in breast milk of mothers taking Lactobacillus GG supplementation that resulted in clinical benefits to the infants.[88]

It appears that atopic children may have bacterial flora different from those of nonatopic children. In one study, significant decreases in the Bifidobacteria-to-Clostridium ratios were found in the GI flora of atopic infants (defined by one positive SPT at 12 months of age) compared with nonatopic infants.[89] In addition, higher Lactobacilli-to-Clostridium ratios in the GI flora of infants were associated with lower prevalences of atopy.[89]

Many studies have investigated the use of probiotics either for treatment or prevention of allergic diseases. Most studies evaluated effects on atopic dermatitis, which is acknowledged as an early manifestation of allergic diseases in children.[90] One randomized, double-blind, placebo-controlled trial involved supplementation of pregnant mothers with Lactobacillus GG 2 to 4 weeks before giving birth and subsequent supplementation of their infants until 6 months of age. This trial revealed lower incidences of atopic dermatitis in infants who received probiotics as compared with infants in the control group through age 2.[91] A similar study involving mothers who received Lactobacillus GG 4 weeks prenatally and 3 months postpartum and their breast-fed infants revealed significantly lower incidences of atopic dermatitis in the active versus placebo groups. Also observed in the study group were significantly higher breast milk concentrations of TGF β2 and a trend toward higher breast milk concentrations of TGF β1.[88]

Using probiotics in the treatment of already established atopic disease has shown promising results, albeit more in infants than adults. A study involving adults with moderate asthma who received *L. acidophilus* in a double-blind cross-over fashion twice daily in yogurt revealed no clinical differences between treatment groups, but the active group showed a trend toward increased serum IFN-γ levels and lower blood eosinophils.[92]

A study investigating the impact of *L. rhamnosus* in adults and adolescents with birch pollen and apple food allergies revealed no benefits in terms of symptom scores during open apple challenge.[93] Another study of infants with atopic dermatitis and cow milk allergies involved a treatment group receiving extensively hydrolyzed whey formula containing Lactobacillus GG. The study revealed significantly decreased atopic dermatitis scores in addition to significant reductions in fecal inflammatory markers (TNF and α1-antitrypsin) in the probiotic group as compared with the placebo group.[94] Similar results were seen in a study involving breast-fed infants with atopic dermatitis in which all infants were switched to extensively hydrolyzed whey formulas with or without the addition of probiotics.[95]

These trials show promise for probiotics in treating allergic diseases, especially atopic dermatitis. However, the data suggest that the probiotics must be introduced early in life to produce optimal benefits. Large controlled trials are needed before any conclusions are reached regarding the use of probiotics in adults and their use in other forms of allergic diseases.

D. Summary

Asthma is a common disease afflicting millions in the United States annually and in rare cases causing death. Current therapies are based on treating preexisting disease and are effective in reducing symptoms for most patients. In order to prevent allergic diseases such as asthma, treatment must be instigated early in life. Dietary alterations may help reduce atopic sensitization early in life, but preliminary data have not demonstrated a significant effect on reducing asthma. It appears unlikely that changes in the diet of a patient who has asthma will significantly improve the disease.

IV. Conclusion

Many potential therapies for allergic respiratory diseases are currently under investigation and include respirable antisense oligonucleotides and inhibitors of transcription factors. Where these and the agents discussed above will fit into the therapy regimens of allergic disorders is unclear and awaits further human studies. Inhibition of critical events in T_H2-driven responses appears a logical approach, but the risk-to-benefit ratio must be carefully scrutinized. Ultimately, better therapeutic options should decrease symptoms, enhance quality of life, improve the course of the disease, reverse pathogenic and physiologic changes, produce low side effects, and be cost effective.

Because of the heterogeneous nature of asthma, specific agents will probably work best for selected types of patients. Ubiquitous treatments will be difficult to develop and most likely will involve agents that target the earliest stages of asthmatic inflammation. Regardless of the obstacles, however, ongoing research into the wide range of therapeutic possibilities should provide new insights into the pathogenesis of allergic respiratory diseases.

References

1. National Heart, Lung, and Blood Institute. Expert Panel Report 2: Guidelines for the Diagnosis and Management of Asthma. National Institutes of Health Publication 97-4051. Bethesda, MD, 1997.
2. Hopfenspirger MT, Parr SK, Hopp RJ, Townley RG, and Agrawal DK. Mycobacterial antigens attenuate late phase airway hyperresponsiveness and bronchoalveolar lavage eosinophils in a mouse model of bronchial asthma. *Int Immunopharmacol* 2001: 1; 1743–1751.

3. Erb KJ, Holloway JW, Sobeck A, Moll H, and Le Gros G. Infection of mice with *Mycobacterium bovis* bacillus Calmette-Guerin (BCG) suppresses allergen-induced airway eosinophilia. *J Exp Med* 1998; 187: 561–569.

4. Herz U, Gerhold K, Gruber C, Braun A, Wahn U, Renz H, and Paul K. BCG infection suppresses allergic sensitization and development of increased airway reactivity in an animal model. *J Allergy Clin Immunol* 1998; 102: 867–874.

5. Shirakawa T, Enomoto T, Shimazu S, and Hopkin JM. The inverse association between tuberculin response and atopic disorder. *Science* 1997; 275: 77–79.

6. Alm JS, Lilja G, Pershagen G., and Scheynius A. BCG vaccination does not seem to prevent atopy in children with atopic heredity. *Allergy* 1998; 53: 537.

7. Alm JS, Lilja G, Pershagen G., and Scheynius A. Early BCG vaccination and development of atopy. *Lancet* 1997; 350: 400–403.

8. Strannegard IL, Larsson LO, Wennergren G, and Strannegard O. Prevalence of allergy in children in relation to prior BCG vaccination and infection with atypical mycobacteria. *Allergy* 1998; 53: 249–254.

9. Marks GB, Ng K, Zhou J, Toelle BG, Xuan W, Belousova EG, and Britton WJ. The effect of neonatal BCG vaccination on atopy and asthma at age 7 and 14 years: historical cohort study in a community with very low prevalence of tuberculosis infection and a high prevalence of atopic disease. *J Allergy Clin Immunol* 2003; 111: 541–549.

10. Hopp RJ, Townley RG, Sueiro R, and Romero T. Pulmonary function and asthma symptom scores following BCG administration in established asthmatics. *J Allergy Clin Immunol* 2003; 111: S297.

11. Hopp RJ, Sueiro R, Romero T, Agrawal DK, and Townley R. Will BCG immunization affect the clinical expression of an established asthmatic? *J Allergy Clin Immunol* 2002; 109: S204.

12. Choi IS and Koh YI. Therapeutic effects of BCG vaccination in adult asthmatic patients: a randomized, controlled trial. *Ann Allergy Asthma Immunol* 2002; 88: 584–591.

13. Shirtcliffe PM, Easthope SE, Cheng S, Weatherall M, Tan PL, Le Gros G, and Beasley R. The effect of delipidated deglycolipidated (DDMV) and heat-killed *Mycobacterium vaccae* in asthma. *Am J Respir Crit Care Med* 2001; 163: 1410–1414.

14. Christodoulopoulos P, Cameron L, Nakamura Y, Lemière C, Muro S, Dugas M, Boulet LP, Laviolette M, Olivenstein R, and Hamid Q. TH2 cytokine-associated transcription factors in atopic and nonatopic asthma: evidence for differential signal transducer and activator of transcription 6 expression. *J Allergy Clin Immunol* 2001; 107: 586–591.

15. Nakamura Y, Ghaffar O, Olivenstein R, Taha RA, Soussi-Gounni A, Zhang DH, Ray A, and Hamid Q. Gene expression of the GATA-3 transcription factor is increased in atopic asthma. *J Allergy Clin Immunol* 1999; 103: 215–222.

16. Nakamura Y, Christodoulopoulos P, Cameron L, Wright E, Lavigne F, Toda M, Muro S, Ray A, Eidelman DH, Minshall E, and Hamid Q. Up-regulation of the transcription factor GATA-3 in upper airway mucosa after *in vivo* and *in vitro* allergen challenge. *J Allergy Clin Immunol* 2000; 105: 1146–1152.

17. Zhang DH, Yang L, Cohn L, Parkyn L, Homer R, Ray P, and Ray A. Inhibition of allergic inflammation in a murine model of asthma by expression of a dominant-negative mutant of GATA-3. *Immunity* 1999; 11: 473–482.
18. Finotto S, De Sanctis GT, Lehr HA, Herz U, Buerke M, Schipp M, Bartsch B, Atreya R, Schmitt E, Galle PR, Renz H, and Neurath MF. Treatment of allergic airway inflammation and hyperresponsiveness by antisense-induced local blockade of GATA-3 expression. *J Exp Med* 2001; 193: 1247–1256.
19. Borish LC and Steinke JW. Cytokines and chemokines. *J Allergy Clin Immunol* 2003; 111: S460–S475.
20. Kuperman, D, Schofield B, Wills-Karp M, and Grusby MJ. Signal transducer and activator of transcription factor 6 (STAT6)-deficient mice are protected from antigen-induced airway hyperresponsiveness and mucus production. *J Exp Med* 1998; 187: 939–948.
21. Henderson WR, Jr, Chi EY, Teo JL, Nguyen C, and Kahn M. A small molecule inhibitor of redox-regulated NF-kappa B and activator protein-1 transcription blocks allergic airway inflammation in a mouse asthma model. *J Immunol* 2002; 169: 5294–5299.
22. Huang TJ, Adcock IM, and Chung KF. A novel transcription factor inhibitor, SP100030, inhibits cytokine gene expression, but not airway eosinophilia or hyper-responsiveness in sensitized and allergen-exposed rat. *Br J Pharmacol* 2001; 134: 1029–1036.
23. Yamaya H, Basaki Y, Togawa M, Kojima M, Kiniwa M, and Marsuura N. Down-regulation of Th2 cell-mediated murine peritoneal eosinophilia by antiallergic agents. *Life Sci* 1995; 19: 1647–1654.
24. Yanagihara Y, Kiniwa M, Ikizawa K, Shida T, Matsuura N, and Koda A. Suppression of IgE production by IPD-1151T (suplatast tosilate), a new dimethylsulfonium agent. 2. Regulation of human IgE response. *Jpn J Pharmacol* 1993; 62: 31–39.
25. Tamaoki J, Kondo M, Sakai N, Aoshiba K, Tagaya E, Nakata J, Isono K, and Nagai A. Effect of suplatast tosilate, a Th2 cytokine inhibitor, on steroid-dependent asthma: a double-blind randomized study. *Lancet.* 2000; 356: 273–279.
26. Yoshida M, Aizawa H, Inoue H, Matsumoto K, Koto H, Komori M, Fukuyama S, Okamoto M, and Hara N. Effect of suplatast tosilate on airway hyperresponsiveness and inflammation in asthma patients. *J Asthma* 2002; 39: 545–552.
27. Shioya T, Satake M, Sano M, Kagaya M, Watanabe A, Sato K, Ito T, Ito N, Sasaki M, and Miura M. Effect of suplatast tosilate, a Th2 cytokine inhibitor, on cough variant asthma. *Eur J Clin Pharmocol* 2002; 58: 171–176.
28. Sano Y, Suzuki N, Yamada H, To Y, Ogawa C, Ohta K, and Adachi M. Effects of suplatast tosilate on allergic eosinophilic airway inflammation in patients with mild asthma. *J Allergy Clin Immunol* 2003; 111: 958–966.
29. Broide DH. Molecular and cellular mechanisms of allergic disease. *J Allergy Clin Immunol* 2001; 108: S65–S71.
30. Dasic G, Juillard P, Graber P, Herren S, Angell T, Knowles R, Bonnefoy JY, Kosco-Vilbois MH, and Chvatchko Y. Critical role of CD23 in allergen-induced bronchoconstriction in a murine model of allergic asthma. *Eur J Immunol* 1999; 29: 2957–2967.

31. Haczku A, Takeda K, Hamelmann E, Loader J, Joetham A, Redai I, Irvin CG, Lee JJ, Kikutani H, Conrad D, and Gelfand EW. CD23 exhibits negative regulatory effects on allergic sensitization and airway hyperresponsiveness. *Am J Respir Crit Care Med* 2000; 161: 952–960.

32. Casale TB, Busse WW, Lizambri PG, Korenblat PE, Schoenwetter WF, Weiler JM, Rosenwasser LJ, Nayak AS, Perea RM, and Totoritis MC. Results of a phase II, multiple-dose, randomized trial of an antiCD23 monoclonal antibody (IDEC) in patients with seasonal allergic rhinitis. *J Allergy Clin Immunol* 2003; 111: S74.

33. Busse WW, Rosenwasser LJ, Lizambri RG, Olejnik TA, and Totoritis MC. Results of a phase I, single-dose-escalating trial of a primatized anti-Cd23 monoclonal antibody (IDEC-152) in patients with allergic asthma. *J Allergy Clin Immunol* 2001; 107: S106.

34. Sharma A, Davis CB, Tobia LA, Kwok DC, Tucci MG, Gore ER, Herzyk DJ, and Hart TK. Comparative pharmacodynamics of keliximab and clenoliximab in transgenic mice bearing human CD4. *J Pharmacol Exp Ther* 2000; 293: 33–34.

35. Kon OM, Sihra BS, Compton CH, Leonard TB, Kay AB, and Barnes NC. Randomising, dose-ranging, placebo-controlled study of chimeric antibody to CD4 (keliximab) in chronic severe asthma. *Lancet* 1998; 352: 1109–1113.

36. Sylvin H, Dahlbäck M, Van Der Ploeg I, and Alving K. The tryptase inhibitor APC-366 reduces the acute airway response to allergen in pigs sensitized to *Ascaris suum*. *Clin Exp Allergy* 2002; 32: 967.

37. Clark JM, Abraham WM, Fishman CE, Forteza R, Ahmed A, Cortes A, Warne RL, Moore WR, and Tanaka RD. Tryptase inhibitors block allergen-induced airway and inflammatory responses in allergic sheep. *Am J Respir Crit Care Med* 1995; 152: 2076–2083.

38. Krishna MT, Chauhan A, Little L, Sampson K, Hawksworth R, Mant T, Djukanovic R, Lee T, Holgate S. Inhibition of mast cell tryptase by inhaled APC 366 attenuates allergen-induced late-phase airway obstruction in asthma. *J Allergy Clin Immunol.* 2001 Jun; 107(6): 1039–1045.

39. Essayan DM. Cyclic nucleotide phosphodiesterases. *J Allergy Clin Immunol* 2001; 108: 671–680.

40. Santing RE, de Boer J, Rohof A, van der Zee NM, and Zaagsma J. Bronchodilatory and anti-inflammatory properties of inhaled selective phosphodiesterase inhibitors in a guinea pig model of allergic asthma. *Eur J Pharmacol* 2001; 429: 335–344.

41. Billah MM, Cooper N, Minnicozzi M, Warneck J, Wang P, Hey JA, Kreutner W, Rizzo CA, Smith SR, Young S, Chapman RW, Dyke H, Shih NY, Piwinski JJ, Cuss FM, Montana J, Ganguly AK, and Egan RW. Pharmacology of N-(3,5-Dichloro-1-oxido-4-pyridinyl)-8-methoxy-2-(trifluoromethyl)-5-quinolone carboxamide (SCH 351591), a novel, orally active phosphodiesterase 4 inhibitor. *J Pharmacol Exp Ther* 2002; 302: 127–137.

42. Hanifin JM, Chan SC, Cheng JB, Tofte SJ, Henderson WR Jr, Kirby DS, and Weiner ES. Type 4 phosphodiesterase inhibitors have clinical and *in vitro* anti-inflammatory effects in atopic dermatitis. *J Invest Dermatol* 1996; 107: 51–56.

43. Brunnee T, Engelstatter R, Steinijans, and Kunkel G. Bronchodilatory effect of inhaled zardaverine, a phosphodiesterase III and IV inhibitor, in patients with asthma. *Eur Respir J* 1992; 5: 982–985.

44. Harbinson PL, MacLeod D, Hawksworth, R, O'Toole S, Sullivan PJ, Heath P, Kilfeather S, Page CP, Costello J, Holgate ST, and Lee TH. The effect of a novel orally active selective PDE4 isoenzyme inhibitor (CDP840) on allergen-induced respones in asthmatic subjects. *Eur Respir J* 1997; 10: 1008–1014.

45. Giembycz MA. Cilomilast: a second generation phosphodiesterase 4 inhibitor for asthma and chronic obstructive pulmonary disease. *Expert Opin Investig Drugs* 2001; 10: 1361–1379.

46. Timmer W, Leclerc V, Birraux G, Neuhauser M, Hatzelmann A, Bethke T, and Wurst W. The new phosphodiesterase inhibitor roflumilast is efficacious in exercise-induced asthma and leads to suppression of LPS-stimulated TNF-alpha *ex vivo*. *J Clin Pharmacol* 2002; 42: 297–303.

47. Schmidt W, Kusma M, Feuring M, Timmer WE, Neuhauser M, Bethke T, Stuck BA, Hormann K, and Wehling M. The phosphodiesterase 4 inhibitor roflumilast is effective in the treatment of allergic rhinitis. *J Allergy Clin Immunol* 2001; 108: 530–536.

48. Gundel RH, Wegner CD, Torcellini CA, Clarke CC, Haynes N, Rothlein R, Smith CW, and Letts LG. Endothelial leukocyte adhesion molecule-1 mediates antigen-induced airway inflammation and late-phase airway obstruction in monkeys. *J Clin Invest* 1991; 88: 1407–1411.

49. Edwards BS, Curry MS, Tsuji H, Brown D, Larson RS, and Sklar LA. Expression and function of P-selectin at low site density promotes selective attachment of eosinophils over neutrophils. *J Immunol* 2000; 165: 4040–4010.

50. Broide DH, Sullivan S, Gifford T, and Sriramarao P. Inhibition of pulmonary eosinophilia in P-selectin- and ICAM-1-deficient mice. *Am J Respir Cell Mol Biol* 1998; 18: 218–225.

51. Kim M-K, Brandley BK, Anderson MB, and Bochner BS. Antagonism of selectin-dependent adhesion of human neutrophils and eosinophils by glycomimetics and oligosaccharide compounds. *Am J Respir Cell Mol Biol* 1998; 19: 836–841.

52. Davenpeck KL, Berens KL, Dixon RAF, Dupre B, and Bochner BS. Inhibition of adhesion of human neutrophils and eosinophils to P-selectin by the sialyl Lewis[x] antagonist TBC1269: preferential activity against neutrophil adhesion *in vitro*. *J Allergy Clin Immunol* 2000: 105: 769–775.

53. He XY, Xu Z, Melrose J, Mullowney A, Vasquez M, Queen C, Vexler V, Klingbeil C, Co MS, and Berg EL. Humanization and pharmacokinetics of a monoclonal antibody with specificity for both E- and P-selectin. *J Immunol* 1998; 160: 1029–1035.

54. Henderson WR, Jr, Chi EY, Albert RK, Chu SJ, Lamm WJ, Rochon Y, Jonas M, Christie PE, and Harlan JM. Blockade of CD49d (α_4 intergrin) on intrapulmonary but not circulating leukocytes inhibits airway inflammation and hyperresponsiveness in a mouse model of asthma. *J Clin Invest* 1997; 100: 3083–3092.

55. Abraham, WM, Ahmed A, Sielczak MW, Narita M, Arrhenius T, and Elices MJ. Blockade of the late-phase airway response and airway hyperresponsiveness in allergic sheep with a small-peptide inhibitor of VLA-4. *Am J Resp Crit Care Med* 1997; 156: 696–703.

56. Abraham WM, Gill A, Ahmed A, Sielczak MW, Lauredo IT, Botinnikova Y, Lin KC, Pepinsky B, Leone DR, Lobb RR, and Adams SP. A small-molecule, tight-binding inhibitor of the integrin alpha(4)beta(1) blocks antigen-induced airway responses and inflammation in experimental asthma in sheep. *Am J Respir Crit Care Med* 2000; 162: 603–611.

57. Heath H, Qin S, Rao P, Wu L, LaRosa G, Kassam N, Ronath PD, and Mackay CR. Chemokine receptor usage by human eosinophils: importance of CCR3 demonstrated using an antagonistic monoclonal antibody. *J Clin Invest* 1997; 99: 178–184.

58. Zhang L, Soares MP, Guan Y, Matheravidathu S, Wnek R, Johnson KE, Meisher A, Iliff SA, Mudgett JS, Springer MS, and Daugherty BL. Functional expression and characterization of macaque C-C chemokine receptor 3 (CCR3) and generation of potent antagonistic anti-macaque CCR3 monoclonal antibodies. *J Biol Chem* 2002; 277: 33799–33810.

59. Chung CD, Kuo F, Kumer J, Motani AS, and Lawrence CE. CCR8 is not essential for the development of inflammation in a mouse model of allergic airway disease. *J Immunol* 2003, 170: 581–587.

60. Goya Í, Villares R, Zaballos Á, Gutiérrez J, Kremer L, Gonzalo JA, Varona R, Carramolino L, Serrano A, Pallares P, Criado LM, Kolbeck R, Torres M, Coyle AJ, Gutierrez-Ramos JC, Martinez-A C, and Marquez G. Absence of CCR8 does not impair the response to ovalbumin-induced allergic airway disease. *J Immunol* 2003; 170: 2138–2146.

61. Warner JA, Jones CA, Jones AC, and Warner JO. Prenatal origins of allergic disease. *J Allergy Clin Immunol* 2000; 105: S493–S498.

62. Kulig M, Bergmann R, Tacke U, Wahn U, and Guggenmoos-Holzmann I. Long-lasting sensitization to food during the first two years precedes allergic airay disease. *Pediatr Allergy Immunol* 1998; 9: 61–67.

63. Armentia A, Banuelos C, Arranz ML, Del Villar V, Martin-Santos JM, Gil FJ, Vega JM, Callejo A, and Paredes C. Early introduction of cereals into children's diets as a risk factor for grass pollen asthma. *Clin Exp Allergy* 2001; 31: 1250–1255.

64. Fergusson DM, Horwood LJ, and Shannon FT. Early solid feeding and recurrent childhood eczema: a 10-year longitudinal study. *Pediatrics* 1990; 86: 541–546.

65. Fergusson DM and Horwood LJ. Early solid food diet and eczema in childhood: a 10-year longitudinal study. *Pediatr Allergy Immunol* 1994; 5: 44–47.

66. Hanrahan JP and Halonen M. Antenatal interventions in childhood asthma. *Eur Respir J Suppl* 1998; 27: 46S–51S.

67. Arshad SH, Matthews S, Gant C, and Hide DW. Effect of allergen avoidance in infancy. *Lancet* 1992; 339: 1493–1497.

68. Hide DW, Matthews S, Matthews L, Stevens M, Ridout S, Twiselton R, Gant C, and Arshad SH. Effect of allergen avoidance in infancy on allergic manifestations at age two years. *J Allergy Clin Immunol* 1994; 93: 842–846.

69. Hide DW, Matthews S, Tariq S, and Arshad SH. Allergen avoidance in infancy and allergy at 4 years of age. *Allergy* 1996; 51: 89–93.

70. Matthews SM, Bateman BJ, and Ashad H. Effect of allergen avoidance in infancy on allergic manifestations at eight years. *J Allergy Clin Immunol* 2001; 107: S300.

71. Calder PC and Grimble RF. Polyunsaturated fatty acids, inflammation and immunity. *Eur J Clin Nutr* 2002; 56: S14–S19.

72. Calder PC. Dietary modification of inflammation with lipids. *Proc Nutr Soc* 2002; 61: 345–358.

73. Arm JP, Thien FC, and Lee TH. Leukotrienes, fish oil and asthma. *Allergy Proc* 1994; 15: 129–134.

74. Thommesen L, Sjursen W, Gasvik K, Hanssen W, Brekke OL, Skattebol L, Holmeide AK, Espevik T, Johansen B, and Laegreid A. Selective inhibitors of cytosolic or secretory phospholipase A2 block TNF-induced activation of nuclear factor-κB and expression of ICAM-1. *J Immunol* 1998; 161: 3421–3430.

75. Calder PC. N-3 polyunsaturated fatty acids and cytokine production in health and disease. *Ann Nutr Metab* 1997; 41: 203–234.

76. Peat JK, Salome CM, and Woolcock AJ. Factors associated with bronchial hyper-responsivenss in Australian adults and children. *Eur Respir J* 1992; 5: 921–929.

77. Thien FC, Atkinson BA, Khan A, Mencia-Huerta JM, and Lee TH. Effect of dietary fish oil supplementation on the antigen-induced late-phase response in the skin. *J Allergy Clin Immunol* 1992; 89: 829–835.

78. Thien FC, Mencia-Huerta JM, and Lee TH. Dietary fish oil effects on seasonal hay fever and asthma in pollen-sensitive subjects. *Am Rev Respir Dis* 1993; 147: 1138–1143.

79. Hodge L, Salome CM and Hughes JM, Liu-Brennan D, Rimmer J, Allman M, Pang D, Armour C, and Woolcock AJ, Effect of dietary intake of omega-3 and omega-6 fatty acids on severity of asthma in children. *Eur Respir J* 1998; 11: 361–365.

80. Mihrshahi S, Peat J, and Marks GB. Eighteen-month outcomes of house dust mite avoidance and dietary fatty acid modification in the childhood asthma prevention study (CAPS). *J Allergy Clin Immunol* 2003; 111: 162–168.

81. Dunstan JA, Mori TA, Barden A, Beilin LJ, Taylor AL, Holt PG, and Prescott SL. Maternal fish oil supplementation in pregnancy reduces interleukin-13 levels in cord blood of infants at high risk of atopy. *Clin Exp Allergy* 2003; 33: 442–448.

82. Rescigno M, Urbano M, Valzasina B, Francolini M, Rotta G, Bonasio R, Granucci F, Kraehenbuhl JP, and Ricciardi-Castagnoli P. Dendritic cells express tight junction proteins and penetrate gut epithelium monolayers to sample bacteria. *Nat Immunol* 2001; 2: 361–367.

83. Warner JA, Jones CA, Jones AC, and Warner JO. Prenatal origins of allergic disease. *J Allergy Clin Immunol* 2000; 105: S493–S498.

84. Christensen H, Frokiaer H, and Pestka JJ. Lactobacilli differentially modulate expression of cytokines and maturation surface markers in murine dendritic cells. *J Immunol* 2002; 168: 171–178.

85. Erickson KL and Hubbard NE. Probiotic immunomodulation in health and disease. *J Nutr* 2000; 130: 403S–409S.

86. Sudo N, Sawamura S, Tanaka K, Aiba Y, Kubo C, and Koga Y. The requirement of intestinal bacterial flora for the development of an IgE production system fully susceptible to oral tolerance induction. *J Immunol* 1997; 159: 1739–1745.

87. Von Der Weid T, Bulliard C, and Schiffrin EJ. Induction by a lactic acid bacterium of a population of CD4+ T cells with low proliferative capacity that produce transforming growth factor β and interleukin-10. *Clin Diag Lab Immunol* 2001; 8: 695–701.

88. Rautava S, Kalliomake M, and Isolauri E. Probiotics during pregnancy and breast feeding might confer immunomodulatory protection against atopic disease in the infant. *J Allergy Clin Immunol* 2002; 109: 119–121.
89. Kalliomaki M, Kirjavainen P, Eerola E, Kero P, Salminen S, and Isolauri E. Distinct patterns of neonatal gut microflora in infants in whom atopy was and was not developing. *J Allergy Clin Immunol* 2001; 107: 129–134.
90. Wahn U and von Mutius E. Childhood risk factors for atopy and the importance of early intervention. *J Allergy Clin Immunol* 2001; 107: 567–574.
91. Kalliomake M, Salminen S, Arvilommi H, Kero P, Koskinen P, and Isolauri E. Probiotics in primary prevention of atopic disease: a randomized placebo-controlled trial. *Lancet* 2001; 357: 1076–1079.
92. Wheeler JG, Shema SJ, Bogle ML, Shirrell MA, Burks AW, Pittler A, and Helm RM. Immune and clinical impact of *Lactobacillus acidophilus* on asthma. *Ann Allergy* 1997; 79: 229–233.
93. Helin T, Haahtela S, and Haahtela T. No effect of oral treatment with an intestinal bacterial strain, *Lactobacillus rhamnosus* (ATCC 53103), on birch-pollen allergy: a placebo-controlled double blind study. *Allergy* 2002; 57: 243–246.
94. Majamaa H and Isolauri E. Probiotics: a novel approach in the management of food allergy. *J Allergy Clin Immunol* 1997; 99: 179–185.
95. Pessi T, Sutas Y, Hurme M, and Isolauri E. Interleukin-10 generation in atopic children following oral *Lactobacillus rhamnosus* GG. *Clin Exp Allergy* 2000; 30: 1804–1810.

26

Regulation of IgE Synthesis

LISA CAMERON and DONATA VERCELLI

University of Arizona
Tucson, Arizona, U.S.A

I. Introduction

This chapter addresses the cellular and molecular mechanisms of IgE regulation. The signals that trigger IgE synthesis are outlined and followed by a detailed description of the molecular events that such interactions induce. Over the past few decades, this molecular approach has allowed immunologists to understand the basic mechanisms of isotype switching to IgE. Finally, potential therapeutic targets of the molecular process of IgE regulation are discussed.

II. Induction of IgE Synthesis: Intercellular Interactions

A. Two-Signal Model

During an immune response, a B lymphocyte can express different immunoglobulin (Ig) heavy chain isotypes sharing the same variable diversity joining (VDJ) region. This process (isotype switching or class switch recombination) allows a single B cell clone to produce antibodies with the same fine specificity but different effector functions. Studies of the molecular events underlying IgE synthesis have provided a novel conceptual framework in which isotype switching is viewed as a two-step process. To switch to a particular isotype, a B cell needs

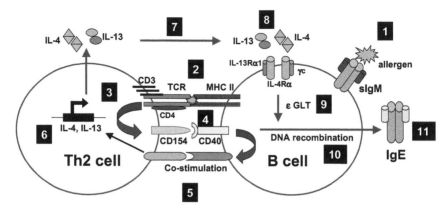

Figure 26.1 T–B cell interactions leading to IgE isotype switching. The signals required for switching are provided to B cells through a complex series of interactions with an antigen (allergen)-specific T cell and a B cell that expresses IgM specific for the allergen (1) binds the allergen via surface immunoglobulin (sIg), processes it, and presents it to an allergen-specific T helper type 2 (Th2) cell, T cells programmed to secrete high IL-4 and low interferon-γ (2). Engagement of the T cell antigen receptor (TCR)–CD3 complex by major histocompatibility complex class II (MHCII) molecules results in rapid expression of CD154 (3) which engages CD40, the counter-receptor constitutively expressed on B cells (4). T–B cell interactions via CD40 and CD154 are further amplified by the up-regulation of other costimulatory molecules on B cells (5) that affect T cell transcription (6) and secretion (7) of IL-4 and IL-13 which bind their heterodimeric receptors (8). At this stage, the B cells receive both signals required for IgE switching. IL-4 and IL-13 trigger germline transcription (GLT) (9), thereby targeting the switch region for recombination. Cross-linking of CD40 by CD40L activates DNA recombination to the targeted switch region (10), leading to IgE isotype switching and IgE secretion (11). IL-13Rα1 = IL-13 receptor alpha chain 1. γc = common cytokine receptor gamma chain.

two signals: signal 1 is cytokine-dependent, results in the activation of transcription at a specific region in the Ig locus, and thus dictates isotype specificity. Signal 2 is CD40-dependent, activates the recombination machinery, and results in DNA switch recombination.

The two signals required for switching to IgE are delivered to B cells by T cells through a complex series of interactions that makes it difficult to establish an unambiguous chronology for the events leading to IgE synthesis. Results obtained by molecular studies clearly point to a hierarchy in the steps to IgE induction and the signals that trigger such steps. The initial event in switching to IgE is the determination of isotype specificity through cytokine (interleukin [IL]-4 and IL-13)-dependent induction of ε germline (GL) transcription, followed by CD40-mediated activation of DNA switch recombination. Amplification circuits involving accessory molecules then lead to high-rate IgE synthesis. The definitions of "signal 1" and "signal 2" used here thus reflect a B cell-centered perspective. However, high-rate cytokine secretion (signal 1) and full B cell activation via CD40/CD40 ligand (CD154) interactions (signal 2) may enhance each other and involve additional ligand–receptor pairs.

B. IL-4 and IL-13 Provide Signal 1

The interaction between IL-4 and the IL-4 receptor (IL-4R) delivers the first signal for switching to IgE. The most compelling evidence for the central role of IL-4 in IgE induction came from gene targeting experiments. Mice in which the IL-4 gene had been knocked out by homologous recombination (IL-4 KO mice) were unable to mount antiparasite IgE responses; their IgG1 responses were also suppressed, although to a lesser extent, whereas production of other isotypes was unaffected.[1]

Another cytokine, IL-13, shares many of the functional properties of IL-4, including the ability to induce IgE synthesis by B cells.[2] Although the sequence homology of IL-13 and IL-4 is only ~30%, all residues that contribute to the hydrophobic core of IL-4 are conserved or have conservative hydrophobic replacements in IL-13.[3] Furthermore, the IL-4Rα chain is a component of both IL-4R (IL-4Rα:γc) and IL-13R (IL-4Rα:IL-13Rα1 and IL-13Rα1:IL-13Rα2).[4] IL-4 and IL-13 and their receptors are by no means identical. IL-13 does not bind to cells transfected with complementary DNA (cDNA) for the IL-4R α and/or γ chain,[5] and most importantly, unlike IL-4, it appears to exert no effect on human T cells.[3]

Marked differences exist in the kinetics of IL-4 and IL-13 production after T cell stimulation through the antigen receptor. IL-4 is secreted in low amounts during the first 24 hours, whereas IL-13 is secreted abundantly for at least 6 days.[6] Furthermore, naïve CD4+CD45RO+ human T cells develop into effector cells that secrete IL-13, IL-5, and interferon (IFN)-γ, but not IL-4, upon T cell receptor cross-linking.[7] These cells can provide efficient help for IgE production.

These findings suggest the intriguing possibility that at least at certain stages of T helper (Th) differentiation, the production of IL-13 and IL-4 may be independently regulated. Comparison of IL-4 and IL-13 single knock-out (KO) mice with animals carrying simultaneous disruptions of both IL-4 and IL-13 demonstrates that only the double KO mice exhibited no IgE in response to challenge with *Schistosoma mansoni*. Unlike IL-4−/− mice, IL-13-null mice fail to clear helminths and recover basal IgE levels after stimulation with IL-4.[8] It is not yet clear to what extent interference with *cis* regulatory elements on the linked allele may have contributed to the phenotypes observed in these experiments.[9]

Genetic linkage analysis has shown that one or more genes within the 5q31.1 region including IL-4, IL-13, IL-5, and IL-9 may be responsible for the

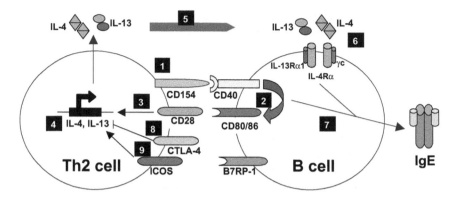

Figure 26.2 T–B cell interactions mediated via CD40 and CD154 are amplified by interactions between costimulatory molecules, particularly the CD28:CD80–CD86 ligand/receptor pair. Once allergen-stimulated T cells express CD154 (1), engagement of CD40 up-regulates CD80–CD86 expression on B cells (2). CD80–CD86 engages CD28 (3), inducing high rate transcription (4) and secretion (5) of IL-4 and IL-13 which will bind their heterodimeric receptors (6). At this stage, the B cells receive both signals required for IgE switching (7). A number of other costimulatory signals have been identified; signaling of CTLA-4 on T cells following interaction with CD80–CD86 has been shown to down-regulate T cell production of IL-4 (8) and reduce IgE synthesis. ICOS interacts with B7RP-1 to induce IL-4 (9) and T cell activation and represents another set of molecules than enhance IgE synthesis.

regulation of overall IgE production.[10] A number of single nucleotide polymorphisms (SNPs) have been identified within these genes and two SNPs in the functionally related α chain of the IL-4R are associated with high IgE levels.[11,12] SNPs in the IL-13 gene have been linked to elevated basal IgE production[13] and asthma.[14]

C. Interaction of CD40 and CD154 Provides Signal 2

The engagement of CD40 on B cells by CD154 expressed on T cells provides the second signal required for switching to IgE. CD154 can be replaced *in vitro* by anti-CD40 monoclonal antibodies (mAbs). Indeed, this was the first system in which the B cell–activating signal for human IgE synthesis could be delivered *in vitro* by antibody-induced engagement of a discrete B cell surface antigen.[15] CD40 is a 50-kD surface glycoprotein belonging to the tumor necrosis factor receptor (TNFR) superfamily. It is expressed on human B lymphocytes, cytokine-activated monocytes, follicular dendritic cells, epithelial cells (including thymic epithelium), but not on T cells, and plays a key role in the survival, growth, and differentiation of B cells.[16]

    The common structural framework of the CD40 extracellular domain is reflected by the ability of the TNFR family members to interact with a parallel family of TNF-related molecules that includes the ligands for CD40, CD27, CD30, OX40, TNF-α, and lymphotoxin. CD154 is a 261-amino acid type 2 membrane glycoprotein expressed transiently on activated, but not on resting, Th1 and Th2 cells. Cells transfected with CD154 induce IgE synthesis by both murine and human B cells in the presence of IL-4.[16] Patients with X-linked hyper-IgM syndrome exhibit defective switching due to mutations in CD154.[17] Furthermore, no IgG, IgA, or IgE responses to thymus-dependent antigens were detectable in CD40[18] and CD154[19] KO mice. Finally, the inability of human newborn B cells to switch and the consequent transient immunodeficiency observed in human neonates have been ascribed to a decrease in both CD154 expression[20] and responses to CD40 agonists.[21]

The interactions between CD40 and CD154 are tightly regulated. T cells become competent only to activate B cells via CD40 after they express CD154, and this in turn requires antigen receptor-dependent T cell activation. A subset of CD4+ memory T cells in germinal centers contains preformed CD154 that is rapidly (within minutes) and transiently expressed on cell surfaces after T cell receptor-mediated activation.[22] The speed at which T cells can express CD154 on their surfaces may be crucial in germinal centers because centrocytes either leave the light zone within a few hours of activation or die *in situ* through apoptosis. The availability of CD154 is drastically limited because the interaction with CD40 induces rapid endocytosis of surface CD154[23] and the release of soluble CD40 by B cells down-regulates CD154 mRNA.[24]

A number of molecules are reported to mimic the function of CD154. BAFF (B cell-activating factor belonging to the TNF family) and APRIL (a proliferation-inducing ligand), expressed mainly by monocytes and dendritic cells, are up-regulated by CD40L[25] and activate a CD40-like pathway that enhances B cell survival through NFκB and BCL-6.[26] These molecules in combination with IL-4 were shown to induce class switch recombination (CSR) to IgE independent of CD40.[25] Additionally, C4-binding protein (C4-BP), a circulating regulatory component of the classical complement pathway, has been found to bind CD40 on B cells and synergize with IL-4 to induce ε GL transcription, CSR to IgE, and IgE protein synthesis.[27]

D. Amplification of Signal 1 and Signal 2 by Costimulatory Molecule Interaction

Several pairs of costimulatory molecules have been shown to participate in interactions of T and B cells conducive to IgE synthesis by complementing and/or up-regulating the T cell-dependent activation of B cells that follows the engagement of CD40 by CD154. A major accessory role is likely to be played by the CD28:CD80–CD86 ligand receptor pairs. Both CD28 on T cells and its B cell counter receptors, CD80 (B7.1) and CD86 (B7.2), are parts of a reciprocal amplification mechanism that amplifies T and B cell interactions mediated via

CD40/CD154. Engagement of CD40 is known to result in expression of CD80 and CD86 on B cells.[28]

Engagement of CD28 results in increased expression of CD154 on T cells.[29] It appears that CD28 activation is required for strong transcriptional activation of the CD154 promoter in response to T cell receptor ligation.[30] Most importantly, both CD28[31] and CD80–CD86[32] KO mice have reduced basal Ig levels, fail to generate antigen-specific antibody responses, lack germinal centers when immunized by a number of routes,[32] and exhibit inhibitions of IL-4 production accompanied by enhanced IFN-γ production.[33] Thus, interactions between CD28 and CD80–CD86 appear critical for both IL-4 secretion and CD40-mediated B cell activation and ultimately will potentiate both signals 1 and 2. CTLA-4 is expressed on activated T cells and acts as a negative feedback regulator of T cell activation.

The inducible costimulator (ICOS) is also a member of the CD28–CD152 receptor family involved in regulating T cell activation. It is up-regulated early on all T cells via the CD28: CD80–CD86 pathway[34] and binds specifically to its counter-receptor B7RP-1, but not to CD80 or CD86.[35,36] *In vivo*, a lack of ICOS results in severely deficient T cell–dependent B cell responses, impaired germinal center formations, low levels of IL-4, and defective class switching to IgE.[37] ICOS may be an important component of the cascade of events required for T cell activation.

E. Amplification of IgE Synthesis by Non-T Cells

Human basophils and mast cells have been reported to secrete IL-4 and IL-13[38,39] and express CD154.[40] While in principle these cells may provide both signal 1 and signal 2 for IgE synthesis, conceivably they play a major role in IgE amplification. The optimal physiologic stimulus for secretion of IL-4 and IL-13 from these cells seems to be allergen-dependent cross-linking of allergen-specific, receptor-bound IgE.[38,39] Cytokine secretion appears to be predicated on the production of allergen-specific IgE. The IgE produced can bind IgE receptors on basophils and mast cells, thus inducing IL-4/IL-13 secretion and CD154 expression. Only at this point may non-T cells trigger an IgE response. Furthermore, and most importantly, IgE responses in IL-4-deficient mice were restored by reconstitution with T cells, but not by non-T cells.[41]

III. Induction of IgE Synthesis: Molecular Events

A. Role of Germline Transcription (GL) Transcription in Isotype Switching

Isotype switching results from a DNA event that juxtaposes different downstream C_H genes to the expressed VDJ gene. Molecular analysis has shown that induction of isotype switching to a particular C_H gene almost invariably correlates with the transcriptional activation of the same gene in GL configuration, that is, in the

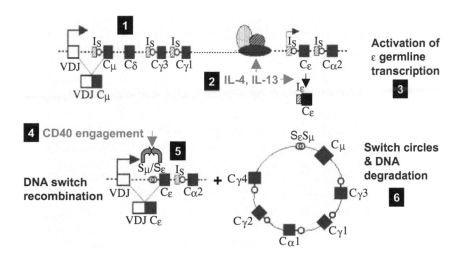

Figure 26.3 Molecular events in IgE isotype switching. Before switching occurs, the IgE locus is in the germline configuration (with all the heavy chain constant genes still unrearranged). VDJ recombination has already occurred, thus determining the antigen specificity of the antibody (1). Stimulation with IL-4 or IL-13 (2) results in the transcriptional activation of the IgE locus, still in the germline configuration (3). Induction and correct splicing of germline transcripts are probably necessary to target the appropriate switch region for recombination and switching. CD40 engagement (4) activates class switch recombination. DNA rearrangement at the targeted S region generates chimeric $S\mu$–$S\varepsilon$ regions composed of the 5' $S\mu$ and 3' portion of the targeted $S\varepsilon$ region (5). During recombination, the region containing the germline promoter and the I exon is deleted as part of a switch circle and subsequently degraded (6).

genomic configuration that exists before class switch recombination leads to deletion of regions targeted by the switching process.[42]

The GL transcripts resulting from this process initiate a few kilobases upstream of the switch (S) region and proceed through one or more short exons (I exons) that are spliced to the first exon of the C_H gene. GL transcripts are also called *sterile transcripts* because the I exon contains multiple stop codons in all three reading frames and is therefore thought to be unable to code for any mature protein of significant length. Although no significant sequence similarity exists between GL transcripts of different isotypes, their overall structure is conserved.[42]

GL transcription is thought to direct switching by modulating the accessibility of a particular S region to a common recombinase. The importance of GL transcription in the regulation of isotype switching was shown by deletion of I exons and their promoters. The result was the inhibition of class switching to the corresponding genes even though the corresponding S regions remained intact.[43] These results indicate that transcription in the I region is necessary to target the appropriate S region for recombination and switching. However, transcription through the region per se is not sufficient because replacement of Iε with a B cell-specific promoter cassette without the Iε splice donor site results in only marginal switch recombination to IgE.[44]

This observation is supported by studies demonstrating that replacement of all known IL-4-inducible elements in the Sγ1 region with the heterologous human metallothionein IIA promoter did not impair γ1 GL transcription or switch recombination to IgG1, provided a 114-bp sequence containing the Iγ1 splice donor site was included in the construct.[45] It is now considered that GL transcription provides the specificity to target distinct S regions by forming stable RNA–DNA hybrid complexes called R loops, leaving the nontemplate strand on its own in a single-stranded state. These R loops have been shown to recruit certain DNA repair endonucleases that cleave the loops in a structure-specific manner.[46,47] In addition to the need for GL transcription to achieve class switch recombination, a linear relationship between the level of GL transcripts and switching efficiency was described. The researchers used a construct containing a constitutively transcribed Sμ region and an Sα region driven by a tetracycline-responsive promoter; deleting the tandem Sμ repeat element in the murine μ heavy chain gene reduced the efficiency of switching.[48]

The 3′ Ig enhancer located several kb downstream of the most 3′ C_H gene contains four DNase I hypersensitive sites (HS3a, HS1,2, HS3b, and HS4),[49] and has been identified as a novel regulatory region that controls GL transcript expression and Ig heavy chain class switching in murine B cells. Insertion of the phosphoglycerate kinase (PGK)–neomycin (neo) cassette in place of the HS1,2, and 3a site down-regulated not only transcription from I promoters of several isotypes but also switching to corresponding isotypes over a 120-kb locus.[49,50]

Although deletion of HS3a by Cre-LoxP gene targeting did not affect switch recombination,[50] joint deletion of HS3b and HS4 was shown to severely impair GL transcription and class switching to most isotypes, indicating that these two HS sites work together.[51] Polymorphisms have been identified within HS 1,2 of the Ig 3′ enhancer and are associated with increased transcriptional strength in reporter gene assays.[52] Furthermore, regulation of ε GL transcription by HS1,2 has recently been suggested to involve specific promoter-enhancer interactions.[53] Based on these data, it has been proposed that sequences within the 3′ Ig enhancer may be essential parts of a locus control region that regulates GL transcription and/or the accessibility of C_H genes.

B. Transcription Factors Regulating ε GL Transcription

Nuclear factors bind specifically to relatively short (10- to 20-bp) DNA sequences, functionally defined as responsive elements. Like all weak promoters, the GL promoters are likely to be limited at multiple steps of the transcription initiation reaction. Thus, different transcription factors impact different limiting steps in the reaction.

Induction of GL transcription is a key step in determining the isotype specificity of the switching event. IL-4 was shown to induce ε GL transcripts in murine[54–56] and human[57,58] B cells. IL-4-dependent ε GL transcription is strongly up-regulated upon CD40 engagement,[59] an effect believed critical for the efficiency of switching.[60] Of note, the synergism between IL-4 and CD40 cross-linking is essential not only for GL transcription, but for the induction of switch recombinase activity as well.[61]

Full activation of the ε GL promoter in response to IL-4 and CD40 engagement requires a constellation of nuclear factors that are expressed constitutively or recruited to the promoter by specific activating signals. Binding elements for STAT6, NF-kB/Rel, and BSAP (β cell-specific activator protein) have been identified in the human ε GL promoter.[62–65] Transduction of the IL-4 signal to the nucleus is critically dependent on the phosphorylation, dimerization, and activation of STAT6. The essential role of this transcription factor in IL-4-dependent ε GL transcription and IgE switching is well established; STAT6-deficient mice do not express IgE.[66–69] NF-kB/Rel proteins bind two distinct sites in the ε GL promoter and play an essential role in IL-4-dependent responses, cooperating with STAT6 for the synergistic activation of human ε GL transcription. Consistent with the well-known ability of CD40 signaling to induce NF-kB activation,[70,71] these nuclear proteins appear to be critical for the CD40-dependent enhancement of IL-4-induced ε GL transcription. Direct STAT6/NF-kB interaction appears necessary for the synergistic activation of transcription from promoters containing both cognate sites.[72,73]

BSAP is specifically expressed in the B cell lineage from the pro-B to the mature B cell stage but is not found in terminally differentiated plasma cells.[74] It binds to a highly conserved region immediately upstream of the major Iε transcription initiation site in both murine[75] and human[64] B cells and plays a role in both IL-4-dependent induction and CD40-mediated up-regulation of human ε GL transcription.[64] It may contribute to the specificity of isotype switching through a differential regulation of GL transcription because over-expression of BSAP under the control of a tetracycline-regulated promoter inhibits α GL transcription and switching to IgA in sIgM+ I.29m cells, but enhances ε GL transcription and switching to IgE.[76]

C. DNA Switch Recombination

Although IL-4 (signal 1) is sufficient for the initiation of transcription through the ε locus, switching and expression of mature Cε transcripts (containing the VDJ region spliced to Cε1-4) require signal 2 (engagement of CD40 by CD154). The role of signal 2 in the induction of IgE switching is complex. In addition to triggering DNA recombination (see below), CD40–CD154 interactions are also critically involved in up-regulating IL-4-induced ε GL transcription.[59,77] Because optimal transcription through the S region is thought to be required for efficient targeting of recombination,[60] this transcriptional effect of CD40 engagement is crucial for switching.

The molecular events that follow the delivery of signal 2 for switching to IgE were characterized only recently.[42,78] Sequencing of chimeric Sμ/Sε switch fragments composed of the 5′ Sμ joined to the 3′ portion of the targeted Sε region or of switch circles, their reciprocal products, formally proved that switch recombination occurs through deletion of intervening DNA. This deletional switch recombination is preceded by point mutations[79] and double-strand breaks in the Sμ as well as the targeted S region.[42] After the DNA is rearranged so that the targeted S region lies adjacent to Sμ, these breaks are repaired by nonhomologous end joining (NHEJ) by Ku proteins — heterodimeric proteins that bind to DNA ends and are members of the DNA–protein kinase complex. Disruption of Ku80 and Ku70 were seen to allow GL transcription but not successful processing of mature Iγ transcripts.[80] Furthermore, mismatch repair mechanisms for processing broken DNA ends also appear to be involved, because the efficiency of isotype switching was reduced in mismatch repair-deficient mice.[81]

For a number of years, the invariable association between GL transcription and switching was taken to support the accessibility model, according to which chromatin opening coupled with transcription allowed the switch recombinase to access its DNA target. However, until the recent discovery of a gene crucial for both class switch recombination and somatic hypermutation, the components of the recombination machinery have remained elusive. Using a murine lymphoma B cell line (CH12F3-2), transfection of DNA constructs containing Sμ and Sα regions constitutively transcribed by separate promoters demonstrated that isotype switching occurred only when the cells were stimulated[61] and could be inhibited by cyclohexamide treatment.[82] This indicates that transgene recombination relies on induction of a new protein, most likely a component of the recombinase. Analysis of the clones identified a novel member of the cytidine deaminase family, activation-induced cytidine deaminase (AID).

Over-expression of AID augmented class switching from IgM to IgA, while AID deficiency abolished isotype switch recombination, even though GL transcription was fully preserved.[83] Although AID was reported initially to be specifically expressed by murine germinal center B cells following *in vitro* stimulation with IL-4 and LPS or CD154,[82] IgD+ human B cells from peripheral blood were shown subsequently to express AID following IL-4 or IL-13 treatment.[84]

Ectopic expression of AID in murine fibroblasts induced CSR in an artificial switch construct, indicating that the presence of this protein is the only B cell-specific factor required for CSR.[85] However, treatment of IgD+ human B cells with IL-4 only, a condition that does not result in substantial class switch recombination,[86] was sufficient to drive AID expression.[84] This suggests that, in addition to AID, recombination requires other substances, most likely CD40-inducible factors, for successful CSR.

AID is closely related to APOBEC-1, a component of the complex that edits apolipoprotein B mRNA by catalyzing the deamination of C6666→U, resulting in altered function,[87] and initially was considered an RNA-editing enzyme. However, AID[−/−] mice failed to accumulate mutations in the S regions[79,88] and the antigen-specific variable region gene[83] that indicates that this protein acts at the DNA level.[89] AID has been shown to deaminate dC DNA nucleotides, creating U/G mismatches repaired by the uracyl–DNA glycosylase (UNG) or mismatch repair pathways,[90,91] ultimately leading to the point mutations characteristic of CSR junction sites.[92] AID appears to act predominantly on single-stranded nontemplate DNA and has been suggested to do so on the strand exposed during the transcription reaction.[93,94] This would explain the observed correlation between the rate of transcription and the rate of CSR.[85] Because production of spliced GL transcripts is normal in AID[−/−] mice,[83] this protein has been speculated to play a role in creating the double-strand breaks (DSBs) and/or the break repairs that join Sμ with one of the downstream S regions.[95] Co-localization of the DNA DSB repair proteins Nbs1/g-H2AX to the IgH locus during CSR was shown to be AID-dependent.[88]

A group of patients with the autosomal recessive form of hyper-IgM syndrome were shown to have mutations in their AID genes.[96] Also, a number of SNPs were identified within the human AID gene and transmission disequilibrium tests showed that the 7888C/T polymorphism may be associated with the pathogenesis of atopic asthma and the regulation of serum IgE levels.[97] While much remains to be learned about the molecular mechanisms that underlie the role of AID in switch recombination and somatic hypermutation, what we know is enough to suggest that AID acts upstream of Sμ and V gene mutation, recruitment of DNA repair proteins, and recombination.

D. Sequential Isotype Switching

Sequential switching and direct switching coexist. Sequencing of switch circles generated in B cells triggered to switch to IgE by IL-4 and anti-CD40 mAb revealed μ–γ–ε switching and even more complex sequential events (μ–α1–γ–ε). However, μ–ε circles representing direct switching events were also found at high frequencies.[98] Likewise, sequence analysis of Sμ–Sε switch fragments from patients with atopic dermatitis showed a predominance of direct Sμ–Sε joining.[99] Of note, some fragments amplified from human B cells stimulated with IL-4 and hydrocortisone contained insertions at the Sμ–Sε junction that were derived from Sγ4.[100] The presence of an Sγ4-derived insertion suggests that some B cells had undergone sequential isotype switching from IgM to IgG4 to IgE.

Indeed, IL-4 has been shown to induce isotype switching to IgG4 as well as to IgE, and single B cells can give rise to clones that secrete IgG4 and IgE.[101] Sequential switching may merely reflect the simultaneous accessibility of two acceptor S regions for switch recombination induced by one cytokine.[102] The apparent dominance of sequential switching observed in the generation of murine IgE-expressing cells after IL-4 stimulation may be due to the parallel activation of Sγ1 and Sε by IL-4, Sγ1 being intrinsically more accessible to recombination with Sμ. Thus, the overall low frequency of IgE switching would be an autonomously determined intrinsic feature of Sε and its control elements. However, data obtained by studying sequential IgG4/IgE switching in humans raise the possibility that the expressed isotype is chosen based on contingent conditions of stimulation, in addition to physical features of the genomic Ig locus.[101]

IV. Modulating IgE Synthesis: Bench to Bedside

As IgE regulation is understood in more detail, several steps in the induction of IgE synthesis emerge as potential targets for therapeutic strategies. A number of approaches — most still at experimental stages — are currently under development. Strategies aimed at blocking signal 1 (cytokines and GL transcription) promise to result in an inhibition of switching that should be relatively IgE isotype-specific. In contrast, targeting of signal 2 (CD40 and recombination) looks more problematic. A blockade of CD40 signaling would in fact be expected to hamper both IgE production and switching to other isotypes. Recent observations, however, suggest that this may not necessarily be the case. Finally, approaches directed at the IgE molecule in the membrane-bound or secreted form are actively pursued because of the well-defined specificity of the target. The strategies that seem most promising in terms of rationale and/or feasibility are discussed briefly below.

IL-4 and IL-13 synthesis is dysregulated in atopic patients.[103] This abnormal commitment to a Th2 response is likely to play a critical role in the pathogenesis of allergic disease. The most common treatment of allergic disorders is glucocorticoid use. *In vitro* glucocorticoids produce complex and paradoxical effects on IgE synthesis, because they actually deliver a potent signal 2 to human B cells and, thus, induce IgE (and IgG4) production in the presence of exogenous IL-4, even though they have no significant direct effects on ε GL transcription.[100,104] However, glucocorticoids strongly suppress IL-4 and IL-13 production[105,106] and therefore block the very first step in IgE induction. Local administration of glucocorticoids has recently been shown to inhibit ε GL transcription and IgE synthesis in the respiratory mucosa. The use of topical corticosteroids with the ability to block IgE production in tissues has contributed significantly to the efficacy of these agents.[107,108]

Another approach for interfering with signal 1 of IgE switching is the use of soluble cytokine receptors. These molecules should inactivate naturally occurring cytokines without mediating cellular activation. Clinical trials show that inhalation of a nebulized soluble recombinant human IL-4R results in significant improvement of lung function in asthmatics[109,110] and in reduction of allergen-induced pulmonary inflammation in mice.[111] Soluble IL-13R also appears to abrogate asthma-like symptoms in mice[112] although it has not yet been studied in humans. Blocking these cytokine pathways may lower IgE levels that may be responsible for the observed clinical improvement, but this remains to be determined.

Because isotype switching to IgE is induced by Th2 cytokines, a number of strategies are aimed at orienting Th cell development toward a Th1 rather than Th2 response. Basic immunology studies suggest that it may be possible to manipulate the cytokine network to shift the Th1–Th2 balance, particularly using IL-12, the cytokine that seems crucial for setting Th1 development in motion *in vitro* and *in vivo*.[113] Unmethylated CpG motifs common in bacterial DNA induce rapid expression of the IL-12 and IFN-γ Th1 cytokines following injection into mice.[114] Synthetic oligonucleotides containing CpG motifs have also been reported to induce Th1 cytokine expression from antigen-specific human CD4+ T cells obtained from atopic donors.[115] In mice primed for Th2 responses, injection with antigen conjugated to CpG-containing oligonucleotides resulted in a *de novo* Th1 response, suppressed IgE synthesis, and higher titers of specific IgG.[116] This conjugate is now undergoing clinical trials.

A number of studies are currently ongoing to evaluate the therapeutic potential of a variety of anti-IgE antibodies.[117] Two different approaches have been proposed: (1) producing antibodies to the portion of IgE that is part of membrane but not secreted IgE, and (2) targeting the IgE binding site for the high-affinity IgE receptor (FcεRI). Although both approaches target the IgE molecule, their rationales are quite different. The first approach is predicated on the existence of a structurally distinct IgE isoform selectively expressed on B cell membranes and is aimed at the ablation of surface IgE-bearing cells. The other relies on extensive analysis of IgE–FcεRI interactions, identification of IgE residues involved in FcεRI binding,[118] and generation of high-affinity humanized antibodies capable of preventing IgE binding to the receptor, such as rhuMab-E25. Clinical trials have demonstrated that E25 is effective in the suppression of allergen-induced symptoms of allergic asthma such as FEV_1 and reduced serum IgE levels[119,120] suspected to be attributed in large part to lower densities of IgE on the surfaces of mast cells and basophils.[121,122] This treatment appears to have some promise for patients with moderate to severe asthma, because it reportedly allows tapering of glucocorticoid dosages.[123]

V. Conclusions

As we learn more about the basic mechanisms that regulate IgE expression and function, it will become possible to design more rational pharmacological antagonists to block this process. In the long term, however, our hope is that a thorough evaluation of the genetic makeup of an allergic individual will complement and orient pharmacological approaches aimed at suppressing the generation of IgE responses.

References

1. Kühn, R., K.R. Rajewsky, and W. Müller. 1991. Generation and analysis of interleukin-4 deficient mice. *Science* 254: 707.
2. McKenzie, A.N.J., J.A. Culpepper, R. de Waal Malefyt, F. Briére, J. Punnonen, G. Aversa, A. Sato, W. Dang, B. G. Cocks, S. Menon, J. E. de Vries, J. Banchereau, and G. Zurawski. 1993. Interleukin 13, a T-cell-derived cytokine that regulates human monocyte and B-cell function. *Proc. Natl. Acad. Sci. USA* 90: 3735.
3. Zurawski, S.M., F. Vega, B. Huyghe, and G. Zurawski. 1993. Receptors for interleukin-13 and interleukin-4 are complex and share a novel component that functions in signal transduction. *EMBO J.* 12: 2663.
4. Nelms, K., A.D. Keegan, J. Zamorano, J.J. Ryan, and W.E. Paul. 1999. The IL-4 receptor: signaling mechanisms and biological functions. *Annu. Rev. Immunol.* 17: 701.
5. Obiri, N.I., W. Debinski, W.J. Leonard, and R.K. Puri. 1995. Receptor for interleukin 13. Interaction with interleukin 4 by a mechanism that does not involve the common γ chain shared by receptors for interleukins 2, 4, 7, 9, and 15. *J. Biol. Chem.* 270: 8797.
6. de Vries, J. 1998. The role of IL-13 and its receptor in allergy and inflammatory responses. *J. Allergy Clin. Immunol.* 102: 165.
7. Brinkmann, V. and C. Kristofic. 1995. TCR-stimulated naïve human CD4[+]45RO[-] T cells develop into effector cells that secrete IL-13, IL-5, and IFN-γ, but no IL-4, and help efficient IgE production by B cells. *J. Immunol.* 154: 3078.
8. McKenzie, G.J., P.G. Fallon, C.L. Emson, R.K. Grencis, and A.N.J. McKenzie. 1999. Simultaneous disruption of IL-4 and IL-13 defines individual roles in T helper cell type 2-mediated responses. *J. Exp. Med* 189: 1565.
9. Guo, L., J. Hu-Li, J. Zhu, C. Pannetier, C. Watson, G.J. McKenzie, A.N. McKenzie, and W.E. Paul. 2001. Disrupting IL-13 impairs production of IL-4 specified by the linked allele. *Nat. Immunol.* 2: 461.
10. Marsh, D.G., J.D. Neely, D.R. Breazeale, B. Gosh, L.R. Freidhoff, E. Ehrlich-Kautzky, C. Schou, G. Krishnaswamy, and T.H. Beaty. 1994. Linkage analysis of IL4 and other chromosome 5q31.1 markers and total serum immunoglobulin E concentrations. *Science* 264: 1152.
11. Hershey, G.K.K., M.F. Friedrich, L.A. Esswein, M.L. Thomas, and T.A. Chatila. 1997. The association of atopy with a gain-of-function mutation in the α subunit of the interleukin-4 receptor. *New Engl. J. Med.* 337: 1720.
12. Ober, C., S.A. Leavitt, A. Tsalenko, T.D. Howard, D.M. Hoki, R. Daniel, D.L. Newman, X. Wu, R. Parry, L.A. Lester, J. Solway, M. Blumenthal, R.A. King, J. Xu, D.A. Meyers, E.R. Bleecker, and N.J. Cox. 2000. Variation in the interleukin 4-receptor alpha gene confers susceptibility to asthma and atopy in ethnically diverse populations. *Am. J. Hum. Genet.* 66: 517.

13. Graves, P.E., M. Kabesch, M. Halonen, C.J. Holberg, M. Baldini, C. Fritzsch, S. Weiland, R.P. Erickson, E. von Mutius, and F.D. Martinez. 2000. A cluster of seven tightly linked polymorphisms in the IL-13 gene is associated with total serum IgE levels in three populations of white children. *J. Allergy Clin. Immunol.* 105: 506.

14. Howard, T.D., P.A. Whittaker, A.L. Zaiman, G.H. Koppelman, J. Xu, M.T. Hanley, D.A. Meyers, D.S. Postma, and E.R. Bleecker. 2001. Identification and association of polymorphisms in the interleukin-13 gene with asthma and atopy in a Dutch population. *Am. J. Respir. Cell Mol. Biol.* 25: 377.

15. Jabara, H.H., S.M. Fu, R.S. Geha, and D. Vercelli. 1990. CD40 and IgE: synergism between anti-CD40 mAb and IL-4 in the induction of IgE synthesis by highly purified human B cells. *J. Exp. Med.* 172: 1861.

16. Banchereau, J., F. Bazan, D. Blanchard, F. Briére, J.P. Galizzi, C. van Kooten, Y.J. Liu, F. Rousset, and S. Saeland. 1994. The CD40 antigen and its ligand. *Annu. Rev. Immunol.* 12: 881.

17. Fuleihan, R., N. Ramesh, R. Loh, H. Jabara, F.S. Rosen, T. Chatila, S.M. Fu, I. Stamenkovic, and R.S. Geha. 1993. Defective expression of the CD40 ligand in X-chromosome-linked immunoglobulin deficiency with normal or elevated IgM. *Proc. Natl. Acad. Sci. USA* 90: 2170.

18. Castigli, E., F.W. Alt, L. Davidson, A. Bottaro, E. Mizoguchi, A.K. Bhan, and R.S. Geha. 1994. CD40-deficient mice generated by RAG-2-deficient blastocyst complementation. *Proc. Natl. Acad. Sci. USA* 91: 12135.

19. Xu, J., T.M. Foy, J.D. Laman, E.A. Elliott, J.J. Dunn, T.J. Waldschmidt, J. Elsemore, R.J. Noelle, and R.A. Flavell. 1994. Mice deficient for the CD40 ligand. *Immunity* 1: 423.

20. Fuleihan, R., D. Ahern, and R.S. Geha. 1994. Decreased expression of the ligand for CD40 in newborn lymphocytes. *Eur. J. Immunol.* 24: 1925.

21. Durandy, A., C. Hivroz, F. Mazerolles, C. Schiff, F. Bernard, E. Jouanguy, P. Revy, J.P. DiSanto, J.F. Gauchat, J.Y. Bonnefoy, J.L. Casanova, and A. Fischer. 1997. Abnormal CD40-mediated activation pathway in B lymphocytes from patients with hyper-IgM syndrome and normal CD40 ligand expression. *J. Immunol.* 158: 2576.

22. Casamayor-Palleja, M., M. Khan, and I.C.M. MacLennan. 1995. A subset of CD4+ memory T cells contains preformed CD40 ligand that is rapidly but transiently expressed on their surface after activation through the T cell receptor complex. *J. Exp. Med.* 181: 1293.

23. Yellin, M.J., K. Sippel, G. Inghirami, L.R. Covey, J.J. Lee, J. Sinning, E.A. Clark, L. Chess, and S. Lederman. 1994. CD40 molecules induce down-modulation and endocytosis of T cell surface T cell–B cell activating molecule/CD40 ligand: potential role in regulating helper effector function. *J. Immunol.* 152: 598.

24. van Kooten, C., C. Gaillard, J.P. Galizzi, P. Hermann, F. Fossiez, J. Bancherau, and D. Blanchard. 1994. B cells regulate expression of CD40 ligand on activated T cells by lowering the mRNA level and through the release of soluble CD40. *Eur. J. Immunol.* 24: 787.

25. Litinskiy, M.B., B. Nardelli, D.M. Hillbert, B. He, A. Schaffer, P. Casali, and A. Cerutti. 2002. DCs induce CD40-independent immunologlobulin class switching through BLyS and APRIL. *Nat. Immunol.* 3: 822.

26. Do, R., E. Hatada, H. Lee, M.R. Tourigny, D. Hillbert, and S. Chen-Kiang. 2000. Attenuation of apoptosis underlies B lymphocyte stimulator enhancement of humoral immune response. *J. Exp. Med.* 192: 953.

27. Brodeur, S., F. Angelini, L.B. Bacharier, A.M. Blom, E. Mizoguchi, H. Fujiwara, A. Plebani, L.D. Notarangelo, B. Dahlback, E. Tsitsikov, and R. Geha. 2003. C4b-binding protein (C4BP) activates B cells through the CD40 receptor. *Immunity* 18: 837.

28. Ranheim, E.A. and T.J. Kipps. 1993. Activated T cells induce expression of B7/BB1 on normal or leukemic B cells through a CD40-dependent signal. *J. Exp. Med.* 177: 925.

29. Klaus, S.J., L.M. Pinchuk, H.D. Ochs, C.L. Law, W.C. Fanslow, R.J. Armitage, and E.A. Clark. 1994. Costimulation through CD28 enhances T cell-dependent B cell activation via CD40–CD40L interaction. *J. Immunol.* 152: 5643.

30. Parra, E., T. Mustelin, M. Dohlsten, and D. Mercola. 2001. Identification of a CD28 response element in the CD40 ligand promoter. *J. Immunol.* 166: 2437.

31. Shahinian, A., K. Pfeffer, K.P. Lee, T.M. Kündig, K. Kishihara, A. Wakeham, K. Kawai, P.S. Ohashi, C.B. Thompson, and T.W. Mak. 1993. Differential T cell costimulatory requirements in CD28-deficient mice. *Science* 261: 609.

32. Borriello, F., M.P. Sethna, S.D. Boyd, A.N. Schweitzer, E.A. Tivol, D. Jacoby, T.B. Strom, E.M. Simpson, G.J. Freeman, and A.H. Sharpe. 1997. B7-1 and B7-2 have overlapping, critical roles in immunoglobulin class switching and germinal center formation. *Immunity* 6: 303.

33. Mark, D.A., C.E. Donovan, G.T. De Sanctis, H.Z. He, M. Cernadas, L. Kobzik, D.L. Perkins, A. Sharpe, and P.W. Finn. 2000. B7-1 (CD80) and B7-2 (CD86) have complementary roles in mediating allergic pulmonary inflammation and airway hyperresponsiveness. *Am. J. Respir. Cell Mol. Biol.* 22: 265.

34. Beier, K.C., A. Hutloff, A.M. Dittrich, C. Heuck, A. Rauch, K. Buchner, B. Ludewig, H. D. Ochs, H.W. Mages, and R.A. Kroczek. 2000. Induction, binding specificity and function of human ICOS. *Eur. J. Immunol.* 30: 3707.

35. Yoshinaga, S.K., J.S. Whoriskey, S.D. Khare, U. Sarmiento, J. Guo, T. Horan, G. Shih, M. Zhang, M.A. Coccia, T. Kohno, A. Tafuri-Bladt, D. Brankow, P. Campbell, D. Chang, L. Chiu, T. Dai, G. Duncan, G.S. Elliott, A. Hui, S.M. McCabe, S. Scully, A. Shahinian, C.L. Shaklee, G. Van, T.W. Mak et al. 1999. T-cell co-stimulation through B7RP-1 and ICOS. *Nature* 402: 827.

36. Aicher, A., M. Hayden-Ledbetter, W.A. Brady, A. Pezzutto, G. Richter, D. Magaletti, S. Buckwalter, J.A. Ledbetter, and E.A. Clark. 2000. Characterization of human inducible costimulator ligand expression and function. *J. Immunol.* 164: 4689.

37. Tafuri, A., A. Shahinian, F. Bladt, S.K. Yoshinaga, M. Jordana, A. Wakeham, L.M. Boucher, D. Bouchard, V.S. Chan, G. Duncan, B. Odermatt, A. Ho, A. Itie, T. Horan, J. S. Whoriskey, T. Pawson, J. M. Penninger, P.S. Ohashi, and T.W. Mak. 2001. ICOS is essential for effective T-helper-cell responses. *Nature* 409: 105.

38. Schroeder, J.T., D.W. MacGlashan, A. Kagey-Sobotka, J.M. White, and L.M. Lichtenstein. 1994. IgE-dependent IL-4-secretion by human basophils: relationship between cytokine production and histamine release in mixed leukocyte cultures. *J. Immunol.* 153: 1808.

39. Burd, P.R., W.C. Thompson, E.E. Max, and F.C. Mills. 1995. Activated mast cells produce interleukin 13. *J. Exp. Med.* 181: 1373.
40. Gauchat, J.F., S. Henchoz, G. Mazzei, J.P. Aubry, T. Brunner, H. Blasey, P. Life, D. Talabot, L. Flores-Romo, J. Thompson, K. Kishi, J. Butterfield, C. Dahinden, and J.Y. Bonnefoy. 1993. Induction of human IgE synthesis in B cells by mast cells and basophils. *Nature* 365: 340.
41. Schmitz, J., A. Thiel, R. Kühn, K. Rajewsky, W. Müller, M. Assenmacher, and A. Radbruch. 1994. Induction of interleukin-4 (IL-4) expression in T helper (Th) cells is not dependent on IL-4 from non Th-cells. *J. Exp. Med.* 179: 1349.
42. Gould, H.J., R.L. Beavil, and D. Vercelli. 2000. IgE isotype determination: epsilon-germline gene transcription, DNA recombination and B-cell differentiation. *Br. Med. Bull.* 56: 908.
43. Stavnezer, J. 2000. Molecular processes that regulate class switching. *Curr. Top. Microbiol. Immunol.* 245: 127.
44. Bottaro, A., R. Lansford, L. Xu, J. Zhang, P. Rothman, and F.W. Alt. 1994. S region transcription *per se* promotes basal IgE class switch recombination but additional factors regulate the efficiency of the process. *EMBO J.* 13: 665.
45. Lorenz, M., S. Jung, and A. Radbruch. 1995. Switch transcripts in immunoglobulin class switching. *Science* 267: 1825.
46. Tian, M. and F.W. Alt. 2000. RNA editing meets DNA shuffling. *Nature* 407: 31.
47. Tian, M. and F.W. Alt. 2000. Transcription-induced cleavage of immunoglobulin switch regions by nucleotide excision repair nucleases *in vitro. J. Biol. Chem.* 275: 24163.
48. Luby, T.M., C.E. Schrader, J. Stavnezer, and E. Selsing. 2001. The mu switch region tandem repeats are important, but not required, for antibody class switch recombination. *J. Exp. Med.* 193: 159.
49. Cogné, M., R. Lansford, A. Bottaro, J. Zhang, J. Gorman, F. Young, H.L. Cheng, and F.W. Alt. 1994. A class switch control region at the 3' end of the immunoglobulin heavy chain locus. *Cell* 77: 737.
50. Manis, J.P., N. van der Stoep, M. Tian, R. Ferrini, L. Davidson, A. Bottaro, and F.W. Alt. 1998. Class switching in B cells lacking 3' immunoglobulin heavy chain enhancers. *J. Exp. Med.* 188: 1421.
51. Pinaud, E., A.A. Khamlichi, C. Le Morvan, M. Drouet, V. Nalesso, M. Le Bert, and M. Cogne. 2001. Localization of the 3' IgH locus elements that effect long-distance regulation of class switch recombination. *Immunity* 15: 187.
52. Denizot, Y., E. Pinaud, C. Aupetit, C. Le Morvan, E. Magnoux, J.C. Aldigier, and M. Cogne. 2001. Polymorphism of the human alpha1 immunoglobulin gene 3' enhancer hs1,2 and its relation to gene expression. *Immunology* 103: 35.
53. Laurencikiene, J., V. Deveikaite, and E. Severinson. 2001. HS1,2 enhancer regulation of germline epsilon and gamma-2b promoters in murine B lymphocytes: evidence for specific promoter-enhancer interactions. *J. Immunol.* 167: 3257.
54. Stavnezer, J., G. Radcliffe, Y.C. Lin, J. Nietupski, L. Berggren, R. Sitia, and E. Severinson. 1988. Immunoglobulin heavy-chain switching may be directed by prior induction of transcripts from constant-region genes. *Proc. Natl. Acad. Sci. USA* 85: 7704.

55. Rothman, P., S. Lutzker, W. Cook, R. Coffman, and F.W. Alt. 1988. Mitogen plus interleukin 4 induction of Cε transcripts in B lymphoid cells. *J. Exp. Med.* 168: 2385.
56. Severinson, E., C. Fernandez, and J. Stavnezer. 1990. Induction of germ-line immunoglobulin heavy chain transcripts by mitogens and interleukins prior to switch recombination. *Eur. J. Immunol.* 20: 1079.
57. Gauchat, J.F., D.A. Lebman, R.L. Coffman, H. Gascan, and J.E. de Vries. 1990. Structure and expression of germline ε transcripts in human B cells induced by interleukin-4 to switch to IgE production. *J. Exp. Med.* 172: 463.
58. Jabara, H.H., L.C. Schneider, S.K. Shapira, C. Alfieri, C.T. Moody, E. Kieff, R.S. Geha, and D. Vercelli. 1990. Induction of germ-line and mature Cε transcripts in human B cells stimulated with rIL-4 and EBV. *J. Immunol.* 145: 3468.
59. Shapira, S.K., D. Vercelli, H.H. Jabara, S.M. Fu, and R.S. Geha. 1992. Molecular analysis of the induction of IgE synthesis in human B cells by IL-4 and engagement of CD40 antigen. *J. Exp. Med.* 175: 289.
60. Lee, C.G., K. Kinoshita, A. Arudchandran, S.M. Cerritelli, R.J. Crouch, and T. Honjo. 2001. Quantitative regulation of class switch recombination by switch region transcription. *J. Exp. Med.* 194: 365.
61. Kinoshita, K., J. Tashiro, S. Tomita, C.G. Lee, and T. Honjo. 1998. Target specificity of immunoglobulin class switch recombination is not determined by nucleotide sequences of S regions. *Immunity* 9: 849.
62. Albrecht, B., S. Peiritsch, and M. Woisetschläger. 1994. A bifunctional control element in the human IgE germline promoter involved in repression and IL-4 activation. *Int. Immunol.* 6: 1143.
63. Messner, B., A.M. Stütz, B. Albrecht, S. Peiritsch, and M. Woisetschläger. 1997. Cooperation of binding sites for STAT6 and NFκB/rel in the IL-4-induced up-regulation of the human IgE germline promoter. *J. Immunol.* 159: 3330.
64. Thienes, C.P., L. De Monte, S. Monticelli, M. Busslinger, H.J. Gould, and D. Vercelli. 1997. The transcription factor B cell-specific activator protein (BSAP) enhances both IL-4- and CD40-mediated activation of the human ε germline promoter. *J. Immunol.* 158: 5874.
65. Mikita, T., M. Kurama, and U. Schindler. 1998. Synergistic activation of the germline ε promoter mediated by Stat6 and C/EBPβ. *J. Immunol.* 161: 1822.
66. Tinnell, S.B., S.M. Jacobs-Helber, E. Sterneck, S.T. Sawyer, and D.H. Conrad. 1998. STAT6, NF-κB and C/EBP in CD23 expression and IgE production. *Int. Immunol.* 10: 1529.
67. Shimoda, K., J. van Deursen, M.Y. Sangster, S.R. Sarawar, R.T. Carson, R.A. Tripp, C. Chu, F.W. Quelle, T. Nosaka, D.A.A. Vignali, P.C. Doherty, G. Grosveld, W.E. Paul, and J.N. Ihle. 1996. Lack of IL-4-induced Th2 response and IgE class switching in mice with disrupted STAT6 gene. *Nature* 380: 630.
68. Takeda, K., T. Tanaka, W. Shi, M. Matsumoto, M. Minami, S.I. Kashiwamura, K. Nakanishi, N. Yoshida, T. Kishimoto, and S. Akira. 1996. Essential role of STAT6 in IL-4 signalling. *Nature* 380: 627.
69. Kaplan, M.H., U. Schindler, S.T. Smiley, and M.J. Grusby. 1996. STAT6 is required for mediating responses to IL-4 and for the development of Th2 cells. *Immunity* 4: 313.

70. Francis, D.A., R. Sen, N. Rice, and T.L. Rothstein. 1998. Receptor-specific induction of NF-κB components in primary B cells. *Int. Immunol.* 10: 285.

71. Lin, S.C., H.H. Wortis, and J. Stavnezer. 1998. The ability of CD40L, but not lipopolysaccharide, to initiate immunoglobulin switching to immunoglobulin G1 is explained by differential induction of NF-κB/Rel proteins. *Mol. Cell. Biol.* 18: 5523.

72. Iciek, L.A., S.A. Delphin, and J. Stavnezer. 1997. CD40 cross-linking induces Igε germline transcripts in B cells via activation of NF-κB: synergy with IL-4 induction. *J. Immunol.* 158: 4769.

73. Shen, C.H. and J. Stavnezer. 1998. Interaction of STAT6 and NF-κB: Direct association and synergistic activation of interleukin-4-induced transcription. *Mol. Cell. Biol.* 18: 3395.

74. Adams, B., P. Dörfler, A. Aguzzi, Z. Kozmik, P. Urbanek, I. Maurer-Fogy, and M. Busslinger. 1992. Pax-5 encodes the transcription factor BSAP and is expressed in B lymphocytes, the developing CNS, and adult testis. *Genes Dev.* 6: 1589.

75. Liao, F., B.K. Birshtein, M. Busslinger, and P. Rothman. 1994. The transcription factor BSAP (NF-HB) is essential for immunoglobulin germ-line ε transcription. *J. Immunol.* 152: 2904.

76. Qiu, G. and J. Stavnezer. 1998. Overexpression of BSAP/Pax5 inhibits switching to IgA and enhances switching to IgE in the I.29μ B cell line. *J. Immunol.* 161: 2906.

77. Warren, W.D. and M.T. Berton. 1995. Induction of germ-line γ1 and ε Ig gene expression in murine B cells. IL-4 and the CD40 ligand–CD40 interactions provide distinct but synergistic signals. *J. Immunol.* 155: 5637.

78. Vercelli, D. 2001. IgE and its regulators. *Curr. Opin. Allergy Clin. Immunol.* 1: 61.

79. Nagaoka, H., M. Muramatsu, N. Yamamura, K. Kinoshita, and T. Honjo. 2002. Activation-induced deaminase (AID)-directed hypermutation in the immunoglobulin Smu region: implication of AID involvement in a common step of class switch recombination and somatic hypermutation. *J. Exp. Med.* 195: 529.

80. Casellas, R., A. Nussenzweig, R. Wuerffel, R. Pelanda, A. Reichlin, H. Suh, X.F. Qin, E. Besmer, A. Kenter, K. Rajewsky, and M.C. Nussenzweig. 1998. Ku80 is required for immunoglobulin isotype switching. *EMBO J.* 8: 2404.

81. Schrader, C.E., W. Edelmann, R. Kucherlapati, and J. Stavnezer. 1999. Reduced isotype switching in splenic B cells from mice deficient in mismatch repair enzymes. *J. Exp. Med.* 190: 323.

82. Muramatsu, M., V.S. Sankaranand, S. Anant, M. Sugai, K. Kinoshita, N.O. Davidson, and T. Honjo. 1999. Specific expression of activation-induced cytidine deaminase (AID), a novel member of the RNA-editing deaminase family in germinal center B cells. *J. Biol. Chem.* 274: 18470.

83. Muramatsu, M., K. Kinoshita, S. Fagarasan, S. Yamada, Y. Shinkai, and T. Honjo. 2000. Class switch recombination and hypermutation require activation-induced cytidine deaminase (AID), a potential RNA editing enzyme. *Cell* 102: 553.

84. Zhou, C., A. Saxon, and K. Zhang. 2003. Human activation-induced cytidine deaminase is induced by IL-4 and negatively regulated by CD45: implication of CD45 as a Janus kinase phosphatase in antibody diversification. *J. Immunol.* 170: 1887.

85. Okazaki, I. M., K. Kinoshita, M. Muramatsu, K. Yoshikawa, and T. Honjo. 2002. The AID enzyme induces class switch recombination in fibroblasts. *Nature* 416: 340.

86. Del Prete, G.F., E. Maggi, P. Parronchi, I. Chretien, A. Tiri, D. Macchia, M. Ricci, J. Banchereau, J.E. de Vries, and S. Romagnani. 1988. IL-4 is an essential factor for the IgE synthesis induced *in vitro* by human T cell clones and their supernatants. *J. Immunol.* 140: 4193.

87. Mehta, A., M. Kintner, N. Sherman, and D. Driscoll. 2000. Molecular cloning of apobec-1 complementation factor, a novel RNA-binding protein involved in the editing of apolipoprotein B mRNA. *Mol. Cell. Biol.* 20: 1846.

88. Petersen, S., R. Casellas, B. Reina-San-Martin, H.T. Chen, M.J. Difilippantonio, P.C. Wilson, L. Hanitsch, A. Celeste, M. Muramatsu, D.R. Pilch, C. Redon, T. Ried, W.M. Bonner, T. Honjo, M.C. Nussenzweig, and A. Nussenzweig. 2001. AID is required to initiate Nbs1/gamma-H2AX focus formation and mutations at sites of class switching. *Nature* 414: 660.

89. Harris, R.S., S.K. Petersen-Mahrt, and M.S. Neuberger. 2002. RNA editing enzyme APOBEC1 and some of its homologs can act as DNA mutators. *Mol. Cell.* 10: 1247.

90. Rada, C., G.T. Williams, H. Nilsen, D.E. Barnes, T. Lindahl, and M.S. Neuberger. 2002. Immunoglobulin isotype switching is inhibited and somatic hypermutation perturbed in UNG-deficient mice. *Curr. Biol.* 12: 1748.

91. Di Noia, J. and M.S. Neuberger. 2002. Altering the pathway of immunoglobulin hypermutation by inhibiting uracil-DNA glycosylase. *Nature* 419: 43.

92. Petersen-Mahrt, S.K., R.S. Harris, and M.S. Neuberger. 2002. AID mutates *E. coli* suggesting a DNA deamination mechanism for antibody diversification. *Nature* 418: 99.

93. Ramiro, A.R., P. Stavropoulos, M. Jankovic, and M.C. Nussenzweig. 2003. Transcription enhances AID-mediated cytidine deamination by exposing single-stranded DNA on the nontemplate strand. *Nat. Immunol.* 4: 452.

94. Bransteitter, R., P. Pham, M.D. Scharff, and M.F. Goodman. 2003. Activation-induced cytidine deaminase deaminates deoxycytidine on single-stranded DNA but requires the action of RNase. *Proc. Natl. Acad. Sci. USA* 100: 4102.

95. Storb, U. and J. Stavnezer. 2002. Immunoglobulin genes: generating diversity with AID and UNG. *Curr. Biol.* 12: R725.

96. Revy, P., T. Muto, Y. Levy, F. Geissmann, A. Plebani, O. Sanal, N. Catalan, M. Forveille, R. Dufourcq-Labelouse, A. Gennery, I. Tezcan, F. Ersoy, H. Kayserili, A.G. Ugazio, N. Brousse, M. Muramatsu, L.D. Notarangelo, K. Kinoshita, T. Honjo, A. Fischer, and A. Durandy. 2000. Activation-induced cytidine deaminase (AID) deficiency causes the autosomal recessive form of the hyper-IgM syndrome. *Cell* 102: 565.

97. Noguchi, E., M. Shibasaki, M. Inudou, M. Kamioka, Y. Yokouchi, K. Yamakawa-Kobayashi, H. Hamaguchi, A. Matsui, and T. Arinami. 2001. Association between a new polymorphism in the activation-induced cytidine deaminase gene and atopic asthma and the regulation of total serum IgE levels. *J. Allergy Clin. Immunol.* 108: 382.

98. Zhang, K., F.C. Mills, and A. Saxon. 1994. Switch circles from IL-4-directed ε class switching from human B lymphocytes — evidence for direct, sequential and multiple step sequential switch from μ to ε Ig heavy chain gene. *J. Immunol.* 152: 3427.

99. van der Stoep, N., W. Korver, and T. Logtenberg. 1994. *In vivo* and *in vitro* IgE isotype switching in human B lymphocytes: evidence for a predominantly direct IgM to IgE class switch program. *Eur. J. Immunol.* 24: 1307.

100. Jabara, H.H., R. Loh, N. Ramesh, D. Vercelli, and R.S. Geha. 1993. Sequential switching from μ to ε via γ4 in human B cells stimulated with IL-4 and hydrocortisone. *J. Immunol.* 151: 4528.

101. Vercelli, D., L. De Monte, S. Monticelli, C. Di Bartolo, and A. Agresti. 1998. To E or not to E? Can an IL-4-induced B cell choose between IgE and IgG4? *Int. Arch. Allergy Immunol.* 116: 1.

102. Jung, S., G. Siebenkotten, and A. Radbruch. 1994. Frequency of immunoglobulin E class switching is autonomously determined and independent of prior switching to other classes. *J. Exp. Med.* 179: 2023.

103. Romagnani, S. 2000. The role of lymphocytes in allergic disease. *J. Allergy Clin. Immunol.* 105: 399.

104. Jabara, H.H., D.J. Ahern, D. Vercelli, and R.S. Geha. 1991. Hydrocortisone and IL-4 induce IgE isotype switching in human B cells. *J. Immunol.* 147: 1557.

105. Rak, S., M.R. Jacobson, R.M. Sudderick, K. Masuyama, S. Juliusson, A.B. Kay, Q. Hamid, O. Lowhagen, and S.R. Durham. 1994. Influence of prolonged treatment with topical corticosteroid (fluticasone propionate) on early and late phase nasal responses and cellular infiltration in the nasal mucosa after allergen challenge. *Clin. Exp. Allergy* 24: 930.

106. Ghaffar, O., S. Laberge, M.R. Jacobson, O. Lowhagen, S. Rak, S.R. Durham, and Q. Hamid. 1997. IL-13 mRNA and immunoreactivity in allergen-induced rhinitis: comparison with IL-4 expression and modulation by topical glucocorticoid therapy. *Am. J. Respir. Cell Mol. Biol.* 17: 17.

107. Durham, S.R., H.J. Gould, C.P. Thienes, M.R. Jacobson, K. Masuyama, S. Rak, O. Lowhagen, E. Schotman, L. Cameron, and Q.A. Hamid. 1997. Expression of epsilon germ-line gene transcripts and mRNA for the epsilon heavy chain of IgE in nasal B cells and the effects of topical corticosteroid. *Eur. J. Immunol.* 27: 2899.

108. Cameron, L.A., S.R. Durham, M.R. Jacobson, K. Masuyama, S. Juliusson, H.J. Gould, O. Lowhagen, E.M. Minshall, and Q.A. Hamid. 1998. Expression of IL-4, C-epsilon RNA, and I-epsilon RNA in the nasal mucosa of patients with seasonal rhinitis: effect of topical corticosteroids. *J. Allergy Clin. Immunol.* 101: 330.

109. Borish, L. C., H. S. Nelson, M. J. Lanz, L. Claussen, J. B. Whitmore, J. M. Agosti, and L. Garrison. 1999. Interleukin-4 receptor in moderate atopic asthma. A phase I/II randomized, placebo-controlled trial. *Am. J. Respir. Crit. Care Med. 160: 1816.*

110. Borish, L.C., H.S. Nelson, J. Corren, G. Bensch, W.W. Busse, J.B. Whitmore, and J.M. Agosti. 2001. Efficacy of soluble IL-4 receptor for the treatment of adults with asthma. *J. Allergy Clin. Immunol.* 107: 963.

111. Henderson, W.R. Jr., E.Y. Chi, and C.R. Maliszewski. 2000. Soluble IL-4 receptor inhibits airway inflammation following allergen challenge in a mouse model of asthma. *J. Immunol.* 164: 1086.

112. Wills-Karp, M., J. Luyimbazi, X. Xu, B. Schofield, T.Y. Neben, C.L. Karp, and D.D. Donaldson. 1998. Interleukin-13: central mediator of allergic asthma. *Science* 282: 2258.

113. Manetti, R., F. Gerosa, M.G. Giudizi, R. Biagiotti, P. Parronchi, M.P. Piccinni, S. Sampognaro, E. Maggi, S. Romagnani, and G. Trinchieri. 1994. Interleukin-12 induces stable priming for IFN-γ production during differentiation of human T helper cells and transient IFN-γ production in established Th2 cell clones. *J. Exp. Med.* 179: 1273.

114. Krieg, A.M., L. Love-Homan, A.K. Yi, and J.T. Harty. 1998. CpG DNA induces sustained IL-12 expression *in vivo* and resistance to *Listeria monocytogenes* challenge. *J. Immunol.* 161: 2428.

115. Parronchi, P., F. Brugnolo, F. Annunziato, C. Manuelli, S. Sampognaro, C. Mavilia, S. Romagnani, and E. Maggi. 1999. Phosphorothioate oligodeoxynucleotides promote the *in vitro* development of human allergen-specific CD4+ T cells into Th1 effectors. *J. Immunol.* 163: 5946.

116. Tighe, H., K. Takabayashi, D. Schwartz, G. Van Nest, S. Tuck, J.J. Eiden, A. Kagey-Sobotka, P.S. Creticos, L.M. Lichtenstein, H.L. Spiegelberg, and E. Raz. 2000. Conjugation of immunostimulatory DNA to the short ragweed allergen amb a 1 enhances its immunogenicity and reduces its allergenicity. *J. Allergy Clin. Immunol.* 106: 124.

117. Jardieu, P.X. 1995. Anti-IgE therapy. *Curr. Opin. Immunol.* 7: 779.

118. Presta, L., R. Shields, L. O'Connell, S. Lahr, J. Porter, C. Gorman, and P. Jardieu. 1994. The binding site on human immunoglobulin E for its high affinity receptor. *J. Biol. Chem.* 269: 26368.

119. Fahy, J.V., H.E. Fleming, H.H. Wong, J.T. Liu, J.Q. Su, J. Reimann, R.B. Fick, Jr., and H.A. Boushey. 1997. The effect of an anti-IgE monoclonal antibody on the early- and late-phase responses to allergen inhalation in asthmatic subjects. *Am. J. Respir. Crit. Care Med.* 155: 1828.

120. Boulet, L.P., K.R. Chapman, J. Cote, S. Kalra, R. Bhagat, V.A. Swystun, M. Laviolette, L.D. Cleland, F. Deschesnes, J.Q. Su, A. DeVault, R.B. Fick, Jr., and D.W. Cockcroft. 1997. Inhibitory effects of an anti-IgE antibody E25 on allergen-induced early asthmatic response. *Am. J. Respir. Crit. Care Med.* 155: 1835.

121. Milgrom, H., R.B.J. Fick, J.Q. Su, J.D. Reimann, R.K. Bush, M.L. Watrous, and W.J. Metzger. 1999. Treatment of allergic asthma with monoclonal anti-IgE antibody. rhuMAb-E25 Study Group. *New Engl. J. Med.* 341: 1966.

122. Saini, S.S., D.W. MacGlashan Jr., S.A. Sterbinsky, A. Togias, D.C. Adelman, L.M. Lichtenstein, and B.S. Bochner. 1999. Down-regulation of human basophil IgE and FC epsilon RI alpha surface densities and mediator release by anti-IgE-infusions is reversible *in vitro* and *in vivo*. *J. Immunol.* 162: 5624.

123. Barnes, P.J. 2000. Anti-IgE therapy in asthma: rationale and therapeutic potential. *Int. Arch. Allergy Immunol.* 123: 196.

Index

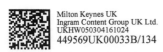

Milton Keynes UK
Ingram Content Group UK Ltd.
UKHW050304161024
449569UK00033B/134